HIV/AIDS

A Guide To Nursing Care

HIV/AIDS

A
Guide To
Nursing Care

SECOND EDITION

Jacquelyn Haak Flaskerud, PhD, RN, FAAN

Professor, School of Nursing
University of California, Los Angeles
Los Angeles, California

Peter J. Ungvarski, MS, RNC

Clinical Nurse Specialist, HIV Infection
VNS Home Care
Visiting Nurse Service of New York
New York, New York

W.B. SAUNDERS COMPANY
Harcourt Brace Jovanovich, Inc.

Philadelphia   London   Toronto   Montreal   Sydney   Tokyo

W. B. SAUNDERS COMPANY
Harcourt Brace Jovanovich, Inc.

The Curtis Center
Independence Square West
Philadelphia, Pennsylvania 19106

Library of Congress Cataloging-in-Publication Data

HIV/AIDS : a guide to nursing care / [edited by] Jacquelyn Haak
Flaskerud, Peter J. Ungvarski. — 2nd ed.
   p.   cm.
   Rev. ed. of: AIDS/HIV infection. 1989
   Includes bibliographical references and index.
   ISBN 0-7216-3718-3
   1. AIDS (Disease)—Nursing. I. Flaskerud, Jacquelyn Haak.
II. Ungvarski, Peter J. III. Title: AIDS/HIV infection.
   [DNLM: 1. Acquired Immunodeficiency Syndrome—nurses' instruction.
WD 308 H6725]
RC607.A26A3473 1992
610.73'699—dc20
DNLM/DLC
                                        91-23674

Editor: Thomas Eoyang

HIV/AIDS: A GUIDE TO NURSING CARE   ISBN 0-7216-3718-3

Printed in Mexico.

Last digit is the print number: 9   8   7   6   5   4   3   2

To John and Jimie
Our longtime companions

Contributors

MARY G. BOLAND, R.N., M.S.N., C.P.N.P.

Associate in Pediatrics, University of Medicine and Dentistry—New Jersey; Director, Children's Hospital AIDS Program, Children's Hospital of New Jersey; Director, National Pediatric HIV Resource Center, Newark, New Jersey

Nursing Care of the Child

W. CAROLE CHENITZ, R.N., Ed.D.

Assistant Clinical Professor, School of Nursing, University of California, San Francisco

Living with AIDS

RICHARD CONVISER, Ph.D.

Consultant, Children's Hospital AIDS Program, Children's Hospital of New Jersey, Newark, New Jersey

Nursing Care of the Child

JACQUELYN HAAK FLASKERUD, Ph.D., F.A.A.N.

Professor, Associate Dean for Academic Affairs, School of Nursing, University of California, Los Angeles

Overview: HIV Disease and Nursing; Psychosocial Aspects; Cofactors of HIV and Public Health Education

CHRISTINE GRADY, R.N., M.S., C.S.

Research Associate, Collaborative Intramural Program, National Center for Nursing Research, National Institutes of Health, Bethesda, Maryland

HIV Disease: Pathogenesis and Treatment; Ethical Aspects

KATHLEEN M. NOKES, Ph.D., R.N.

Associate Professor, Hunter College—Bellevue School of Nursing, City University of New York; Project Director, Nursing of Persons with HIV/AIDS, New York, New York

Community-Based and Long-Term Care; HIV Infection in Women

NANCY B. PARRIS, R.N., M.P.H.

Assistant Clinical Professor, School of Nursing, University of California, Los Angeles; Director, Hospital Infection Control, and Nurse Epidemiologist, University of California, Los Angeles, Medical Center, Los Angeles, California

Infection Control

JO ANNE STAATS, R.N., M.S.N., A.N.P.

HIV Clinical Scholar, St. Vincent's Hospital and Medical Center, New York, New York

Chemical Dependency

PETER J. UNGVARSKI, M.S., R.N.

Clinical Nurse Specialist, HIV Infection, Visiting Nurse Service of New York; Grant Associate, Nursing Persons with AIDS, Hunter College—Bellevue School of Nursing, City University of New York, New York, New York

Clinical Manifestations of AIDS; Nursing Management of the Adult Client; Community-Based and Long-Term Care

Preface

HIV disease is an individual and public health problem in which nurses and nursing care play a vital role. This text grew out of a need among nurses for information about AIDS and HIV infection. The content of the first edition of the book was based on a national survey of nurses in which they identified (1) their needs for information about HIV/AIDS; (2) the groups to which they were providing counseling, education, and referrals for HIV infection, and (3) the resources they used or preferred to use to gain knowledge of HIV disease. The second edition addresses additional concerns identified in a survey of nurses who read and evaluated the first edition of the text. These nurses made valuable suggestions for improving the scope of the book. The second edition constitutes a greatly expanded and detailed guide to nursing, human service, and medical care, including the care of women, children, and intravenous drug users. As in the first edition, the focus of the text remains on clinical practice. The book provides a comprehensive view of the spectrum of HIV disease to assist the nurse in clinical practice, whether that practice be in primary, secondary, or tertiary prevention of HIV. It serves also as an in-depth text for students learning the practice of nursing or specializing in a nursing clinical area. All health and human service workers who use a case management approach to HIV care will find the book invaluable.

Chapters 1 and 2 provide a context into which the HIV epidemic and the consequent demands on nursing care can be placed:

- An overview of the history of the epidemic, the sociodemographic distribution of AIDS in the United States, nurses' knowledge and attitudes, and strategies for changing these.

- A description of the characteristics of HIV and how it affects the immune system; the effects of HIV on organ systems.

Nurses' needs for information about the care of persons infected with HIV are addressed in Chapters 3 through 6 and in Chapters 11 and 12. These chapters provide guidelines for nursing care that can be applied in the hospital or in the community.

- A comprehensive delineation of common infections and neoplasms associated with AIDS and their medical treatment (a summary of drugs commonly in use and their side effects is provided in Appendix I).

- An in-depth nursing care plan for managing the adult client with HIV disease through primary, secondary, and tertiary prevention measures; the plan is based on symptom assessment and organized by nursing diagnosis.

- A multifaceted look at the nursing care of children with HIV/AIDS; current treatments available, home care, and the changing needs of children and their families.

- The psychosocial and spiritual needs of persons with HIV disease, their families, lovers, spouses, and friends, and the nurses caring for them; guidelines for HIV antibody testing and counseling.

- Infection control guidelines applicable to both the hospital and the community; information on risk to health care workers and household contacts.

- The ethical concerns of nurses regarding HIV disease; access to care, obligation to treat, confidentiality, and decisions about treatment.

Information that will assist nurses in counseling, education, referrals, and community care are provided in Chapters 7 through 10.

- The various community activities that occur surrounding HIV disease: education, counseling, referrals, home care, and hospice care organized from a case management perspective.

- A detailed account of cofactors of HIV infection and disease expression with attention to the levels of prevention.

- Issues and nursing care specific to persons with chemical dependencies: substance abuse, transmission, and treatments available.

- The special problems of women with HIV/AIDS: prevention, transmission, presenting diagnoses, pregnancy.

Finally, bringing together and giving meaning to much of the information presented in other chapters, a nurse shares her personal experience of living with AIDS (Chapter 13).

Readers of this text should be aware of two phenomena associated with the burgeoning literature on HIV/AIDS. First, information on HIV disease is constantly developing. For example, as we go to press, the Centers for Disease Control (CDC) has announced that it will expand the definition of AIDS to include diseases common to women and intravenous drug users. The new definition will rely also on laboratory evidence, specifically T4 cell counts, to identify the AIDS caseload. Knowledge of infection and the disease may also change on a day-to-day basis. This information will affect the care and teaching that nurses provide. Nurses should be cognizant of this constant change and keep themselves up-to-date through continuing education courses and by reading the voluminous literature on HIV/AIDS.

Second, because of the vast amount of literature available, there is a diversity of opinion on risk of infection, transmission, and disease expression. This diversity is common to all areas of knowledge that are developing and constantly changing but is exaggerated in the case of AIDS because of the high rate of mortality associated with the disease and because of the social stigma and moral disapproval associated with the largest transmission groups. There are currently many unknowns regarding HIV/AIDS. This is partially due to the constant change in information and partially to the differences in human nature. Opinion on what current information means can reflect attempts to exploit public fear for personal or political gain, competition in the scientific community, public policy and political expediency, professional vs. lay opinion, individual pessimism vs. optimism, and the focus of one discipline as opposed to another. A current example is the conflicting opinions about the transmissibility of HIV from infected health care workers to their patients. Public concern fueled by media publicity of this issue has persuaded the CDC to release new recommendations for health care workers involved in invasive procedures. However, professional organizations representing health care workers believe universal precautions are adequate to protect both patients and health care workers from infection. It is important that nurses stay well informed and abreast of information on HIV disease so that they can sift through the diversity of opinion, give informed care to their clients, and allay their own fears and those of the public. It is in this spirit and with confidence in the intelligence, sensitivity, intentions, and motivation of nurses that the book was written.

Several persons and organizations made important contributions to the development of this second edition. The survey of nurses' information needs and staff support for the project was funded by the National Institute of Allergy and Infectious Diseases. Special appreciation goes to John Fahey, Director of the Center for Interdisciplinary Research in Immunology and Diseases (CIRID) at UCLA, for his belief in and support of the value of the project and his constant encouragement, interest, and ideas. Diana Shin, Cecilia Rush, and CIRID staff members provided valuable assistance and support. The contributing authors were spirited, cooperative, and inspiring—an intelligent and knowledgeable group with whom it was an honor to work. Our editor Thomas Eoyang facilitated this project through his constant belief in it and his unflagging attention, assistance, and string-pulling. Thanks to our friends and family for encouragement, valued critiques, and suggestions. And finally a special thank you to our best friends John Flaskerud and Jimie Rottner for their good cheer, love, and dedication to the detail, excellence, and completion of this project.

Contents

Appendix IV

Overview: HIV Disease and Nursing

Jacquelyn Haak Flaskerud

At this writing, more than 160,000 cases of acquired immunodeficiency syndrome (AIDS) have been documented in the United States and 1 million people are believed to be infected by the virus. No cure has been found, and predictions are that AIDS will be with us until the twenty-first century (CDC, 1988, 1991; Coolfont Report, 1986; Osmond & Moss, 1989; Staff, *JAMA*, 1990).

WHAT IS HIV DISEASE?

To speak knowledgeably and to understand the disease known as AIDS, it is necessary to define the problem in all its complexity. AIDS is the most severe disease state yet observed in the continuum of illness related to human immunodeficiency virus type 1 (HIV-1) infection. The virus was known in the past as human T-cell lymphotropic virus type III or lymphadenopathy-associated virus. HIV infection and AIDS are not synonymous terms. HIV infection ranges from asymptomatic infection to the full-blown clinical disease AIDS. The clinical presentation of HIV infection varies. In the past, published classification schemes for HIV infection stratified various HIV-related illnesses into separate syndromes such as AIDS-related complex and lymphadenopathy syndrome. These different presentations of HIV disease are now considered a continuum of host response to HIV infection and not separate syndromes (Abrams, 1986, 1987, 1990; Najera et al., 1987; Osmond, 1990).

PRIMARY HIV INFECTION

In many people the primary HIV infection is subclinical; that is, they have no symptoms but become seropositive for antibodies to HIV. In some cases, however, the HIV infection is manifested as an acute illness that occurs 2 to 6 weeks after infection. Signs and symptoms may include fever, rigors, arthralgias, and myalgias lasting 2 to 3 weeks. Rashes, abdominal cramps, diarrhea, and acute meningitis may also occur. Immunologic abnormalities during primary illness may include mild leukopenia, lymphopenia, thrombocytopenia, elevated erythrocyte sedimentation rate, and relative monocytosis (Abrams, 1987).

HIV SEROPOSITIVITY

Persons who have had a primary HIV infection will be seropositive according to a blood test for antibodies to HIV. Commonly used tests are the enzyme-linked immunosorbent assay (ELISA) and the enzyme immunoassay (EIA); the Western blot assay and immunofluorescence assay (IFA) are used to confirm positive results. Performed correctly and repeatedly, these tests together can identify previous exposure to the virus and avoid false-positive results. In some situations an error might occur, but in general these tests are more than 99% accurate (Ascher & Francis, 1987; Menitove, 1990). A test for the p24 part of HIV antigen can detect HIV infection when tests for the HIV antibody are negative. However, the practical utility of the test might not match its theoretic importance given the accuracy of repeated antibody tests (Menitove, 1990).

AIDS-RELATED COMPLEX

As noted earlier, HIV infection encompasses a range of conditions from asymptomatic infection to various expressions of disease. The term "AIDS-related complex (ARC)" was used in the past to describe certain clusters of symptoms. This term is no longer considered useful from either a clinical or a public health perspective (Institute of Medicine, 1988). However, since the term is still used infrequently, it is defined here. The term "ARC" was used when a person infected by HIV had at least two well-developed symptoms of immunodeficiency with at least two laboratory abnormalities. The term was used to describe a disease that did not fit the criteria for AIDS according to the Centers for Disease Control (CDC) but was clearly a "disease" in HIV-infected persons. Symptoms such as fever, drenching night sweats, weight loss, fatigue, and lymphadenopathy in the absence of an opportunistic infection or Kaposi's sarcoma were known formerly as ARC. It was thought that ARC might be a prodrome (precursor) to AIDS, a mild form of AIDS, or the dominant pattern of HIV disease. No data on the number of ARC cases or the life expectancy of persons with ARC are available, and no prospective cohort studies that would shed light on the course of ARC have been published (Scitovsky, 1989).

LYMPHADENOPATHY SYNDROME OR PERSISTENT GENERALIZED LYMPHADENOPATHY

Lymphadenopathy syndrome (LAS) is a term that was used to designate another syndrome associated with HIV seropositivity. LAS described a chronic, diffuse, noncancerous lymph node enlargement. When accompanied by fever, it was often called lymphadenopathy fever syndrome. These terms were used when lymph nodes in at least two extrainguinal sites were swollen to more than 1 cm for 3 months or longer. In addition to the swollen, sometimes painful nodes, symptoms included fever, night sweats, weight loss, and an enlarged spleen. Prospective studies of persons with clinical signs and symptoms of LAS report rates of progression to AIDS similar to those of asymptomatic HIV-seropositive persons. Based on estimates and prospective studies, the current median incubation period from HIV infection until the emergence of AIDS is 9 to 10 years (Abrams, 1987; Osmond, 1990).

ACQUIRED IMMUNODEFICIENCY SYNDROME

AIDS is the life-threatening complications of HIV infection, defined as (1) the presence of reliably diagnosed disease at least moderately indicative of underlying cellular immunodeficiency (Kaposi's sarcoma in a patient under 60 years of age, *Pneumocystis carinii* pneumonia or other opportunistic infection, dementia, emaciation, or wasting) and (2) the absence of known causes of underlying immunodeficiency and of any other reduced resistance reported to be associated with the disease (CDC, 1986). (Dementia and wasting as indicators of AIDS were added to the CDC definition in 1987.) This classification scheme may be expanded in the future to include T4 cell counts and diseases common to women and IV drug users (see Chapters 2, 3, 9, and 10).

HISTORY OF AIDS

The history of the AIDS epidemic in the United States is very recent (Abrams, 1986, 1987; CDC, 1981a,b, 1985; Najera et al., 1987; *Time*, Feb. 16, 1987, Apr. 13, 1987). The name "AIDS" dates back only to 1982. In June 1981 the first description of what would soon be referred to as AIDS appeared in the CDC's *Morbidity and Mortality Weekly Report*. This report described the occurrence of *P. carinii* pneumonia (PCP) in five previously healthy, sexually active, young homosexual men from Los Angeles. This was quickly followed by case reports of an unusual and extremely rare tumor, Kaposi's sarcoma (KS) in a male homosexual population in New York City.

Both of these conditions occur infrequently. PCP is seen almost exclusively in immunosuppressed individuals. It is a protozoan infection that produces an atypical pneumonia. KS in its classic form is a relatively rare, systemic, multicentric, neoplastic, angiomatous growth of unknown origin composed of proliferating vascular and fibroelastic elements. Classic Kaposi's sarcoma occurs in an indolent form predominantly in elderly men of black, Italian, and Jewish origin. A more aggressive form of the disease has been seen in young African men. Both the indolent and aggressive forms occur in immunosuppressed persons (Abrams, 1986; Ungvarski, 1983).

Throughout the summer of 1981, similar cases were reported to the CDC in increasing numbers. The numbers of cases initially were doubling every 6 months. In addition to PCP and KS, other unusual viral, fungal, and parasitic infections were being diagnosed in young homosexual men. Again, these diseases had previously been seen only in severely immunosuppressed individuals. Laboratory studies of patients with these opportunistic infections and cancers revealed that all of them had severe immunologic deficiencies; clinically they deteriorated and died of these unusual infections quickly.

At first only homosexual and bisexual men were thought to be affected, and some aspect of the gay life-style was hypothesized to be the probable cause of the immune deficiency. The disease was named gay-related immune deficiency at that time. However, as the complex of diseases became more widely recognized, other cases reported to the CDC made it obvious that AIDS was not a disease limited to homosexuals. The same infections and tumors were reported in heterosexual intravenous (IV) drug users; Haitian immigrants; persons with hemophilia; spouses, sexual partners, and children of persons with AIDS or at risk for AIDS; and recipients of blood or blood components from persons infected with AIDS. With the exception of Haitian immigrants, in whom infections were found to be related to the other modes of transmission, these other groups became and remain among the major transmission groups for AIDS. It soon became apparent that AIDS was transmitted through an exchange of body fluids, principally blood and semen.

Persons at increased risk of contracting HIV infection are those who have unprotected sex with multiple partners, share needles, receive blood or blood products from HIV-infected individuals, or are the sexual partners or children of these persons. Transmission occurs through both heterosexual and homosexual contacts, but currently the largest transmission group in the United States is bisexual and homosexual men and the next largest is IV drug users (both males and females). These two groups account for 88% of persons with AIDS nationwide; 89% of patients with AIDS are males (CDC, 1991). The World Health Organization (WHO) has designated this pattern of transmission as pattern 1. However, the proportion of IV drug users among those with newly diagnosed infection is increasing, especially along the Eastern Seaboard (Joseph, 1987; Ron & Rogers, 1989). The proportion of cases related to each transmission group varies significantly among the geographic regions of the United States. These differences are addressed later in this chapter.

While the number of cases was mounting in the United States, AIDS started appearing in Europe, where an interesting phenomenon was observed. Although in many European countries transmission patterns were similar to those in the United States (pattern 1 transmission), a sizable number of cases were occurring in immigrants from central Africa or in Europeans who traveled the major trade routes in central and east Africa. When investigators turned their attention to Africa, they discovered an epidemic that could be traced through serologic studies to 1959 (von Reyn & Mann, 1987). A quite different aspect of the epidemic in Africa was that it affected men and women equally and was widespread in the heterosexual population (WHO designation, pattern 2). The disease has spread to 54 countries in Africa and has been transmitted principally through sexual contact with multiple partners, including prostitutes (Quinn, 1990; Staff, AIDS/HIV Record, 1990). In Africa, in addition to HIV-1, retroviruses designated HIV-2 and HTLV-IV have been isolated in patients (Najera et al., 1987; Quinn, 1990). HIV-2 has transmission patterns and clinical features similar to those of HIV-1 (Quinn, 1990).

HIV-1 was identified and named in stages. Not until early 1983 in France was there any indication that a virus first discovered in 1980, human T-cell leukemia/lymphotropic virus (HTLV), might be the causative agent. In the United States in 1984 investigators at the National Institutes of Health reported the isolation of a group of cytopathic retroviruses and antibodies against those viruses in persons with AIDS. They termed their discovery human T-lymphotropic virus type III (HTLV-III). Scientists at the Institut Pasteur in France had called theirs lymphadenopathy-associated virus (LAV). For the sake of standardization and communication, the virus is now known worldwide as human immunodeficiency virus type 1 (HIV-1). Identification of the virus led to development of a test for HIV antibody in the blood. This test made it possible to determine which persons carried HIV antibody and therefore had been infected by HIV; it also permitted the screening of blood and blood products to prevent transmission by blood transfusion (Abrams, 1986; Najera et al., 1987).

Since 1981 the AIDS epidemic has assumed major proportions; if progress is not made against it, it will rank with history's greatest killers.

According to WHO (Staff, *AIDS/HIV Record*, 1990), AIDS has been reported in more than 160 countries. WHO officials estimate that 10 million people in the world carry the virus and that as many as 100 million will become infected in the next 10 years. WHO also estimates that by 1991 AIDS will have developed in between 500,000 and 3 million infected people since the beginning of the epidemic. In the United States more than 160,000 cases have been reported and about 1 million people are estimated to carry the virus (CDC, 1991; Osmond & Moss, 1989; Staff, *JAMA*, 1990). The Public Health Service projects that by the end of 1992 the cumulative number of AIDS cases in the United States will total 365,000 with 263,000 deaths (Staff, *Caring*, 1989).

WHO estimates that 3 to 5 million people in Africa are infected, that more than 100,000 cases of AIDS have occurred in the countries of central Africa, and that at least 50,000 Africans have already died of the disease. If a vaccine is not found, 1.5 million more may become ill. In major cities in some African countries (Tanzania, Uganda, Zaire), 50% of the adult population is affected. In Nairobi, Kenya, a study of prostitutes showed that 88% carried the AIDS virus. Epidemiologists have predicted that some African countries could lose 25% of their populations if a cure is not found (Quinn, 1990; *Time*, Feb. 16, 1987; Weisman, 1990).

When the first edition of this text was published in 1989, the progress made against the disease from 1981 to that time was summarized: the probable causative agent of AIDS had been discovered, the virus had been cloned, a blood screening program had been implemented, work on the development of a vaccine had begun, and therapies that extend life had been identified. In the last 2 years many major changes have occurred in the progression and epidemiology of the disease, treatment and nursing care, and the delivery of care. These changes are outlined here and addressed in detail in the following chapters.

Understanding of the disease has grown in the last 2 years. Kaposi's sarcoma as a presenting diagnosis has been declining (Lifson et al., 1990; Scitovsky, 1989), possibly because of an increased percentage of IV drug users among the new cases. The HIV infection rate has slowed substantially, especially among homosexual men (Osmond & Moss, 1989). Both the Public Health Service and independent investigators (Osmond & Moss, 1989) have revised the estimates of the prevalence of HIV infection in the United States. These revised estimates are lower and are based on the rate of progression to clinical AIDS in seropositive persons. Estimates range from about 600,000 to 1 million HIV-infected persons in the United States.

Some of the previously identified cofactors of HIV acquisition or disease progression, such as the use of nitrite inhalants, the presence of pregnancy, and disease outcomes based on transmission group are examples of cofactors to infection or disease progression that have recently been challenged and are now thought to be less important than originally hypothesized (Jason et al., 1989; Lifson et al., 1988; Nanda & Minkoff, 1989). Moreover, HIV strain type has been suggested as a cofactor that might explain widely differing longevity in persons with HIV infection (Gail et al., 1990; Jason et al., 1989; Lifson et al., 1988; Najera et al., 1987).

Changes in behavioral cofactors to acquisition of infection have been reported among homosexual men and IV drug users (Becker & Joseph, 1988). Condom use, fewer sexual partners, and a decline in anal receptive sexual practices have been reported among gay men in San Francisco, New York City, Chicago, and London. Among IV drug users, changes in behavior include decreasing or stopping needle sharing, attempting to sterilize needles, and stopping IV drug use (Becker & Joseph, 1988). However, changes in high-risk behavior for women and adolescent and young adult male heterosexuals have not been observed. Urban black and Latino populations are also experiencing less behavioral change. Cofactors of all types (agent, host, and environmental) are discussed in detail in Chapter 8.

Survival following diagnosis of AIDS has improved in recent years, primarily among persons with P. carinii pneumonia (Lemp et al., 1990; Rothenberg et al., 1987). Therapy with zidovudine (azidothymidine [AZT]) may be partly responsible for these recent improvements (Gail et al., 1990; Lemp et al., 1990). Zidovudine is also being evaluated in asymptomatic HIV-infected persons and as a prophylactic to infection in persons at risk, notably health care workers with occupational exposure and unborn fetuses with HIV-infected mothers (see Chapters 5 and 11).

The effect of such agents as zidovudine on the natural history of HIV infection will be determined in current and future clinical trials. In addition, prophylactic antibiotics, such as inhaled pentamidine and trimethoprim-sulfamethoxazole, are being tested to determine whether they can prevent certain manifestations of HIV disease, such as P. carinii pneumonia. Several vaccines against the virus are also being tested (see Chapter 2). The clinical presentation and treatment of the opportunistic infections and neoplasms are addressed in depth in Chapter 3.

Nursing care and treatment protocols for persons with HIV disease have shifted to a minimum of acute care hospital time and a maximum of extended care, home care, and hospice time (Scitovsky, 1989; Shulman & Mantell, 1988). Recent data indicate that the average hospital length of stay for persons with AIDS (PWAs) is decreasing. Nursing management, including community-based care, of PWAs is discussed in Chapters 4, 5, 7, 9, and 10. The nursing and medical community has become more knowledgeable and comfortable in treating PWAs on an ambulatory basis. However, long-term care facilities still resist accepting PWAs, and finding stable housing for PWAs is a major problem in many cities where AIDS is prevalent.

The cost of AIDS care has been variously estimated and differs by geographic region and transmission group (Scitovsky, 1989; Shulman & Mantell, 1988). Serious gaps in information remain, including an almost total lack of data on the number and medical costs of HIV-infected persons who are asymptomatic or who have symptoms and conditions other than AIDS (Scitovsky, 1989). Their medical costs might escalate sharply if prophylactic drug treatment turns out to be promising and the demands for treatment by asymptomatic seropositive persons increase. The costs of care could skyrocket just from the use of zidovudine treatment for seropositive persons without AIDS. In addition, the costs of testing for HIV would increase as more people sought tests or were required by the government to have them. Currently legislation is pending in over half the state legislatures that would require premarital serologic tests for HIV (Brandt, 1988). These costs have yet to be factored in to the cost of HIV health care. In addition to the costs of testing, the ethics of testing may undergo change. The ethics of mandated testing and of testing in an environment that offers life-sustaining treatment are discussed in Chapter 12.

The epidemiology of AIDS and nurses' knowledge, attitudes, and practices related to the disease have changed. The epidemiology of AIDS for special populations is discussed in Chapters 9 and 10. An overview of epidemiologic changes is given here. Risks to nurses and other health care workers, as well as nurses' practices in relation to universal precautions, are addressed in Chapter 11. An overview of nurses' knowledge, attitudes, and practices is given later in this chapter.

CHANGES IN EPIDEMIOLOGY OF HIV

The sociodemographic characteristics of persons with HIV disease differ with geographic region in the United States. These differences have become more pronounced during the last 2 years and have come to characterize the population with AIDS in each region. The national statistics often do not adequately reflect the sex, ethnicity, or route of transmission of PWAs in a particular city or region. To mount effective prevention and treatment programs, nurses must be aware of the sociodemographic characteristics of their own region. The demographics of the 10 Standard Metropolitan Statistical Areas (SMSAs) and 10 states or commonwealths with the most AIDS cases is presented in Table 1–1.

The statistics for transmission groups, sex, and ethnicity in the Eastern Seaboard states and SMSAs differ from the national statistics and those in the Midwest and West. Infection of IV drug users, women, and ethnic or racial subgroups is greater in the East. Infection of IV drug users (IVDUs), based on 92 seroprevalence studies of this group in the United States, is highest in the Northeast (10% to 65%) and Puerto Rico (45% to 59%);

TABLE 1–1. Demographics of Total AIDS Cases

TEN LEADING SMSAs	% OF TOTAL CASES	TEN LEADING STATES OR COMMONWEALTHS	% OF TOTAL CASES
New York City	19.0	New York	22.0
Los Angeles	7.0	California	19.0
San Francisco	6.0	Florida	8.0
Houston	3.0	Texas	7.0
Washington, D.C.	2.8	New Jersey	6.5
Newark	2.7	Illinois	3.0
Chicago	2.4	Puerto Rico	2.9
Miami	2.4	Pennsylvania	2.8
Philadelphia	2.0	Georgia	2.6
Atlanta	2.0	Massachusetts	2.0
Combined % of total	49.3	Combined % of total	75.8

Statistics from Centers for Disease Control (1991, April). *AIDS Weekly Surveillance Report.* United States AIDS Program, Atlanta.
SMSA, Standard Metropolitan Statistical Area.

lower in the South Atlantic states (7% to 29%) and in the metropolitan areas of Atlanta (10%), Detroit (7% to 13%), and San Francisco (7% to 13%); and 5% or less in other areas of the West, Midwest, and South (Hahn et al., 1989).

Infection of women, based on seroprevalence data from reproductive health clinics and delivery room settings, is highest in the urban areas of New Jersey (290 per million female population), New York (270 per million), the District of Columbia (216 per million), and Florida (138 per million). States or commonwealths with 40 or more cases of AIDS per million female population include those just listed plus Rhode Island, Delaware, Connecticut, Massachusetts, Maryland, and Puerto Rico. States with 20 to 39 cases per million female population include Pennsylvania, Virginia, South Carolina, Georgia, Mississippi, Louisiana, Colorado, Arizona, Nevada, California, Alaska, and Hawaii (Shapiro et al., 1989).

Infection rates of blacks and Hispanics are also higher along the Eastern Seaboard. For example, the racial breakdown of cases in New York City is 37% white, 34% black, 28% Hispanic/Latino and 1% others. This compares with a New York City population distribution of 52% white, 24% black, 20% Hispanic, and 4% other. Another way of expressing this is that the cumulative incidence of AIDS per million population is 1110 for whites, 1600 for blacks, and 1500 for Hispanics/Latinos (Friedman et al., 1987). The racial distribution of the AIDS epidemic is related to the proportion of infected drug users (Ron & Rogers, 1989) and the proportion of infected women (Landesman, 1989). Race, gender, and IV drug use are interrelated and associated with the proportion of individuals who are infected in a specific geographic region. Table 1–2 presents the transmission group, gender, and racial distribution of AIDS cases by geographic region compared with the national distribution of cases in these categories.

As can be noted from the table, transmission groups differ widely between the East Coast and both the Midwest and West, with higher percentages of IV drug users among the total cases in the East and South. The number of new cases of AIDS among IV drug users has been increasing yearly, with Eastern Seaboard states reporting an increase of 43% between

TABLE 1–2. Geographic Distribution of AIDS Cases (in Percent)

	UNITED STATES	NEW YORK STATE	NEW YORK CITY	NEW JERSEY	DADE CO., FL
Transmission Group					
Homosexual or bisexual male	60	46	48	27	47
IV drug user	21	39	38	55	18
Homosexual male and IV drug user	7	4	4	4	4
Hemophilia	1	0	0	1	0
Heterosexual	5	5	6	9	18
Transfusion	2	1	1	2	3
Other	3	4	3	2	10
Age and Gender					
Adult*	98	98	98	97	96
Male	91	86	86	79	85
Female	9	14	14	21	15
Children†	2	2	2	3	4
Age and Race or Ethnic Group					
Adults					
White	56	38	37	34	26
Black	27	35	34	54	44
Hispanic	16	27	28	12	30
Other	1	1	1	0	0
Children					
White	22	9	8	20	2
Black	52	55	55	59	90
Hispanic	25	34	37	20	8
Other	1	1	0	1	0

Statistics based on surveillance data provided by the Centers for Disease Control and the states and cities listed as of Spring 1990.
IV, intravenous; NR, None reported.
*Includes all patients 13 years of age and older.
†Includes all patients under 13 years of age.

1988 and 1989. The number of new cases of AIDS in sexual partners of IV drug users increased 58% during this same period in the East. In geographic areas where IV drug users make up a greater percentage of the total AIDS cases, the numbers of African Americans and Hispanics also make up a greater percentage. The ranges in the distribution of cases by transmission groups and the ethnic/racial makeup of these groups call for new knowledge, prevention, and treatment approaches among nurses. Chapter 9 deals with these topics.

SAN JUAN, P.R.	CHICAGO	HOUSTON	DALLAS	LOS ANGELES	SAN FRANCISCO
18	75	80	82	81	85
60	12	4	4	4	3
8	5	9	11	8	10
0	1	1	0	1	1
8	3	1	1	1	0
2	2	2	2	2	1
4	3	3	1	3	0
96	99	100	100	99	99
83	95	98	98	97	99
17	5	2	2	3	1
4	1	NR	0	1	1
0	51	74	82	64	82
0	36	14	12	16	7
99	13	11	6	18	8
0	0	0	0	2	2
0	13	NR	38	26	50
0	45	NR	63	32	38
100	42	NR	0	38	12
0	0	NR	0	4	0

Gender of HIV-infected persons also differs regionally and is closely related to cases of AIDS in children. As a greater proportion of women make up the total AIDS cases, predictably the proportion of infected children also rises. The proportion of AIDS cases among women and children who are black or Latino is particularly striking. The proportion of ethnic and racial minority women with AIDS closely parallels the percentages among children with AIDS as depicted in Table 1–2. For example, of Dade County, Florida, women with AIDS, 84% are black, 9% white, 7% Hispanic/Latina, and 1% other. In New York City women with AIDS are 53% black, 33% Latina, and 14% white. In contrast, women with AIDS in San Francisco are 53% white, 31% black, 8% Latina, and 8% other. Despite these differences between the East and West coasts, the proportion of cases of AIDS among minorities has been increasing steadily on both coasts. For instance, in Los Angeles County the proportion of whites among persons with AIDS has decreased from 68% in 1986 to 59% in 1988 to 54% in 1990. During this period the percentages of blacks have increased from 14% in 1986 to 21% in 1990, and of Latinos from 14% in 1986 to 24% in 1990. The danger of the spread of AIDS in the African American and Latino communities cannot be overstated. This is especially true among women and children. Chapters 5 and 10 deal with HIV infection in children and women, respectively.

Early in the epidemic it was predicted that by 1991 most people in major U.S. cities would know someone who has AIDS. As the epidemiology of AIDS makes clear, providing health care services in those cities is virtually impossible without knowledge of AIDS and the groups it affects most.

The explosion of knowledge about AIDS has been phenomenal. Nurses and other health care workers need in-depth and up-to-date knowledge of AIDS to practice. Nurses have close and constant contact with PWAs in a variety of settings, and nursing is one of the principal professions involved in AIDS education and prevention.

NURSES' NEEDS FOR KNOWLEDGE ABOUT AIDS AND HIV INFECTION

With few exceptions the management of AIDS and the care of PWAs become the responsibility of nurses in secondary and tertiary care centers. In acute care hospitals nurses provide constant, direct care to patients with AIDS with exacerbations of their disease. To do so, they need knowledge regarding nursing management of the alterations in health status caused by the disease and precautions to prevent transmission in the workplace.

In home health settings, as well as intermediate- and long-term care settings, nurses are often the only professionals involved daily with patients in the remission or chronic phase of their disease. Knowledge regarding prevention, precautions, infection control in the home, nutrition, transmission among household contacts, and safer sexual practices is necessary.

Schoolchildren, their parents, and teachers sometimes request information from nurses on how HIV infection is spread to allay their fears of having a child with AIDS in the classroom. In addition, teenagers need information on safer sexual practices and the dangers of drug use to reduce the likelihood of transmission.

In primary care settings nurses are in positions to screen and counsel populations at risk for HIV infection and AIDS and to assist in the identification of cases. Nurses need knowledge of sexual and drug use practices to assess these in their clients. They also need knowledge of sexual and drug use counseling. Nurses have contact with HIV-infected persons and their families in a variety of nursing care and occupational settings and may assume one or more roles in the prevention or treatment of HIV infection. Nurses working in occupational health settings or as independent practitioners need assessment skills to determine whether referral for HIV testing is needed.

Nurses in acute care or mental health settings must be familiar with the psychosocial and neuropsychiatric aspects of HIV disease, since they may have to deal with the depression and anxiety that accompany a diagnosis of HIV infection or AIDS and with the dementia associated with AIDS. Knowledge of HIV disease is necessary for counseling persons in any stage of infection, as well as the "worried well." Mental health nurses, hospital nurses, community health nurses, and nurses working in hospices need knowledge of supportive therapies to deal with death and dying.

Community health nurses need information on prevention, transmission, risk assessment and case finding, HIV antibody testing, and psychosocial support to be of service to their clients. In addition, they must know the sexual and life-style practices of various subcultures in the United States to work effectively and to educate. Nurses are commonly the source of referrals for PWAs and their families and friends in dealing with many of the problems associated with AIDS. They provide information about AIDS to the general public.

Nurses need knowledge about HIV infection, AIDS, and management of the disease because they have a greater range of contact with AIDS patients and their families than does any other health care professional group. Nurses are also frequently consulted about AIDS by laypersons and community groups. Finally, to give safe and sensitive care to PWAs, nurses must understand the disease, its effects on patients, transmission, precautions for avoiding infection, and the supportive care of persons with HIV infection. Questions have been raised about whether nurses have adequate knowledge of HIV disease and the care of infected persons and whether their attitudes interfere with sensitive, supportive, and safe care.

NURSES' KNOWLEDGE AND ATTITUDES AND THEIR EFFECT ON PRACTICE

Often knowledge and attitudes are interrelated in the care of persons with HIV infection. Anxiety, fear, discomfort, embarrassment, and negative social attitudes usually decrease as knowledge of the disease and its transmission and experience working with PWAs increase. Fear of the disease and its transmissibility has been an overriding concern of nurses and physicians. As a result of this fear, some nurses have left their jobs, refused to care for PWAs, or given only minimal care to these patients. Nurses have sometimes used inappropriate precautions and isolation techniques with patients who have AIDS.

Early studies of nurses' knowledge of AIDS and attitudes toward PWAs showed that knowledge was inadequate and attitudes were sometimes negative. In February 1986 the American Nurses' Association released a survey of state nurses' associations' responses to a questionnaire on AIDS that addressed a variety of issues. Twenty-eight state nurses associations and eight state affiliates of the Emergency Nurses Association responded. Fourteen associations or affiliates reported instances in which registered nurses refused to care for AIDS patients. These were isolated events that occurred early in the AIDS epidemic; education and information about transmission alleviated fears. In nine states employees were permitted to request reassignment to avoid caring for persons with AIDS; this was not allowed in eight states. If allowed to request reassignment, the employee had to meet certain requirements such as pregnancy or immunosuppressed condition. Only two state associations reported that disciplinary action was necessary. In most cases nurses backed down on threats to resign when told that refusal to care for persons with AIDS would result in termination of employment. At the time of the survey all hospitals and health care facilities in one state were adopting specific guidelines regarding care of PWAs and employee protection from exposure, most hospitals and facilities in seven states were doing so, and some hospitals and facilities in fifteen states were doing so.

Nurses' knowledge of AIDS and its transmission, as well as clear institutional policies regarding obligation to provide treatment, appears to influence attitudes toward caring for PWAs. Knowledge, however, might be inaccurate and inadequate. In January 1986 the Veterans Administration Medical Center in Washington, D.C., and the National Institutes of Health surveyed knowledge of AIDS in 1194 hospital employees (including nurses) of a large hospital in that city. Significant findings included the following inaccurate beliefs and information about AIDS and consequent effects on the care of patients with AIDS:

1. Fifty percent believed that AIDS could be spread through casual contact.
2. Twenty percent believed AIDS could be spread through coughing and sneezing.
3. More than fifty percent said they would wear a gown and mask when caring for an AIDS patient.
4. Forty-nine percent said they spent less time with AIDS patients than with other patients.
5. Thirty-five percent reported actively avoiding involvement with patients with AIDS (Macks, 1986).

A survey of 1019 nurses in California demonstrated other areas of deficient knowledge about AIDS and consequent behavior toward persons with AIDS (van Servellen et al., 1988). About half of these nurses had cared for a patient with AIDS in the preceding 6 months, and two thirds cared for patients at risk for or concerned about contracting AIDS; 62% of the sample were general staff nurses. Knowledge and practice deficits occurred in correctly identifying the symptoms of AIDS (88% could not) and in taking a sexual history (91% did not). However, 69% were able to identify the groups at risk for AIDS, and 82% knew the correct infection control procedures. The effect on patient care could be inferred from the findings: 23% said they absolutely would not care for patients with AIDS, and 54% said that nurses should be allowed to refuse to care for patients having or suspecting of having HIV infection. Nurses who had recently cared for patients with AIDS and those at risk and who had attended lectures and education forums on AIDS were more likely to know AIDS symptoms, groups at risk, and necessary precautions. They were also more willing to give care to PWAs. Early in the AIDS epidemic the nursing community believed that knowledge would increase and attitudes would improve with adequate education.

The past 2 years has seen many more studies of nurses' knowledge and attitudes about AIDS and the effect of these on the nurses' practice. In many cases the results have not been encouraging and do not show the changes that were anticipated earlier. A random sample of 581 registered nurses in Erie County, N.Y., revealed that about half feared contracting the disease, worried that they might put friends and family at risk, and were concerned that they would be unable to meet the intense physical and psychologic needs of PWAs (Scherer et al., 1989). Furthermore, about half believed that they had the right to refuse care to a PWA. Influencing their attitudes toward PWAs were feelings of hopelessness about the prognosis of the disease and negative attitudes toward homosexuals. D'Augelli (1989) reported similar findings in a sample of 144 nurses attending an

AIDS conference in rural central Pennsylvania. Respondents generally had correct knowledge about AIDS and its transmission, but one third harbored irrational fears about transmission from restaurant waiters and one half feared sharing meals and utensils. Participants held negative views of homosexuals; homophobic attitudes correlated significantly with AIDS phobia. In both of these studies the investigators suggested targeted intervention strategies for nurses, including additional AIDS education that dealt with the illness, its transmission, and affective issues.

A high level of knowledge of AIDS is not always related to positive attitudes. In a comparison of 42 nurses in a teaching hospital and 48 nurses in a religious-affiliated community hospital, knowledge of AIDS was uniformly high in both settings (Damrosch et al., 1990). Attitudes of teaching hospital nurses were more favorable than those of community hospital nurses, but a sizable proportion of both groups (45% and 65%, respectively) indicated that they would refuse to care for a PWA. Those refusing had higher levels of concern about acquiring AIDS through occupational exposure and negative attitudes toward homosexuals and PWAs.

The issue of occupational exposure surfaces in most studies. Wiley and colleagues (1990) found that of 323 nurses surveyed in a large medical center in Chicago, 64 (20%) reported HIV exposure. Reported exposure was significantly related to concerns about becoming HIV infected, considerations of changing profession to avoid infection, and beliefs that nurses should be involved in formulating institutional HIV policies. These investigators raised questions about the high percentage of nurses who claimed HIV exposure, since only seven such cases had been reported to the Occupational Health Department since 1985. If indeed the number of HIV exposures claimed was accurate, these nurses needed to be more accountable for following the agency's HIV infection control policies and procedures. The authors suggested that nurses need more information about HIV infection control and seroconversion rates of HIV-exposed nurses.

A study by Gruber and colleagues (1989) underscores the concerns and recommendations of the previous study. These investigators found that knowledge of HIV infection and universal precaution practices was not related to nurses' implementation of universal precautions. Knowledge scores were high among 213 nurses studied in a northeastern medical center, yet few nurses were wearing gowns when changing the linen of incontinent patients or wearing goggles and masks when suctioning the airways of patients with tracheostomies. Significantly, 62% did not notify their immediate supervisor after an accidental blood exposure, in direct conflict with hospital policy. A similar lack of compliance was found at San Francisco General Hospital, where employees attributed their noncompliance to inadequate AIDS education and supplies at the hospital.

In the study by Gruber and associates, nurses gave as their reasons for failure to follow policy the unavailability of supplies, habit, frequent changes in CDC directives, and weak or nonspecific directives by agencies. These investigators noted the need for interventions that would motivate nurses to implement universal precautions. They suggested that these interventions should have both psychosocial and educational components.

Other studies have shown that accurate knowledge about AIDS is significantly correlated with lower anxiety, willingness to work with PWAs, and appropriate professional behavior toward the PWAs (Christ & Wiener, 1985; Macks, 1986). Lawrence and Lawrence (1989) compared knowledge and attitudes about AIDS among registered nurses, baccalaureate nursing students, and nurses with graduate degrees. They found that higher levels of education were associated with more favorable attitudes and greater knowledge of AIDS. Knowledge of AIDS was positively correlated with more favorable attitudes toward AIDS in all comparison groups. In general, accurate and regular in-service education on transmission and infection control, clear and consistent institutional policies on precautions for health care workers, and clear and consistent institutional guidelines on the obligation to treat have decreased the fears and inappropriate behaviors of nurses working with HIV-infected persons (Malik-Nitto & Plantemoli, 1986).

Several studies report the effects of continuing education conferences or workshops and experience working with PWAs on nurses' knowledge and attitudes. The findings are generally positive. In a review of literature about the effects of AIDS education on health care workers' knowledge and anxieties, All (1989) identified essential aspects of educational intervention strategies for changing nurses' knowledge and attitudes. These were (1) accurate information on precautions and infection control guidelines and perceived risk, (2) experience in sexual history taking and counseling patients on transmission, and (3) psychosocial support to reduce stress related to the intense physical and psychologic demands of caring for PWAs. Other researchers have suggested involving nurses in establishment of institutional policies about HIV exposure and developing programs with affective components to deal with homophobia (Wiley et al., 1990; Young et al., 1989).

Flaskerud and colleagues (1989) reported the effects of a 1-day continuing education conference in Southern California on nurses' knowledge and attitudes. The conference included all of the components identified by All (1989) and the other investigators noted, as well as current information on AIDS regional epidemiology, etiology, and legal and ethical issues. The 125 participants were pretested, posttested, and retested after 2 to 3 months on their attitudes and knowledge. Significant pretest-posttest differences occurred in both knowledge and attitudes, and these were retained on retest. Experience in caring for a PWA and increasing attendance at AIDS workshops were factors related to greater knowledge and more positive attitudes.

In a study with similar results, Young et al. (1989) measured changes in knowledge and attitudes toward AIDS and homosexuality after an all-day educational program on AIDS. The participants were 56 nurses from rural New York and Pennsylvania. The program content was similar to that recommended by All (1989). Pretest, posttest, and retest (after 3 months) measures revealed significant positive changes in knowledge and attitudes. Participants were less fearful and more willing to care for PWAs 3 months later. These changes were correlated with differences in attitudes toward the disease and homosexuality. The investigators attributed attitude change to the program's affective component (dialogue and reassessment of values about homosexuality, sexual behaviors, and sexual history taking). These findings are congruent with a previous study (1988) in which Young found that an affective teaching method promotes short-term changes in nurses' attitudes about homosexuality.

Three studies of nursing students offer the best evidence of the positive effects of direct care experience with PWAs on knowledge and attitudes. Klisch (1990) identified the reactions of 11 nursing students to giving nursing care to an HIV-infected person in each of the four phases of the nurse-patient relationship. Students progressed from moderate or severe anxiety to fear and depersonalization of the patient, to identifying with the patient, to feeling close to the patient. The students' knowledge of AIDS also increased while they were caring for PWAs. The students perceived the experience of providing direct care to such patients as positive and growth producing. They recommended that all students have the opportunity to care for PWAs.

Matocha (1990) described similar results with nine students caring for HIV-seropositive persons. Students progressed from fear, ambivalence, and considerations of refusing the assignment or leaving the profession to an identification of the nurse's supportive role in providing care to HIV-infected persons, to actually providing that care. Positive outcomes reported by the students included the opportunity to experience a rewarding nurse-patient relationship and the opportunity to review their value judgments.

Cassels and Redman (1989) added confirming data on the attitudes and knowledge of new baccalaureate graduates. Of the 427 new graduates responding to their survey, two thirds indicated that if given a choice of patient assignment, they would readily provide direct care for a person with HIV disease and would take appropriate precautions. Students in these studies differed in attitudes and knowledge from their more practiced colleagues in studies described earlier in this chapter.

OCCUPATIONAL RISKS, HOMOPHOBIA, AND ATTITUDES

The studies of nurses' attitudes and knowledge suggest that fear of occupational exposure to HIV may be one cause for negative attitudes toward caring for HIV-infected persons. For some time now, evidence has indicated that the risk to health care workers is small and that the precautions recommended for health care personnel are adequate. In addition, the CDC's prospective study (1987) of percutaneous injuries to health care workers caring for patients with AIDS should lessen nurses' fears about acquiring AIDS in the workplace. The risk to health care workers has not changed in the last 2 years; it remains small. A prospective cohort study of 270 health care workers (including nurses) at San Francisco General Hospital evaluated the risk of occupational transmission of HIV, hepatitis B virus (HBV), and cytomegalovirus (CMV) to health care workers with intensive exposure to HIV-infected patients for at least 1 year before the study (Gerberding et al., 1987). These subjects were examined for antibody at enrollment and 10 months later; a follow-up at 9 to 12 months was planned. None of the subjects had developed antibody, and no evidence of increased risk for HBV or CMV was obtained. These results indicate that health care workers are at minimal risk for HIV, HBV, and CMV even when exposure to infected patients is intensive. However, reducing the hazard from exposure is a realistic goal for any employee health program and can be accomplished by relatively simple infection control measures (Gerberding, 1989).

Some nurses and physicians continue to believe that the government, their hospital, researchers, or the CDC is withholding information on the transmission of AIDS (Ostrow & Gayle, 1986; Wallack, 1989). This attitude is more prevalent among minority physicians and nurses, many of whom are foreign born. Approximately two thirds of the 239 subjects in Wallack's study (1989) believed that they were at significant risk of becoming infected with HIV despite following hospital infection control guidelines. More than 60% also distrusted information about their safety provided by national experts. Infection control procedures and universal precautions are addressed in depth in Chapter 11. The issue of occupational exposure to HIV among nurses is raised here to consider the relationship between fear of exposure and nurses' attitudes toward PWAs. If fear of HIV exposure is behind nurses' negative attitudes, a comprehensive intervention strategy dealing with that fear is needed to change their attitudes. However, fear of occupational exposure is often accompanied by negative attitudes toward homosexuals. In Wallack's survey (1989) 48% of the physicians and nurses reported feeling angry at the homosexual population and blamed homosexual promiscuity for causing an epidemic that now threatens the heterosexual population.

Wallack's finding focuses attention on the problem of health care workers making moral and social judgments about the worth and value of HIV-infected persons. In several studies referred to earlier, nurses said they should be allowed to refuse to care for clients with AIDS (Damrosch et al., 1990; van Servellen et al., 1988; Wiley et al., 1990). This belief was accompanied by negative attitudes toward the sexual behaviors and life-styles of some groups, such as homosexuals, IV drug users, and prostitutes. In the study by van Servellen and colleagues (1988), about half the nurses surveyed thought that the average nurse was uncomfortable discussing sexual matters with male homosexual patients and 38% indicated moderate to great discomfort when caring for these patients. These nurses were more likely to believe that they should be allowed to refuse to care for patients with AIDS, to think that they were at high risk for contracting AIDS, and to use overly cautious isolation techniques. They were also less knowledgeable about AIDS symptoms, transmission groups, and correct precautions.

Among medical students surveyed in New York City, more than 48% believed that they should have the prerogative of declining to care for patients with AIDS (Imperato et al., 1988). They also held inaccurate perceptions of their risks of acquiring HIV disease. These beliefs were influencing both their career choices and their site of residency training. A survey of a probability sample of 473 primary care physicians in New York City yielded similar findings: more than one third said they would refer an asymptomatic HIV-positive patient elsewhere rather than treat the patient themselves, and more than half had concerns about contracting HIV infection from a patient (Gemson et al., 1989). Physicians with less favorable attitudes toward homosexual men were less knowledgeable and less willing to care for HIV-positive patients.

Several studies of health care workers' attitudes toward homosexuals have assessed homophobia among physicians and nurses. Kelly and colleagues (1987a,b, 1988) used an experimental design that tested the separate and combined effects of an AIDS diagnosis and gay sexual preference on participants' evaluations of patients described in vignettes. Separate samples of nurses, medical students, and physicians were found to be significantly biased against PWAs (as compared with leukemia patients). In addition, the nurses and medical students showed evidence of bias against homosexuals. In Wallack's study (1989), 18% of physicians and 33% of nurses believed that homosexual men with HIV disease had only themselves to blame. Underscoring the homophobia among health care workers apparent in these studies is evidence that the public's attitude toward homosexuals has become more negative during the last 2 years. Reports of gay-bashing have increased. A survey of college students found that attitudes toward homosexuals became significantly more negative from 1986 to 1988 (Sheehan et al., 1990). Men reported more negative attitudes and fears than women. With this backdrop the task of changing nurses' knowledge and attitudes appears formidable.

NURSE-IDENTIFIED AIDS INFORMATIONAL NEEDS

As the AIDS epidemic spreads and takes form across the United States, all nurses will need information about HIV infection to provide optimal care for their clients. The content of the first edition of this book was based on an assessment of nurses' needs for AIDS information. A national survey of 832 nurses was conducted to identify nurses' AIDS informational needs, the groups of clients to whom they were providing care, and their preferred educational resources for information about HIV. When the first edition was published, a random sample of 200 nurses from the original survey was selected. These nurses received a copy of the book and a questionnaire to use in evaluating the text; 162 (81%) of the sample completed and returned the evaluation. The nurses responding had worked in their present nursing occupation for an average of 11 years; their primary work settings were hospitals (29%), community agencies (25%), and schools (19%); the majority (61%) had cared for a PWA within the preceding 6 months. The questionnaire items for evaluation of the book were similar to the items used in the first survey. In this case, however, nurses were asked whether the book met their needs for information in a particular area and not whether they had needs for information in that area (the original question). On these items more than 90% said that the book met their needs for information. A second set of items asked respondents to indicate in which areas they needed more information about AIDS. The nurses identified the following areas:

1. Current treatment   60%
2. Drugs in use   65%
3. Symptom assessment   70%
4. Precautions for health care workers   68%
5. Transmission in the workplace   66%
6. Sexual history taking   60%
7. Sexual counseling   70%
8. Prevention   65%
9. Psychosocial aspects   73%
10. Ethical issues   75%

The respondents also expressed an interest in information on special topics: 95% were interested in epidemiologic trends in the United States; 89% desired information on IV drug users; about three fourths wanted information on the differences in HIV infection among women (75%) and children (79%); 97% were interested in changes in treatment of HIV disease; and 85% wanted to learn about changes in the virus and virus strains. Change in general was of particular interest to the nurses. They recognized that the AIDS arena changes rapidly and that their needs for information require constant updating. The respondents also expressed interest in an annual AIDS update for nurses that would focus on changes in HIV epidemiology, disease, medical treatment, nursing care, and the needs of special populations.

Based on these data, the content of this second edition of the text was developed. The major focus is on nursing practice to meet the needs and interests of nurses working with PWAs. In developing the content areas, nurses' needs for AIDS information were inferred also from the studies of nurses' knowledge and attitudes reviewed in this chapter. Several implications for nursing educational efforts may be drawn from these two sources of data.

PLANNING EDUCATIONAL INTERVENTIONS

Nurses planning educational programs for their peers or for nursing students may be guided by researchers' findings in addressing nurses' knowledge and attitudes. In general, investigators have found that nurses' knowledge of AIDS is high. Therefore nursing education should now be directed at changes in information rather than at basic AIDS information. Nurses are interested in changes in the virus and new virus strains; in treatment and experimental uses of zidovudine; in nursing assessment of symptoms and effective nursing care (skin care, mouth care, nutrition planning, treatment of diarrhea, and so forth); and in antibiotic and antiviral drugs and their effectiveness against the various opportunistic infections and neoplasms. They are also interested in areas that were not explored in depth in the past: the components of a neuropsychiatric examination, the care of IV drug users, differences in HIV disease in women, current prognosis of the disease, and treatment of children. Changes in the epidemiology of the disease are also of interest because of differences in the major transmission groups in the various parts of the United States. These changes identify the groups to whom nurses will be providing care.

Many areas of patient education are of interest to nurses: What is the latest information on early intervention? What are the roles of cofactors? How can persons with HIV infection get themselves enrolled in research protocols? What alternative therapies are available and what is their effectiveness? How is partner notification handled? What community resources are available to PWAs? What resources are available for long-term care and home care? Topics of educational programs for nurses to increase knowledge are listed in Table 1–3.

Several areas of knowledge are related to feelings of anxiety and in-

TABLE 1–3. Components of a Nursing Educational Program to Increase Knowledge

CONTENT	STRATEGIES
Immunology, viral strains	Provide information
Treatment, uses of azidothymidine	
Specific antibiotic and antiviral therapies for specific opportunistic infections and neoplasms	
Regional epidemiology	
HIV in drug users	
HIV in women	
HIV in children	
Nursing assessment of symptoms	Provide information
Neuropsychiatric assessment	Provide practice for skill attainment
Effective nursing care: mouth care, skin care, nutrition, diarrhea, providing a safe environment	Provide demonstration
Client education	Provide information
Information on early intervention	Include service providers as sponsors and resources
Role of cofactors	
Enrolling in research protocols	
Alternative therapies	
Partner notification	
Community resources	

security among nurses. Foremost among these are occupational exposure to HIV, transmission in the workplace, and precautions for health care workers. For nurses' fears to be allayed, they must frequently be given up-to-date information on risks to nurses and infection control procedures. As noted in the review of research on nurses' knowledge and attitudes, nurses are skeptical of information on transmission in the workplace given to them by national experts. Some believe that new strains of the virus have developed and require new precautions. Repeated information on the documented risk to health care workers and the effectiveness of universal precautions may calm nurses' fears in this regard. However, a second area of concern is nurses' apparent failure to use universal precautions even when these are well known and a matter of hospital policy. Educational efforts with an affective component (opportunity for dialogue, expression of feelings in a nonthreatening atmosphere) may help motivate nurses to change behaviors and thus reduce their risk.

Group discussions of institutional policies with a knowledgeable leader may be an effective means of educating nurses about universal precautions and other areas of AIDS care. Group discussions give nurses practice and information for involvement in institutional policymaking. A comprehensive institutional policy should include direction on reporting HIV exposure, information on the care and treatment of health care workers who are exposed, clear and relatively stable information on universal precautions, a commitment to provide adequate equipment for implementing precautions, psychosocial support services for health care personnel working with HIV-infected persons, and legal and ethical support services for health care workers.

Anxiety, insecurity, and discomfort among nurses arise in response to a lack of knowledge about sexual practices, sexual history taking, and sexual counseling. Information in these areas followed by practice in the form of role playing may provide education and allay anxieties, insecurities, and discomfort with topics of sexuality. The same is true of drug use behavior. Most nurses know little about assessing drug use behavior, counseling about drug use, and resources in the community for treating and rehabilitating drug users. Again, a combination of education and behavioral strategies such as role playing may reduce anxiety and discomfort with this topic (Table 1–4).

Changing nurses' attitudes requires more than just providing more information or education about AIDS. As noted previously, attitudes are influenced by fears of infection and anxiety associated with a lack of information and skills in some areas such as sexual behavior and drug use. However, attitudes are also formed by deeply held negative social and moral judgments about homosexuals and homosexuality, IV drug use, and promiscuity. Nurses share these attitudes with other health care workers and the public. The studies reviewed in this chapter indicate that nurses' attitudes have not changed substantially in the last 2 years and that education alone does not motivate attitude change. The most effective educational strategies for influencing attitudes have a strong affective component in which feelings can be expressed openly and in a nonthreatening atmosphere. This includes negative feelings about homosexuals and IV

TABLE 1–4. Components of a Nursing Educational Program to Increase Knowledge and Change Attitudes

CONTENT	STRATEGIES
Occupational exposure	Provide information
Transmission in the workplace	Group discussions with knowledgeable
Precautions for health care workers	leaders (infection control nurses)
Failure to use universal precautions	
Hospital and institutional HIV policies	Provide practice in designing comprehensive policy
Sexual practices and drug use	Provide information
Sexual practices, history taking, and counseling	Provide practice by role playing
	Include service providers as sponsors and resources
Drug use practices, history taking, counseling, and referral	

drug users, about various sexual practices, and about hospitals forcing nurses to care for PWAs against their wishes. It also includes identifying what angers or frightens nurses about homosexuality, drug use, or caring for a PWA.

Expressing negative feelings and identifying fears and hostilities cannot be the only components of an affective educational program. Researchers have reported that nurses with positive attitudes share a number of characteristics: they have a homosexual friend or family member; they have cared for a person with AIDS; they have more knowledge of AIDS, sexuality, and drug use; they are younger; they are more educated; they are United States born and white; and they have no religion or belong to a religious group that does not condemn homosexuality. Educational program planners can enhance these characteristics among participants when possible, compensate for their lack by providing supplemental information when feasible, and design specific interventions for nurses based on their social and cultural differences. For example, involving gay men, PWAs, and drug users in educational programs for health care workers gives participants in these programs a chance to meet and engage in a dialogue with people they have not known previously. A positive group experience with PWAs, drug users and gay men assists respondents in knowing and understanding transmission behaviors a little better. Providing information about AIDS and practice in developing skills in areas in which nurses are less knowledgeable and comfortable (e.g., sexual history taking and counseling) may also affect their attitudes. Role playing and practice tend to normalize behaviors that program participants might at first consider abnormal. Programs with different emphases might have to be developed for nurses who are, for instance, foreign born and United States born. Distrust of government (e.g., CDC) statements on transmission, unfounded fears of risks from casual contact, and moral disapproval and denial of care to homosexuals and drug users by some groups of nurses are issues that might require specific educational programs for nurses in some communities. Programs or group discussions led by a knowledgeable nurse whose social and cultural background is similar to the participants' may significantly reduce feelings of distrust and skepticism. On the other hand, the group makeup does not have to be homogeneous. The value of discussion with persons who hold differing social and moral positions should not be minimized for its role in producing individual growth and understanding. Educational programs that bring nurses together to discuss their various views can facilitate their acceptance and understanding of their patients and each other.

The part that religion plays in condemning homosexuals, drug users, and sexually promiscuous persons should not be underestimated in its influence on nurses' attitudes toward PWAs. However, most religions have at their core a commitment to charity and goodwill that can be cited to

TABLE 1–5. Components of a Nursing Educational Program to Change Attitudes

CONTENT	STRATEGIES
Homosexuality	Provide information
Drug use	Exploration of feelings in small group format
Sexual promiscuity	Provide knowledgeable group leaders who share participants' social, cultural background (include black, Hispanic, Asian and foreign born nurses)
	Include gay men, drug users, PWAs in discussion groups
	Include clergy and religious representatives in discussion groups

persuade nurses of the worth of PWAs and other stigmatized groups. In fact, in some religions the highest good can be achieved by service to those society considers to have the least worth. Many dedicated clergy and representatives from religious groups of all the major religions have been involved in providing care to PWAs. Whenever possible, such religious leaders should be included in program and group discussions. Such persons can be role models for nurses who share their religious affiliation. In addition, frank group discussions of religious beliefs may remind nurses of the commitments to charity and compassion that characterize most major religions (Table 1–5).

Educational workshops and conferences can no longer focus on "AIDS 101"; nurses now need and are looking for something more. The literature on nurses' knowledge and attitudes that has been published in the last 2 years provides a basis for planning educational offerings that meet nurses' current needs. This literature also provides a conceptual framework for the development of educational intervention strategies.

SUMMARY

Many changes in HIV disease and the AIDS epidemic have occurred in the last 2 years. This chapter provides an overview of those changes and refers the reader to subsequent chapters in which current information is presented in depth. Two areas of change not addressed elsewhere are covered here: the changing regional epidemiology of HIV infection and changes in nurses' knowledge and attitudes. Suggestions are given for planning nursing education workshops and conferences to improve nursing knowledge, skills, and attitudes in the care of persons with HIV disease.

Information about HIV infection is changing so rapidly that it is impossible to publish anything that is completely up to date. For this reason it is especially important for nurses to remain aware of new developments and changes in information about HIV. Close attention to AIDS- and HIV-related research, conferences, and information in the popular media can help nurses keep up with issues and information about HIV disease and the AIDS epidemic.

References

Abrams, D.I. (1986). AIDS: Battling a retroviral enemy. *California Nursing Review, 8*(6), 10–16, 36–37, 44.

Abrams, D.I. (1987). AIDS: A search for hope. *California Nursing Review, 9*(1), 4–7, 11–13, 38–40.

Abrams, D.I. (1990). Definition of ARC. In P.T. Cohen, M.A. Sande, & P.A. Volberding (Eds.), *The AIDS knowledge base* (pp. 1-4.1.3 to 3-4.1.3). Waltham, MA: Medical Publishing Group.

All, A. (1989). Health care workers' anxieties and fears concerning AIDS: A literature review. *Journal of Continuing Education in Nursing, 20*(4), 162–165.

American Nurses Association (1986, February). Survey of state nurses' associations. Questionnaire on AIDS. Kansas City, MO.

Ascher, M.S., Francis, D.P. (1987). Is the blood supply safe from AIDS? *California Physician, 4*(7), 18–19.

Becker, M.H., Joseph, J.G. (1988). AIDS and behavioral change to reduce risk: A review. *The American Journal of Public Health, 78*(4), 394–410.

Brandt, A.M. (1988). AIDS in historical perspective: Four lessons from the history of sexually transmitted diseases. *The American Journal of Public Health, 78*(4), 367–371.

Cassells, J.M., Redman B.K. (1989). New baccalaureate graduates in care of AIDS patients: Perceptions of preparedness and information accessibility. *The Journal of Continuing Education in Nursing, 20*(4), 156–161.

Centers for Disease Control (1981a). *Pneumocystis* pneumonia—Los Angeles. *Morbidity and Mortality Weekly Report, 30*, 250–253.

Centers for Disease Control (1981b). Kaposi's sarcoma and *Pneumocystis* pneumonia among homosexual men—New York City and California. *Morbidity and Mortality Weekly Report, 30*, 305–309.

Centers for Disease Control (1985). WHO workshop: Conclusions and recommendations on AIDS. *Morbidity and Mortality Weekly Report, 34*, 275.

Centers for Disease Control (1986). Classification system for human T-lymphotropic virus III/lymphadenopathy–associated virus infections, *Morbidity and Mortality Weekly Report, 35*, 335.

Centers for Disease Control (1987). Update: Human immunodeficiency virus infections in health care workers exposed to blood of infected persons. *Morbidity and Mortality Weekly Report, 36*(19), 285–289.

Centers for Disease Control (1988). Human immunodeficiency virus infection in the United States: A review of current knowledge. *Morbidity and Mortality Weekly Report, 36*(suppl 6), 15.

Centers for Disease Control (1991, April). *AIDS Weekly Surveillance Report,* 1–18. United States AIDS Program, Atlanta.

Christ, G.H., Wiener, L.S. (1985). Psychosocial issues in AIDS. In V.T. DeVita Jr. (Ed.), *AIDS etiology, diagnosis, treatment and prevention* (pp. 275–297). Philadelphia: J.B. Lippincott.

Coolfont Report (1986). A PHS plan for prevention and control of AIDS and the AIDS virus. *Public Health Report, 101*, 341–348.

Damrosch, S., Abbey, S., Warner, A., et al. (1990). Critical care nurses' attitudes toward, concerns about, and knowledge of the acquired immunodeficiency syndrome. *Heart and Lung, 19*, 395–400.

D'Augelli, A.R. (1989). AIDS fears and homophobia among rural nursing personnel. *AIDS Education and Prevention, 1*(4), 277–284.

Flaskerud, J.H., Lewis, M.A., Shin, D. (1989). Changing nurses' AIDS-related knowledge and attitudes through continuing education. *The Journal of Continuing Education in Nursing,* 20(4), 148–154.

Friedman, S.R., Sotheran, J.L., Abdul-Quader, A., et al. (1987). The AIDS epidemic among blacks and Hispanics. *The Milbank Quarterly,* 65(2), 455–499.

Gail, M.H., Rosenberg, P.S., Goedert, J.J. (1990). Therapy may explain recent deficits in AIDS incidence. *Journal of Acquired Immune Deficiency Syndromes,* 3(4), 296–306.

Gemson, D.H., Colombotos, J., Elinson, J., et al. (1989). The role of the physician in AIDS prevention: A survey of primary care physicians in New York City. Final report. New York: Columbia University School of Public Health and New York City Department of Health.

Gerberding, J.L. (1989). Risks to health care workers from occupational exposure to hepatitis B virus, human immunodeficiency virus, and cytomegalovirus. *Infectious Disease Clinics of North America,* 3(4), 735–743.

Gerberding, J.L., Bryant-LeBlanc, C.E., Nelson, K., et al. (1987). Risk of transmitting the human immunodeficiency virus, cytomegalovirus, and hepatitis B virus to health care workers exposed to patients with AIDS and AIDS-related conditions. *Journal of Infectious Diseases,* 156(1), 1–8.

Gruber, M., Beavers, F.E., Johnson, B., et al. (1989). The relationship between knowledge about acquired immunodeficiency syndrome and the implementation of universal precautions by registered nurses. *Clinical Nurse Specialist,* 3(4), 182–185.

Hahn, R.A., Onorato, I.M., Jones, T.S., et al. (1989). Prevalence of HIV infection among intravenous drug users in the United States. *Journal of the American Medical Association,* 261(18), 2677–2684.

Imperato, P.J., Feldman, J.G., Nayeri, K., et al. (1988). Medical students' attitudes toward caring for patients with AIDS in a high incidence area. *New York State Journal of Medicine,* 88, 223–227.

Institute of Medicine/National Academy of Sciences (1988). Confronting AIDS: Update 1988. *Journal of Acquired Immune Deficiency Syndromes,* 1(2), 173–186.

Jason, J., Lui, K., Ragni, M.V., et al. (1989). Risk of developing AIDS in HIV-infected cohorts of hemophilic and homosexual men. *Journal of the American Medical Association,* 261(5), 725–727.

Joseph, S.C. (1987). AIDS in New York City: Moving ahead on effective public health approaches. *New York State Journal of Medicine,* 87(5), 257–258.

Kelly, J., St. Lawrence, J., Hood, H., et al. (1988). Nurses' attitudes toward AIDS. *Journal of Continuing Education in Nursing,* 19, 78–83.

Kelly, J., St. Lawrence, J., Smith, S., et al. (1987a). Medical students' attitudes toward AIDS and homosexual patients. *Journal of Medical Education,* 62, 549–556.

Kelly, J., St. Lawrence, J., Smith, S., et al. (1987b). Stigmatization of AIDS patients by physicians. *American Journal of Public Health,* 77, 789–791.

Klisch, M.L. (1990). Caring for persons with AIDS: Student reactions. *Nurse Educator,* 15(4), 16–20.

Landesman, S.H. (1989). Human immunodeficiency virus infection in women: An overview. *Seminars in Perinatology,* 13(1), 2–6.

Lawrence, S., Lawrence, R. (1989). Knowledge and attitudes about acquired immunodeficiency syndrome in nursing and non-nursing groups. *Journal of Professional Nursing,* 5, 92–101.

Lemp, G.F., Payne, S.F., Neal, D., et al. (1990). Survival trends for patients with AIDS. *Journal of the American Medical Association,* 263(3), 402–406.

Lifson, A.R., Darrow, W.W., Hessol, N.A., et al. (1990). Kaposi's sarcoma in a cohort of homosexual and bisexual men. *American Journal of Epidemiology,* 131(2), 221–231.

Lifson, A.R., Rutherford, G.W., Jaffe, H.W. (1988). The natural history of human immunodeficiency virus infection. *Journal of Infectious Diseases,* 158(6), 1360–1367.

Macks, J. (1986). The Paris AIDS conference: Psychosocial research. *Focus,* 1(10), 1–2.

Malik-Nitto, S., Plantemoli, L. (1986). A strategic plan for the management of patients with AIDS. *Nursing Management,* 17(6), 46–48.

Matocha, L.K. (1990). Student clinical experience with persons who are HIV-positive or have ARC/AIDS: A model of success. *Journal of Nursing Education,* 29(2), 90–92.

Menitove, J.E. (1990). Current risk of transfusion-associated human immunodeficiency virus infection. *Archives of Pathology and Laboratory Medicine, 114,* 330–334.

Najera, R., Herrera, M.I., de Andres, R. (1987). Human immunodeficiency virus and related retroviruses. *Western Journal of Medicine, 147,* 694–701.

Nanda, D., Minkoff, H.L. (1989). HIV in pregnancy—transmission and immune effects. *Clinical Obstetrics and Gynecology, 32*(3), 456–466.

Osmond, D. (1990). Progression to AIDS in persons testing seropositive for antibody to HIV. In P.T. Cohen, M.A. Sande, & P.A. Volberding (Eds.), *The AIDS knowledge base* (pp. 1-1.1.6 to 8-1.1.6). Waltham, MA: Medical Publishing Group.

Osmond, D.H., Moss, A.R. (1989). The prevalence of HIV infection in the United States: A reappraisal of the public health service estimate. In P. Volberding & M.A. Jacobson (Eds.), *AIDS clinical review 1989* (pp. 1-17). New York: Marcel Dekker.

Ostrow, D.G., Gayle, T.C. (1986, August). Psychosocial and ethical issues of AIDS health care programs. *Quality Review Bulletin, 12,* 284–294.

Quinn, TC. The global epidemiology of the human immunodeficiency virus. Paper presented Aug. 9, 1990, at the Clinical Care and Management of the HIV-Infected Patient Conference at the Medical College of Ohio, Toledo, OH.

Ron, A., Rogers, D.E. (1989). AIDS in New York City: The role of intravenous drug users. *Bulletin of the New York Academy of Medicine, 65*(7), 787–800.

Rothenberg, R., Woelfel, M., Stoneburner, R., et al. (1987). Survival with the acquired immunodeficiency syndrome. *New England Journal of Medicine, 317*(21), 1297–1302.

Scherer, Y.K., Haughy, B.P., Wu, Y.B. (1989). AIDS: What are nurses' concerns? *Clinical Nurse Specialist, 3*(1), 48–54.

Scitovsky, A.A. (1989). The cost of AIDS: An agenda for research. *Health Policy, 11,* 197–208.

Shapiro, C.N., Schulz, S.L., Lee, N.C., et al. (1989). Review of human immunodeficiency virus infection in women in the United States. *Obstetrics and Gynecology, 74*(5), 800–808.

Sheehan, E.P., Ambrosio, A., McDevitt, T.M., et al. (1990). A study of change in AIDS-related knowledge, attitudes, and behaviors over a two-year period. Paper presented at the Western Psychological Association conference, April 1990, Los Angeles, CA.

Shulman, L.C., Mantell, J.E. (1988). The AIDS crisis: A United States health care perspective. *Social Science and Medicine, 26*(10), 979–988.

Staff (November 1989). AIDS update. *Caring, 8*(11), 50.

Staff (March 16, 1990). HIV prevalence, projected AIDS case estimates: Workshop, October 31—November 1, 1989. *Journal of the American Medical Association, 263*(11), 1477.

Staff (April 30, 1990). From the World Health Organization. *AIDS/HIV Record, 4*(1), 10.

Time (Feb. 16, 1987). The big chill, fear of AIDS: "You haven't heard anything yet"; In the grip of the scourge. pp. 56–59.

Time (April 13, 1987). Yalta of AIDS. p. 60.

Ungvarski, P. (1983). Acquired immune deficiency syndrome. *Nursing Mirror, 157,* 17–20.

van Servellen, G.M., Lewis, C.E., Leake, B. (1988). Nurses' responses to the AIDS crisis: Implications for continuing education programs. *Journal of Continuing Education in Nursing, 19,* 4–8.

von Reyn, C.F., Mann, J.M. (1987). Global epidemiology. *Western Journal of Medicine, 147,* 694–701.

Wallack, J.J. (1989). AIDS anxiety among health care professionals. *Hospital and Community Psychiatry, 40*(5), 507–510.

Weisman, J. (1990, August). American Foundation for AIDS Research, International Research and Education Fund, Solicitation letter from the Chair. Los Angeles, CA.

Wiley, K., Heath, L., Acklin, M., et al. (1990). Care of HIV-infected patients: Nurses' concern, opinions, and precautions. *Applied Nursing Research, 3*(1), 27–33.

Young, E.W. (1988). Nurses' attitudes toward homosexuality: Analysis of change in A workshops. *Journal of Continuing Education in Nursing, 19,* 9–12.

Young, E.W., Koch, P.B., Preston, D.B. (1989). AIDS and homosexuality: A longitudinal of knowledge and attitude change among rural nurses. *Public Health Nursing, 6*(4) 196.

2

HIV Disease: Pathogenesis and Treatment

Christine Grady

HIV is the causative agent of a syndrome characterized by a progressive, gradual, irreversible, and disabling deterioration of the human immune system (Bowen et al., 1985). The resulting profound immunosuppression ultimately is clinically manifested by the infected host's susceptibility to a wide range of opportunistic infections (OIs) and malignancies. When the OIs and malignancies and other signs and symptoms of more advanced immunosuppression occur, the infected person's condition is diagnosed as AIDS according to the surveillance definition of the Centers for Disease Control (CDC). Since the identification of HIV as the causative agent of AIDS and AIDS-related conditions (Barre-Sinoussi et al., 1983; Gallo et al., 1984), it has become apparent that HIV begins its attack on the immune system long before the development of clinical signs and symptoms (Rosenberg & Fauci, 1989a). Infection with HIV may result in a spectrum of clinical consequences, including but not limited to the constellation of diseases defined as AIDS. The CDC (1986) has classified the spectrum of HIV-related clinical manifestations into distinct groups (Table 2–1). Another classification scheme, the Walter Reed Staging Classification, groups infected persons according to laboratory parameters (specifically the T4 cell count and the delayed-type hypersensitivity reaction) and some clinical information (Redfield & Burke, 1988). The CDC classification scheme of 1986 follows.

Group I—Acute Infection. This group includes a subset of recently infected persons who experience a complex of flulike symptoms, including fever, malaise, lymphadenopathy, fatigue, and myalgias, sometimes accompanied by skin rash or neurological symptoms. The symptoms generally occur about 14 to 21 days after exposure to the virus and resolve within a week or so, followed in most patients by seroconversion to positive antibody to HIV (Abrams, 1988).

TABLE 2–1. Centers for Disease Control Classification System for HIV Infection

Group I. Acute infection
Group II. Asymptomatic infection
Group III. Persistent generalized lymphadenopathy
Group IV. Other disease
        Subgroup A. Constitutional disease
        Subgroup B. Neurologic disease
        Subgroup C. Secondary infectious diseases
          Category C-1. Diseases as specified in Centers for Disease Control surveillance definition for AIDS
          Category C-2. Other specified infectious diseases
        Subgroup D. Secondary cancers
        Subgroup E. Other conditions

From Centers for Disease Control (1986). Classification system for human T-lymphotropic virus III/lymphadenopathy–associated virus infections. *Morbidity and Mortality Weekly Report*, 35, p. 335.

Group II—Asymptomatic. This group includes all HIV-infected individuals who have no clinical symptoms. The largest number of HIV-infected persons is believed to fall within this group (Abrams, 1988; Heyward & Curran, 1988).

Group III—Persistent Generalized Lymphadenopathy. Group III comprises infected individuals with persistent generalized lymphadenopathy (PGL) and no other clinical symptoms. PGL is defined as palpable lymphadenopathy persisting longer than 3 months, with greater than 1 cm enlargement at more than one extrainguinal site, and with no other causal explanation for the lymphadenopathy.

Group IV—Other Disease. Group IV includes HIV-infected persons with other clinical symptoms or opportunistic diseases. Group IV is divided into five subgroups; an individual may be in one or more subgroups at any given time.

    Subgroup A—Constitutional Disease. This group includes persons with one or more of the following: persistent fever for more than 1 month, involuntary weight loss of more than 10% of body weight, or diarrhea for more than 1 month, and the absence of a concurrent illness other than HIV infection to explain these symptoms.

    Subgroup B—Neurologic Disease. Infected persons are in this group if they have dementia, myelopathy, or peripheral neuropathy in the absence of concurrent illness other than HIV infection.

    Subgroup C—Secondary Infectious Diseases. This subgroup is further divided into two categories. Category C-1 includes persons with one of the opportunistic infections listed in the CDC surveillance definition of AIDS (see Chapter 3). Category C-2 includes patients with one of the following invasive diseases: oral hairy leukoplakia, multidermatomal herpes zoster, recurrent *Salmonella* bacteremia, nocardiosis, tuberculosis, or oral candidiasis (CDC, 1986).

Subgroup D—Secondary Cancers. This group includes HIV-infected individuals with certain types of malignancies as listed in the CDC definition of AIDS. These include Kaposi's sarcoma, non-Hodgkin's lymphoma, and primary lymphoma of the brain.

Subgroup E—Other. This is a catch-all group for any clinical findings or diseases that are not classifiable in the other groups, but are perhaps attributable to HIV infection or indicative of cell-mediated immunodeficiency. Examples are chronic interstitial pneumonitis and thrombocytopenia.

In the CDC classification scheme each group is distinct; a person can be classified in only one group at a time although the person's classification can be expected to change with time (this is not true of the group IV subgroups). The classification scheme is also hierarchic; a person can move from group I only to group II, III, or IV, and from group II only to III or IV but not back to group I or II, and so on (CDC, 1986). The order of this hierarchy reflects the progression of immunologic changes occurring in infected persons with time, even though this classification scheme itself contains no immunologic parameters. The common denominator throughout the spectrum is infection with HIV.

This chapter focuses on the characteristics of the virus itself, the damage it does to human lymphocytes and other human cells, and some of the therapeutic strategies being studied for controlling or eliminating HIV in infected individuals.

CHARACTERISTICS OF HIV

HIV is simply genetic material wrapped in a protein capsid and further encased in an envelope. HIV is a ribonucleic acid (RNA) virus, meaning the genomic material is RNA. HIV is composed of two strands of RNA surrounded by a 24,000 dalton molecular weight protein capsid or cylindrical core, usually referred to as the p24 *gag* protein or the core. This is further surrounded by an outer lipid envelope. The envelope has a balloonlike outer surface antigen called gp120 (glycoprotein of 120,000 daltons), which is anchored to a transmembrane segment referred to as gp41. Figure 2–1 illustrates the proposed mechanism for HIV infection of a cell. The envelope is sometimes referred to in its entirety as gp160. The genome of HIV has been well mapped. Structural genes include *gag,* which codes for the p24 core protein (as well as p15 and p17); *env,* which codes for the envelope (gp41 and gp120); and *pol,* which codes for the

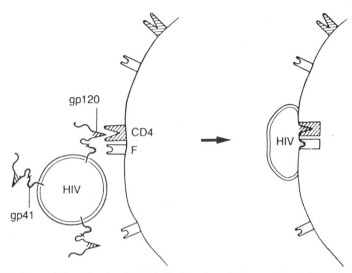

FIGURE 2-1. Proposed mechanism for HIV infection of a cell. The outside viral envelope protein, gp 120, attaches to a cell surface receptor, most likely the CD4 antigen. The external portion of the transmembrane protein, gp41, attaches to a specific fusion receptor on the cell surface. Either receptor may permit viral entry into the cell, but both together would make this event more efficient.

viral polymerases (reverse transcriptase, integrase, and protease). At least six other regulatory genes play an important part in the pathogenesis of HIV infection. These include *tat, rev, nef, vif, vpr,* and *vpu* (Rosenberg & Fauci, 1989b).

The HIV virion (viral particle) cannot replicate until it gets inside a cell and exploits the biosynthetic apparatus of the cell to reproduce. HIV is a retrovirus and so has a unique way of infecting and reproducing in cells. Only a few retroviruses are known to infect humans, including human lymphotrophic virus type I (HTLV-I); HTLV-II; human immuno-deficiency virus type 1 (HIV-1), the cause of AIDS and the subject of this chapter; and HIV-2, a second human retrovirus that causes an immuno-deficiency similar to that caused by HIV-1. Retroviruses contain a group of enzymes referred to as reverse transcriptase. These enzymes facilitate the reverse transcription of viral genomic RNA into DNA, which can then integrate itself into the cell genome as "proviral DNA," subsequently al-lowing virus to be passed from parent cell to progeny cells during meiosis. This is referred to as vertical or nuclear spread. HIV shares certain features, such as morphology and nucleotide sequences, with members of the non-transforming and cytopathic lentiviruses of the retrovirus family (Fauci, 1988; Ho et al., 1987).

HIV is transmitted by sexual contact, by infected blood or blood products, and from an infected mother to the fetus or neonate during the perinatal period (Heyward & Curran, 1988). HIV enters the body and infects predominantly cells that express a surface membrane CD4 molecule, the most numerous of which are T4 lymphocytes. Other CD4-positive cells that are targets for HIV infection include certain cells of the monocyte-macrophage lineage, dendritic cells, Langerhans' cells, promyelocytic cell lines, Epstein-Barr virus (EBV)–transformed B cells, and microglial cells (Fauci, 1988; Rosenberg & Fauci, 1989b; Vlahov, 1989).

The gp120 of the HIV binds avidly and specifically to the CD4 molecule, which acts as a receptor on the cell. After binding, the virus fuses with the cell membrane and is uncoated, and the HIV RNA enters the cell (Bowen et al., 1985; Fauci, 1988; Ho et al., 1987; Margolick et al., 1987). Once inside the cell the retroviral RNA is transcribed into DNA by the viral polymerase, reverse transcriptase (RT). This reverse transcription is a unique feature of RT-containing retroviruses. Some of the newly formed viral DNA is integrated into the cellular DNA in the cell nucleus with the help of another viral enzyme, integrase. The nuclear integrated viral DNA is referred to as the "provirus" (Fauci, 1988; Ho et al., 1987; Rosenberg & Fauci, 1989b). A substantial amount of remaining viral DNA remains unintegrated in the cellular cytoplasm (Ho et al., 1987; Rosenberg & Fauci, 1989b; Weber & Weiss, 1988). The replication of HIV in the cell is restricted at this stage until the infected cell is activated. Once activated, the proviral sequence in the cell nucleus can transcribe messenger and genomic RNA, leading to the synthesis of new viral proteins (Fauci, 1988; Ho et al., 1987; Weber & Weiss, 1988). The viral proteins and RNA assemble at the cell surface and bud out as mature virions (Ho et al., 1987; Rosenberg & Fauci, 1989b; Shaw et al., 1988; Weber & Weiss, 1988). The cell remains infected for its lifetime with viral DNA in its genome, and as it replicates and divides during normal cell division, it produces progeny cells that also contain the proviral sequence (Fauci, 1988; Ho et al., 1987; Weber & Weiss, 1988). For this reason, unless therapy that can eliminate the virus is found, an infected person will remain infected and infectious for life (Ho et al., 1987).

Once infected, a cell can remain intact with latent or low-level production of virus for long and variable periods (Bowen et al., 1985; Fauci, 1988; Ho et al., 1987; Margolick et al., 1987; Rosenberg & Fauci, 1989b, 1990). When an appropriate stimulus activates or stimulates an infected cell, there is active production of virus, which has been shown in vitro to contribute to the rapid destruction and death of the T4 cell (Fauci, 1988; Ho et al., 1988; Rosenberg & Fauci, 1989b; Shaw et al., 1988). Transcription of the provirus also results in expression of viral proteins, such as gp120, on the cell surface (Vlahov, 1989). Because of this, HIV not only is cytopathic for its target cells, but also causes syncytium or multinucleated giant cell formation between infected and uninfected cells. The cells that make up the syncytium then develop ballooning cytoplasm and die quickly (Ho et al., 1987; Vlahov, 1989).

The stimuli that provoke activation of the infected cell and rapid expression of virus fall under the broad category of cofactors. Several classes of factors involved in the activation of infected cells that may upregulate HIV expression have been identified. These include mitogens; antigens; heterologous viruses such as cytomegalovirus (CMV), herpes simplex virus (HSV), EBV, hepatitis B virus (HBV), and human herpesvirus type 6 (HHV-6); cytokines such as interleukin-6 (IL-6), granulocyte-macrophage colony stimulating factor (GM-CSF), and tumor necrosis factor–alpha; (TNF-alpha); and physical agents such as heat and ultraviolet light (Rosenberg & Fauci, 1989b, 1990).

IMMUNE RESPONSE TO HIV

People infected with HIV generate an impressive immune response to the virus. The existence of antibodies to HIV was noted early in the AIDS epidemic (Rosenberg & Fauci, 1989b). Infected individuals produce antibody to most of the major proteins of the virus, including gp120, gp160, gp41, and p24. Many studies have suggested that the titer of p24 antibody is highest early in HIV infection and lowest in the late stages of disease (Rosenberg & Fauci, 1989b). This may inversely correlate with the levels of measurable p24 antigen in the serum. Although neutralizing antibodies are present at varying titers in most infected persons, whether these antibodies can inhibit the spread of HIV infection in vivo is unclear. In addition to antibody formation, in vitro evidence shows that cell-mediated cytotoxicity (CMC), antibody-dependent cellular cytotoxicity, (ADCC), and natural killer cell activity can all participate in the immune response to HIV infection. Despite this potentially effective immune response, HIV is able to persist and cause relentlessly progressive damage to the immune system.

How HIV can evade the host's immune responses and persist in the infected individual for long periods is not known. One explanation may be the generation of antigenic variants. Variation exists throughout the genome, but the region of greatest variability is the *env* gene (Rosenberg & Fauci, 1989b). Perhaps because of these structural changes in the envelope region, the virus is able to escape an immune response and the infected person is unable to generate sustained protection. There is evidence that numerous genetic and biologic variants of HIV can develop with time in vivo and coexist in a single individual (Shaw et al., 1988).

TESTING FOR HIV

The simplest and most readily available laboratory test for HIV infection is the determination of the presence of antibody to HIV. As suggested previously, infected individuals almost always mount a substantial immune response to HIV and produce antibodies to the antigenic components of the major viral proteins (Vlahov, 1989). Unfortunately, these antibodies do not appear to provide lasting protection in an infected individual.

Tests for HIV antibody were first developed to screen blood before transfusion. Detection of HIV antibody indicates that a person has been exposed to HIV and has mounted an immune response. The presence of antibody (except in neonates) is an indication that the person is infected and infectious (Sandler et al., 1988). A negative antibody test does not, however, guarantee that the person is not infected, especially if exposure to the virus was recent. The enzyme-linked immunosorbent assay (ELISA) is the most widely used antibody test. It is used for screening, early diagnosis, and surveillance. The ELISA measures antibody to the whole virus. Because the ELISA was designed to detect contaminated blood in an effort to prevent transfusion-related infection, it is a very sensitive test (Sandler et al., 1988). False-positive results are particularly common in multiparous women, recipients of multiple blood transfusions, and others with high levels of circulating antibodies. The rate of false-positive results is higher when low-prevalence populations are tested. Because of this high degree of sensitivity, a reactive ELISA should always be repeated. If a person's blood is reactive in two or more ELISA tests, a confirmatory test is performed. The most commonly used confirmatory test is the Western blot analysis. Other tests, which are used less frequently and are less well established, are the immunofluorescence assay (IFA), and the radioimmune precipitation assay (RIPA). The Western blot is a more specific test than the ELISA. It confirms that the antibody in question is specifically reactive with HIV by detecting antibody reactivity to individual components of the virus. If a person's serum has antibody to two or more of the major viral proteins, the test is considered positive (Sandler et al., 1988).

HIV infection can also be detected by growing HIV on cultures of infected cells (HIV coculture), detecting viral antigens in blood (p24 antigen assay), amplifying HIV genes (polymerase chain reaction), and other techniques. Tests for antigen, viral culture, and gene amplification are research methods used primarily to monitor the effectiveness of antiviral agents in clinical trials. Many of these tests for virus are still in development, and the techniques of performance and interpretation of results have yet to be standardized (Poiesz et al., 1988).

IMMUNOPATHOGENESIS OF HIV

As previously stated, HIV selectively infects human cells that display a CD4 antigen on their surface. The majority of human cells that express CD4 antigens are T4 lymphocytes, although cells of the monocyte-macrophage family, EBV-transformed B cells, dendritic cells, and microglial cells also express a CD4 protein and are sometimes infected. HIV infection of T4 lymphocytes has a great impact because these cells either directly or indirectly induce virtually every other response of the human immune system (Fauci, 1988; Roitt et al., 1989; Stites et al., 1987; Vlahov, 1989). Of particular note, the recognition and elimination of certain antigens, including viruses in infected cells, is a major function of T cell immunity and is initiated and orchestrated by the T4 lymphocytes (Roitt et al., 1989; Stites et al., 1987). By selectively infecting T4 cells, the virus damages and ultimately leads to the destruction of the very cell that would normally ensure the destruction and elimination of the virus (Rosenberg & Fauci, 1989b).

The selective infection of T4 lymphocytes and their subsequent gradual and progressive destruction and depletion are the ultimate basis for the immunologic abnormalities and clinical consequences of HIV disease. It is HIV's uncanny ability to become intimately intertwined with the normal functioning of the immune system that not only leads to the devastating clinical and immunologic consequences, but also creates an enormous challenge to therapy and vaccine development.

T Cells. The most conspicuous immunologic abnormality associated with HIV infection is a striking quantitative deficiency of T4 cells (Fauci, 1988; Rosenberg & Fauci, 1989b). HIV infects and is cytopathic for T4 cells. When the infected T4 cell is stimulated, HIV is rapidly produced and the cell is destroyed (Ho et al., 1987; Rosenberg & Fauci, 1989b). The number of T4 cells drops significantly in the first few weeks after initial infection with HIV, then rises again to approach, but not usually to attain, preinfection levels within the first 3 months. After this, a gradual decline in number occurs over an extended period, with the rate of loss accelerating as disease progresses (Rosenberg & Fauci, 1990). In time a depletion in the number and percentage of measurable T4 cells is seen.

In addition to direct destruction of infected T4 cells by HIV, the dramatic depletion seen may also be the consequence of HIV infection of T cell precursors or cells that secrete factors stimulating the propagation of the entire lymphoid cell pool (Fauci, 1988; Rosenberg & Fauci, 1989b). In an immunologically intact individual the number of T4 cells measurable in the peripheral blood ranges from 600 to 1200 cells/mm^3. In someone with advanced HIV disease, it is not uncommon to find fewer than 10 T4 cells/mm³; some individuals with AIDS have undetectable numbers of T4 cells in peripheral blood.

The number of T4 cells can be correlated with the clinical course of HIV infection and disease. A person with fewer than 200 T4 cells/mm³, for example, is much more vulnerable to an opportunistic disease than someone with 400 or more T4 cells/mm³ (Kovacs & Masur, 1988). However, from the time of initial infection many years may elapse before the level of T4 cells drops low enough to permit the development of opportunistic infections or malignancies (Rosenberg & Fauci, 1990). The numerical depletion of T4 cells can be observed by noting increasing lymphopenia on a complete blood cell count (CBC) with a differential count. Quantification of T cell subsets, usually accomplished by cytofluorimetric (FACS) analysis, shows that the lymphopenia is actually a selective depletion of T4 cells with a relative sparing of T8 cells. Other useful measures to monitor the quantity of T4 cells include the T4 cell percentage and the ratio of T4 cells to T8 cells (T4/T8 ratio).

In addition to progressive T4 depletion, persons with HIV disease develop functional impairment in virtually every component of their immune system (Fauci, 1988; Rosenberg & Fauci, 1989a). HIV causes a qualitative defect in the function of T4 cells. The T4 cells of infected individuals have a defect in their responsiveness to specific antigen stimulation (Fauci, 1988; Margolick et al., 1987). This occurs even in asymptomatic HIV-infected persons. A T cell unable to be stimulated by antigen is also unable to perform its antigen-induced T cell functions, such as production and release of lymphokines, mediators that carry the inductive signal from the T4 cell to other cells in the host defense system (Bowen et al., 1985; Fauci, 1988; Lane & Fauci, 1985; Margolick et al., 1987). Thus defective immune responses occur over the entire spectrum of the antigen-specific T cell repertoire.

In vitro tests of T4 cells from infected individuals demonstrate decreased production of lymphokines such as interleukin-2 (IL-2), decreased expression of IL-2 receptors, decreased T cell colony formation, decreased cell-mediated cytotoxicity, decreased help to B cells for immunoglobulin synthesis, and a decreased ability to proliferate in a mixed lymphocyte culture (done to test for alloreactivity). Probably all these deficiencies are due at least in part to the lack of an adequate inductive signal from the T4 lymphocytes (Bowen et al., 1985; Fauci, 1988; Margolick et al., 1987; Rosenberg & Fauci, 1989a,b).

The lack of induction of other host defense mechanisms by the T cell is most likely due to both the quantitative and qualitative defects in the T4 lymphocyte. Many of the T cell abnormalities observed, such as decreased delayed-type hypersensitivity reaction, decreased lymphocyte blast transformation to mitogens, and decreased cytotoxic activity, result directly from the reduction in T4 cell number (Rosenberg & Fauci, 1989a).

The lack of a proliferative response to soluble antigen is not due predominantly to a low number of T4 cells but rather to an intrinsic defect in the remaining T4 cells. Furthermore, HIV selectively, but not exclusively, infects the antigen-responsive "memory" subset of T4 cells (Schnittman et al., 1990). This occurs even in asymptomatic HIV-infected individuals with normal or near normal T4 cell numbers (Lane et al., 1985b). These abnormalities of T cell or cell-mediated immunity are manifested clinically as lymphopenia, an altered T4/T8 cell ratio (because of the low number of T4 cells), anergy or decreased delayed hypersensitivity reaction to skin tests with common antigens, and a susceptibility to diseases against cell-mediated immunity, which usually provides protection. These opportunistic diseases are directly responsible for most of the morbidity and mortality associated with HIV infection.

B Cells. In addition to abnormalities in T cell–mediated immunity, abnormalities develop in other parts of the immune system, such as in B cell or humoral immunity. Since normally the function of the B cell is closely integrated with and dependent on induction by the T4 cell, many of the B cell abnormalities seen in HIV infection are probably due to lack of induction and regulation by the infected T4 cell. In addition, B cells demonstrate polyclonal hyperactivity, which results in hypergammaglobulinemia in most HIV-infected adults (Rosenberg & Fauci, 1989a,b).

HIV-infected adults often have high levels of circulating immune complexes. Some persons manifest immune complex–type symptoms or diseases. For example, certain of the thrombocytopenias seen in HIV-infected individuals are believed to result from immune complex phenomena in which platelets are destroyed as "innocent bystanders" (Ho et al., 1987). At the same time that B cells are erratically producing polyclonal immunoglobulin, they demonstrate a decreased ability to mount an antibody response to a *new* antigen (Bowen et al., 1985; Lane & Fauci, 1985; Margolick et al., 1987). Because of this, the effectiveness of immunizations in infected persons, for example, with the influenza vaccine is questionable. The reliability of serologic diagnosis for certain infections is also doubtful (Fauci, 1988). The most serious consequences of a reduced B cell ability to mount an antibody response to a new antigen are seen in infants and children who have not had previous exposure to a variety of pathogenic bacteria and must rely on a primary antibody response for adequate defense (Fauci, 1988).

Monocytes and Macrophages. Monocyte and macrophage function is also abnormal in HIV-infected persons. This, too, may result from lack of induction from the T4 cell, coupled with the fact that some monocytes and macrophages are themselves directly infected with HIV (Rosenberg & Fauci, 1990). In vitro, macrophages from HIV-infected individuals exhibit decreased chemotaxis, decreased expression of class II HLA antigens, and decreased production of IL-1 (Fauci, 1988). The ability of macrophages to be cytotoxic and protective against certain pathogens is also compromised, which presumably contributes to the increased susceptibility to parasitic and other intracellular infections (Bowen et al., 1985). Although many of these defects may be explained by the lack of gamma-interferon and other stimulating lymphokines from the defective T4 cell repertoire, direct infection of certain macrophages may also play a role (Fauci, 1988). Infected macrophages may also secrete increased amounts of IL-1 and TNF-a. Both of these monokines may contribute to the fevers and wasting syndrome that occur in many persons with AIDS.

The outcome of HIV-infected monocytes and macrophages differs in several important ways from that of infected T4 cells. First, many functions of the infected monocytes and macrophages remain unaltered (Rosenberg & Fauci, 1990). Second, infection of monocytes and macrophages appears to be persistent and does not result in significant cell death or syncytium formation. Also, HIV in infected monocytes and macrophages predominantly buds and accumulates intracellularly within intracytoplasmic vesicles rather than from the plasma membrane (Rosenberg & Fauci, 1990; Meltzer et al., 1990). HIV within the intracytoplasmic vesicles is sheltered from the immune response in vivo. Because of this ability to sequester virus, monocytes and macrophages may function as a reservoir of virus and play a major role in the pathogenesis of HIV infection (Fauci, 1988; Meltzer et al., 1990).

In contrast to T4 cells, infected macrophages are normal in number, phenotype, and many functions even in the late stages of HIV disease, while at the same time the infected macrophage represents an important source and reservoir of HIV that remains hidden from the host's immune system (Fauci, 1988; Meltzer et al., 1990). In addition, infected monocytes and macrophages may be responsible for transporting HIV to the lung or brain (Meltzer et al., 1990). HIV-infected macrophages are found in the brain, lymph nodes, and lung, but not in other tissues, such as the Kupffer cells of the liver (Meltzer et al., 1990). Infected macrophages may release toxic substances that are harmful to surrounding tissues, such as brain cells (Ho et al., 1987; Price et al., 1988).

Precursor Cells. Hematologic abnormalities, including lymphopenia, anemia, thrombocytopenia, and myelodysplasia, are common in patients with AIDS. Studies have suggested that hematologic abnormalities may be the result of HIV infection of bone marrow precursor cells (Rosenberg & Fauci, 1989b). The infection of bone marrow progenitor cells is similar to infection in monocytes and macrophages; that is, it is noncytopathic and replicates with intracellular budding. Bone marrow may also function as a reservoir of HIV infection in the body (Rosenberg & Fauci, 1989b). A recent study has demonstrated that thymic precursor cells may be infected with HIV in vitro (Schnittman et al., 1990). This may help to explain the inability of the T4 cell pool to regenerate itself in HIV-infected individuals, even during effective antiretroviral therapy.

EFFECTS OF HIV ON OTHER ORGAN SYSTEMS

Neurologic System. Central nervous system complications have been common in people with AIDS throughout the epidemic and can be grouped as (1) opportunistic infections, such as toxoplasmosis encephalitis, cytomegalovirus encephalitis, and cryptococcal meningitis, (2) central nervous system tumors, such as primary brain lymphoma, and (3) HIV encephalopathy or AIDS dementia complex (ADC). Evidence is substantial that this third group, found in up to two thirds of people with AIDS, is a direct result of HIV infection (McArthur et al., 1988; Price et al., 1988). HIV has been isolated in large amounts from both the brains and the cerebrospinal fluid of patients with ADC (Ho et al., 1987; McArthur et al., 1988; Price et al., 1988). In the brain the cells infected by HIV are predominantly the CD4-positive cells of the monocyte-macrophage lineage (including microglial cells), and it is these cells that are believed to play the central role in the pathogenesis of ADC (Ho et al., 1987). Probably factors other than cellular damage directly caused by HIV are involved. For example, HIV infection is postulated to cause the release of toxins or lymphokines that result in cellular dysfunction or interfere with neurotransmitter function (McArthur et al., 1988).

Clinical characteristics of ADC include a progressive loss or decline in cognitive function and motor and behavioral changes. Symptoms include apathy, memory impairment, inability to concentrate, depression, and psychomotor retardation (Ho et al., 1987; McArthur et al., 1988; Price et al., 1988). Focal motor abnormalities and behavioral changes may also occur. In the majority of patients who show symptoms of ADC, the symptoms progress rapidly and full-blown dementia complex usually develops within a year.

In addition to ADC, HIV may be responsible for other common neurologic complications in patients with AIDS, including peripheral neuropathy (with painful dysthesias and paresthesias) and vacuolar myelopathy (vacuolar degeneration of the spinal cord) (Price et al., 1988).

Renal System. HIV-associated nephropathy was first described in 1984 (Gardenswartz et al., 1984; Pardo et al., 1984; Rao et al., 1984). These reports were of heavy proteinuria or the nephrotic syndrome and a rapid progression to end-stage chronic renal failure. The etiology of renal disease is diverse and includes renal invasion by a variety of opportunistic pathogens (e.g., CMV, *Cryptococcus, Candida, Pneumocystis,* mycobacteria) and neoplasms (e.g., lymphoma and Kaposi's sarcoma) (Bourgoignie, 1989). In addition, disturbances in extracellular fluid volume (e.g., from vomiting, diarrhea, or inadequate intake) may result in a hemodynamic contribution to renal dysfunction (O'Regan et al., 1990). Also, many nephrotoxic drugs (such as pentamidine, amphotericin B, sulfadiazine, and foscarnet) are used in the management of AIDS-related OIs. More recently a characteristic form of aggressive focal segmental glomerulosclerosis, termed HIV-associated nephropathy (HIVN or HIVAN) has been described. HIVN may be an early manifestation of HIV disease because almost half of reported cases occurred in people who did not have AIDS by definition (Bourgoignie, 1989; Carbone et al., 1989). HIVN is a nonspecific glomerulopathy and tubulopathy with a spectrum of clinical manifestations ranging from modest proteinuria and mildly decreased renal function to a full-blown nephrotic syndrome with chronic renal insufficiency or failure (Bourgoignie, 1989). Most patients with HIVN are black and from metropolitan areas in the eastern United States, especially New York City and Miami (Bourgoignie, 1989; Carbone et al., 1989; O'Regan et al., 1990). The prevalence is distinctly low in white homosexual men. Although HIVN is also more common in intravenous drug users (IVDU), it does not seem to be necessarily related to intravenous drug use because it is prevalent in women, children, and Haitian blacks who have little history of drug use (O'Regan et al., 1990).

The pathogenesis of HIVN is unknown. Possibilities include (1) OI, but HIVN does occur in patients without OI; (2) immune complex nephritis, although no evidence has been found for this; (3) hemodynamic glomerulopathy as a result of primary or compensatory intraglomerular hemodynamic alterations; or (4) mediation by local lymphokines with activity on capillary permeability (Bourgoignie, 1989). The ultrastructural changes seen in renal tissue are compatible with a viral etiology, and although no viral particles or virions have been identified, HIV genome has been found in tubular epithelia, leaving open the question of direct infection of renal tissue with HIV (Cohen et al., 1989).

Ocular System. Ocular lesions in AIDS have been described since early in the epidemic. Studies have shown that between 40% and 90% of patients with AIDS have some ocular involvement (Holland, 1985; Marsh, 1989; Palestine et al., 1984), and some have shown ocular changes in earlier stages of HIV infection (Humphry et al., 1987). Ocular changes may be accompanied by severe morbidity and in some cases blindness. Krieger and Holland (1988) grouped the ophthalmologic complications of AIDS into four categories: (1) primary retinal microvascular disease, (2) OI of the eye and adnexa (especially CMV, HSV, and varicella-zoster virus [VZV]); (3) neoplasms of the eye (Kaposi's sarcoma), and (4) neuro-phthalmic abnormalities (such as those seen with ADC or OI of the central nervous system).

Although severe morbidity is frequently associated with OIs of the eye, especially CMV retinitis, primary retinal microvascular disease may be the most common ophthalmic condition. It is characterized by bilateral, usually transitory cotton-wool spots and less commonly by retinal hemorrhage, microaneurysm, and other abnormalities (Marsh, 1989). Although HIV antigen and particles have been found in the capillary endothelial cells (Pomerantz et al., 1987), evidence suggests that these abnormalities are the result of the deposition of immune complexes obstructing the capillary lumen, rather than directly a result of HIV infection.

Cardiac System. A wide variety of cardiac abnormalities, sometimes without associated signs or symptoms, have been reported in people with AIDS. These abnormalities include ventricular dysfunction, neoplastic involvement, nonbacterial endocarditis, myocarditis, dilated cardiomyopathy, and pericardial effusion. Although the incidence of cardiac abnormalities may be as high as 73% (Nyamathi, 1989; Valle & Lemberg, 1987), cardiac disease has not played a major role in the clinical course of most HIV-infected patients. In fact, many of the abnormalities have been found at autopsy or by invasive exploration (Acierno, 1989; Coplan & Bruno, 1989). The large number of patients who have myocarditis at autopsy but who had no clinical evidence of heart disease suggests that cardiovascular problems may become more prominent in AIDS if the therapeutic efficacy for noncardiac disease continues to improve and prolong survival (Acierno, 1989; Coplan & Bruno, 1989).

Of particular interest is myocarditis not found to be associated with any particular opportunistic infection or duration of illness. Usually unaccompanied by clinical symptoms, it is estimated to occur in up to 60% of patients with AIDS (Anderson et al., 1986). The cause is unknown, but possibilities include (1) immunologic mechanisms (Keriakis & Parmley, 1984), (2) certain opportunistic infections such as CMV (Cohen et al., 1986), and possibly (3) direct viral pathogenesis from HIV (Calabrese et al., 1987). HIV has been isolated in cultures of endomyocardial tissue from a patient with congestive cardiomyopathy (Calabrese et al., 1987). The symptoms of myocarditis may range from nonexistent or obscured ("silent") myocarditis to strikingly severe with full-blown congestive heart failure or disabeling arrhythmias or both (Acierno, 1989).

AIDS-related heart disease has been considered an end-stage manifestation of chronic disease in a dying patient or the result of another opportunistic pathogen infecting the patient. Drugs taken by HIV-infected persons may cause cardiac disease, for example, cardiomyopathy associated with alpha-interferon therapy. The findings of Levy and colleagues (1989) demonstrated, however, that even HIV-infected patients without AIDS, any active opportunistic infection, or any debilitation sometimes had cardiac abnormalities, suggesting that HIV might be a cardiac pathogen. HIV may damage mononuclear cells in the heart by direct infection and ultimate cytolysis or by "innocent bystander destruction." The latter mechanism is similar to that of HIV damage in neuroglial cells; that is, as HIV replicates within lymphocytes and macrophages, enzymes and lymphokines toxic to surrounding tissue are released (Levy et al., 1989).

Gastrointestinal System. Patients with AIDS experience a wide variety of symptoms that can adversely affect their nutritional status. Also, people with AIDS frequently have infections or other disease in the gastrointestinal (GI) tract. The symptoms and malnutrition may lead to functional disabilities, exacerbate immune dysfunction, contribute to disease progression, and cause morbidity and death (Chlebowski et al., 1989; Kotler et al., 1989). Even HIV-infected patients without AIDS often have GI dysfunction, especially anorexia, weight loss, and diarrhea. In fact, HIV wasting syndrome (wasting with HIV infection and no superimposed opportunistic enteric infection) is a defining condition for the diagnosis of AIDS (Crocker, 1989) (see Chapter 3).

The entire GI tract is a major target for HIV disease. Clinical and pathologic changes have been found in the oral cavity, esophagus, stomach, liver, small and large intestines, and rectum. The scope of GI pathology is broad. In a given individual with HIV-related GI dysfunction, the etiology is likely to be multifactorial (Cuff, 1990). GI dysfunction in HIV disease may be caused by (1) opportunistic pathogens especially *Candida, Cryptosporidium,* CMV, *Mycobacterium avium, M. isospora,* and *Microsporidium;* (2) neoplasms (Kaposi's sarcoma invades the GI tract in approximately 50% of those with the tumor; lymphomas have been reported in the bowel, esophagus, and small intestine of HIV-infected persons); (3) adverse effects of medications; and (4) unknown causes. Conceivably direct HIV infection of lymphoid and monocytoid cells in the gut could lead indirectly to GI dysfunction.

A common finding is AIDS enteropathy with persistent diarrhea, weight loss, malabsorption, and malnutrition in the absence of an identifiable etiologic agent. Biopsies of the small intestine have shown pathologic structural changes, including villous atrophy, crypt hyperplasia, an increased number of intraepithelial lymphocytes, and the presence of spherical intracellular viruslike particles (Cello, 1989). These findings suggest HIV infection of the enterocytes with an associated immune response. Although AIDS enteropathy is common, the *majority* of patients with diarrhea and weight loss have identifiable infections (Cello, 1989). Organ-specific symptoms, particularly dysphagia, postprandial emesis, hematemesis, biliary colic, increased abdominal girth, and small-volume diarrhea, may be definitively diagnosed and respond to therapy (Cello, 1989). More research is needed to elucidate the etiology, contributing factors, and effective interventions for HIV enteropathy.

CHEMOPREVENTION AND TREATMENT OF HIV

An extraordinary amount of scientific information about HIV, its structure, characteristics, life cycle, and pathogenesis has accumulated in a short time, creating a valuable foundation for the development of therapies and vaccines. Several important strategies for controlling or stopping the damage done by HIV are being studied.

First, ongoing research is concerned with interventions to prevent a person exposed to HIV from becoming infected. Vaccination that elicits sufficient immunity to prevent infection on exposure is one example. Phase I clinical trials are evaluating the safety and immunogenicity of several anti-HIV vaccine candidates. Chemoprophylaxis with zidovudine (azidothymidine [AZT], Retrovir) of health care workers exposed to HIV-infected blood by percutaneous injury is another example of an attempt to prevent infection following exposure.

Another major strategy being intensively studied is the use of anti-retroviral drugs or agents to interfere with the infectivity, replication, or production of HIV and treat infected individuals at various stages of HIV infection. Zidovudine works in this way and is approved for all HIV-infected persons with fewer than 500 T4 cells/mm^3. Several other antiviral drugs that interfere with the life cycle of HIV are being investigated.

A third strategy under investigation is reconstitution or repair of the immune system damaged by HIV. Several agents in clinical trials can potentially reconstitute or enhance immune function at least transiently in an HIV-infected, immunosuppressed person.

In addition to these strategies for controlling or eliminating virus and the immune damage it inflicts, considerable research is aimed at developing treatment and prophylactic agents for opportunistic infections and other diseases that occur in patients with AIDS as a consequence of the severe immunosuppression (see Chapter 3).

Anti-HIV Vaccines. The purpose of a vaccine is to introduce the antigen to the host for the first time in a harmless form and induce an immune response, so that on subsequent exposures to the same antigen the host's immune response will be rapid, targeted, and sufficient to prevent infection and clinical disease. The development of an anti-HIV vaccine continues to be a high research priority because of the global prevalence of HIV. There are, however, several obstacles to the development and evaluation of an anti-HIV infection. These include the way HIV integrates into the cellular genome, hides inside the cell, and remains somewhat dormant; the diversity of various isolates of HIV; the lack of an adequate animal model for HIV disease; the lack of understanding of what constitutes protective immunity against HIV; the possibility that HIV transmission can occur via infected cells; and the numerous ethical difficulties in conducting phase II and III vaccine trials (Fauci et al., 1989; Fischinger, 1989).

Despite the obstacles, much has been accomplished in vaccine research. A number of vaccines have been developed and tested in animals, and several are being evaluated in phase I clinical trials. At the end of 1990 at least 10 clinical trials of candidate HIV vaccines were being conducted (Koff & Fauci, personal communication, 1990). The most extensive experience with any experimental vaccine being tested in humans is with a recombinant gp160 vaccine made in a baculovirus vector by Micro-GeneSys (West Haven, Conn.) A phase I trial of this recombinant envelope product began in 1987 at the National Institutes of Health. Since then more than 150 volunteers in two independent sites have been vaccinated with doses ranging from 40 to 1320 μg. Volunteers received a booster at 1 month, 6 months, and/or 12 months. Data show that the vaccine has minimal, tolerable adverse reactions and that both humoral and cell-mediated immune responses to gp160 were elicited at the higher doses (Koff & Fauci, 1989; Kovacs, personal communication, November 1990).

At least three separate vaccine trials using the simian immunodeficiency virus (SIV) in monkeys have established that protection against challenges with live SIV could be achieved by vaccination with whole killed virus (Desrosiers et al., 1989; Gardner, 1990; Murphy-Corb et al., 1989). These studies have established the feasibility of protective immunity induced by vaccine in an animal model closely analogous to humans.

Antiretroviral Therapy. Elimination or suppression of HIV itself is critical to any strategy for control, remission, or cure of HIV infection. Understanding the characteristics and life cycle of HIV has enabled investigators to develop anti-HIV therapies that interfere with or interrupt specific steps in the process. Some agents being developed, screened, or tested reportedly have the ability to (1) prevent viral attachment, (2) inhibit reverse transcriptase or the transcription of viral RNA to DNA, (3) inhibit the transcription of DNA to messenger or genomic RNA, and (4) inhibit viral component synthesis, assembly, or the budding of mature virions (Broder et al., 1990; Johnson & Schooley, 1989; Richman, 1988; Yarchoan & Broder, 1988; Yarchoan et al., 1988) (Table 2–2).

To date only one antiretroviral drug, zidovudine (azidothymidine [AZT], Retrovir), has been approved and is widely available for HIV-infected people. Zidovudine is a dideoxynucleoside analogue of thymidine (one of the building blocks of DNA). In the cell, zidovudine triphosphate competes with thymidine triphosphate as a substrate for DNA polymerase. In this way zidovudine inhibits viral reverse transcriptase, terminates DNA chain elongation, or does both.

Zidovudine clearly prolongs survival and reduces morbidity; in addition, in some individuals it decreases measurable p24 antigen and in-

**TABLE 2–2. Antiretroviral Agents with Activity Against
HIV (in Clinical Trials, September 1990)**

MECHANISM	AGENTS IN CLINICAL TRIAL
Inhibitors of binding to CD4	Peptide T
	Lipid compounds (e.g., AL-721)
	Dextran sulfate
	Anti-Leu-3a
	Soluble rCD4
	CD4-IgG
	Castanospermine
	Butyl deoxynojirmycin (DNJ)
	Pentosan
	Sulfated polyvinyl alcohols (PVAs)
Inhibitors of reverse transcriptase; DNA chain terminators	Zidovudine (AZT)
	Dideoxycytidine (ddC)
	Didanosine (ddI)
	Azidouridine (AzdU)
	D4T
	Foscarnet
	TIBO
	Pentosan
Inhibitors of posttranscription processing and translation of mRNA	Ribaviran
	Ampligen (?)
	Interferons (?)
Inhibitors of HIV protein synthesis, assembly, and release	Alpha-interferon
	Hypericin (HY)
	Pseudohypericin
	Protease inhibitors

Data from American Foundation for AIDS Research (1990), Mossinghoff (1989), Polsky and Armstrong (1988), and Yarchoan and Broder (1988).

creases T4 cells. Originally zidovudine was approved for people with advanced HIV infection. Currently its use is approved for all HIV-infected persons with fewer than 500 T4 cells/mm³. This change in indications approved by the Food and Drug Administration came about in March 1990 as a result of two studies showing that zidovudine delayed progression to AIDS or symptomatic disease in infected individuals who were either without symptoms (Volberding et al., 1990) or mildly symptomatic (Fischl et al., 1990). Recommended doses (according to the package insert) are (1) for persons with symptomatic disease, 200 mg every 4 hours, reducible to 100 mg every 4 hours after 1 month, and (2) for infected persons with asymptomatic disease, 100 mg every 4 hours while awake.

Although zidovudine can prolong lives and prevent adverse events in infected persons, it is also toxic and expensive. Major toxic effects are anemia and leukopenia, often severe enough to necessitate dose adjustment or cessation of the drug. Subjective toxic effects include headache, nausea, insomnia, and irritability. Long-term zidovudine therapy might also cause proximal muscle myopathy in some patients. All of the toxic effects occur more frequently in advanced disease. HIV-infected individuals with no symptoms have fewer and less severe side effects. Lower doses are also less toxic than the originally approved 250 mg every 4 hours. Concurrent administration of other marrow-toxic drugs increases the possibility and severity of dose-limiting hematologic toxic effects. For example, some of the drugs used to treat opportunistic infections such as *Pneumocystis* infection, toxoplasmosis, CMV, or mycobacterial diseases, as well as treatment for lymphoma and other malignancies, also have hematologic toxicity that may necessitate the discontinuation of zidovudine.

Zidovudine is approved for HIV-infected children between the ages of 3 months and 12 years at a dosage of 120 to 180 mg/m² every 6 hours. Studies have shown that HIV-infected children receiving zidovudine not only have clinical and immunologic improvement, but may have a dramatic reduction in neuropsychiatric symptoms (Blanche et al., 1988; Pizzo et al., 1988).

Zidovudine continues to be tested at different dosages and in combination with other therapies. For example, clinical trials are evaluating the combination of zidovudine with acyclovir, with alpha-interferon, with IL-2, with dideoxycytidine, and with other agents (American Foundation for AIDS Research, 1990).

Health care workers are being given zidovudine after exposure to HIV-contaminated blood through a percutaneous injury or extensive mucosal contact. In 1989 the National Institutes of Health started an open-label study of zidovudine as prophylaxis for health care workers with substantial exposure. Participants begin to take zidovudine within hours after exposure and take 100 mg every 4 hours for 6 weeks. The rationale for this approach comes from animal studies in which early administration of AZT following retroviral exposure seems to prevent the establishment of infection.

Two other nucleoside analogues, didanosine (dideoxyinosine [ddI], Videx) and dideoxycytidine (ddC), have recently received considerable attention. The antiviral mechanism of both is through action as a substrate for and inhibitor of viral reverse transcriptase. Both are potent inhibitors of HIV in vitro. In early trials evaluating high doses of ddC, painful and persistent peripheral neuropathy was a frequent and dose-limiting side effect. Current clinical trials are studying lower doses of ddC alone and in combination with other agents or alternating with other antiviral drugs such as zidovudine or didanosine. In phase I and II studies didanosine produced sustained clinical, immunologic, and virologic improvement for 9 months or more in most subjects (Merigan et al., 1989). Dose-limiting side effects included pancreatitis, peripheral neuropathy, and hepatitis, all of which occurred more frequently at higher doses. More than 11,000 HIV-infected persons have taken didanosine through an expanded access program in which the drug is provided to patients who are ineligible for clinical trials of didanosine and who are intolerant of or have failed to improve with zidovudine. Expanded access to ddC for those who have failed to improve with or are intolerant of zidovudine is also available.

Alpha-interferon, a naturally occurring monokine, is a potent anti-proliferative agent that may induce a partial or complete tumor response in 30% to 40% of patients with Kaposi's sarcoma. In addition, alpha-interferon has a significant antiretroviral effect, which may be heightened by combination with other agents. Alpha-interferon acts by inhibiting transcription and translation of mRNA, as well as by inhibition of viral protein synthesis and assembly of mature virions (Lane et al., 1990a).

Many other antiviral compounds effective in inhibiting HIV replication in vitro are being studied in clinical trials. None has yet been proved effective (see Table 2–2).

Immunomodulation. Because of the multiple and progressive immune defects caused by infection with HIV, as well as the resulting susceptibility to opportunistic disease, therapies aimed at halting or repairing immune damage may have an important role in treatment of HIV-infected persons (Lane, 1989). Repair of the immune system can theoretically be accomplished by reconstitution of the system or by enhancement of existing immune components and responses (Lane, 1989).

The immune system can be reconstituted through transfusion of mature, competent, histocompatible lymphocytes or transplantation of bone marrow. Both technologies are limited by histocompatibility restrictions and graft-versus-host reactions. Early attempts at bone marrow transplantation in persons with AIDS did not achieve clinical or lasting immunologic improvement, probably because the transplanted marrow became infected by persistent HIV. Later studies combined the use of antiretroviral therapies (such as suramin and later zidovudine) with bone marrow transplantation and lymphocyte transfusions in identical twins. At least partial reconstitution was seen in several of these patients, but the effect was only transient (Lane et al., 1990b).

The immune system in HIV infection could potentially be enhanced by any of a number of immunomodulating substances. Some of these are naturally occurring substances known as cytokines, such as IL-2, GM-CSF, and interferon-gamma (Lane, 1989). So far none of the agents evaluated for their ability to enhance the function of an infected person has demonstrated significant enhancement (Lane, 1989). The search for a potent in vivo immunomodulator with minimal toxic effects continues; such an agent may ultimately be an important component of treatment for HIV-related disorders.

SUMMARY

HIV, a retrovirus, progressively and severely damages the human immune system. This immune damage leaves the infected host susceptible to a wide range of opportunistic diseases that cause substantial morbidity and ultimately death. In addition, HIV may be pathogenic in other human tissues, either through direct infection of cells expressing a CD4 surface protein or through immune-mediated damage in the area. The control and eradication of HIV disease depend on a complete understanding of how this menacing virus operates and on the development of therapies that stop the replication and reproduction of HIV in vivo.

References

Abrams, D. (1988). The pre-AIDS syndromes. *Infectious Disease Clinics of North America,* 2(2), 343–351.
Acierno, L. (1989). Cardiac complications in AIDS. *Journal of the American College of Cardiology,* 13(5), 1144–1154.
American Foundation for AIDS Research (1990). *AIDS/HIV Experimental Treatment Directory,* 4(2).
Anderson, D., Virmani, R., O'Leary, T., et al. (1986). Dilated cardiomyopathy and myocarditis in the acquired immunodeficiency syndrome. *Circulation, 74,* II–142.
Barre-Sinoussi, F., Chermann, J., Rey, F., et al. (1983). Isolation of a T-lymphotropic retrovirus from a patient at risk for the acquired immunodeficiency syndrome. *Science, 220,* 868–871.
Bestetti, R. (1989). Cardiac involvement in the acquired immunodeficiency syndrome. *International Journal of Cardiology,* 22:143–146.
Blanche, S., Caniglia, M., Fischer, A., et al. (1988). Zidovudine therapy in children with AIDS. *American Journal of Medicine, 85,* 203–207.
Bourgoignie, J. (1989). AIDS related renal disease. *Klinische Wochen-schrift, 67,* 889–894.
Bowen, D., Lane, H., Fauci, A. (1985). Immunopathogenesis of the acquired immunodeficiency syndrome. *Annals of Internal Medicine,* 5(103), 704–709.
Broder S., Mitsuya, H., Yarchoan, R., and Pavlakis, G. (1990). Antiretroviral therapy in AIDS. *Annals of Internal Medicine,* 113(8), 604–618.
Calabrese, L., Proffitt, M., Yen-Lieberman, B., et al. (1987). Congestive cardiomyopathy and illness related to AIDS and isolation of retrovirus from myocardium. *Annals of Internal Medicine, 107,* 691–692.
Carbone, L., D'Agati, V., Cheng, J., Appel, G. (1989). Course and prognosis of HIV associated nephropathy. *The American Journal of Medicine,* 87(4), 389–395.
Cello, J. (1989). GI manifestations of HIV infection. In M. Sande & P. Volberding (Eds.), *Medical management of AIDS* (pp. 141–151), Philadelphia: W.B. Saunders.
Centers for Disease Control (1986). Classification system for human T-lymphotropic virus type III/lymphadenopathy–associated virus infection. *Morbidity and Mortality Weekly Report 35,* 334–336.
Chlebowski, R., Grosvenor, M., Bernhard, N., et al. (1989). Nutritional status, GI dysfunction, and survival in patients with AIDS. *American Journal of Gastroenterology,* 84(10), 1288–1293.
Cohen, A., Sun, N., Shapshak, P. (1988). HIV associated nephropathy: Direct viral infection of kidneys? *Laboratory Investigation, 58,* 19A.
Cohen, A., Sun, N., Shapshak, P., Imagaura, D. (1989). Immune complex glomerulonephritis in HIV infected patients: Lack of HIV antigens in immune complexes. *Laboratory Investigation, 60,* 18A.

Cohen, I., Anderson, D., Virmani, R., et al. (1986). Congestive cardiomyopathy in association with AIDS. *New England Journal of Medicine, 315,* 628–630.

Coplan N., Bruno, M. (1989). AIDS and heart disease: The present and the future. *American Heart Journal, 117*(5), 1175–1177.

Crocker, K. (1989). Gastrointestinal manifestations of the acquired immunodeficiency syndrome. *Nursing Clinics of North America, 24*(2), 395–406.

Cuff, P. (1990). Acquired immunodeficiency syndrome and malnutrition: The role of GI pathology. *Nutrition in Clinical Practice, 5,* 43–53.

Desrosiers, R.C., Wyand, M.S., Kodama, T., et al. (1989). Vaccine protection against simian immunodeficiency virus infection. *Proceedings of the National Academy of Sciences of the United States of America, 86,* 6353–6357.

Fauci, A. (1988). HIV: Infectivity and mechanisms of pathogenicity. *Science, 239,* 617–622.

Fauci, A., Gallo, R., Koenig, S., et al. (1989). Development and evaluation of a vaccine for HIV infection. *Annals of Internal Medicine, 110*(5), 373–385.

Fischinger, P. (1989). Progress in vaccine development against AIDS. *AIDS Update, 2*(4): 1–10.

Fischl, M., Richman D., Nansen N., et al. (1990). The safety and efficacy of zidovudine in the treatment of subjects with mildly symptomatic HIV-1 infection: A double blind placebo-controlled trial. *Annals of Internal Medicine, 112*(11), 727–737.

Gallo, R., Salahuddin, S., Popovic, M., et al. (1984). Frequent detection and isolation of cytopathic retroviruses (HTLV-III) from patients with AIDS and at risk for AIDS. *Science, 224,* 500–503.

Gardenswartz, M., Lerner, C., Seligson, G., et al. (1984). Renal disease in AIDS: A clinicopathologic study. *Clinical Nephrology, 21*:197–204.

Gardner, M.B., McGraw, T., Luciw, P., Carlson, J. (1990). SIV vaccine protection of rhesus macaques. *International Conference on AIDS, June 20-23, 1990* (abstract # 2H.A.342). San Francisco, CA.

Glassock, R., Cohen, A., Danovich, G., Parsa, P. (1990). HIV infection and the kidney. *Annals of Internal Medicine, 112*(1), 35–49.

Grady, C. (1988). HIV: Epidemiology, immunopathogenesis, and clinical consequences. *Nursing Clinics of North America, 23*(4), 683–696.

Grady, C. (1990). HIV infection: Prospects for therapy and chemoprevention. In T. Green, T. Knobf, & S. Hubbard, (Eds.), *Current issues in cancer nursing practice,* (pp. 49–58). Philadelphia: J.B. Lippincott.

Heyward, W., Curran, J. (1988). The epidemiology of AIDS in the United States. *Scientific American, 259*(4), 72–81.

Ho, D., Pomerantz, R., Kaplan, J. (1987). Pathogenesis of infection with HIV. *New England Journal of Medicine, 317,* 278–286.

Holland, G. (1985). Ocular manifestations of the acquired immunodeficiency syndrome. *International Opthalmology Clinics, 25,* 179–187.

Humphry, R., Weber, J., Marsh, R. (1987). Ophthalmic findings in a group of ambulatory patients infected by HIV: A prospective study. *British Journal of Opthalmology, 71,* 565–569.

Johnson, R., Schooley, R. (1989). Update on antiviral agents other than zidovudine. *AIDS, 3*(suppl 1), S145–S151.

Keriakis, D., Parmley, W. (1984). Myocarditis and cardiomyopathy. *American Heart Journal, 108,* 1318–1321.

Koff, W., Fauci, A. (1989). Human trials of AIDS vaccines: Current status and future directions. *AIDS, 3*(supp 1), S125–S129.

Kotler, D., Tierney, A., Wang, J., Pierson, R. (1989). Management of body-cell-mass depletion and the timing of death from wasting in AIDS. *American Journal of Clinical Nutrition, 50,* 444–447.

Kovacs, J., Masur, H. (1988). Opportunistic infections. In V. DeVita, S. Hellman, & S. Rosenberg, (Eds.), *AIDS: Etiology, diagnosis, prevention, and treatment* (2nd Ed.) (pp. 199–225). Philadelphia: J.B. Lippincott.

Krieger, A., Holland, G. (1988). Ocular involvement in AIDS. *Eye, 2,* 496–505.

Lane, H., Fauci, A. (1985). Immunologic abnormalities in the acquired immunodeficiency syndrome. *Annual Review of Immunology, 3,* 477–500.

Lane, H., Depper, J., Greene, W., et al. (1985). Qualitative analysis of immune function in patients with the acquired immunodeficiency syndrome: Evidence for a selective defect in soluble antigen recognition. *New England Journal of Medicine, 313*, 79–82.

Lane, H.C., (1989). The role of immunomodulators in the treatment of patients with AIDS. *AIDS, 3*(suppl 1), S181–S185.

Lane, H.C., Darcy, V., Kovacs, J., et al. (1990a). Interferon alpha in patients with asymptomatic HIV infection. *Annals of Internal Medicine, 112*(11), 805–811.

Lane, H.C., Zunich, K., Wilson, W., et al. (1990b). Syngeneic bone marrow transplantation and adoptive transfer of peripheral blood lymphocytes combined with zidovudine in human immunodeficiency virus infection. *Annals of Internal Medicine, 113*(7), 512–519.

Levy, W., Simon, G., Rios, J., Ross, A. (1989). Prevalence of cardiac abnormalities in HIV infection. *American Journal of Cardiology, 63*(1):86–89.

Margolick, J., Lane, H., Fauci, A. (1987). Immunopathogenesis of HTLV-III/LAV infection. In *Viruses and human cancer* (pp 59–79). New York: Alan R. Liss.

Marsh, R. (1989). Ocular manifestations of AIDS. *British Journal of Hospital Medicine, 42*(3), 224–230.

McArthur, J., Palenicek, J., Bowersox, L. (1988). Human immunodeficiency virus and the nervous system. *Nursing Clinics of North America, 23*(4), 823–842.

Meltzer, M., Skillman, D., Hoover, D., et al. (1990). Macrophages and the human immunodeficiency virus. *Immunology Today, 11*(6), 217–223.

Merigan, T., Skowron, G., Bozzette, S., et al. (1989). Circulating p24 antigen levels and responses to dideoxycytidine in HIV infection. *Annals of Internal Medicine, 110*, 189–194.

Mossinghoff, G. (1989). AIDS medicines in development. *AIDS Patient Care, 3*(5):4–8.

Murphy-Corb, M., Martin, L.N., Davison-Fairburn, B., et al. (1989). A formalin-inactivated whole SIV vaccine confers protection in macques. *Science, 246*, 1293–1297.

Newsome, D. (1989). Noninfectious ocular manifestations of AIDS. *International Ophthalmology Clinics, 29*(2), 95–97.

Nyamathi, A. (1989). AIDS related heart disease: A review of the literature. *Journal of Cardiovascular Nursing, 3*(4), 65–76.

O'Regan, S., Russo, P., Lapointe, N., Rousseau, E. (1990). AIDS and the urinary tract. *Journal of Acquired Immunodeficiency Syndrome, 3*:244–251.

Palestine, A., Rodrigues, M., Macher, A., et al. (1984). Ophthalmic involvement in the acquired immunodeficiency syndrome. *Ophthalmology, 91*, 1092–1099.

Pardo, V., Aldana, M., Cotton, R., et al. (1984). Glomerular lesions in the acquired immunodeficiency syndrome. *Annals of Internal Medicine, 101*, 429–434.

Pizzo, P., Eddy, J., Falloon, J., et al. (1988). Effects of continuous intravenous infusion of zidovudine in children with symptomatic HIV infection. *New England Journal of Medicine, 319*, 889–896.

Polsky, B., Armstrong, D. (1988). Other agents in the treatment of AIDS. In V. DeVita, S. Hellman, & S.A. Rosenberg (Eds). *AIDS: Etiology, diagnosis, treatment, and prevention* (pp. 295–303). Philadelphia: J.B. Lippincott.

Poiesz, B., Ehrlich, G., Papsidero, L., et al. (1988). Detection of human retroviruses. In V. DeVita, S. Hellman, & S. Rosenberg (Eds). *AIDS: Etiology, diagnosis, treatment, and prevention* (pp. 137–154). Philadelphia: J.B. Lippincott.

Pomerantz, R., Kurutzkes, D., DeLa Monte, S., et al. (1987). Infection of the retina by HIV-1. *New England Journal of Medicine, 317*, 1643–1647.

Price, R., Brew, B., Sidtis, J., et al. (1988). The brain in AIDS: Central nervous system HIV-1 infection and AIDS dementia complex. *Science, 239*, 586–591.

Rao, T., Fillippone, E., Nicastri, A., et al. (1984). Associated focal and segmental glomerulonephritis in the acquired immunodeficiency syndrome. *New England Journal of Medicine, 310*, 669–673.

Redfield, R., Burke, D. (1988). HIV infection: The clinical picture. *Scientific American, 259*(4), 90–99.

Richman, D. (1988). The treatment of HIV infection. *AIDS, 2*(suppl 1), S137–S142.

Roitt, I., Brostoff, J., Male, D. (1989). *Immunology* (2nd Ed.). St. Louis: C.V. Mosby.

Rosenberg, Z., Fauci, A. (1989a). Immunology of AIDS: Approaches to understanding the immunopathogenesis of HIV infection. *Research in Clinical Laboratories, 19*, 189–209.

Rosenberg, Z., Fauci, A. (1989b). The immunopathogenesis of HIV infection. *Advances in Immunology, 47*, 377–431.

Rosenberg, Z., Fauci, A. (1990). Activation of latent HIV infection. *Journal of NIH Research, 2*, 41–45.

Sandler, S., Dodd, R., Fang, C. (1988). Diagnostic tests for HIV infection: Serology. In V. DeVita, S. Hellman, S. Rosenberg (Eds.), *AIDS: Etiology, diagnosis, treatment, and prevention* (2nd Ed.) (pp. 121–136). Philadelphia: J.B. Lippincott.

Schnittman, S., Denning, S., Greenehouse, J., et al. (1990). Evidence for susceptibility of intrathymic T cell precursors and their progeny carrying T cell antigen receptor for phenotypes TCR alpha-beta and TCR gamma-delta to human immunodeficiency virus infection: A mechanism for CD4 + lymphocyte depletion. *Proceedings of the National Academy of Sciences, 87*, 7727–7731.

Shaw, G., Wong-Stoll, F., Gallo, R. (1988). Etiology of AIDS: Virology, molecular biology, and evolution of HIV. In V. DeVita, S. Hellman, & S. Rosenberg (Eds.), *AIDS: Etiology, diagnosis, treatment, and prevention* (2nd Ed.) (pp. 11–32). Philadelphia: J.B. Lippincott.

Shay, L., Thomas, R., Wyvill, K., et al. (1990). New drug therapy for patients with HIV. *Cancer Nursing, 13*(5), 269–277.

Stites, R., Stobo, J., Wells, J. (1987). *Basic and clinical immunology* (6th Ed.). Los Altos, CA: Lange Medical Publishers.

Valle, B., Lemberg, L. (1987). The Miami vices in the CCU. II. Cardiac manifestations of AIDS. *Heart Lung, 16*, 584–589.

Vlahov, D. (1989). AIDS: Overview, immunology, virology, and informational needs. *Seminars in Oncology Nursing, 5*(4), 227–235.

Volberding, P., Cohen, P. (1990). Indications for the use of HIV antibody testing. In P. Cohen, M. Sande, & P. Volberding (Eds.), *The AIDS knowledge book* (pp. 2.1.1-1 to 2.1.1-9). Waltham, MA: Medical Publishing Group.

Volberding, P., Lagakos, S., Koch, M. et al. (1990). Zidovudine in asymptomatic human immunodeficiency virus infection: A controlled trial in persons with less than 500 CD4 positive cells per cubic mm. *New England Journal of Medicine, 322* (14), 941–949.

Weber, J., Weiss, R. (1988). HIV infection: The cellular picture. *Scientific American, 259*(4), 100–109.

Yarchoan, R., Broder, S. (1988). Pharmacologic treatment of HIV infection. In V. DeVita, S. Hellman, and S. Rosenberg (Eds.), *AIDS: Etiology, diagnosis, treatment, and prevention* (2nd Ed.) (pp. 277–294). Philadelphia: J.B. Lippincott.

Yarchoan, R., Mitsuya, H., Broder, S. (1988). AIDS therapies. *Scientific American, 259*(4), 110–119.

3

Clinical Manifestations of AIDS

Peter J. Ungvarski

In the early years of the AIDS epidemic the disease was considered essentially fatal and emphasis was placed on compassionate, low-technology care aimed at improving the quality, rather than the length, of life (Cotton, 1989). Individuals who participated in low-risk behaviors were discouraged from undergoing HIV antibody testing, since virtually no treatment was available for HIV disease and since its consequences, development of opportunistic diseases, was inevitable. All this has changed because of the development of antiviral agents, such as zidovudine, and improved therapies, not only for treating but in some cases for preventing the AIDS-related diseases. See the drug guide in Appendix I.

At present HIV disease is considered one in which cure may not be possible but in which early intervention might improve survival (Cotton, 1989). HIV disease is now viewed as a long-term disease that requires health care planning and management along a chronic disease continuum. Volberding (1989) suggested that previously used diagnostic terms such as AIDS-related complex (ARC) and AIDS are obsolete and should be replaced with the broad diagnostic term "HIV disease" with early, middle, and late stages. The diagnosis of AIDS is not as representative of late stages of HIV disease as some individuals may be led to believe. For example, Kaposi's sarcoma can occur even in a relatively good state of health in an HIV-infected person, who may remain asymptomatic for years. The antithesis is the AIDS-related disease progressive multifocal leukoencephalopathy, which usually results in death within months after being diagnosed. Within the next few years the definition of AIDS will be revised. The latest proposed revision includes persons with a T4 count of 200/mm^3 or less. This chapter deals with the most frequently encountered AIDS-indicator diseases (Table 3–1).

TABLE 3–1. Frequently Diagnosed AIDS-Indicator Diseases

I. Constitutional disease
   A. HIV wasting syndrome
II. Neurologic disease
   A. HIV encephalopathy
III. Infections
   A. Bacterial infections
      1. *Mycobacterium tuberculosis* (TB)
      2. *Mycobacterium avium* complex disease (MAC)
      3. Salmonellosis
   B. Fungal infections
      1. Candidiasis
      2. Cryptococcosis
      3. Histoplasmosis
      4. Coccidioidomycosis
   C. Protozoan infections
      1. Pneumocystosis
      2. Cryptosporidiosis
      3. Toxoplasmosis
      4. Isosporiasis
   D. Viral infections
      1. Herpes simplex virus (HSV) disease
      2. Cytomegalovirus (CMV) disease
      3. Progressive multifocal leukoencephalopathy (PML)
IV. Neoplasms
   A. Kaposi's sarcoma
   B. Non-Hodgkin's lymphoma (NHL)

Nurses caring for people infected with HIV and those diagnosed as having AIDS face a challenging situation. They must possess a clinical knowledge base of not only HIV disease but also the AIDS-related opportunistic infections and malignancies. These diseases are strange sounding, to say the least, and new to the nurse, who often feels powerless when confronted with providing nursing care in the presence of the unknown (Ungvarski, 1987). For example, how many nurses have cared for a person with progressive multifocal leukoencephalopathy? Therefore the goal of this chapter is to provide the information nurses require to care competently and comfortably for persons with AIDS-indicator diseases.

To understand the clinical aspects of the development of opportunistic infections (OIs) associated with AIDS, the reader should be aware of some generalizations that can be made about their presence in an HIV-infected person (Glatt et al., 1988; National Institute of Allergy and Infectious Diseases, 1990). OIs are caused by a diverse spectrum of pathogens, many of which are ubiquitous in nature and rarely cause disease in normal hosts (persons with an intact immune system). In many cases these infections are a secondary appearance of a previous primary infection or, in other words, reactivation of a previously acquired pathogen. The OIs associated with AIDS are rarely curable and at best can be controlled during an acute episode; they require long-term suppressive therapy to prevent recurrence. Complicating the issue of long-term therapy is the resistance to standard therapies that some opportunistic pathogens develop.

A single OI is rare in persons with AIDS; concurrent or consecutive infections with different organisms are common. Infections associated with HIV, because of the coexisting immunodeficiency, are often severe and difficult to treat and require extended initial treatment regimens. Furthermore, many infections become disseminated with a high density of organisms in the affected tissues. By understanding the epidemiologic characteristics of certain pathogens, the nurse can provide clients with information on preventing some of these infections. Progress in research on AIDS-related OIs has led to the development of medical treatment to prevent some infections.

Approximately 95% of the neoplasms associated with AIDS are either Kaposi's sarcoma or non-Hodgkin's malignant lymphoma (Levine, 1987). Other malignancies, which are not AIDS defining or considered part of the spectrum of HIV disease but which have been reported, include: Hodgkin's disease; squamous carcinoma of the head, neck, and anus; melanoma; plasmacytoma; adenocarcinoma of the colon; small cell carcinoma of the lung; germ cell (testicular) carcinoma; and basal cell carcinoma (Kaplan, 1990a).

In 1987 the CDC revised the case definition for AIDS and added two AIDS-indicator diseases that were neither OIs nor malignancies. These new diseases were HIV wasting and HIV encephalopathy, both consequences of progressive HIV disease (CDC, 1987a). This chapter focuses on the clinical manifestations of AIDS and the most frequently diagnosed AIDS-indicator diseases.

HIV WASTING SYNDROME

From the earliest descriptions of AIDS in the United States, weight loss has been an initial complaint of a significant number of HIV-infected persons (CDC, 1981b). In addition to Kaposi's sarcoma and opportunistic infections, a diarrhea-wasting syndrome has characterized AIDS in Africa (Quinn et al., 1986). In fact, wasting in Africans with AIDS is so pronounced that AIDS is often referred to there as "slim disease" (Greene, 1988). As mentioned previously, in 1987 the CDC included HIV wasting syndrome as an indicator disease of AIDS in the revised surveillance case definition.

Epidemiology. In 1989 HIV wasting syndrome was reported in 19%

of the adult and adolescent cases and 16% of the pediatric cases of AIDS (CDC, 1990a). According to King (1990), prospective and retrospective investigations have shown that 91% to 100% of people with AIDS lose weight. In a detailed report published in 1990, the Federation of American Societies for Experimental Biology (FASEB) concluded that wasting and malnutrition were common occurrences in HIV disease; however, the extent of specific nutrient deficiencies was unclear and required further research. The FASEB report cited several mechanisms of malnutrition and weight loss, including reduced food intake, malabsorption of nutrients, and altered metabolism of nutrients.

Factors contributing to reduced food intake include anorexia, oral or esophageal lesions, nausea and vomiting, diarrhea, and neurologic or psychologic complications (FASEB, 1990). Additional factors related to reduced food intake may include the presence and severity of fatigue and its impact on the client's ability to obtain and prepare food; lack of money to buy food; unavailability of a stove or refrigerator, or even electricity; lack of knowledge of nutrition in general or of nutritional needs in HIV disease; disinterest in nutritional status and weight loss; and side effects of medications.

Nutritional malabsorption is related to small intestine injury, but disease of other digestive organs such as the stomach, liver, gallbladder, and pancreas contributes. Kotler (1989) identified three categories of intestinal disease: primary infection of the enterocytes, secondary involvement from systemic or otherwise disseminated disorders, and a syndrome of inflammatory bowel disease. In AIDS, primary enterocyte infection such as cryptosporidiosis and isosporiasis produces a clinical picture resembling short bowel disease. Systemic or disseminated infections caused by pathogens, such as cytomegalovirus or *Mycobacterium avium-intracellulare*, or by multifocal malignancies, such as Kaposi's sarcoma, result in secondary involvement of the intestinal tract. Many individuals with HIV disease have inflammatory bowel disease that is unrelated to any identifiable pathogen or cancer and may be due to intestinal infection by HIV itself (Kotler, 1989).

Wasting, characterized by loss of lean body mass seen in cachexia related to cancer or chronic infection, differs from weight loss in starvation, in which adaptive mechanisms preserve lean body mass relative to fat. These adaptive mechanisms are primarily reflected as either an increase or a decrease in the basal metabolic rate or resting energy expenditure (FASEB, 1990). Persons with clinically stable AIDS, in the absence of active infection or disease, conserve lean body mass even with small losses of body weight caused by malabsorption (Kotler et al., 1990). However, patients with AIDS who have active disease, such as OI with fever, commonly are hypermetabolic and burn excess calories, resulting in wasting (FASEB, 1990). Kotler and associates (1990) reported metabolic rates 20% to 60% above predicted values in HIV-infected persons with acute systemic illness or with chronic infection. Hommes and co-workers (1989) reported that even in the absence of acute illness, persons infected with HIV had higher rates of resting energy expenditure resulting in weight loss.

Kotler and colleagues (1989) studied the impact of malnutrition on survival of persons with AIDS and found that death from wasting in AIDS is related to the magnitude of tissue depletion and is independent of the underlying cause of wasting. They concluded that attempts to maintain body mass could prolong survival in persons with AIDS.

Pathogenesis. Early in the HIV epidemic, important similarities in the immunodeficiencies associated with AIDS and those found in protein-calorie malnutrition (PCM) were noted, including multiple opportunistic infections of viral, bacterial, protozoal, and fungal origin and the presence of Kaposi's sarcoma and lymphoma (Gray, 1983). Among the most significant immunologic changes that result from either HIV infection or PCM are deficiencies in cellular immunity, including decreases in the absolute number of T4 helper cells, as well as decreases in T4 activity; inverted helper to suppressor cell ratios; anergy; and decrease in lymphokine production (FASEB, 1990). Humoral immune deficiencies seen in both include increased levels of serum immunoglobulins, the presence of immune complexes in serum, diminished primary antibody response, decreased antibody affinity, and increased numbers of circulating immunoglobulin-secreting B cells (FASEB, 1990).

Documented relationships between specific nutrients and the immune function in HIV disease indicate that deficiencies in vitamins A, C, and B_6, selenium, and zinc increase the susceptibility to infection (FASEB, 1990). Scevola and colleagues (1989) found a relationship between nutritional status and the rate of incidence of opportunistic infections in persons with AIDS, suggesting that nutritional status is an important determinant of infection.

Malnutrition related to HIV disease may influence morbidity and mortality in several ways: (1) muscle wasting results in a decrease in cardiac and respiratory functions; (2) loss of body cell mass, increases in total body water, and other changes in body composition can alter the pharmacokinetic and pharmacodynamic responses to drug therapy; (3) malnutrition leads to weakness and the need for care and assistance, increasing length of stay in the hospital, and greater need for home care services; and (4) undernourished, hypermetabolic persons with AIDS may be inactive, apathetic, and listless, all of which reflect a poorer quality of life (FASEB, 1990).

Clinical Presentation. Common symptoms of HIV wasting syndrome include weight loss, although the client perceives caloric intake to be adequate; anorexia; fever; and diarrhea (Greene, 1988). Careful nutritional history taking is a key to detecting inadequate protein and caloric intake. Greene (1988) emphasized the need for a food diary and careful dietary history to uncover such problems as a calorically sparse macrobiotic diet or a belief that megavitamin therapy can be substituted for adequate nutritional intake. Early satiety may indicate a visceral disorder such as hepatomegaly, splenomegaly, or infiltrative disease of the gastrointestinal tract (e.g., Kaposi's sarcoma or infection with *M. avium* complex) (Greene, 1988).

The presence of polyuria, polydypsia, polyphagia, and visual problems along with neuropathy may indicate diabetes-induced weight loss. In some persons with AIDS this is a consequence of systemic pentamidine isethionate therapy for *Pneumocystis carinii* pneumonia (Anderson et al., 1986; Bouchard et al., 1982; Greene, 1988; Stahl-Bayliss et al., 1986).

Anorexia can be related to clinical depression, anxiety, neurosis, frank psychosis, or AIDS dementia complex (Greene, 1988). Adrenal insufficiency in HIV disease can also cause anorexia and weight loss, which may be manifested along with hyponatremia, hyperkalemia, hyperpigmentation, and orthostatic hypotension (Greene, 1988; Hilton et al., 1988; Merenich et al., 1990).

Many of the drugs used to treat opportunistic infections or malignancies associated with AIDS can cause anorexia and weight loss. Major adverse gastrointestinal effects of zidovudine therapy include dyspepsia, nausea, and vomiting (Burroughs-Wellcome Company, 1990).

Disease of the upper gastrointestinal tract, such as candidiasis or lesions caused by herpes simplex virus or cytomegalovirus, also results in anorexia. Bloating, distention, or colicky pain often occurs 30 to 60 minutes after eating in patients with disseminated mycobacterial infection or Kaposi's sarcoma and can lead to avoidance of food (Greene, 1988).

Fever and weight loss can be related to the chronic viremia of HIV, opportunistic infections, or malignancies associated with AIDS. Diarrhea and weight loss can be associated with enteric infection, neoplasm, or HIV-related enteropathy. Other common gastrointestinal complaints in persons with HIV disease include dysphagia, odynophagia, dysgeusia (altered sense of taste), lactose intolerance, and steatorrhea (fatty stools) (Crocker, 1989). Steatorrhea may be associated with fat malabsorption caused by enteric infection or pancreatic insufficiency. Evidence of pancreatitis includes increased amylase level, abdominal pain, history of chronic alcohol abuse, and pancreatic calcifications (Friedman, 1990).

Diagnosis. The CDC (1987a) in revising its case definition for AIDS included HIV wasting syndrome (emaciation or "slim disease"), with laboratory evidence of HIV disease, as a definitive diagnosis for AIDS. The diagnostic criteria include (1) findings of profound involuntary weight loss, defined as greater than 10% of the baseline body weight, *plus* either chronic diarrhea, defined as at least two loose stools per day for more than 30 days, or chronic weakness and documented fever that is present either intermittently or constantly; and (2) the absence of concurrent illness or condition other than HIV disease that could explain the findings, for example, cancer, tuberculosis, cryptosporidiosis, or other specific enteritis (CDC, 1987a).

Adequate nutritional assessment includes evaluation of voluntary inadequate intake, especially with restricted dietary regimens; early satiety; drug side effects and drug-nutrient interactions; anorexia resulting from neuropsychiatric, endocrinologic, and gastrointestinal conditions; fever and infection; and diarrhea and malabsorption (Greene, 1988).

Treatment. Nutritional counseling and education should be provided as soon as HIV disease is diagnosed. Emphasis on protein and calorie intake and the appropriate servings of the basic four food groups should serve as the basis for nutritional teaching. In later stages of HIV disease, nutritional support should be emphasized. Counseling the person about food safety considerations to prevent foodborne infections is equally important (see Chapter 4).

Megestrol acetate, a synthetic progesterone, is under study to determine its safety and efficacy in promoting weight gain in HIV-associated cachexia (Friedman, 1990; von Roenn et al., 1988). Friedman (1990) attributed weight gain in persons taking zidovudine to improved immune function and reduced frequency of opportunistic infections. The Burroughs-Wellcome Company (1990) reported weight maintenance as a benefit of zidovudine therapy. Medications to control such symptoms as painful oral lesions, nausea, vomiting, and diarrhea make oral intake easier. Treatment of intestinal parasitic infections or corticosteroid therapy for adrenal insufficiency should control the weight loss associated with these problems.

Oral and enteral nutritional supplements may alleviate weight loss, but formulas that have a high carbohydrate or fat content, contain lactose, or have high osmotic loads can exacerbate gastrointestinal problems (Crocker, 1989). The Task Force on Nutrition Support in AIDS recommended enteral tube feedings in the following circumstances: (1) When appetite is so poor or anorexia is so profound that nutrient intake is inadequate or weight loss occurs, tube feedings of calorically dense formula may be used to supplement oral intake. (2) If oral intake is impaired by oral symptoms, intermittent or continuous tube feeding of a balanced formula should be considered. (3) If nausea and vomiting are expected to reduce oral intake for 2 weeks or more (e.g., for drug therapy) or significant unintentional weight loss has occurred, an enteral formula introduced into the small intestine and adjusted for osmolality should be used. (4) When diarrhea cannot be managed by modification of diet, enteral feeding is appropriate except in total small bowel disease. (5) When nutritional needs cannot be met orally in persons with infection and sepsis, an isoosmolar formula is suggested. Because of the risk, expense, and inconvenience, parenteral nutrition is usually considered a final option except for severe malnutrition associated with disease involving the entire small intestine and malabsorption, in which case total parenteral nutrition is indicated (Task Force on Nutrition Support in AIDS, 1989).

Considerations for Nursing. Weight loss and generalized wasting should not be casually accepted as a consequence of HIV disease or AIDS. Kotler and colleagues (1989) provided important evidence that maintaining body mass can prolong survival in AIDS. Detailed diet histories should be obtained, and nutritional teaching should, as much as possible, be based on the client's current intake patterns rather than introducing a whole new menu. The client's cultural preferences, cooking and storage facilities, and financial resources should also be taken into consideration.

Information about community-based services that provide "buddies" or volunteers to shop for food or prepare meals, as well as agencies that deliver free meals, should be included in teaching plans. While the client is in the hospital, significant others and families should be taught how to prepare high-protein, high-calorie diets and encouraged to bring the client a casserole instead of flowers. The same applies to friends who visit people with AIDS at home. Those preparing food gifts benefit from the satisfaction of participating in the plan of care.

The plan of care for a person with HIV disease and weight loss requires a multidisciplinary approach. The multifactorial causes of weight loss are identified and treated by the physician, nurse, and clinical dietitian, as well as the client and significant others. Concrete, realistic goals should be based on objective data: desired weight measurements should be established even if the best result achievable is only a slowing of weight loss. Failure to achieve these goals should result in a redesign of the care plan.

Related Nursing Care. See the discussions of weight loss, fatigue, diarrhea, dry painful mouth, and fever in Chapter 4.

HIV ENCEPHALOPATHY

By 1982 the University of California, Los Angeles, School of Medicine had reported that three of four persons with AIDS had some degree of neurologic involvement (Gapen, 1982). In 1983 the first comprehensive description of neurologic complications appeared in the literature (Snider et al., 1983). Most cases described were associated with opportunistic infections or neoplasms related to AIDS, but in a small number of patients the cause of central nervous system disease was unknown, although cytomegalovirus infection was suspected. Levy and associates (1985) reported that in an unselected group of 318 patients, 124 or 39% had neurologic symptoms and 35 had subacute encephalitis with an unclear etiology. In the same year Ho and associates and Resnick and colleagues provided evidence that HIV was not only lymphotropic, but also neurotropic.

Nervous system disease is responsible for the initial symptoms in 10% of persons with AIDS; at autopsy neuropathologic abnormalities are found in more than 80% of adults with AIDS (Gabuzda & Hirsch, 1987; Levy et al., 1990). An estimated 40% of people with AIDS will at some time have major neurologic symptoms, caused by HIV disease or an opportunistic infection or neoplasm of the central nervous system (Levy et al., 1988).

Primary central nervous system syndromes associated with HIV include aseptic meningitis, vacuolar myelopathy, progressive HIV encephalopathy of childhood, and chronic HIV encephalopathy in adults (Dalakas et al., 1989). Discussion here is limited to the AIDS-defining condition HIV encephalopathy.

Epidemiology. Chronic HIV encephalopathy is a major cause of neurologic dysfunction in HIV-infected adults (Dalakas et al., 1989). In the literature HIV encephalopathy is also referred to as subacute encephalopathy, HIV or AIDS dementia, and AIDS dementia complex (ADC). The precise incidence of ADC is uncertain for a variety of reasons. First, the neurotropic effects of HIV were not discovered until 1985. Second, most data accumulated thus far have been obtained through retrospective pathologic studies rather than population-based prospective analysis (Price et al., 1988). Third, the CDC did not include ADC as an AIDS-indicator disease for surveillance reporting until 1987. Fourth, AIDS-related neurologic involvement is probably grossly underdiagnosed because the initial symptom presentation is so subtle (Levy & Bredesen, 1988).

Most accumulated data support the hypothesis that cognitive deficits are uncommon in HIV-seropositive, otherwise asymptomatic individuals when compared with seronegative controls (Levy & Bredesen, 1989; McArthur et al., 1989). However, the presence of neurologic, cognitive, or affective symptoms becomes more apparent as the disease progresses and the other symptoms of AIDS-related complex appear (Janssen et al., 1989). In contrast, Koralnik and associates (1990) reported that electroencephalographic testing revealed neurologic abnormalities are common in HIV asymptomatic persons. Fitzgibbon and colleagues (1989) found that neurotropic effects of HIV, even in asymptomatic individuals, did reduce fine motor control (cause motor slowing).

Pathogenesis. The cell type predominantly infected with HIV in the brain is the monocyte-macrophage; however, the mechanisms by which these cells mediate neurologic dysfunction and destruction remain unclear (Ho et al., 1989). HIV has been identified in deep gray matter structures, including the basal ganglia and thalamus, and in the white matter, with cortical infection less common (Gartner et al., 1986; Price et al., 1988; Stoler et al., 1986).

Recent reports from San Francisco and Stockholm indicate that HIV in blood and cerebrospinal fluid from the same infected individual may differ and that the HIV in the brain may be a special subgroup (Cheng-Mayer et al., 1989; Chiodi et al., 1989). The differences noted were in replicative capacity in different cell lines, cytopathic effect, and protein profile.

Price and associates (1988) proposed that neuroinfection with HIV and the development of ADC correspond directly with increasing severity of immunosuppression. That is, asymptomatic or mild ADC in the initial period of HIV disease progresses to severe ADC as the disease progresses to AIDS.

Clinical Presentation. Price and colleagues (1988) recommended replacing the earlier term "AIDS dementia" with "AIDS dementia complex (ADC)" for the following reasons: (1) *AIDS*, because of the neurologic relationship to HIV disease and AIDS; (2) *dementia*, because cognitive impairment, or dyslogia, is the most notable and most disabling aspect of the disorder; and (3) *complex* because of the associated neurologic manifestations such as organic psychosis and progressive paraparesis related to myelopathy.

Clinical symptoms of ADC include cognitive dysfunction (inability to concentrate, decreased memory, slowness in thinking), motor deficits (leg weakness, ataxia, clumsiness), and behavioral changes (apathy, reduced spontaneity, social withdrawal) (Ho et al., 1989; Price et al., 1988; Weisberg & Ross, 1989).

In a small number of patients the initial or predominant feature of ADC is agitated organic psychosis ranging from irritability, hyperactivity, and anxiety without an identifiable cause to mania or delirium (Price et al., 1988). Boccellari and colleagues (1988) reported hyperactivity, euphoria, and grandiose delusions, increasing the possibility of a secondary mania in persons with ADC and no previous psychiatric history.

Left undiagnosed or untreated, ADC progresses slowly as a predominant component and the individual becomes increasingly apathetic and indifferent to his or her illness. Progression of motor abnormalities can lead to paraparesis and bladder and bowel incontinence. At the end stages, the person with ADC usually lies in bed with a vacant stare, little response to the environment, incontinence, and inability to walk (Price et al., 1988).

Diagnosis. Diagnosis of ADC may initially be overlooked, especially in an acute care setting where examination of the mental status of a person with AIDS is not a priority given the plethora of physical problems requiring attention. In addition, a differential diagnosis is required to distinguish ADC from opportunistic infections or neoplasms of the central nervous system and metabolic encephalopathies. ADC may also be confused with multiple sclerosis, Parkinson's disease, or Alzheimer's disease (Price et al., 1988; Weiler et al., 1988). Weiler (1989) pointed out that ADC in the elderly may increase significantly in the coming years because of a greater number of patients with AIDS over 50 years of age. This author also noted a tendency to discount AIDS as a possible diagnosis because of a patient's age.

Diagnosis of ADC begins with a history, presence of neurologic signs and symptoms indicating cognitive, motor, and behavioral dysfunction, and serologic evidence of exposure to HIV. Computed tomography and magnetic resonance imaging should be performed to look for cerebral atrophy and white matter disease, and cerebrospinal fluid analysis can show elevated protein levels and pleocytosis, as well as rule out other infections or neoplasms (Price et al., 1988).

Treatment. Thus far the most dramatic response to treatment has been with zidovudine. Persons with HIV disease and AIDS treated with zidovudine have shown improvement in cognitive functions, including memory, attention, and general mental speed, as well as improved motor skills (Schmitt et al., 1988; Yarchoan et al., 1988). The possibility that zidovudine may prevent ADC by inhibiting viral replication may explain the declining incidence of ADC since widespread use of this drug began in some countries (Portegies et al., 1989). Fernandez and associates (1988) noted improvement in cognitive function with the use of psychostimulants such as methylphenidate and dextroamphetamine. Cognitive stimulation therapy should be provided along with medication.

Considerations for Nursing. Because of the time spent with HIV-infected clients in the provision of nursing care, nurses are key clinicians in detecting the subtle signs and symptoms of ADC. Clients with HIV disease commonly complain about problems with memory, concentration, and maintaining their train of thought. Nurses begin to notice this when they find themselves repeating information previously discussed with the client or when the client cannot pay attention to conversations with them.

Simple numerical calculations can be difficult for clients and can lead to financial miscalculations and errors in self-medication; this should not be confused with a lack of basic arithmetic skills resulting from a limited education or learning disabilities. Clients may take longer to complete routine activities of daily living and may omit details, resulting in a disheveled appearance. They may watch television less and read less because of inability to follow the plot or characters or to interpret written meanings. The nurse may recognize problems with memory and comprehension when an evaluation of the outcomes of teaching shows that minimal or no learning has taken place.

Nurses in community-based settings or clinics may notice missed appointments or inability to comply with prescribed medication regimens. The latter can be especially problematic if the client is supposed to take zidovudine every 4 hours to control and reduce ADC or is receiving antibiotic therapy for infectious processes such as tuberculosis.

Many clients are aware of changes in cognitive abilities and become embarrassed or ashamed. In an attempt to hide symptoms they may talk less and withdraw socially. Lovers, spouses, and significant others are helpful in noticing these behaviors, especially in individuals who deny the existence of any problem. Suicide risk increases with the development of dementia (Glass, 1988).

Early motor impairment may be discrete, and patients may not notice that they frequently drop things or that hand activities such as eating and writing are slower and less precise. Significant changes in writing a signature can lead to problems with checks and legal documents. Disturbances in gait, coordination, and balance can lead to tripping and falling. Initially this may be passed off as clumsiness; however, the nurse will notice the client reflexively exercising more caution when walking.

In the case of clients who cannot take or do not respond to zidovudine, the nursing care plan should include client safety and preparing the significant others for the cognitive, motor, and behavioral changes that will occur. Health teaching should be directed toward the care partner, and the care plan should include respite for the care partner to prevent physical and psychologic exhaustion. Referrals for home care and emotional support should also be made.

Related Nursing Care. See the discussions of impaired cognition, impaired mobility, and weight loss in Chapter 4.

MYCOBACTERIAL TUBERCULOSIS

In the United States, tuberculosis (TB) is becoming a disease of racial and ethnic minorities and the foreign born (Bloch et al., 1989). Among non-Hispanic whites TB is predominantly seen in the elderly, whereas in racial and ethnic minority populations and the foreign born it is concentrated in young adults. Current surveillance data support the hypothesis that the spread of HIV disease has increased the risk of TB.

Although neolithic and pre-Columbian skeletons, as well as early Egyptian remains, show evidence of spinal TB, TB was not recognized as a major health problem until crowded urban living conditions were created early in the industrial revolution (DesPrez & Heim, 1990). In 1882 Koch demonstrated the tubercle bacillus and its pathogenicity (DesPrez & Heim, 1990). By 1890 TB was the leading infectious disease causing death in the United States (Schechter, 1990).

With the advocacy of rest in open air and special care in sanitoriums during the first half of the twentieth century, a steady decline in TB began (DesPrez & Heim, 1990; Schechter, 1990). This reduction was accelerated by the introduction of streptomycin in 1946 (D'Esopo, 1982; DesPrez & Heim, 1990). A temporary halt in the decline occurred in 1980 with the immigration to the United States of refugees from Indochina (Rieder et al., 1989). Between 1984 and 1986, with the concomitant rise in the number of individuals infected with HIV, the United States had a 2.6% increase in the number of cases of TB, with the largest increases noted in New York, New Jersey, Michigan, Arkansas, Florida, and North Carolina (CDC, 1988). The relationship between the incidence of TB, as well as other mycobacterial diseases, and immunosuppression in HIV is now well established (Bloch et al., 1989; CDC, 1989a; Dunagan, 1990; Modilevsky et al., 1989; Tenholder et al., 1988).

Epidemiology. Factors that contribute to the rapid spread of TB are crowded living conditions, favoring airborne spread of infection, and individuals with little native resistance (DesPrez & Heim, 1990). Unsurprisingly, the dual diagnosis of TB and HIV disease frequently occurs among the inner city poor such as racial and ethnic minorities and intravenous drug users (CDC, 1989a; Fertel & Pitchenik, 1989; Schechter, 1990). Detailed demographic information on the association of TB with HIV disease and AIDS in New York City, Florida, and Newark, New Jersey, revealed that blacks and Hispanics accounted for 80%, 90%, and 100% of the cases, respectively (CDC, 1989a). In San Francisco, where HIV disease occurs predominantly in white homosexual and bisexual men, the dual diagnosis of TB and AIDS is found in white men who do not use intravenous drugs, but at a much lower incidence (Schechter, 1990).

TB has always been a problem in correctional institutions, where the environment is crowded and conducive to airborne transmission of infection among inmates, staff, and visitors (CDC, 1989b). Braun and coworkers (1989) reported that in some correctional facilities in New York State the incidence of TB among inmates increased from 15.4 cases per 100,000 in 1976 through 1978 to 105.5 cases per 100,000 in 1986. The same study revealed that the majority (56%) of inmates with a diagnosis of TB reported in 1985 and 1986 also had HIV disease or AIDS.

DiPerri et al. (1989) reported a nosocomial epidemic of active tuberculosis among HIV-infected patients; active disease developed in 8 of 18 HIV-infected individuals exposed to *Mycobacterium tuberculosis*. Both health care workers and patients may be at risk for exposure to TB in settings where cough-inducing procedures, such as aerosolized administration of medications, sputum induction, and bronchoscopy, are performed on patients with TB (CDC, 1989c).

The finding that TB often precedes, by 1 to 2 months, the development of AIDS as specified by the national surveillance definition was confirmed in two large studies in Florida and New York City (CDC, 1986, 1987b). The recognition of TB as a sentinel disease has led to the inclusion of TB clinics in HIV serosurveys (CDC, 1989a). TB can occur at any time through-out the spectrum of HIV illness (Hopewell, 1989).

Further study is needed to detect the concomitant presence of TB and HIV disease in other settings where TB is an actual or potential problem, such as shelters for the homeless, residential care facilities, drug detox-ification and treatment centers, adult homes, psychiatric facilities, and community-based congregate living facilities for populations with special needs (Nardell, 1989; Selwyn et al., 1989).

Pathogenesis. M. tuberculosis is an aerobic, obligate parasite, acid-fast bacillus. Almost all infections are spread by the respiratory route through inhalation of droplet nuclei that are aerosolized by coughing, sneezing, or talking. A cough or talking for 5 minutes can produce 3000 infectious droplet nuclei, which can remain suspended in the air for a long time (DesPrez & Heim, 1990). Infection usually requires prolonged exposure to an infectious environment; brief contact produces little risk (DesPrez & Heim, 1990). Once inhaled by a susceptible individual, the infectious particles settle in the terminal air passages where they multiply unimpeded and infection begins.

In an individual with HIV disease and impaired cell-mediated im-munologic function, tuberculous infection continues unchallenged and becomes progressive. The immunodeficiency caused by HIV disease may increase the risk of TB by two possible mechanisms. HIV-related immu-nodeficiency could increase susceptibility to new infection and permit that infection to progress rapidly to clinically apparent disease, or im-munodeficiency could allow a previously latent TB infection to progress to clinically apparent disease (CDC, 1987b). According to Chaisson and Volberding (1990) and Jacobson (1988), the majority of TB cases in HIV-infected people represent reactivation of latent M. tuberculosis infection acquired in the past.

Clinical Presentation. Clinically apparent TB can precede, coincide with, or follow a diagnosis of AIDS. Consistent with the nature of clinical problems associated with HIV disease, the clinical features vary with the degree of immunosuppression; the more severe the T4 lymphopenia, the more atypical the clinical presentation (Chaisson & Volberding, 1990).

Fever, weight loss, night sweats, and fatigue may be the initial com-plaints, but these symptoms, along with lymphadenopathy, are present in other diseases associated with HIV disease. While dyspnea, chills, hemoptysis, and chest pain may occur with pulmonary TB infection, extrapulmonary disease occurs in 40% to 75% of individuals with a dual diagnosis of HIV disease and TB (CDC, 1989a). Extrapulmonary sites or fluids that may show evidence of TB in HIV-positive persons include lymph nodes, bones, joints, bone marrow, liver, spleen, cerebrospinal fluid, skin, gastrointestinal mucosa, central nervous system, mass lesions (tuberculoma), urine, and blood or tuberculosis bacteremia (Jacobson, 1988; Schechter, 1990).

Diagnosis. Intradermal tuberculin testing may be unreliable in an HIV-infected person, since the underlying cell-mediated immunodeficiency results in anergy or a false-negative reaction (CDC, 1989a; Chaisson et al., 1987; Hanson & Reichman, 1989; Schechter, 1990). To establish a diagnosis, the clinician may need to obtain a variety of specimens for mycobacterial culture, including respiratory secretions, bronchial washings, gastric lavage, lung tissue, pleural fluid, lymph node tissue, bone marrow, blood, urine, stool, brain tissue, and cerebrospinal fluid (CDC, 1989a). Specimens should be examined microscopically to demonstrate acid-fast bacilli (AFB). The classic radiographic manifestations of pulmonary TB may be atypical in an HIV-infected person (Jacobson, 1988).

Treatment. Anti-TB chemotherapy should be started whenever AFB are seen in a specimen from the respiratory tract of a person with HIV disease, or from a person at increased risk for HIV disease whose HIV antibody status is unknown and who declines to be tested. CDC (1989a) recommendations for an adult with known or suspected HIV disease include isoniazid, rifampin, and pyrazinamide during the first 2 months of therapy. Persons taking rifampin who are also taking methadone should have their methadone dosage increased to avoid withdrawal symptoms resulting from interaction between the two drugs (CDC, 1989a). The half-life of methadone is reduced through enhancement of hepatic metabolism by rifampin (Farr & Mandell, 1990). Ethambutol should be part of the initial treatment regimen of individuals with central nervous system or disseminated TB or when isoniazid resistance is suspected.

The continuation phase, after the first 2 months, should include at least isoniazid and rifampin. Treatment should be continued for a minimum of 9 months and for at least 6 months beyond culture-documented conversion. Iseman (1987) suggested that individuals with a dual diagnosis of TB and HIV disease or AIDS be maintained with lifelong isoniazid therapy. Kavesh and associates (1989) conducted a retrospective study of the combined toxicity of zidovudine and antimycobacterial agents and concluded that persons receiving concurrent therapy can tolerate it without unacceptable toxic effects.

Tuberculosis Screening and HIV Disease. All persons with or at risk for HIV disease should be given a Mantoux skin test with 5 tuberculin units of tuberculin purified protein derivative. If the skin reaction shows 5 mm induration or more, a chest roentgenogram should be obtained and the patient should be examined for evidence of extrapulmonary disease. All HIV-positive persons with advancing disease and related diagnosis, including AIDS, should undergo chest roentgenography and be examined for pulmonary TB, regardless of the skin test reaction. Populations known to be at higher risk for HIV disease, such as inmates of correctional facilities and clients in drug treatment programs, should be routinely screened for TB, as well as offered HIV testing and counseling.

The benefits and risks of Calmette-Guerin bacillus (BCG) vaccination of HIV-infected persons remain largely undocumented. Neither the CDC nor the World Health Organization advocates the use of BCG in the United States at present. Disseminated *Mycobacterium bovis* infection developed in one person with AIDS who had been given a BCG vaccination (CDC, 1985a).

Considerations for Nursing. TB should be considered in the differential diagnosis of persons with HIV disease and unexplained pulmonary symptoms, and appropriate precautions, including AFB isolation, should be followed (CDC, 1983). In the acute care setting this includes a private room, with special ventilation and the door closed; a mask for the health care worker or visitor if the client does not reliably cover his or her mouth when coughing; and gowns if gross contamination of clothing is likely (gowns are usually unimportant because TB is rarely spread by fomites). Because a significant number of HIV-infected persons concomitantly have extrapulmonary TB, as well as atypical mycobacterial infection, meticulous handwashing is important and gloves should be worn when body secretions and excretions are handled.

During the initial diagnostic period the determination of the specific isolation precautions to be employed, that is, for *M. tuberculosis* or atypical mycobacterial disease such as *M. avium-intracellulare*, is complicated by the fact that only a provisional diagnosis is established by specimen stains for AFB. The determination of the actual type of mycobacterial infection takes 6 to 8 weeks until organism culture results are final. AFB precautions should be maintained until the client shows a clinical response to therapy and the sputum smear is negative for TB organisms. Receiving drug therapy for the specified number of days does not ensure that the desired response is being achieved, nor does it validate that the sputum is AFB negative and the person is no longer infectious.

AFB precautions are most important during and immediately after procedures that may induce coughing, such as bronchoscopy, sputum collection, aerosol induction of sputum, and administration of aerosolized medications such as pentamidine. If procedures that might expose staff and other HIV-positive persons to airborne transmission are needed, they should be carried out in rooms or booths with negative air pressure in relation to adjacent rooms or hallways, and with air exhausted directly to the outside and away from intake sources. During the time between patients, a number of air exchanges (6 per hour) should take place in the room (CDC, 1989a).

Community-based health care workers such as home care nurses, hospice nurses, and clinic nurses may be required to care for persons with HIV disease in areas where TB infection is also prevalent. They should be aware of the symptoms and airborne transmission of TB and should employ appropriate precautions. All health care staff who have contact with TB patients should participate in a TB screening program.

The essential ingredient to the successful treatment of TB is compliance with the prescribed medication regimen. Most individuals require assistance not only adjusting to the diagnosis of TB but also getting started with the routine of taking medications. Before the client is discharged from the hospital, follow-up by clinic appointments, appointments with a private physician or nurse-practitioner, or home visits from a visiting nurse should be arranged. This is especially necessary for the individual who has impaired cognitive function because of the neurotropic effects of HIV, profound fatigue, and a history of alcohol or drug abuse and is not in treatment. In recent reports, TB that is drug-resistant has been associated with noncompliance related to alcohol and drug addiction or to a belief that TB is incurable and that medications are ineffective (CDC, 1990d).

Persons with pulmonary TB, including those with HIV disease, are potentially infectious until a satisfactory clinical and bacteriologic response to therapy is achieved. All cases of TB must be reported to local health departments so that standard procedures for TB contact investigation can be implemented. Community-based nurses should be familiar with local health department policies for reporting and tracing noncompliant clients.

The CDC (1990e) has recently developed special recommendations for high-risk groups in addition to HIV-infected persons. These groups include close contacts of persons with known or suspected TB sharing the same household or other environments; persons with medical conditions known to increase the risk of disease if infection has occurred; foreign-born persons from countries with high TB prevalence; medically underserved low-income populations, including high-risk racial or ethnic minority populations (e.g., blacks, Hispanics, and Native Americans); alcoholics and intravenous drug users; and residents of long-term care facilities, correctional institutions, mental institutions, nursing homes or facilities, and other residential facilities for long-term care. All nurses should become familiar with these recommendations.

Related Nursing Care. See the discussions of fever, cough, shortness of breath, weight loss, and compliance in Chapter 4.

MYCOBACTERIUM AVIUM COMPLEX DISEASE

Until the 1950s the role of *Mycobacterium* species, other than the etiologic agents of TB and leprosy, remained widely unrecognized (Sanders & Horowitz, 1990). This was primarily due to the practice of diagnosing

TB on the basis of acid-fast smears and usually without species identification by culture. Current practice usually allows for a presumptive diagnosis of mycobacterial infection after AFB smears and initial microbiologic study. After the receipt of culture results, which takes an average of 6 to 8 weeks, a definitive diagnosis of infection with *M. avium-intracellulare* is made.

From the first reports of AIDS in 1981, physicians at the UCLA Center for the Health Sciences, Los Angeles, identified the presence of disseminated infection with *M. avium-intracellulare* complex (MAC) in persons with AIDS (Zakowski et al., 1986). Before this, MAC was rarely found to cause disseminated disease. By the mid-1980s, autopsy reports indicated MAC infection in more than 50% of the cases and suggested that a substantial rate of undetected infection was present in the AIDS population (Wallace & Hannah, 1988).

Microorganisms of the *M. avium* and *M. intracellulare* groups are so similar that they are usually dealt with collectively. Although they can be distinguished serologically, this is of little benefit in the overall medical management of the infected individual (Sanders & Horowitz, 1990).

Epidemiology. *M. avium-intracellulare* is ubiquitous and has been isolated from soil, water, animals, birds, and footstuffs such as eggs and unpasteurized dairy products. *M. avium-intracellulare* is often referred to as atypical mycobacterial infection and is noncommunicable with little evidence of person-to-person transmission (Sanders & Horowitz, 1990).

Related studies have shown that *M. avium-intracellulare* can be aerosolized in significant numbers near water, which suggests that inhalation may be a mode of transmission in humans (O'Brien, 1989; Sanders & Horowitz, 1990). Since MAC can be isolated from both chlorinated and unchlorinated water supplies, duMoulin and colleagues (1988) suggested that drinking water and hot water aerosols encountered when taking a shower are possible methods of transmission. Since nontuberculous mycobacterial infection is uniformly distributed throughout the different transmission groups of HIV-infected individuals, Chaisson and Volberding (1990) proposed that MAC infection is probably a newly acquired, or primary, infection rather than reactivation of a previous infection. These investigators also suggested that the longer an individual survives with HIV disease, the greater the likelihood that MAC infection will develop.

M. avium-intracellulare is distributed worldwide. Although accurate information on its geographic distribution is not available, since disease reporting of MAC infection is not mandatory, its prevalence is generally considered greatest in the southeastern United States (Sanders & Horowitz, 1990). Källenius and associates (1989) hypothesized that the requirement for general vaccination with BCG in Sweden may offer protection from MAC infection as well as TB, since MAC infection develops in only 10% of people with AIDS in their country.

Pathogenesis. Data collected by Wallace and Hannah (1988) showed that in persons with AIDS and widespread MAC infection, no consistent pattern of inflammatory response or tissue damage was present. Small and Hopewell (1990) concluded that although MAC infection may contribute to a general discomfort and disability in persons with AIDS, it may not be the cause of specific organ failure.

MAC is acquired orally or inhaled, with the gastrointestinal or respiratory tract, respectively, acting as the portal of entry. MAC can cause infection in the bone marrow, liver, spleen, gastrointestinal tract, lymph nodes, lungs, skin, brain, adrenal glands, and kidneys (Chaisson & Volberding, 1990). More recently discovered MAC infections in persons with HIV disease include endophthalmitis, endobronchial polypoid lesions, and pericarditis (Cohen & Saragas, 1990; Mehle et al., 1989; Woods & Goldsmith, 1989).

In nonimmunocompromised hosts MAC infection is manifested predominantly in the respiratory tract. In immunosuppressed persons with HIV the usual clinical course is hematogenous spread of the disease to various body sites. Barbaro and co-workers (1989) reported localization of MAC in skin abscesses in persons with AIDS taking zidovudine. They concluded that zidovudine was responsible for localized presentation of MAC infection in HIV-infected persons rather than the usual disseminated clinical course.

Clinical Presentation. In HIV disease the symptoms attributed to MAC infection are multiple and nonspecific and are consistent with systemic illness: fevers, fatigue, weight loss, anorexia, night sweats, abdominal pain, and diarrhea (Chaisson & Volberding, 1990; Connolly et al., 1989; Gray & Rabeneck, 1989; MacDonell & Glassroth, 1989; Small & Hopewell, 1990). In HIV-infected persons MAC infection is usually disseminated rather than localized in the lungs, so respiratory symptoms are uncommon (Small & Hopewell, 1990).

Physical examination shows emaciation, generalized lymphadenopathy, and other signs of immunodeficiency, such as thrush; abdominal examination may reveal diffuse tenderness and hepatosplenomegaly (Chaisson & Volberding, 1990). Laboratory findings are usually nonspecific and difficult to ascribe to MAC infection and include anemia, leukopenia, and thrombocytopenia (Chaisson & Volberding, 1990; Small & Hopewell, 1990; Wallace & Hannah, 1988).

Diagnosis. The diagnosis of MAC is established by isolation of the organism in cultures of blood, bone marrow, liver, or lymph nodes, as well as stool in persons with disseminated disease (Small & Hopewell, 1990). Special blood culture techniques now available for isolating mycobacteria yield a sensitivity of 100% (Jacobson, 1988). The importance of isolating MAC in sputum is uncertain. Jacobson (1988) found that in most patients with AIDS the isolation of MAC from sputum represents colonization and not dissemination.

Treatment. Definitive recommendations for treatment have always been difficult because drug resistance is common and susceptible strains vary widely (Sanders & Horowitz, 1990). The decision to treat an individual with HIV disease and MAC is highly individualized and takes into account several factors: the severity of the illness, the general state of health, the potential for drug adverse effects or intolerance, the presence of concurrent infections or diseases and the required therapy; and potential adverse reactions with incompatible agents (Sanders & Horowitz, 1990; Small & Hopewell, 1990). Clement (1990) recommended that individuals with constitutional symptoms, bacteremia, bone marrow dysfunction, gastrointestinal disease, or active pulmonary disease be treated and that persons with terminal disease, hepatic or renal dysfunction, or no symptoms be excluded from treatment.

Treatment regimens vary and can include anywhere from two to six drugs, including amikacin, clofazimine, ethambutol, ciprofloxacin, rifampin, rifabutin, cycloserine, and ethionamide (Sanders & Horowitz, 1990; Small & Hopewell, 1990). Hoy and associates (1990) recently reported clearing of mycobacteremia caused by MAC and symptom resolution in 22 of 25 patients treated with quadruple-drug therapy (rifabutin, clofazimine, isoniazid, and ethambutol). Small and Hopewell (1990) recommended the basic therapeutic principle of using as benign a regimen as possible to treat patients whose symptoms are attributable to MAC. Serious adverse drug events leading to death have been reported in persons receiving didanosine (ddI; Videx) for AIDS and concurrently receiving rifabutin and clofazimine to treat MAC infection (Bristol-Myers Squibb Company, personal communication, June 4, 1990). In persons who are not being treated for MAC or who cannot tolerate treatment, nonsteroidal antiinflammatory drugs or acetaminophen may be used for relief of constitutional symptoms (Clement, 1990a).

Considerations for Nursing. Many health care workers are unaware that the genus *Mycobacterium* is one of the most widely distributed bacterial genera and contains approximately 19 medically important species, of which MAC is one (Sanders & Horowitz, 1990). Therefore it is not unusual for staff members hearing the word *Mycobacterium* to institute AFB precautions that would prevent person-to-person airborne transmission, which is appropriate with *M. tuberculosis* but unnecessary with MAC infection. Staff education is essential so that unnecessary isolation precautions are not instituted. Explaining to the staff that MAC is not spread from person to person and is often referred to as atypical, noncommunicable disease may help.

Staff members may question why a person with MAC is not receiving specific antimycobacterial chemotherapy. Because of poor response to therapy and cure failure, relatively asymptomatic HIV-positive persons with MAC are commonly not given therapy. The hepatotoxic nature of the drugs, as well as preexisting systemic problems such as anemia, leukopenia, and thrombocytopenia, may preclude treatment.

Washing fruits and vegetables well before eating, avoiding unpasteurized dairy products, and drinking bottled liquids when traveling should be incorporated in the plan of care. DuMoulin and colleagues (1988) suggested bathing in a tub instead of showering to avoid hot water aerosols. Before implementing this practice, however, the nurse should assess carefully for chronic skin lesions such as herpes and candidiasis, since tub bathing could reseed infection to other body sites.

Related Nursing Care. See the discussions of fever, fatigue, weight loss, and pain in Chapter 4.

SALMONELLOSIS

The classification of *Salmonella* is in transition as a result of DNA studies (Hook, 1990). What were previously referred to as serotypes are now named as species, for example, *S. typhi*. Since the beginning of AIDS, *Salmonella* has been identified as a common pathogen causing severe bacteremic salmonellosis (Chaisson et al., 1990). Disseminated infections with *S. typhimurium, S. enteritidis, S. arizona, S. dublin*, and other *Salmonella* species (serotypes) have been diagnosed in persons with AIDS at a prevalence greatly exceeding that in the general population (Chaisson et al., 1990; Glaser et al., 1985; Jacobs et al., 1985; Smith et al., 1985). Although salmonellosis can occur at any time throughout the spectrum of HIV illness, the recurrent presence of nontyphoidal *Salmonella* septicemia is considered an indicator disease for the diagnosis of AIDS (CDC, 1987a).

Epidemiology. In humans *Salmonella* is usually acquired by ingestion of contaminated food or water (Hook, 1990). Other reported modes of acquisition include ingestion of contaminated medications or diagnostic agents; direct fecal-oral spread, especially with sexual activities that include anilingus with an infected person; transfusion of contaminated blood products; and inadequately sterilized fiberoptic instruments used in upper gastrointestinal endoscopic procedures (Hook, 1990; Janoff & Smith, 1988).

Although *Salmonella* may be transmitted from person to person, infection in animals is the principal source of nontyphoidal *Salmonella* in humans. *Salmonella* has been found in chickens, turkeys, ducks, cows, pigs, turtles, cats, dogs, mice, guinea pigs, hamsters, doves, pigeons, parrots, starlings, sparrows, cowbirds, sheep, seals, donkeys, lizards, and snakes (Hook, 1990). With the exclusion of S. *typhi*, of which humans are the only known reservoirs, almost all *Salmonella* species produce disease in both animals and humans. Significant sources of human infection are chickens, turkeys, ducks, and their eggs, which may contain not only surface contamination but also infected yolks (Hook, 1990). In 1990 the CDC reported dramatic increases in S. *enteritidis* infection associated with contaminated eggs in New England and the mid-Atlantic states (CDC, 1990b).

Meats, especially beef and pork, and raw and powdered milk are often implicated in outbreaks of *Salmonella* infection (Hook, 1990). In 1985 salmonellosis occurred in between 150,000 and 200,000 individuals in Illinois and was associated with pasteurized low-fat (2%) milk contaminated with S. *typhimurium* (Ryan et al., 1987). This was the largest epidemic of salmonellosis ever reported in the United States. Spika and colleagues (1987) reported outbreaks of S. *newport* in California traced to contaminated ground beef. Both of these outbreaks resulted from animal resistance to antimicrobial agents used in animal feed. Major sources of infection among animals are feeds containing *Salmonella*, contaminated fishmeal, or by-products of the meat-packing industry (Hook, 1990). Raw meat and poultry, purchased in retail markets, are frequently contaminated with *Salmonella*, and food handlers are more likely to be asymptomatic carriers of *Salmonella* than are members of the general population (Hook, 1990).

Telzak and associates (1990) studied the largest nosocomial outbreak of salmonellosis in the United States, which took place in 1987. In the hospital affected, salmonellosis developed in 404 patients (9 died) who ate tuna fish salad containing mayonnaise made with raw eggs at the hospital. As a result, the New York State Department of Health issued recommendations to eliminate raw or undercooked eggs from the diets of persons who were institutionalized, elderly, or immunocompromised.

Other sources of *Salmonella* include pets, especially turtles; waterborne outbreaks involving S. *typhi*, also called typhoid fever; ingested items contaminated with animal manure (this caused a marijuana-associated outbreak in 1981); nosocomial spread from person to person by the hands or clothing of hospital staff; and fomites such as dust, patient care equipment, and furniture (Hook, 1990).

Hidden culprits in disease transmission may include cultural beliefs and practices. Riley and colleagues (1988) reported salmonellosis in Hispanic persons ingesting rattlesnake capsules. The ingestion of rattlesnake meat or dried powder is a well-described Mexican folk remedy. *Farmacias* in Hispanic neighborhoods in Mexico and southern California sell the capsules under a variety of names: *vibra de cascabel*, *pulvo de vibora*, and *carne de vibora*.

Pathogenesis. The development of disease after *Salmonella* ingestion is related to the virulence of the organism, inoculum size, and the host defenses. In HIV-infected individuals with severe cell-mediated immunodeficiency, infection can become disseminated. *Salmonella* passes through the stomach and begins multiplying in the small intestine. Small inocula of *Salmonella* may be inactivated by gastric pH, but larger inocula may survive and cause infection (Chaisson et al., 1990). *Salmonella* can then pass through the intestinal mucosa to the large lymphatics and through hematogenous spread can infect any organ. Jacobs and colleagues (1985) isolated *Salmonella* in cultures of specimens from lungs, heart, brain, liver, spleen, kidneys, and bone marrow of persons with AIDS and salmonellosis. Destruction of the gastrointestinal mucosa in persons with AIDS, resulting from concurrent lesion-producing infections such as cytomegalovirus, *Candida*, and herpes simplex, can also provide easy access for salmonellae to enter the bloodstream (Chaisson et al., 1990).

Clinical Presentation. In immunocompetent individuals, *Salmonella* symptoms are most often confined to the gastrointestinal tract, but persons with HIV disease appear to lack localizing signs indicating salmonellosis (Chaisson et al., 1990). Nonspecific signs and symptoms include fever (seen in virtually all cases), chills, sweats, weight loss, diarrhea, and anorexia (Chaisson et al., 1990).

Diagnosis. Diagnosis of *Salmonella* infection is based on bacterial culture. Since many persons with HIV disease and salmonellosis have *Salmonella* bacteremia, routine blood cultures can provide the diagnosis. Stool cultures may yield the organism in individuals with blood cultures negative for *Salmonella*. Despite treatment, cultures may continue to yield the organism (Chaisson et al., 1990). Recurrent *Salmonella* bacteremia despite appropriate treatment has been reported (Nadelman et al., 1985).

Treatment. Although treatment of nontyphoid salmonellosis is usually unnecessary in immunocompetent individuals, it is required in persons with HIV disease (Chaisson et al., 1990). Antibiotic selection depends on drug sensitivities; however, ampicillin and chloramphenicol are most often used. Despite the efficacy of trimethoprim and sulfamethoxazole, Chaisson and colleagues (1990) recommended that they not be used because of the possibility of allergic reactions and the potential need for them later to treat *P. carinii* pneumonia. Other agents employed to treat salmonellosis in HIV disease include third-generation cephalosporins, amoxicillin, ciprofloxacin, and nonfloxacin. Since chronic infection and relapse are common in persons with HIV disease, suppressive therapy, usually with the above-named antibiotics, is necessary to prevent recurrence. Some individuals, even while continuing suppressive therapy, may have recurrent infection and require retreatment with intravenous antibiotic therapy.

Considerations for Nursing. Since *Salmonella* infection is preventable, HIV-positive persons should be taught how to avoid infection as soon as the diagnosis of HIV disease is known. Some basic precautions include drinking only bottled liquids when away from home; avoiding fast-food restaurants, delicatessens, and other places where many people handle food; washing all fresh food items brought into the home before cooking or consuming; cooking meats and fish until well done and avoiding ingestion of raw or uncooked meats and fish; consuming only pasteurized dairy products; consuming eggs that are cooked well and avoiding foods that may contain partially cooked eggs such as meringue or hollandaise or béarnaise sauces, as well as foods containing raw eggs such as home-made eggnog or Caesar salad; washing hands and food preparation surfaces well when handling fresh, uncooked foods; wearing gloves when cleaning up pet excreta and washing hands afterward; and avoiding handling turtles. When taking a health history the nurse should include cultural practices that may expose the client to pathogens, such as exposure to animal blood or ingestion of raw animal products.

Nurses should be aware of the need to wear gloves and practice meticulous handwashing when handling fecal material, especially from HIV-infected persons with diarrhea of unknown etiology. They should also be aware of the role clothing may have in *Salmonella* transmission and should wear a plastic apron or disposable gown when providing care to a client with fecal incontinence. The plan of care should include environmental cleaning to reduce the potential for fomite transmission. Although enteric precautions are employed when the diagnosis is known, the potential problem of *Salmonella* infection exists before the definitive diagnosis. Therefore barrier precautions should be practiced routinely.

Related Nursing Care. See the discussion of fever, weight loss, diarrhea, and dry skin in Chapter 4.

CANDIDIASIS

The first written description of oral lesions that were probably thrush date to the time of Hippocrates (Edwards, 1990). Although the fungal etiology of *Candida* infection was established during the nineteenth century, most of the investigative work began in the 1940s, when antibiotics were introduced. At present approximately 100 synonyms are used for *Candida albicans*; the most widely used is *Monilia albicans* (Edwards, 1990).

The increasing incidence of *Candida* infections is due not only to the widespread use of antibiotics, but also to medical advances such as organ transplantation and internal prosthetic devices (Edwards, 1990). *C. albicans* is the etiologic agent for the most prevalent type of fungal infection in persons with HIV disease.

Epidemiology. *Candida* organisms are yeasts, that is, fungi that exist predominantly in unicellular forms (Edwards, 1990). *C. albicans* is ubiquitous in nature and has been found in soil, food, inanimate objects, and hospital environments. *Candida* is a commensal organism that can be found on teeth, gingiva, and skin and in the oropharynx, vagina, and large intestine.

The majority of infections caused by *Candida* are endogenous and related to interruption of normal defense mechanisms. Examples of increased infection potential include naturally occurring immunocompromise with diseases such as diabetes mellitus; damaged or diseased skin or mucous membranes; invasive procedures such as insertion of intravenous cannulating devices and infusion-pressure monitoring equipment, Foley catheters, and drainage systems; immunosuppression related to drug therapy such as steroids, antibiotics, and antineoplastics; illicit intravenous use of drugs such as heroin; and acquired immunosuppression caused by disease such as HIV disease (Chernoff & Sande, 1990a; Edwards, 1990).

Human-to-human transmission is possible. Examples include congenital transmission in babies, in whom thrush develops after vaginal delivery; development of balanitis in uncircumcised men who did not wear a condom during intercourse with a woman who had *Candida* vaginitis; and nosocomial spread in hospital settings (Edwards, 1990).

Pathogenesis. The likelihood of mucosal *Candida* infection increases with the progressive cellular immunodeficiency associated with HIV disease and is often associated with a decreased number of circulating T4 lymphocytes (Chaisson & Volberding, 1990; Tindall et al., 1989). Most clinicians now believe that oral candidiasis is an accurate predictor of disease progression and the development of other AIDS-related infections (Barone et al., 1990; Greenspan et al., 1988).

The frequent use of broad-spectrum antibiotics to treat infections associated with HIV disease suppresses normal bacterial flora and allows *Candida* to proliferate, especially in the gastrointestinal tract (Chernoff & Sande, 1990a; Edwards, 1990). Skin alterations caused by poor nutrition, dehydration, poor hygiene, or indwelling catheters can also provide a portal of entry for *Candida*.

Clinical Presentation. When discussing the clinical presentation of *Candida* in persons with HIV disease, Chernoff and Sande (1990a) divided *Candida* infection into two categories: mucocutaneous, a very common site of infection, and systemic, a very rare site of infection. Clinical presentation depends on the site of infection and may include the mouth, esophagus, skin, nails, and vagina, as well as disseminated infection.

By far the most prevalent form of *Candida* infection in persons with HIV disease is pseudomembranous candidiasis, more commonly referred to as thrush. The clinical presentation is creamy, curdlike, yellowish patches, surrounded by an erythematous base, found on the buccal mucosa and tongue surfaces. The patches can be wiped off, leaving an erythematous or even bleeding mucosal surface. An atrophic form, seen occasionally, appears as smooth red patches on the hard or soft palate, buccal mucosa, or dorsal surface of the tongue (Greenspan et al., 1988). Thrush can be accompanied by angular cheilitis, which produces erythema, cracks, fissures, and maceration at the corners of the mouth (Berger, 1990).

Another oral form of candidiasis is candidal leukoplakia, which appears as white lesions on the buccal mucosa, tongue, or hard palate and cannot be wiped off (Greenspan et al., 1988). This can be confused with hairy leukoplakia. Oral candidiasis can be superimposed on other oral lesions such as herpes simplex and cause secondary infections.

Complaints of dysphagia in the individual with HIV disease are most commonly associated with C. albicans (Cello, 1988). Thrush and esophageal candidiasis are not necessarily present concurrently; therefore absence of thrush does not preclude the possibility that an HIV-infected person may have Candida esophagitis (Chernoff & Sande, 1990a; Gould et al., 1988). Cello (1988) defined the dysphagia associated with Candida esophagitis as difficulty swallowing with a sensation of food sticking. Although pain on swallowing (odynophagia) and episodic retrosternal pain without swallowing may be present with the complaint of dysphagia, they are more commonly associated with ulcerations of the esophagus caused by herpesvirus or cytomegalovirus (Cello, 1988; Gould et al., 1988).

Intertrigo can occur in any site where the proximity of skin surfaces provides a warm, moist environment. This cutaneous form of candidiasis can involve the groin, axillary vault, or areas surrounding the breasts and appears as a vivid red, slightly eroded eruption with a wrinkled surface coated by a white membrane (Berger, 1990; Edwards, 1990). Candida can proliferate in urine-soaked diapers and adult incontinence garments and underpads, beneath occlusive and wet dressings and condom catheters, around draining stomas and fistulas, and anywhere the skin stays moist continuously (Cuzzell, 1990). Clients with cutaneous candidiasis usually complain of burning and itching.

Candida infection of the nails is usually manifested as paronychia (inflammation of the tissues surrounding the nails) but can also involve the nail itself (Berger, 1990; Edwards, 1990). In addition to the inflamed appearance, the patient complains of tenderness in the area. Frequent exposure to water is a significant predisposing factor in Candida nail infection.

Candida is the most common cause of vaginitis and is frequently associated with diabetes mellitus, antibiotic therapy, and pregnancy (Rein, 1990). Characterized by intense pruritus of the vulva and a curdlike vaginal discharge, this infection usually results in an erythematous vagina and labia and may extend into the perineum. Chronic refractory vaginal candidiasis may be an initial symptom of HIV disease. Women with HIV disease and unexplained oral and vaginal candidiasis are at risk for other opportunistic infections (Rhoads et al., 1987).

According to Chernoff and Sande (1990a), disseminated candidiasis is rare unless other identified risk factors are present, such as the use of steroids, cytotoxic agents to treat malignancies, or prolonged antibiotic therapy. As survival increases among persons with AIDS, the need for lifetime antibiotic therapy to treat or prevent certain opportunistic infections could increase the number of cases of disseminated candidiasis. Candidiasis in the presence of HIV disease has also been reported to cause peritonitis in persons receiving continuous ambulatory peritoneal dialysis, as well as meningitis (Dressler et al., 1989; Ehni & Ellison, 1987).

Diagnosis. Definitive diagnosis of candidiasis is made by gross inspection by endoscopy or at autopsy, or by microscopy on a specimen of affected tissues. Diagnosis by culture is unreliable because the distinction between infection and colonization, in body sites where *Candida* is normally present, is not always clear. Isolation of *Candida* from blood may also be questionable in a patient with an indwelling intravenous catheter, since transient candidemia is possible and often clears without treatment once the device is removed (Chernoff & Sande, 1990a).

Treatment. Traditional treatment of candidiasis includes nystatin suspension and clotrimazole troches for thrush; nystatin suspension or pastilles, clotrimazole troches, or oral ketoconazole for esophagitis; topical treatment with clotrimazole, miconazole, or ketoconazole for cutaneous candidiasis; topical imidazole or oral ketoconazole or both for candidiasis of nails; clotrimazole or miconazole topical agents (creams, tablets, vaginal suppositories) or oral ketoconazole for vaginitis; and amphotericin B with or without 5-flucytosine for disseminated candidiasis (Chernoff & Sande, 1990a; Rein, 1990). In some patients ketoconazole may lose its effectiveness because antacids, hydrogen blockers such as cimetidine or ranitidine, and alkaline foods such as milk inhibit absorption by reducing stomach acidity, which is required for absorption; because drugs such as rifampin inhibit the action of ketoconazole by causing rapid metabolism and thereby decreasing drug levels in the blood; or because long-term use of ketoconazole may result in resistant organisms (Clement, 1989). Fluconazole is a promising new drug recently approved for the treatment of oropharyngeal and esophageal candidiasis.

Considerations for Nursing. Candidiasis should be considered a sentinel disease, and its presence without a plausible explanation should alert nurses to take careful histories and explore the possibilities of HIV disease. Nurses should be aware that mucocutaneous candidiasis is rarely cured and often becomes chronic or recurrent; therefore continual assessment for its presence is warranted. Equally important is the need to assess the client during each contact for cutaneous manifestations of candidiasis, especially in genital and perianal regions and under skinfolds.

Nursing measures directed at preventing severe *Candida* infections include establishing an effective, routine regimen of oral hygiene; keeping skin surfaces dry and exposed to air as much as possible; teaching the client how to detect early signs and symptoms of infection; meticulously taking precautions, such as use of gloves, handwashing techniques, and extreme care when handling and manipulating intravenous therapy equipment; and evaluating carefully the risk/benefit potential when using occlusive dressings.

Related Nursing Care. See the discussions of stomatitis, dry skin and skin lesions, and fever in Chapter 4.

CRYPTOCOCCOSIS

Human natural resistance to *Cryptococcus neoformans* is so strong that in Europe cryptococcosis is often referred to as *malade signal*, indicating that it is usually a sign of an underlying disease (Davis, 1986). Examples of underlying conditions associated with cryptococcosis are steroid therapy, sarcoidosis, lymphoreticular malignancies (especially Hodgkin's disease), and diabetes mellitus (Diamond, 1990). In the 1980s a significant increase in cryptococcosis developed in association with AIDS, making it the fourth most common life-threatening infection after *P. carinii* pneumonia, cytomegalovirus infection, and mycobacterial infection (Diamond, 1990). *C. neoformans* is the most common life-threatening fungal pathogen infecting persons with AIDS (Dismukes, 1988).

Epidemiology. *C. neoformans* is a yeastlike fungus that is ubiquitous in nature and can be found worldwide. The organism is found in pigeon droppings and can be retrieved in nesting places, soil, fruit, and fruit juices. *C. neoformans* can remain viable for up to 2 years in desiccated pigeon feces (Davis, 1986). Neither person-to-person nor animal-to-person transmission has been documented. The disease is naturally acquired from the environment where the organism is aerosolized and inhaled. The severe cell-mediated immunodeficiency associated with HIV disease permits cryptococcosis to develop, causing meningitis or pneumonia or both in most cases (Grant & Armstrong, 1988). Infection with *C. neoformans* is more common among intravenous drug users and ethnic minorities with AIDS and in the south central United States (Chaisson & Volberding, 1990).

Pathogenesis. After being inhaled, the fungus settles in the lungs, where it can remain dormant or spread to other parts of the body, particularly the central nervous system. In a host with an intact immune system, the infection is usually contained, but an immunodeficiency increases the potential for extrapulmonary spread. Chernoff and Sande (1990b) speculated that cryptococcal infections in persons with AIDS probably result from reactivation of latent infection as the immune system is progressively destroyed.

Anticryptococcal factors present in normal serum are absent in cerebrospinal fluid, which therefore is a good growth medium for cryptococci and explains why the central nervous system is the predominant focus of infection (Diamond, 1990). Since the fungus usually infects the brain as well as the meninges, this disease is more appropriately referred to as cryptococcal meningoencephalitis than as meningitis. *Cryptococcus* is responsible for three forms of infection: pulmonary, central nervous system, and disseminated.

Clinical Presentation. Pulmonary cryptococcosis may coexist with central nervous system and disseminated cryptococcal infection. Clark and colleagues (1990) suggested that the incidence of this form is high. Pulmonary infection may go undetected because initially it is often subclinical and asymptomatic (Chernoff & Sande, 1990b). Wasser and Talavera (1987) reported that the clinical presentation of five patients with AIDS and primary pulmonary cryptococcosis included fever, cough, dyspnea, and pleuritic chest pain. Pleural effusion in cryptococcosis has also been reported (Katz et al., 1989; Newman et al., 1987). In its most severe form, cryptococcosis can cause adult respiratory distress syndrome (Murray et al., 1988; Similowski et al., 1989).

The clinical presentation of CNS cryptococcosis is similarly elusive because of its characteristic waxing and waning course and insidious onset. No signs or symptoms are sufficiently characteristic to distinguish cryptococcal meningitis from other infections seen with AIDS (Chuck & Sande, 1989). In addition, most cases of CNS cryptococcosis do not appear with classic signs of meningitis. In a study of 89 patients with AIDS and cryptococcal meningitis, Chuck and Sande (1989) found symptoms present in the following percentages of patients: fever, 65%; malaise, 76%; headaches, 73%; stiff neck, 22%; nausea or vomiting, 42%; photophobia, 18%; altered mentation, 28%; focal deficits, 6%; seizures, 4%; cough or dyspnea, 31%; and diarrhea, 21%. In the same group of patients they found a temperature above 38.4° C (102° F) in only 56%, meningeal signs in 27%, alterations in mentation in 17%, and focal deficits in 15%.

Cryptococci can infect other organs and tissues. Cutaneous infection occurs in 10% to 15% of persons with cryptococcosis and may precede clinical signs of central nervous system disease (Hernandez, 1989). Painless skin lesions can appear as macules, papules, pustules, subcutaneous swellings, or shallow cutaneous ulcers (Chernoff & Sande, 1990b). Clinical presentation of cutaneous cryptococcosis has also been reported to mimic molluscum contagiosum and Kaposi's sarcoma (Concus et al., 1988; Jones et al., 1990; Miller, 1988). Other unusual presentations of cryptococcosis in patients with AIDS include oral lesions, placental infection, myocarditis, prostatic infection, optic neuropathy with visual loss associated with arachnoiditis, abdominal cryptococcoma, infected semen, rectal abscess and anal fistula, and massive peripheral and mediastinal lymph node infection (Glick et al., 1987; Kida et al., 1989; Lafont et al., 1987; Larsen et al., 1989; Lipson et al., 1989; Lynch & Naftolin, 1987, 1990; Scalfano et al., 1988; Staib et al., 1989; Torres, 1987; Van Calck et al., 1988).

Diagnosis. The diagnosis of cryptococcal meningitis can be made by visualizing the fungus in cerebrospinal fluid (CSF) with an India ink stain, detecting cryptococcal antigen in CSF, urine, or serum, and culturing the fungus (Chernoff & Sande, 1990b). According to Chuck and Sande (1989) the most reliable methods of diagnosis are determining cryptococcal antigen titers and culturing blood and CSF. Computed tomography of the head should be performed to rule out hydrocephalus and to look for focal lesions such as cryptococcomas, toxoplasmosis, or lymphoma (Chuck & Sande, 1989; Dismukes, 1988).

The client should be carefully examined for *Cryptococcus* in other parts of the body such as the eye or skin. Chest roentgenograms are helpful in detecting cryptococcal pneumonia, especially in clients who have culture-positive sputum or bronchoscopic specimens (Chernoff & Sande, 1990b).

Treatment. Primary therapy for the initial cryptococcal infection includes amphotericin B, with or without flucytosine, or fluconazole. For the past decade amphotericin B, administered intravenously for 6 to 8 weeks, has been the drug of choice to treat cryptococcosis. Administration of amphotericin B intrathecally has been used in place of, or in combination with, intravenous amphotericin B in patients failing to respond to standard intravenous therapy. In some cases the combination of amphotericin B and 5-flucytosine has demonstrated synergism against cryptococci. However, this combination does not seem to provide any benefit over amphotericin B alone; 5-flucytosine is not administered alone because of the development of drug resistance (Chernoff & Sande, 1990b).

By 1990, clinical trials had demonstrated the efficacy and safety of a new antifungal agent, fluconazole. Fluconazole is less toxic and better tolerated than amphotericin B (Clement, 1990b).

As with many of the opportunistic infections associated with AIDS, initial treatment of the acute infection does not cure the patient; therefore suppressive therapy is necessary. Until fluconazole was approved, the only effective agent available was amphotericin B. This necessitated intermittent home infusion therapy and in most cases insertion of an indwelling central venous catheter. Regardless of whether the initial intravenous treatment of cryptococcal meningitis is with amphotericin B or fluconazole, the National Institute of Allergy and Infectious Diseases recommends oral fluconazole for maintenance suppressive therapy (Clement, 1990b).

Considerations for Nursing. Because of the insidious onset of cryptococcal infection, as well as the waxing and waning presentation, persons with HIV disease often postpone medical evaluation. It may be significant others, family, or friends who notice personality or behavioral changes or cognitive impairment. Undetected CNS cryptococcosis can lead to seizures before help is sought. Without encouraging hypervigilant or hypochondriac behaviors, health care workers should stress to patients early in the course of HIV disease that it is infinitely better to ask questions or seek evaluation when symptoms appear than wait until symptom severity increases.

For the person with concurrent AIDS and cryptococcosis, neuropsychiatric evaluation should be performed to detect often subtle symptoms of cognitive impairment. Problems with short-term memory or calculations may lead to noncompliance with medication regimens and recurrence of infection. This is especially important now, since many individuals are taking oral fluconazole rather than receiving intravenous maintenance therapy.

The evaluation process associated with long-term suppressive therapy commonly includes lumbar punctures. Clients often experience fear and emotional trauma related to this procedure. Nurses should prepare clients adequately and support them during the procedure.

Cryptococcus is ubiquitous in nature, and infection is probably a reactivation of latent pulmonary foci. However, HIV-positive individuals should avoid places where exposure to *C. neoformans* is likely, such as pigeon roosts and areas where pigeons and other birds congregate in numbers (Chernoff & Sande, 1990b).

Related Nursing Care. See the discussions of impaired cognition, fever, stomatitis, cough, and dyspnea in Chapter 4.

HISTOPLASMOSIS

Darling first identified *Histoplasma capsulatum* in a human being in Panama in 1905, and for 40 years thereafter histoplasmosis was regarded as a rare fatal disease (Loyd et al., 1990). By 1945 histoplasmosis was known to be a common benign infection that accounted for pulmonary calcifications previously thought to result from tuberculosis. By 1956 it had been demonstrated that *H. capsulatum* was present in the soil where bird and bat excrement collected and that the spores of this fungus caused acute pulmonary disease in some individuals.

Epidemiology. *H. capsulatum* exists in its native habitat, the soil, and forms spores that are readily airborne and of such size that they readily reach the bronchioles and alveoli when inhaled (Loyd et al., 1990). The major endemic areas in the United States are the middle, central, and south central states, with the highest concentrations in the Ohio and

Mississippi river basins. According to Loyd and associates (1990), the most likely sources of soil contamination in endemic areas are blackbird roosts, pigeon roosts, chicken houses, chicken manure, fertilizer, and sites frequented by bats such as caves, attics, old buildings, and hollow trees. Disturbance of such sites, as through wind or construction, raises spores and causes exposure.

Areas where *H. capsulatum* infection is endemic have a higher incidence of progressive disseminated histoplasmosis as an opportunistic infection in persons with HIV disease (Kurtin et al., 1990). Johnson and colleagues (1986) reported disseminated histoplasmosis as the most common AIDS-defining opportunistic infection in endemic areas. Disseminated histoplasmosis has also been reported in persons from nonendemic areas such as New York City in individuals long removed from endemic areas such as the Caribbean or South America (Salzman et al., 1988).

Pathogenesis. After inhalation the spores settle in the small bronchioles and alveoli where they germinate. In the primary infection the yeast form of the fungus proliferates locally and then disseminates through the blood. In an immunocompetent host with no previous exposure, the immune response to the organism occurs within 24 to 48 hours and results in minimal proliferation of the yeast and asymptomatic infection (Chernoff, 1990; Loyd et al., 1990).

The two most important factors affecting the severity of infection are the ability of cell-mediated immunity to control infection and the quantity of the inoculum (Loyd et al., 1990). According to Fels (1988), most epidemiologic evidence suggests that disseminated histoplasmosis in persons with HIV disease is caused by secondary infection (reactivation of latent infection). Chernoff (1990) however, pointed out that persons with HIV disease who live in endemic areas are at increased risk for disseminated disease because of frequent environmental exposure. This may account for reports of a fulminant disease course in persons with AIDS in endemic areas and a prolonged, subacute course in comparable persons in nonendemic areas (Loyd et al., 1990).

Clinical Presentation. Johnson and associates (1989) in a review of 61 cases of progressive disseminated histoplasmosis (PDH) identified fever; weight loss; enlargement of the liver, spleen, or lymph nodes; and anemia as the most common signs and symptoms. Loyd and co-workers (1990) noted a fulminant course in endemic areas to include advanced hematologic abnormalities such as thrombocytopenia, leukopenia, disseminated intravascular coagulation, and respiratory failure, whereas in nonendemic areas patients had the vague nonspecific complaints of fever, weight loss, and lassitude. Less common manifestations include diarrhea, cerebritis, chorioretinitis, meningitis, oral and cutaneous lesions, and gastrointestinal mucosal lesions causing bleeding, (Anaissie et al., 1988; Chernoff, 1990; Freeman et al., 1989; Greenberg & Berger, 1989; Huber et al., 1989; Ibanez & Ibanez, 1989).

Diagnosis. Histoplasmosis underscores the need to include travel in the health history of a person with HIV disease. Smith and colleagues (1989), in their presentation of the first case of disseminated histoplasmosis in a person with AIDS in Europe, emphasized the importance of a detailed history, including travel, in clinical evaluation.

According to Johnson and co-workers (1989), bone marrow biopsy and culture, examination and culture of pulmonary tissue and secretions, and blood culture were the most common initial means of establishing a diagnosis. Chest roentgenograms are unreliable and have been normal in up to 30% of individuals with disseminated histoplasmosis. In an HIV-positive person, disseminated histoplasmosis at a site other than or in addition to the lungs or cervical or hilar lymph nodes fulfills the CDC criteria for a diagnosis of AIDS (CDC, 1987a).

Treatment. In an immunologically normal host, acute pulmonary histoplasmosis requires no specific treatment. For disseminated histoplasmosis the drug of choice is amphotericin B. Since the initial treatment does not cure histoplasmosis in a person with AIDS, lifelong suppressive therapy with either amphotericin B or ketoconazole is indicated. Trials of itraconazole for suppressive therapy are under way (American Foundation for AIDS Research, 1990).

Considerations for Nursing. The diagnosis of histoplasmosis can be delayed if travel history of an HIV-infected person is not documented. Clients who were born in or have lived in endemic areas or who have relocated to large cities such as New York, Boston, or San Francisco may be overlooked for latent histoplasmosis infection. It seems prudent, based on epidemiologic data, to advise HIV-positive individuals against travel for pleasure to endemic areas.

Related Nursing Care. See the discussions of fever, fatigue, weight loss, cough, dyspnea, and impaired vision in Chapter 4.

COCCIDIOIDOMYCOSIS

The first description of coccidioidomycosis was provided by Posada in 1892, in Buenos Aires, Argentina (Stevens, 1990). The organism was originally thought to be a protozoan and in 1896 was named *Coccidioides* ("resembling the protozoan *Coccidia*") *immitis* ("not mild") (Stevens, 1990). Approximately 10 years later it was identified as a fungus and the lungs were identified as the portal of entry. Further study of this fungus during the 1930s identified it as the etiologic agent of a self-limited disease seen frequently in California, known as San Joaquin Valley fever or valley fever.

Epidemiology. *Coccidioides* exists in the soil and fragments into spores that become airborne. Coccidioidomycosis is endemic in certain areas of North, Central, and South America. Stevens (1990) estimated that 100,000 people in the United States are infected annually, primarily in southwestern states, and that medical costs approximate $6.4 million each year. Outside endemic areas the disease occurs in travelers to endemic areas, in former residents of endemic areas, and as infections acquired from fomites such as fruit, cotton, or a landfill (Stevens, 1990). Bronnimann and associates (1987) noted that the rate of infection of disseminated coccidioidomycosis in persons with AIDS in Tucson, Arizona, approximated the incidence of positive coccidioidin skin tests in that area.

Coccidioidomycosis has been found in persons whose exposure was only a few hours (Stevens, 1990). Although this is an infectious disease, it is not a contagious one. The only reported instance of person-to-person transmission occurred when attention was not paid to the fungus's ability to revert from a tissue infection to its airborne spore form (Stevens, 1990). A patient had coccidioidomycosis in purulent drainage under a cast. When the cast was opened or removed, the spores became airborne and infected the health care worker removing the cast.

Pathogenesis. After the spores are inhaled, the lungs become the primary site of infection. In the acute phase, purulent pulmonary infection may be present, followed by lesion fibrosis. As in tuberculosis, caseation may occur (Stevens, 1990). In an immunocompetent person coccidioidomycosis is usually subclinical or associated with subacute respiratory symptoms that are indistinguishable from ordinary upper respiratory infections (Stevens, 1990).

C. immitis is more invasive in immunodeficient persons with HIV disease and usually results in a combination of diffuse pulmonary disease and widespread dissemination (Bronnimann et al., 1987). According to Minamoto and Armstrong (1988), disseminated coccidioidomycosis in persons with AIDS results predominantly from reactivation of latent infection. However, some cases may be due to primary infection, as evidenced by disseminated disease occurring in persons with AIDS shortly after they moved to Tucson, Arizona, from nonendemic areas (Bronnimann et al., 1987).

Clinical Presentation. Clinical symptoms of coccidioidomycosis are usually nonspecific and include malaise, fever, weight loss, cough, and fatigue (Minamoto & Armstrong, 1988). Infection of the meninges, brain, and cerebellum, as well as peritonitis, has been reported (Byrne & Dietrich, 1989; Levy & Bredesen, 1988). Cutaneous manifestations are rare. Joint effusions and bone destruction, often seen with disseminated disease, have not been reported in persons with AIDS (Minamoto & Armstrong, 1988). In endemic areas coccidioidomycosis is the leading cause of death among pregnant women, with a survival rate of only one in eight infected women (Stevens, 1990).

Diagnosis. The major problem in diagnosing coccidioidomycosis in persons with AIDS is the lack of suspicion of the disease (Stevens, 1990). As mentioned previously, this disease emphasizes the need to include questions regarding travel in the clinical history taking of a person at risk for or with HIV disease. Persons with HIV disease who reside in or have traveled to endemic areas, as well as persons who have had positive skin tests for previous exposure, should be considered at risk for coccidioidomycosis. In the United States endemic areas include Arizona, California, Nevada, New Mexico, Utah, and western Texas. Outside the United States, particular attention should be given to travel or previous residence in Mexico and Central and South America.

Definitive diagnosis of coccidioidomycosis is made by microscopy, culture, or direct examination of affected tissues or fluid from those tissues, including bronchoscopic specimens, blood, bone marrow, lymph node, urine, and liver specimens.

Treatment. As with most opportunistic infections associated with AIDS, treatment is not curative and lifelong suppressive therapy is required. For the initial phase of treatment the drug of choice is usually amphotericin B, followed by a suppressive regimen with either amphotericin B or ketoconazole (Ampel et al., 1989; Armstrong, 1989; Minamoto & Armstrong, 1988). Problems with treatment of coccidioidomycosis in persons with AIDS include delayed diagnosis and a lack of effective and relatively nontoxic drugs (Armstrong, 1989).

Considerations for Nursing. Nurses should be aware of the geographic distribution of *C. immitis* and anticipate possible development of coccidioidomycosis in HIV-infected individuals who live in, have previously lived in, or may have traveled to these states. The importance of including travel and previous locales of residence in the history of clients at risk for or with HIV disease is self-evident in the case of coccidioidomycosis. HIV-positive persons should be advised against travel for pleasure to endemic areas.

Related Nursing Care. See the discussions of fever, fatigue, weight loss, and dyspnea in Chapter 4.

PNEUMOCYSTOSIS

Carlos Chagas first identified *Pneumocystis carinii* in the lungs of guinea pigs in Brazil in 1909 (Glatt & Chirgwin, 1990). A few years later the species was named after Carini, another Brazilian investigator, who further described the organism after discovering it in the alveoli of rats. *P. carinii* was not implicated as a pathogen in human disease until the

1940s, when it was found to cause pneumonia in premature or protein-calorie malnourished infants (Glatt & Chirgwin, 1990; Hopewell, 1990; Walzer, 1990). In the 1950s, *P. carinii* was identified as the cause of disease in adults, as well as children, and in persons with lymphoid malignancies.

According to Hopewell (1990), between 1955 and 1967 only 130 cases of *P. carinii* pneumonia (PCP) were reported in the American literature, and until 1981 cases were sporadic, primarily involving persons who had hematologic or lymphoreticular malignancies or were receiving immunosuppressive therapy. The incidence of PCP changed drastically in 1981, when it became one of the first opportunistic infections identified in the AIDS epidemic (CDC, 1981a).

The taxonomy of *P. carinii* has remained uncertain, since the organism's life cycle has similarities to those of both protozoa and fungi (Henry & Thurn, 1990; Hopewell, 1990). According to Walzer (1990), most investigators have classified *P. carinii* as a protozoan based on its morphologic structure, but more recent study of the ribosomal RNA sequences indicates that this organism bears a closer relationship to fungi than to protozoa. In most major texts *P. carinii* continues to be classified as a protozoan.

Epidemiology. *P. carinii* is a ubiquitous organism with a worldwide distribution. It exists in human lungs and has been identified in the lungs of rats, rabbits, guinea pigs, dogs, mice, goats, sheep, cattle, monkeys, foxes, shrews, swine, and cats (Hughes, 1982). Although the organism can be found in the air, on food, and in water, transmission appears to be by the airborne route (Hughes, 1982; Walzer, 1990). Seroepidemiologic studies have indicated that most healthy children have acquired *P. carinii* infection by 4 years of age (Hopewell, 1990; Hughes, 1982; Walzer, 1990).

Since the beginning of the HIV-AIDS epidemic, PCP has been the most common life-threatening opportunistic infection in persons with AIDS. PCP has been the first AIDS-indicator opportunistic infection in 60% of persons with HIV disease and has occurred in an additional 20% of individuals with AIDS diagnosed because of other indicator diseases (Glatt et al., 1988; Murray et al., 1984). The increasing use of PCP prophylaxis in the HIV population is showing results; the incidence of PCP in cases of AIDS reported to the CDC in 1989 decreased to 53% of cases in adults and adolescents and 36% of cases in children (CDC, 1990a).

Pathogenesis. According to Walzer (1990), *P. carinii* has such low virulence that the initial infection in an immunocompetent person is suppressed by normal host defense mechanisms and causes no observable damage. In immunocompromised hosts PCP is usually a reactivation of a latent infection, often from a childhood exposure (Hopewell, 1990). Hughes (1982) demonstrated that the organism is communicable and that horizontal transmission may occur from sources of infection to susceptible persons (e.g., persons who are immunodeficient).

Since *P. carinii* is not considered a particularly pathogenic organism, a severe immunodeficiency must be present for this microbe to cause disease. In the case of HIV disease the natural history of progressive T4 cell depletion results in development of PCP in the majority of cases. The likelihood of PCP in an HIV-positive person increases significantly as the T4 cell count falls below 200 cells/mm^3 (Hopewell, 1990). Knowledge of the pathogenesis of HIV disease and PCP has led to the development of measures to prevent an initial episode of PCP in HIV-positive persons with a T4 cell count of less than 200 cells/mm^3 and to suppress and prevent subsequent episodes in individuals who have had at least one bout of PCP (CDC, 1989d).

Although *P. carinii* infection is generally confined to the lungs, extrapulmonary pneumocystosis can occur. Hematogenous dissemination from a pulmonary site has been reported to cause adrenal, bone marrow, cutaneous, otic, retinal, thyroid, hepatic, renal, and splenic involvement (Cote et al., 1990; Coulman et al., 1987; Gallant et al., 1988; Heyman & Rasmussen, 1987; Lubat et al., 1990; Macher et al., 1987; Pilon, 1990; Ravalli et al., 1990; Rossi et al., 1990).

Clinical Presentation. According to Hopewell (1990), clients usually have fever, fatigue, and weight loss for several weeks to months before respiratory symptoms develop. Thrush indicative of severe immunocompromise is usually present, along with a T4 cell count less than 200 cells/mm^3. The initially mild presentation and insidious onset are characteristic of PCP in persons with HIV disease (Levine & White, 1988). The most common symptoms are fever; shortness of breath, usually manifested initially as dyspnea on exertion, later noted also at rest; and cough, which usually starts out dry and nonproductive and later becomes productive (Glatt & Chirgwin, 1990; Hopewell, 1990; Levine & White, 1988).

The initial cough may be productive in clients who smoke or have a bacterial bronchitis or pneumonia (Hopewell, 1990). In the presence of severe immunocompromise the body's host defense mechanisms are severely impaired and fever may not be present. Kales and colleagues (1987), in a review of 140 patients with AIDS and PCP, noted the presence of fever in 86%. In 6% to 7% of the clients the initial presentation of PCP is asymptomatic (Levine & White, 1988).

Although PCP prophylaxis with inhaled pentamidine has proved successful, it does not always eliminate the development of *P. carinii* infection (Golden et al., 1989). Upper lobe PCP and disseminated pneumocystosis have been reported in persons receiving aerosol therapy (Abd et al., 1988; Conces et al., 1989; Cote et al., 1990; Hagopian & Huseby, 1989; Ravalli et al., 1990). Glatt and Chirgwin (1990) in a review of the literature cited failure rates with pentamidine aerosol ranging from 13% to 85%. However, Hopewell (1990) pointed out that PCP in clients who received pentamidine aerosol prophylaxis is less severe and easier to treat.

Pulmonary tissue damage caused by PCP can be extensive and cause necrosis, cavitation, pneumothorax, and pneumomediastinum (Bevan et al., 1990; Masur et al., 1990; Saldana & Mones, 1989; Villalona-Calero et al., 1989). Another complication of PCP is acute respiratory failure. Montaner and colleagues (1989) reviewed 136 cases of AIDS-related PCP and found that acute respiratory failure developed in 21%.

Diagnosis. Hopewell (1990) pointed out that HIV-positive persons who have not been under routine health care and do not readily seek medical attention may have advanced pneumonia and marked symptoms when first examined. Emphasis on symptom presentation is extremely important. In 5% to 10% of individuals with AIDS-related PCP the chest roentgenogram appears normal (Glatt & Chirgwin, 1990; Hopewell, 1990). Israel and co-workers (1987) noted that hypoxemia can be present with a normal chest roentgenogram. Arterial blood gas studies may reveal hypoxemia, hypocarbia, and an increase in the alveolar/arterial oxygen gradient, especially with exercise (Hopewell, 1990).

Pulmonary function studies usually reveal reductions in the vital capacity, total lung capacity, and single breath diffusing capacity for carbon monoxide. Hopewell (1990) noted that abnormal chest roentgenograms and abnormal pulmonary function studies are not uncommon in intravenous drug users and can confound the evaluations of these individuals. Gallium lung scanning is sensitive for the presence of PCP and is especially helpful when the chest roentgenogram is normal.

Since the majority of persons with AIDS-related PCP have a nonproductive cough, sputum induction may yield samples with positive findings and preclude the need for bronchoscopy. Although techniques for identifying the organism in expectorated sputum are improving, a negative result is not considered sufficient to exclude a diagnosis of PCP (Glatt & Chirgwin, 1990). Henry and Thurn (1990) noted that potential for identifying *P. carinii* in induced sputum is significantly reduced in individuals who are receiving PCP prophylaxis but in whom this pneumonia may be developing. Bronchoalveolar and transbronchial biopsies have proved highly sensitive in identifying pulmonary pathogens in persons with AIDS. Hopewell (1990) recommended that even if these techniques fail to establish a definitive diagnosis, a second bronchoscopic procedure be performed, leaving open-lung biopsy via thoracotomy as a last resort.

The CDC (1987a), in the revision of the surveillance case definition of AIDS, allowed presumptive diagnosis of PCP with laboratory evidence for HIV disease, according to the following guidelines: (1) a history of dyspnea on exertion or nonproductive cough of recent onset (within the past 3 months) *and* (2) chest x-ray evidence of diffuse bilateral interstitial infiltrates or gallium scan evidence of diffuse bilateral pulmonary disease *and* (3) arterial blood gas analysis showing an arterial oxygen tension of less than 70 mm Hg or a low respiratory diffusing capacity (less than 80%

of predicted values) or an increase in the alveolar/arterial oxygen tension gradient and (4) no evidence of bacterial pneumonia. Miller and colleagues (1989) found that empiric treatment for PCP can be performed accurately and can spare the client from bronchoscopy.

The detection of P. carinii in extrapulmonary sites is difficult, and even repeated biopsies may fail to yield a definitive diagnosis (Ravalli et al., 1990). Henry and Thurn (1990) raised the concern that prophylaxis or therapeutic interventions targeting only the lungs may result in a greater morbidity from extrapulmonary disease caused by P. carinii.

Treatment. Etinger (1990) noted that response to treatment for PCP is usually slow and that a worsening of arterial oxygenation, slower respiratory rate, and dyspnea, lasting 3 or more days, may occur initially after treatment is started. In addition, a delayed response to therapy, in some cases as long as 10 days and combined with a worsening appearance in the chest roentgenogram initially, should be expected and does not necessarily indicate treatment failure. Current standard therapy for PCP includes either intravenous pentamidine isethionate or trimethoprim-sulfamethoxazole (TMP-SMX) given orally or intravenously.

According to Masur and colleagues (1989), TMP-SMX is the preferred therapy, since the efficacy is at least as good as that of parenteral pentamidine and TMP-SMX is better tolerated. Oral administration of TMP-SMX also appears to be as effective as the intravenous route and, unless there are reasons to doubt gastrointestinal absorption or compliance, is the preferred route for mild cases of PCP.

Controlled studies have demonstrated that the toxic effects of TMP-SMX and pentamidine are usually tolerable and not life threatening even when the drugs are continued for the full 21-day course of treatment (Sattler et al., 1988). The same study demonstrated that a reduced dosage was better tolerated without compromising efficacy. Concurrent therapy with intravenous pentamidine in persons receiving didanosine (ddI; Videx) appears to increase the risk of pancreatitis (Bristol-Myers Squibb Company, personal communication, Nov. 5, 1990).

A third choice of conventional therapy is pyrimethamine-sulfadiazine. Experimental agents to treat PCP include (1) pentamidine aerosol, (2) trimethoprim-dapsone, (3) dapsone, (4) trimetrexate, (5) piritrexim, (6) clindamycin-primaquine, and (7) difluorome-thylornilthine (DFMO) (Masur et al., 1989). Early adjunctive therapy with corticosteroids decreases the risks of respiratory failure and death (Bozzette et al., 1990; Gagnon et al., 1990).

Although often avoided, intubation and mechanical ventilation may improve the chance of survival for persons who have AIDS and PCP with respiratory failure (Efferen et al., 1989). An alternative to intubation for mechanical ventilation is provision of positive airway pressure by face mask (Gregg et al., 1990).

Zidovudine alone does not prevent PCP, but zidovudine and aerosol pentamidine together have greater levels of protection than those provided by either drug alone (Girard et al., 1989; Leoung et al., 1990). Clinical studies of combined therapy have shown that aerosol pentamidine and zidovudine do not have additive toxicity (Hopewell, 1990).

Either primary or secondary prophylaxis against PCP is a therapeutic necessity in all HIV-positive persons. Primary prophylaxis refers to therapy provided to HIV-positive persons considered at risk for PCP (those whose T4 count is in the 200 to 300 cells/mm³ range) to prevent an initial episode of infection. Secondary prophylaxis refers to therapy to prevent recurrence or relapse in persons who have already had PCP. Current CDC guidelines recommend either pentamidine aerosol or TMP-SMX for prophylactic PCP therapy (CDC, 1989d).

Considerations for Nursing. PCP illustrates the major improvements in the treatment of AIDS in its first decade. Many nurses can recall first hearing about PCP in 1981 and then discovering that the recommended diagnostic strategy was open-lung biopsy. Many witnessed persons with AIDS-related PCP going to surgery and being cared for postoperatively in intensive care units with chest tubes and mechanical ventilators. Significant numbers of these patients had respiratory failure secondary to treatment failure, since clinicians were unaware that aggressive drug therapy beyond 10 to 14 days was required. Today diagnosis without invasive techniques is possible, and zidovudine and PCP prophylaxis can prevent or at least decrease the severity of illness. PCP prevention and treatment are a concrete example of why individuals should be tested for HIV and seek medical follow-up early in the course of disease.

Nurses should understand clearly that PCP or disseminated pneumocystosis may still develop in persons receiving primary or secondary PCP prophylaxis. Therefore HIV-positive individuals should be taught to pay attention to signs and symptoms of infection development, even when they are afebrile, and to seek medical advice. Nurses assisting individuals with pentamidine aerosol therapy should be aware that this treatment is affected by many variables, including particle size generated by the nebulizer, length of nebulizer tubing, and the client's ventilatory pattern, and that not all nebulizer systems have comparable efficacy (Corkery et al., 1988; Masur et al., 1989; Smaldone et al., 1988). Using equipment, dosages, or techniques for aerosol therapy that have not been recommended by the CDC and Food and Drug Administration (excluding approved research protocols) may not only be of limited benefit to the client, but also represent failure to meet established standards of care. (See Appendix II for the procedure for aerosolized pentamidine prophylaxis.)

Related Nursing Care. See the discussions of cough, shortness of breath, fever, and fatigue in Chapter 4.

CRYPTOSPORIDIOSIS

In 1907 Tyzzer first described a coccidian parasite in the gastric glands of laboratory mice and named it *Cryptosporidium* (Soave & Weikel, 1990). Although this parasite was known to be present in a variety of animal species, often without causing symptoms, it was not until 1971 that cryptosporidiosis was identified in cattle and it became clear that this disease might pose a threat to livestock (Armstrong, 1987). Cryptosporidiosis was not identified in humans until 1976, and until 1982 only seven cases were reported in the literature (CDC, 1984). By November 1982, 21 cases of cryptosporidiosis had been identified in persons with AIDS (CDC, 1982a).

Because of the lack of clinical data about human infection, cryptosporidiosis was initially thought to occur only among animal handlers who came in contact with infected animals, especially calves. With the onset of disease primarily in homosexual men with AIDS, it was thought to be transmitted through sexual practices such as anilingus and fellatio with infected individuals (New York City Department of Health, 1983). In 1983, however, Jokipii and colleagues noted that *Cryptosporidium* occurs frequently in travelers, suggesting that endemic regions might exist.

Epidemiology. The name *Cryptosporidium* denotes an organism with spores. Various species have been identified in mammals, birds, reptiles, and fish (Soave & Weikel, 1990). *Cryptosporidium* is now well recognized as a pathogen in both immunologically intact individuals and compromised hosts, such as persons with HIV disease. In addition to animal-to-human transmission, person-to-person transmission has been documented in attendees of day care centers, household contacts of infected persons and hospital patients and health care workers (Armstrong, 1987; Reif et al., 1989; Skeels et al., 1990; Soave & Weikel, 1990; Wofsy, 1990a).

Waterborne transmission has been implicated as a source of cryptosporidial diarrhea in travelers, as well as a potential problem relating to contamination of community water supplies, since chlorination does not kill *Cryptosporidium* (Gallaher et al., 1989; Hamoudi et al., 1988; Hayes et al., 1989; Jokipii & Jokipii, 1986; Jokipii et al., 1983; Rolston, 1990; Soave & Weikel, 1990; Tzipori, 1988; Wofsy, 1990a). *Cryptosporidium* has been found in rivers and other surface water in Arizona, Washington, Texas, Colorado, Oregon, Ohio, and Utah (Hamoudi et al., 1988; Soave & Weikel, 1990). Other possible modes of transmission are through food contaminated with mouse or rat excreta and through airborne exposure to coughing of infected animals (New York City Department of Health, 1983; Soave & Weikel, 1990; Wofsy, 1990a).

The *Cryptosporidium* oocyst is hardy and resistant to a number of disinfectants, including iodophor, cresylic acid, 3% sodium hypochlorite, benzalkonium chloride, sodium hydroxide, and 5% formaldehyde (Soave & Weikel, 1990; Wofsy, 1990a). Fomites are a hazard; Reif and associates

(1989) reported that a woman acquired cryptosporidiosis through handling her husband's contaminated clothing when doing the wash.

Although the parasite is known to be distributed throughout the world, the incidence of cryptosporidiosis in persons with AIDS varies. In the United States in 1989 cryptosporidiosis was reported as an indicator disease in 2% of the adult and 3% of the pediatric cases of AIDS, while in Haiti and Africa more than 50% of persons with AIDS have this disease (CDC, 1990a; Soave & Weikel, 1990).

Pathogenesis. After ingestion of the organism the most common site of infection is the small intestine, although in immunocompromised individuals cryptosporidia have been found throughout the gastrointestinal tract, including the pharynx, esophagus, stomach, duodenum, small intestine, appendix, colon, rectum, gallbladder, pancreas, bile, and pancreatic ducts, and in the respiratory tract as well (Ma et al., 1984; Soave & Weikel, 1990).

Wofsy (1990a) proposed that the symptoms and chronicity are related to the degree of immunocompromise. This position is supported by reports of symptom resolution and failure to detect cryptosporidia in previously infected individuals given zidovudine (Chandrasekar, 1987; Connolly et al., 1988; Greenberg et al., 1989).

Clinical Presentation. Human cryptosporidiosis is characterized by profuse watery diarrhea, abdominal cramping, flatulence, weight loss, anorexia, and malaise and may also be associated with fever, nausea, vomiting, and myalgia. In immunocompetent hosts the disease is self-limited with a 2- to 14-day incubation period, an illness usually lasting 10 to 14 days, and spontaneous recovery (Jokipii & Jokipii, 1986; Soave & Weikel, 1990). However, the occysts may continue to be excreted in stool even after recovery (Jokipii & Jokipii, 1986).

The same constellation of symptoms is present in cryptosporidiosis in persons with AIDS, with the addition of weight loss averaging more than 10 pounds, dehydration, malabsorption, electrolyte disturbances, and voluminous diarrhea that often reaches 10 to 15 L/day (Rolston, 1990). In atypical AIDS cases the infection may resolve spontaneously, and asymptomatic patients may show evidence of *Cryptosporidium* in specimens (Smith & Janoff, 1988; Wofsy, 1990a).

Diagnosis. Until the late 1980s the principal method of diagnosis was histologic examination of biopsy specimens. Today *Cryptosporidium* oocysts can be identified in fresh stool specimens or formalin-preserved specimens by a variety of staining techniques (Rolston, 1990).

Treatment. No effective anticryptosporidial therapy exists. In immunocompetent individuals the disease is self-limited and does not require therapy. Refractory cryptosporidiosis, as occurs in most persons with AIDS, usually results in death from profound malabsorption, electrolyte imbalances, malnutrition, and dehydration. Anticryptosporidial agents currently include spiramycin and eflornithine. The efficacy of spiramycin remains controversial (Moskovitz et al., 1988; Pilla et al., 1987; Rolston, 1990; Wofsy, 1990a). Eflornithine has been found to produce either complete resolution of diarrhea or reduction of symptoms in some patients with cryptosporidiosis, but the many untoward effects, including bone marrow suppression, hearing impairment, and gastrointestinal intolerance, limit its use (Rolston et al., 1989). Other agents being evaluated include hyperimmune bovine colostrum, cow's milk globulin, bovine transfer factor, trimetrexate, recombinant interleukin-2, and somatostatin (Rolston, 1990; Soave & Weikel, 1990; Wofsy, 1990a).

Patients receiving zidovudine have had the most immediate promising responses, presumably as a result of improved immunologic status (Chandrasekar, 1987; Connolly et al., 1988; Greenberg et al., 1989). Perhaps a combination of antiretroviral and anticryptosporidial agents will reduce the morbidity and mortality of cryptosporidiosis and AIDS. At present most medical therapy is palliative and directed toward symptoms, focusing on fluid replacement, occasionally total parenteral nutrition, correction of electrolyte imbalances, and the prescription of analgesic, antidiarrheal, and antiperistaltic agents.

Considerations for Nursing. Since palliation and symptom control are effective therapy, cryptosporidiosis in the person with AIDS calls for intensive nursing care. Nursing goals include measures to minimize the physical discomforts associated with continuous explosive diarrhea: skin breakdown in the perianal, genital, gluteal, and upper thigh regions, and pain, as well as measures to help the patient cope with significant alterations in body image as a result of malnutrition, dehydration, and weight loss. Nurses caring for this client population need emotional support themselves to deal with such frustrations as never getting the bed clean for longer than a few minutes or having to leave the client lying in fecal material to get medications.

Infection control measures should be carefully planned to prevent person-to-person transmission or fomite transmission, not only in hospitals but in the home as well. Protective clothing, wearing gloves during care, proper waste disposal, and meticulous handwashing, along with instructions to staff and significant others on enteric precautions, are imperative to proper care. Keeping the fecal waste contained is a never-ending challenge.

In institutions, environmental cleaning with prescribed disinfectants should be performed regularly. At home the usual household bleach containing 5.25% sodium hypochlorite may be ineffective against *Cryptosporidium*. However, the infectivity of *Cryptosporidium* is destroyed by ammonium, which can be used in solution to clean the patient's immediate environment and bathroom (Wofsy, 1990a).

Some clients are confronted with the decision of whether to accept insertion of indwelling infusion devices and total parenteral nutrition. Although some clients find this therapeutic modality initially attractive, it may prove frustrating to them once the therapy is initiated. Many soon discover that they are confined with the equipment, supplies, and an infusion pump and that getting to the toilet with the equipment can be especially difficult.

Prevention of cryptosporidiosis in HIV-infected persons includes early teaching regarding a low-microbe diet and avoidance of unbottled drinking water when away from home. Counseling about such sexual practices as anilingus should be provided.

Related Nursing Care. See the discussions of diarrhea, fatigue, weight loss, fever, dry skin, pain, and stomatitis in Chapter 4.

TOXOPLASMOSIS

Toxoplasma gondii is an obligate protozoan that causes toxoplasmosis in humans and domestic animals. According to McCabe and Remington (1988), the tragedy of toxoplasmosis is that although it can be prevented and is known to cause disease that leads to blindness and psychomotor retardation in children, it has never concerned the medical community in the United States as much as in Europe. Toxoplasmosis is a major cause of encephalitis in persons with AIDS.

Epidemiology. Infection with *T. gondii* occurs worldwide, and the organism infects herbivorous, carnivorous, and omnivorous animals. Although the definitive hosts of *Toxoplasma* are members of the cat family, not all cats are infected. McCabe and Remington (1990) noted that excretion of *Toxoplasma* oocysts has been reported in approximately 1% of the cats in diverse parts of the world. Although cats are considered of primary importance in transmission of the infection, toxoplasmosis has been found in locales without cats and a low prevalence of infection has been reported in areas with cats (McCabe & Remington, 1990).

The prevalence of *Toxoplasma* tissue cysts in meat consumed by humans is high. Although tissue cysts are rarely found in beef, as much as 25% of lamb and pork samples tested have been shown to contain them (McCabe & Remington, 1990). Cockroaches, flies, earthworms, snails, and slugs may serve as transport hosts for the oocyst, and ingestion of vegetables containing cysts probably accounts for *Toxoplasma* seropositivity in vegetarians (McCabe & Remington, 1990). Oocysts have also been found in unpasteurized goat's milk and eggs. The major means of transmission of *Toxoplasma* in humans is through ingestion of meats and vegetables containing oocysts (McCabe & Remington, 1990; Miller, 1986).

The only evidence of human-to-human transmission is from mother to fetus when the mother acquires infection during pregnancy. The risk of a woman of childbearing age becoming infected with *Toxoplasma* is related to the geographic area of residence and the number of people in that area who have been previously infected, as well as the rate of primary infection (McCabe & Remington, 1990). Moving from an area of low prevalence to an area of high prevalence increases risk; for example, in New York City the prevalence of infection among women of childbearing age is 15%, and in Paris among the same population it is 70% (McCabe & Remington, 1990). The overall seroprevalence increases with age; in the United States more than 50% of adults have been infected with *Toxoplasma* (Reinis-Lucey et al., 1990).

Rarer documented sources of infection include accidental self-inoculation by laboratory workers, transfusion of infected whole blood or white blood cells, and organ transplantation (McCabe & Remington, 1990).

Pathogenesis. Toxoplasmosis in a person with HIV disease is almost always a secondary appearance of chronic latent infection with *T. gondii* (Holliman, 1988; Israelski & Remington, 1988; McCabe & Remington, 1990). However, serologic studies of AIDS patients in France, a high-prevalence area for *Toxoplasma*, suggest that their infections were recently acquired (Reinis-Lucey et al., 1990). Although serologic studies of an individual with acute toxoplasmosis cannot always distinguish between primary active and latent infection, evidence indicates that an HIV-infected person who is seropositive for *Toxoplasma* antibodies is at considerable risk for toxoplasmosis (Israelski & Remington, 1988). Whether infection is primary or secondary, the cell-mediated immunodeficiency associated with HIV disease renders the individual defenseless against the progression of infection by *T. gondii*.

After entering the body, usually by ingestion, *Toxoplasma* replicates, disseminates via the blood and lymphatics, and causes asymptomatic or mildly symptomatic infection in an immunocompetent host. In an immunodeficient host, such as a person with HIV disease, regardless of whether the infection is primary or secondary (reactivation), it rapidly causes focal or diffuse meningoencephalitis with cellular necrosis, progresses unchecked to the lungs, heart, and skeletal muscle, and can result in death (McCabe & Remington, 1990; Reinis-Lucey et al., 1990).

When congenital transmission of *T. gondii* from an immunocompetent mother occurs, usually the mother acquired the organism after conception. McCabe and Remington (1990) cited one case in which an immunocompetent mother, having acquired infection 2 months before conception, gave birth to an infected child. An immunodeficient mother with chronic *Toxoplasma* infection can transmit the infection regardless of whether she is symptomatic or asymptomatic (McCabe & Remington, 1990). The outcome of such a pregnancy can be spontaneous abortion, stillbirth, or severe disease in the newborn.

Clinical Presentation. Despite the severity of infection, the symptoms of toxoplasmosis in a person with AIDS may be vague and nonspecific and are sometimes ignored (Reinis-Lucey et al., 1990). In a review of the literature by Israelski and Remington (1988), 44% to 56% of the patients complained of headache and 60% had altered mental status manifested as confusion, lethargy, delusional behavior, frank psychosis, global cognitive impairment, anomia, and coma; the presence of fever varied from a low of 10% of the cases to 74%. The most common focal neurologic deficit is hemiparesis; others include aphasia, ataxia, visual field loss, cranial nerve palsies, dysmetria, and motor disorders. In approximately one third of AIDS patients with toxoplasmosis, seizures are the initial reason for seeking medical attention (Israelski et al., 1990). Other sites of *Toxoplasma* infection in persons with AIDS include the heart, lungs, skin, stomach, abdomen, testes, and spinal cord (Crider et al., 1988; Derouin et al., 1989; Haskell et al., 1989; Herskovitz et al., 1989; Hirschmann & Chu, 1988; Israelski et al., 1988; Mendelson et al., 1987; Smart et al., 1990; Tawney et al., 1986).

In congenital toxoplasmosis, signs and symptoms may be nonspecific, may mimic disease caused by herpes simplex, cytomegalovirus, or rubella, and may include chorioretinitis, strabismus, blindness, epilepsy, psychomotor or mental retardation, anemia, jaundice, rash, petechiae caused by thrombocytopenia, encephalitis, pneumonitis, microcephaly, intracranial calcification, hypothermia, and nonspecific illness (McCabe & Remington, 1990). Congenital cardiac toxoplasmosis has also been reported (Medlock et al., 1990).

Diagnosis. In the presence of HIV disease the appearance of neurologic symptoms can suggest any number of opportunistic infections and neoplastic processes. The physician must direct the clinical diagnosis not only toward establishing the presence of toxoplasmosis, but also toward clearly ruling out other infections such as cryptococcal meningitis, progressive multifocal leukoencephalopathy, herpes simplex encephalitis, mycobacterial encephalitis, HIV disease of the central nervous system, and neoplasms such as primary lymphoma of the brain and Kaposi's sarcoma.

Until 1987 the CDC required that diagnosis of an AIDS-indicator disease be definitive, and in the case of toxoplasmosis this meant the diagnosis of AIDS could be achieved only by brain biopsy. In 1987 the CDC made a major change in the diagnosis of AIDS to be more consistent with the current diagnostic practices. This change permitted the presumptive diagnosis of certain indicator diseases in patients with laboratory confirmation of HIV disease. This was particularly important for the diagnosis of toxoplasmosis, since many clients and physicians avoided neurosurgical brain biopsy because of the associated risks and because lesions visualized by neuroradiologic procedures were often in surgically inaccessible regions of the brain.

In most cases toxoplasmosis in clients with laboratory-confirmed HIV disease is diagnosed presumptively according to suggested guidelines. These guidelines include (1) recent onset of a focal neurologic abnormality consistent with intracranial disease or a reduced level of consciousness; (2) brain imaging evidence of a lesion having a mass effect (on computed tomography [CT] or nuclear magnetic resonance imaging) or whose radiographic appearance is enhanced by injection of contrast medium; and (3) serum antibody to toxoplasmosis or successful response to therapy for toxoplasmosis (CDC, 1987a).

Treatment. The mainstay of therapy for toxoplasmosis in persons with AIDS has been the combination of sulfadiazine (or trisulfapyrimidines) and pyrimethamine. Symptoms usually diminish within 8 to 10 days, and CT abnormalities resolve between the first and fourth weeks of therapy (Reinis-Lucey et al., 1990). Adjunctive therapy may include decadron for abscesses associated with a severe mass effect, dilantin for infection-induced seizures, and folinic acid to ameliorate the bone marrow toxicity of pyrimethamine (Israelski & Remington, 1988; Reinis-Lucey et al., 1990). Israelski and Remington (1988) emphasized that folic acid should not be used, since it inhibits the action of pyrimethamine (i.e., destruction of *Toxoplasma* by blocking folic acid metabolism of the organism).

Persons with AIDS who take sulfadiazine and pyrimethamine for toxoplasmosis have a high incidence of adverse reactions. Severe adverse reactions necessitating discontinuation of this regimen during the initial treatment phase may occur in 40% to 60% of the patients (Haverkos, 1987; Israelski & Remington, 1988; McCabe & Remington, 1990). Either the dose is adjusted or an alternative regimen is selected. Alternative regimens include cessation of sulfadiazine and continuation of pyrimethamine alone or with the addition of clindamycin. Dannemann and associates (1988) found clindamycin either alone or in combination with pyrimethamine to be effective therapy for toxoplasmosis encephalitis in persons with AIDS. Although clindamycin appears to be effective for toxoplasmosis chorioretinitis, it does not penetrate the central nervous system well and should not be used alone for central nervous system toxoplasmosis (Reinis-Lucey et al., 1990). Other agents that have been used include spiramycin, trimetrexate, trimethoprim, and sulfamethoxazole. Prospective controlled studies are needed to assess the role of alternative drugs such as clindamycin and trimetrexate in the treatment of central nervous system toxoplasmosis (Tuazon, 1989). Empiric therapy, frequently employed in association with presumptive diagnosis of CNS toxoplasmosis, has proved satisfactory (Cohn et al., 1989).

As with most opportunistic infections in persons with AIDS, suppressive therapy is necessary because cure is not possible. Agents employed are pyrimethamine with or without sulfadiazine, pyrimethamine-sulfadixine, and clindamycin.

Considerations for Nursing. Whether infection with *T. gondii* in a person with AIDS is due to primary or secondary infection (reactivation of latent infection) is often unknown. Since the *Toxoplasma* antibody status of most persons with HIV disease is unknown and probably some have not been infected, and since toxoplasmosis is a preventable disease, clients should be taught about prevention of *Toxoplasma* infection as early as possible in the course of HIV disease. Key elements in prevention are cooking meat until it is well done, washing fruits and vegetables, wearing gloves when gardening or disposing of cat litter (if these tasks cannot be avoided) (McCabe & Remington, 1988). Freezing to $-20°$ C ($-4°$ F) kills cysts in meat, but most home freezers do not achieve or maintain this temperature (Remington & McLeod, 1986). Boiling water and dry heat greater than 66° C (151° F) render the cysts noninfectious. Cooking meat to destroy infectivity means reaching an internal temperature of 60° C (140° F) for at least 10 minutes (Reinis-Lucey et al., 1990).

For the person with AIDS and toxoplasmosis, emphasis on health teaching, follow-up, and evaluation of compliance with a suppressive therapy regimen is essential to prevent relapse. Factors that may impede compliance, such as cognitive impairment or continuation or resumption of alcohol or drug use, should be assessed when individualized follow-up is planned. Often a significant other is asked to assume some responsibility for suppressive therapy, since the client may be unable to do so.

Any residual neurologic deficits, especially vision loss, aphasia, and motor impairment (e.g., hemiparesis) should be evaluated in relation to the individual's ability to perform activities of daily living and communicate. Many clients with toxoplasmosis benefit significantly, both emotionally and physically, from physical, occupational, or speech therapy to increase their functional abilities.

Related Nursing Care. See the discussion of impaired vision and motor dysfunction in Chapter 4.

ISOSPORIASIS

First described by Woodstock and Wenyon in 1885, human isosporiasis remains a poorly understood disease (Soave & Weikel, 1990). Only 500 cases of gastrointestinal isosporiasis were reported between 1948 and 1974 (Wofsy, 1990b). In the early 1980s there were sporadic reports of *Isospora belli* infection in persons with AIDS in the United States, and in 1985 isosporiasis was included in the revised case definition of AIDS (CDC, 1985b). Although isosporiasis is diagnosed in less than 1% of AIDS patients in the United States, in Haiti 15% of persons with AIDS have this disease (DeHovitz et al., 1985; Pape et al., 1989).

Epidemiology. *I. belli* is a coccidian protozoan parasite that is more common in tropical climates and causes endemic disease in South America, Africa, and Southeast Asia (Soave & Weikel, 1990). Sorvillo and colleagues (1990) reported a 25% increase in 1989 in cases of isosporiasis in persons with AIDS, primarily Hispanic immigrants from Mexico and Central America. Although not documented, transmission of *Isospora* is thought to occur through sexual contact (anilingus) with infected humans and by means of environmental contaminants such as water (Pape et al., 1990; Soave & Weikel, 1990; Wofsy, 1990b). Although *I. belli* is ubiquitously distributed in the animal kingdom, no evidence of animal-to-human transmission has been reported (Wofsy, 1990b).

Pathogenesis. After ingestion, *Isospora* cysts infect the small intestine and result in malabsorption and a nonbloody, watery diarrhea. Restrepo and associates (1987) reported disseminated, extraintestinal isosporiasis in a person with AIDS.

Clinical Presentation. The clinical features of isosporiasis resemble those of cryptosporidiosis with the exception of less frequent bowel movements: 8 to 10 per day in isosporiasis compared with 6 to 26 per day in cryptosporidiosis (Wofsy, 1990b). Characteristics of this illness include profuse watery, nonbloody diarrhea, cramping abdominal pain, nausea, anorexia, weight loss, weakness, occasionally vomiting, and a low-grade fever (Smith & Janoff, 1988; Wofsy, 1990b). Clinical illness ranges from self-limiting enteritis or chronic diarrhea in immunocompetent individuals to chronic or relapsing disease in persons with AIDS (Soave & Weikel, 1990). Severe debilitating dehydration may occur (Pape et al., 1989). Steatorrhea (fat in the feces) caused by malabsorption can be seen in stool specimens.

Diagnosis. Diagnosis of isosporiasis is by identification of the *Isospora* oocysts in fecal specimens. Several specimens, as well as specimen concentration techniques, may be required to confirm the diagnosis, since *Isospora* oocysts may be shed only intermittently and in small numbers (Soave & Weikel, 1990). Pape and colleagues (1989) recommended that a minimum of four stool examinations be performed for persons with AIDS and chronic diarrhea.

Treatment. Pape and co-workers (1989) found a 10-day course of trimethoprim-sulfamethoxazole to be as effective as the previously recommended 31-day course of treatment for persons with AIDS and isosporiasis. They found that diarrhea ceased within a mean of 2.5 days of the initiation of therapy and that *Isospora* oocysts could not be detected in the stools of infected persons after 2 days of trimethoprim-sulfamethoxazole.

Since relapse and recurrent infection is well documented in persons with AIDS, continuation of a suppressive prophylactic regimen in necessary. Suppressive therapy includes either trimethoprim-pyrimethamine or sulfadoxine-pyrimethamine; pyrimethamine can be prescribed for persons allergic to sulfonamides (Pape et al., 1989).

Considerations for Nursing. Food and water precautions should be advised for all HIV-positive persons to avoid infection such as isosporiasis (Sorvillo et al., 1990; Ungvarski, 1989). This is especially important with travel to tropical and subtropical climates. Additional health teaching for persons with isosporiasis includes avoidance of sexual practices such as anilingus that may predispose others to infection with *Isospora* or reexpose the client. The importance of indefinite continuation of suppressive therapy must also be emphasized.

Although nosocomial transmission has not been reported, the use of gloves and other barrier precautions, along with meticulous handwashing, is essential to prevent health care workers and significant others from acquiring isosporiasis. Frequent routine cleaning of the infected person's environment using standard disinfectant and cleaning agents is essential.

Related Nursing Care. See the discussion of diarrhea, fatigue, weight loss, dry skin, and pain in Chapter 4.

HERPES SIMPLEX VIRUS

Viruses have the distinction of being the oldest recorded etiologic agents of disease (e.g., rabies), as well as some of the most recently identified (e.g., HIV disease) (Tyler & Fields, 1990). Although the yellow fever virus was the first disease-causing virus discovered, the modern era of virology began in the late 1940s and early 1950s with the culture and vaccine development of the poliovirus and the development of electron microscopy (Tyler & Fields, 1990).

Most people think of herpes as a synonym for a cold sore or genital lesion. However, the name is derived from a family of viruses called Herpesviridae, which has seven members. The herpesviruses and some commonly related diseases are (1) herpes simplex virus type 1 (HSV-1) causing cold sores and eye infections; (2) herpes simplex virus type 2 (HSV-2) causing genital herpes; (3) varicella-zoster virus (VZV) causing chickenpox and shingles; (4) Epstein-Barr virus (EBV) causing infectious mononucleosis; (5) cytomegalovirus (CMV) causing mononucleosis; (6) human herpes virus type 6 causing roseola; and (7) herpes B virus (sometimes referred to as human herpes virus type 7 or simian herpes B virus) causing skin lesions or brain infection (Straus, 1990).

A major biologic feature of the herpesviruses is the phenomenon of latency and reactivation. After initial or primary infection with any of the seven herpesviruses, they remain lifelong latent viruses in humans and have the potential to be reactivated, producing recurrent infections. Sites of latency include sensory nerve ganglia for HSV-1, HSV-2, and VZV; monocytes, neutrophils, or lymphocytes for CMV; B lymphocytes and salivary glands for EBV; lymphocytes for human herpesvirus 6; and sensory nerve ganglia for herpes B virus (Straus, 1990).

Herpesviruses are fragile and do not survive for prolonged periods in the environment (Straus, 1990). HSV-1, HSV-2, VZV, and herpes B virus are transmitted by direct contact with infected lesions. Oral-genital contact and sexual intercourse transmit HSV-1, HSV-2, CMV, and possibly EBV (saliva is the major route of EBV transmission), and all human herpesviruses can cause congenital and neonatal infections (Straus, 1990). The following discussion is limited to herpes simplex virus infection and its relationship to HIV disease.

Epidemiology. Herpes simplex viruses are ubiquitous and have a worldwide distribution. Humans appear to be the only natural host. The principal mode of transmission is contact with oral secretions for HSV-1 and contact with genital secretions for HSV-2. Transmission of HSV-1 can occur in the genital area by oral-sexual contact or autoinoculation (i.e., touching a cold sore, then touching the genitals), and HSV-2 can be transmitted orally by similar modes. Although transmission is facilitated during contact with a person with active infection, it can also occur from asymptomatic excretors (Hirsch, 1990; Rooney et al., 1986).

Spread of HSV-1 from oral secretions can be an occupational hazard for dentists and respiratory care personnel, causing primary herpetic finger infections referred to as herpetic whitlow (Hirsch, 1990). Cutaneous infection with HSV in wrestlers and rugby players has occurred through skin-to-skin contact with lesions and is referred to as herpes gladiatorum (CDC, 1990c). Other names seen in the literature include herpes oralis for HSV-1 and herpes genitalis for HSV-2.

Serologic studies indicate that exposure to HSV-1 commonly occurs in early childhood and that the risk of infection is related to socioeconomic conditions such as overcrowding (Corey & Spear, 1986; Erlich & Mills, 1990). A different pattern of infection occurs with HSV-2. Except in infants born to mothers with vaginal lesions, HSV-2 infection risk usually begins at puberty with the onset of sexual activity and increases with the number of different sexual partners (Corey & Spear, 1986; Erlich & Mills, 1990). Higher rates of HSV-2 prevalence have been found in prostitutes, sexually active homosexual men (who have higher rates than sexually active heterosexual men), adults of lower socioeconomic status, and persons attending sexually transmitted disease clinics (Corey & Spear, 1986). In HIV-infected persons the progressive immunosuppression induced by HIV permits recurrent or chronic HSV infection.

HSV-2 has been implicated as a risk factor for HIV disease in both homosexuals and heterosexuals, not only in relation to an increased num-

HSV encephalitis. Since clinical diagnosis of HSV encephalitis is usually impossible, and a brain biopsy is usually required for definitive diagnosis but often refused, an empiric trial of intravenous acyclovir may be used (Erlich & Mills, 1990). Oral acyclovir, suspension or capsules, may be used for either acute HSV infection or long-term suppressive therapy. Acyclovir has been shown in cell culture to have greater antiviral activity against HSV-1 than HSV-2 (O'Brien & Campoli-Richards, 1989). Topical acyclovir ointment is used to relieve subjective symptoms of skin lesions and to reduce viral shedding.

By 1989 several cases of acyclovir-resistant HSV-2 infection had been reported (Erlich et al., 1989b; Marks et al., 1989; Norris et al., 1988). Engel and colleagues (1990) reported success in treating acyclovir-resistant HSV-2 infection in persons with AIDS by administering high-dose, continuous-infusion acyclovir for 6 weeks. This was done after treatment failure when acyclovir had been given orally and intravenously in traditional divided doses. Alternative drugs for acyclovir-resistant HSV are foscarnet and vidarabine. Favorable results have been reported with foscarnet (Erlich et al., 1989a; MacPhail et al., 1989; Sall et al., 1989; Youle et al., 1988). Randomized trials comparing foscarnet and vidarabine are under way (American Foundation for AIDS Research, 1990).

Considerations for Nursing. Health history of an HIV-positive person is important to determine the potential for recurrent HSV infection. The individual's knowledge of HSV transmission, as well as prevention related to specific sexual behaviors, such as condom use and oral sex, should be assessed. Practicing safer sex should be reviewed with all HIV-positive persons to prevent transmission or acquisition of sexually transmitted diseases. HIV-positive clients sometimes assume that if they have sex with another HIV-positive person, they can do whatever they want and no longer need to practice safer sex. Health teaching should stress that the rate of HSV infection is high in HIV-positive persons and that even if no HSV lesions are visible, asymptomatic excretors can pass on the virus (Hirsch, 1990).

Nursing care of external lesions is directed at preventing secondary infections and autoinoculation, especially from genital and perianal lesions to other parts of the body. This is a problem especially in persons with HIV disease, who for any number of reasons may have impaired cognitive function. The burning, itching, and tingling sensations associated with mucocutaneous lesions invite scratching. Acyclovir ointment can reduce these sensations. When acyclovir ointment is used on an area that will be covered with clothing or that comes in direct contact with bed linens, the area should be covered with an impervious dressing so that the ointment is not absorbed by clothing and stays on the lesion(s). Dressing the lesions of confused and disoriented individuals may be necessary to prevent autoinoculation.

The risk of nosocomial transmission of HSV-1 and HSV-2 from infected patients, most often causing herpetic whitlow, is well documented (Henderson, 1990). Nurses should wear gloves during physical examination of a new client, since they cannot predict what types of mucocutaneous lesion may be present. Gloves should also be worn for any procedures that involve oral or genital secretions, such as mouth care, suctioning, urinary catheter procedures, or vaginal care. Meticulous handwashing should be performed, and skin-to-lesion contact should be avoided as much as possible.

Related Nursing Care. See the discussions of dry skin and skin lesions, fever, fatigue, and dry and painful mouth in Chapter 4.

CYTOMEGALOVIRUS

In 1881 Ribbert first described what he called protozoan-like cells in the kidney of a stillborn child. By 1925, 25 cases of cytomegalic inclusion disease had been described (Ho, 1990). In the late 1950s, Weller and his associates first isolated human cytomegalovirus (CMV) and gave the organism its name, replacing the term "cytomegalic inclusion disease" (Ho, 1990). By the 1970s scientists had detected both antigens and the virus in body fluids, including blood, semen, cervical secretions, and urine (Vinters & Ferreiro, 1990).

CMV shares with the other herpesviruses the phenomenon of latency and reactivation, or as Ho appropriately stated, "Once infected, always infected" (1990, p. 1159). In this respect CMV, and all herpesviruses, are true opportunists that remain dormant in tissues of a previously infected person, waiting to be reactivated and to cause infection. CMV is one of two etiologic agents of mononucleosis (the other is the Epstein-Barr virus).

Epidemiology. Infection with CMV is widely distributed throughout the world and is usually inapparent. Depending on the socioeconomic conditions of the population, the prevalence of antibodies indicating previous infection ranges from 40% to 100% in adults. According to Pomeroy and Englund (1987), seroprevalence ranges from 30% to 40% in middle-class communities to nearly 100% in lower socioeconomic urban groups and in underdeveloped nations. A wide variation exists in the United States; for example, the seroprevalence rate is 45% in Albany, New York, and 79% in Houston (Ho, 1990).

According to Ho (1990), the potential for infection is increased during two periods: the perinatal period through the preschool years, and later during the sexually active years. In the first period CMV can be acquired as intrauterine or congenital infection, via vaginal delivery through a contaminated cervix, from human milk by breast feeding or from banked milk, by transmission from child to child in nurseries or day care centers, or among children within a family. Infected children carry the virus in the respiratory tract and urine for long periods (Ho, 1990).

Drew and Erlich (1990a) identified several factors supporting heterosexual transmission in adults: (1) CMV does not spread from adults by ordinary, nonsexual contact; (2) the virus has been isolated from semen and cervical secretions; (3) the prevalence of CMV antibody more than doubles between the ages of 15 and 35, the years of the highest sexual activity; and (4) bidirectional transfer (men to women and women to men) has been documented. Kissing and spread through saliva are also a probable means of CMV transmission (Pagano & Lemon, 1986). Little information is available on CMV transmission and specific sexual practices, such as heterosexual cunnilingus or fellatio, and virtually no studies of CMV transmission between lesbians have been reported. With the AIDS epidemic, specific activities between men have received considerable attention.

In 1981 investigators found a higher prevalence rate of CMV infection in homosexual men than in heterosexual men (Drew & Erlich, 1990a). This finding was confirmed in 1987 by Collier and associates. Of the numerous sexual practices among homosexual men studied, only receptive anal intercourse correlated with a higher incidence of CMV antibody or seroconversion. In 1988 Rabinowitz and colleagues reported for the first time a case of CMV proctitis in an immunocompetent HIV-negative woman after anal intercourse. This finding emphasizes that it is sexual practices, not sexual orientation, that may result in transmission of the disease.

Largely because information about reducing the risk of AIDS was disseminated among the gay communities across the United States early in the 1980s, changes in sexual behavior began to occur. In 1987 Martin reported that the frequency of homosexual episodes involving the exchange of body fluids and mucous membrane contact had declined by an average of 70% and also that condom use during anal intercourse had increased. Becker and Joseph (1988) in a review of the literature reported that changes in sexual behavior, especially among homosexual and bisexual men, were occurring because of the threat of AIDS. Presumably this change in sexual behavior has contributed to the decline of CMV transmission among homosexual men (Drew et al., 1988).

Drew and Erlich (1990b) pointed out that reexposure, as by receptive anal intercourse without a condom, in a man with long-standing seropositivity can result in reinfection with exogenous strains of CMV (coexisting different isolates of CMV have been found in persons with AIDS). Double infections with CMV do occur in patients with AIDS. Alternative routes of CMV transmission include transfusion of blood products and transplantation of organs or tissues. Immunosuppressive drugs, corticosteroids, and cytotoxic drugs such as cyclophosphamide or azathioprine can permit reactivation of latent disease (Ho, 1990).

Pathogenesis. CMV causes disease in three ways: by directly destroying tissue in sites such as the brain, lungs, retina, and liver; by causing immunologic responses resulting in hemolytic anemia and thrombocytopenia; and by facilitating neoplastic transformation (Straus, 1990). According to Ho (1990), the site of latency is not precisely known but probably includes leukocytes. In immunologically normal adults CMV is not detectable except in cervical secretions of some women and the semen of some men, with a higher incidence in homosexual men (Ho, 1990). Immunocompetent individuals may continue to shed the virus in body fluids for several months after recovering from acute CMV infection. Carriers, often chronic, include individuals with congenital or perinatal infection and immunocompromised hosts such as transplant recipients and persons with HIV disease.

Drew and Erlich (1990b) suggested that CMV may be a cofactor in the acquisition or expression of HIV disease based on the following: (1) CMV infection is associated with decreased proliferation of lymphocytes and defects in the cytoxic cell response; (2) prior infection with CMV may facilitate subsequent infection by HIV; (3) alternately, CMV infection of cells could reactivate a latent HIV disease. CMV along with other viruses has been investigated as a possible cause of Kaposi's sarcoma, but the findings have been inconsistent (Beral et al., 1990; Drew et al., 1988).

Clinical Presentation. In immunocompetent normal adults, CMV infection, or more appropriately CMV mononucleosis, is clinically similar to Epstein-Barr virus mononucleosis, also referred to as infectious mononucleosis. Fever and fatigue are the only characteristic clinical findings. Although rare, complications can occur in immunocompetent individuals and include interstitial pneumonitis, hepatitis, Guillain-Barré syndrome, meningoencephalitis, myocarditis, thrombocytopenia, hemolytic anemia, and cutaneous lesions (Ho, 1990). Persons with HIV disease who have active CMV infection can remain asymptomatic or exhibit various clinical manifestations such as chorioretinitis, pneumonitis, encephalitis, adrenalitis, colitis, esophagitis, cholangitis, and hepatitis (Drew et al., 1990).

Clients with ocular infection usually complain of painless visual loss, ranging from loss of a portion of the visual field to blurred vision, or of floaters, either unilaterally or bilaterally (Bloom & Palestine, 1988; Drew et al., 1990; Vinters & Ferreiro, 1990). Impaired vision is frequently the first sign of disseminated CMV infection in a person with HIV disease. Other reported ocular manifestations of CMV infection include panuveitis and conjunctivitis (H. H. Brown et al., 1988; Daicker, 1988).

Pulmonary CMV infection is usually seen in combination with other opportunistic disease such as *P. carinii* pneumonia, *Mycobacterium avium* complex infection, pyogenic bacterial infection, or *Cryptococcus neo-*

formans infection (Wallace & Hannah, 1987). Drew and associates (1990) noted that many of these clients respond to therapy directed at the concurrent infection (e.g., *Pneumocystis carinii* pneumonia), which raises the question of the actual pathogenicity of pulmonary CMV. CMV pulmonary infection in a person with AIDS is often manifested as progressive shortness of breath, dyspnea on exertion, and a dry nonproductive cough, with or without fever (Drew et al., 1990; Jacobson & Mills, 1988). Other respiratory manifestations of CMV infection reported in persons with AIDS include fever and wheezing in a client with CMV bronchiolitis and hoarseness in a client with CMV infection of the laryngeal nerve (Small et al., 1989; Vasudevan et al., 1990).

Although the effects of congenital CMV infection on the central nervous system can be severe, postnatal CMV infection is rare even in immunodeficient individuals (Ho, 1990). CMV is not considered a postnatal neurotropic virus, although cases of AIDS and CMV central nervous system infection have been reported (Fuller et al., 1989a; Masdeu et al., 1988; Vinters et al., 1989). What was earlier thought to be subacute encephalitis caused by CMV is now considered a common clinical central nervous syndrome caused by HIV and is encompassed by the diagnosis AIDS dementia complex (Ho, 1990). When CMV and HIV coexist in the brain of a person with AIDS, the in vivo interaction may be the cause of the encephalitis (Wiley & Nelson, 1988). Regardless of whether HIV or CMV is causing the encephalitis, the clinical presentation is similar: personality changes, cognitive impairment, and motor impairment. Other central nervous system pathologic processes attributable to CMV include radiculomyelitis, ascending myelitis, and necrotizing spinal lesions (Behar et al., 1987; Borgstein et al., 1989; Fuller et al., 1989b; Jacobson et al., 1988; Mahieux et al., 1989).

Virtually all parts of the gastrointestinal tract, from the oral cavity to the perianal area, have been reported as infected with CMV (Francis et al., 1989; Kanas et al., 1987). Esophageal ulceration with CMV is most often associated with odynophagia and dysphagia (Cello & Wilcox, 1988; Gould et al., 1988). CMV colitis is usually associated with weight loss, anorexia, and fever (Drew et al., 1990). The feces should be monitored regularly for hematochezia (blood), since the potential for hemorrhage, infarction, and perforation of the gastrointestinal tract exists (DeRiso et al., 1989; Houin et al., 1987; Spiller et al., 1988; Tucker et al., 1989; Wajsman et al., 1989; Wexner et al., 1988). Other gastrointestinal sites reported to be infected with CMV in persons with AIDS include the liver, gallbladder, and pancreas (Aaron et al., 1988; Jacobson et al., 1988; Joe et al., 1989; Ong et al., 1989; Vinters & Ferreiro, 1990).

CMV infection of the adrenal gland in persons with AIDS can produce such manifestations as postural hypotension and sodium deficits (Bleweiss et al., 1986; Lortholary et al., 1990; Vinters & Ferreiro, 1990).

CMV infection of the thyroid and pituitary glands has also been reported (Ferreiro & Vinters, 1988; Frank et al., 1987).

Vascular infection caused by CMV includes thrombophlebitis, cerebral venous thrombosis, and vascular cutaneous lesions that can be mistaken for Kaposi's sarcoma (Abrams & Farhood, 1989; Bourn'erias et al., 1989; Meyohas et al., 1989; Peterson & Stahl-Bayliss, 1987). Genitourinary CMV infection reported in persons with AIDS includes cystitis, endometritis, and infections of the cervix and testes (Benson et al., 1988; Brodman & Deligdisch, 1986; Brown et al., 1988; Lucas et al., 1989; Nistal et al., 1990).

Diagnosis. Drew and Erlich (1990c) noted that CMV infection must be distinguished from CMV disease, since CMV can be isolated from blood, urine, semen, cervical secretions, or other body fluids in the absence of clinical illness. The diagnosis of CMV disease is based on microscopic identification of CMV inclusion bodies or positive cultures from specific organs such as the brain, lung, liver, and adrenal glands, or both, in the absence of other infectious agents.

The presumptive diagnosis of CMV chorioretinitis is usually based on loss of vision and characteristic findings of serial ophthalmoscopic examinations in a person with definitively diagnosed HIV disease. The diagnosis of CMV adrenalitis is usually presumptive, based on the identification of adrenal insufficiency and isolation of CMV from the blood (New York Statewide Professional Standards Review Council Inc., 1990).

Treatment. In June 1989 the Food and Drug Administration licensed ganciclovir for the treatment of sight-threatening CMV retinitis. Ganciclovir is an antiviral agent with virostatic therapeutic effects that suppress rather than cure CMV infection.

The success of intravenous ganciclovir for CMV retinitis is well documented. The drug has been reported to cause clinical improvement, disease stabilization, or slowing of disease progression (Holland et al., 1989; Jabs et al., 1989). Kotler and associates (1989) noted also weight gain, repleted body cell mass and body fat, and increased serum albumin in persons with AIDS and CMV infection treated with ganciclovir. Despite lifelong therapy, blindness related to disease progression, retinal detachment, or ganciclovir-resistant CMV infection has been reported (Erice et al., 1989; Holland et al., 1989; Jabs et al., 1989).

Neutropenia is the most common dose-limiting toxic effect of ganciclovir and limits the concomitant use of zidovudine (American Foundation for AIDS Research, 1990). For individuals unable to tolerate systemic ganciclovir therapy because of severe neutropenia, catheter-induced sepsis, or the need to continue zidovudine, intravitreal injections of ganciclovir are an effective alternative (Cantrill et al., 1989; Heinemann, 1989; Henry et al., 1987).

Intravenous foscarnet is under investigation as an alternative therapy for CMV retinitis. It suppresses CMV retinitis and can be used in combination with zidovudine (Fanning et al., 1990; Jacobson et al., 1989). Additional studies are needed to determine the optimal dosage for maintenance therapy. The major dose-limiting toxicity is nephrotoxicity (Jacobson & O'Donnell, 1991).

Other drugs that have been used to treat CMV retinitis include acyclovir, alpha-interferon, and combination therapy with ganciclovir and immune globulin (Drew et al., 1990c; Vinters & Ferreiro, 1990). Treatment of CMV infection, other than retinitis, in persons with HIV disease is still under investigation.

Considerations for Nursing. For the client with HIV disease who has been receiving zidovudine therapy and has newly diagnosed CMV retinitis, a crisis can occur in deciding between zidovudine and ganciclovir. Simply stated, the individual is asked to choose between continuing zidovudine and thus living longer with fewer symptoms of HIV disease but possibly going blind, or selecting ganciclovir in an attempt to prevent blindness but possibly having a shortened life expectancy and more symptoms of HIV disease. Guyer and colleagues (1989) reported regression in CMV retinitis in a 55-year-old person with AIDS who declined ganciclovir therapy in favor of zidovudine. Demands for answers and the need for support will prevail throughout the decision-making process. Should the client select ganciclovir and, despite maintenance therapy, still go blind from disease progression or retinal detachment, regrets and anger will surface along with depression.

Investigators hope that research on combination therapy either with ganciclovir and didioxyinosine or with foscarnet and zidovudine will find a safe way of treating CMV and HIV concomitantly. Irrespective of the agents or combinations, continuous infusion therapy will be necessary, since both ganciclovir and foscarnet require intravenous administration.

Throughout the HIV epidemic, concern has been expressed about the risk that health care workers, especially pregnant women, caring for persons with AIDS will acquire CMV infection. Balfour and Balfour (1986) studied graduates and nursing students caring for clients with a known high rate of CMV infection in renal transplant and hemodialysis services and neonatal intensive care units and found that nurses who practice good personal hygiene are no more likely to acquire CMV than their peers in the community. Balcarek and colleagues (1990) studied employees at a children's hospital and found the incidence of CMV among them similar to the rate expected for the general population. Finally, Gerberding and colleagues (1987) and Gerberding (1989) found no evidence of increased risk for acquiring CMV from occupational exposure to persons with AIDS, even when exposure was for a long period. In fact, Gerberding (1989) pointed out that although the issue of CMV as an occupational hazard has stimulated controversy, occupational CMV transmission has yet to be documented in a health care worker and advises that pregnant health care workers and sexual partners of pregnant women can safely provide care to persons with CMV infection by complying with the universal infection control guidelines.

Related Nursing Care. See the discussion of impaired vision, diarrhea, weight loss, fever, and fatigue in Chapter 4.

PROGRESSIVE MULTIFOCAL LEUKOENCEPHALOPATHY

Astrom and associates first described progressive multifocal leukoencephalopathy (PML) in 1958 when they discovered demyelinative lesions in the brains of two elderly women who had died of progressive cerebral disease late in the course of chronic lymphocytic leukemia (Richardson, 1988). One year later, cases of PML in association with immunodeficiencies were reported from Great Britain and a virus was proposed as the etiologic agent. Although viral particles were identified by electron microscopy in 1965, not until 1971 was the virus recovered (Chaisson & Griffin, 1990). In that year Padgett and Walker at the University of Wisconsin in Madison cultivated and named it J.C. virus, after the initials of the patient whose cultures grew the virus (Richardson, 1988). The J.C. virus causing PML should not be confused with Jacob-Creutzfeldt disease, a totally different disease entity.

The Papovaviridae are a family of viruses that contains two genera, papillomavirus and polyomavirus. Papillomavirus is associated with infection of surface epithelia, producing benign tumors or warts (Dix & Bredesen, 1988; Lehrich, 1990). Polyomaviruses include three types: the J.C. virus, the B.K. virus, and simian virus 40 (SV40). The J.C. virus is associated with PML, and the B.K. virus, also named for the patient from whom it was first isolated, causes hemorrhagic cystitis in immunocompromised individuals (Chaisson & Griffin, 1990). SV40, which causes asymptomatic latent infection in rhesus monkeys, was accidentally introduced into large numbers of people immunized against poliovirus between 1955 and 1961 (Chaisson & Griffin, 1990; Dix & Bredesen, 1988). No evidence that this exposure produced illness has been found, although seroconversion to SV40 was detectable in 20% of vaccine recipients (Chaisson & Griffin, 1990; Dix & Bredesen, 1988). Thus far SV40 has been recovered from the brains of two patients with PML, neither of whom had received the SV40-contaminated polio vaccine or been exposed to monkeys (Dix & Bredesen, 1988).

Epidemiology. The J.C. virus is distributed worldwide. Both the J.C. and B.K. viruses cause childhood infection without a recognized disease syndrome, as evidenced by the fact that 50% of children by 6 years of age demonstrate seroconversion to these viruses (Chaisson & Griffin, 1990). By 9 years of age essentially all people have been infected by the B.K. virus, and by middle adulthood 80% to 90% of the population has become infected with the J.C. virus (Chaisson & Griffin, 1990). Evidence suggests that the appearance of PML in persons with HIV disease is associated with the phenomenon of latency and reactivation of the J.C. virus related to immunosuppression. This is the same phenomenon associated with other opportunistic infections, such as herpesviruses. One major question that remains to be answered is why, if the majority of persons with HIV disease have serologic evidence of previous infection with J.C. virus, PML is so rare in AIDS. By 1990 PML had been diagnosed in only 1% of the adults and adolescents and 1% of the children with AIDS (CDC, 1990a). Lehrich (1990) proposed as an alternative explanation to reactivation of latent infection, that PML occurs as a primary infection in adults who fail to acquire immunity during childhood.

Pathogenesis. The kidney is considered the site of latent J.C. virus infection as evidenced by the presence of the virus in urine; hematogenous spread by lymphocytes to the brain is suspected (Chaisson & Griffin, 1990). The possibility that brain cells are infected with primary infection during childhood also exists.

PML is a subacute demyelinating disease of the central nervous system. Multiple lesions develop in white matter of the cerebrum and sometimes the brainstem or cerebellum, resulting in focal neurologic deficits. The disease progresses rapidly, often leads to dementia, blindness, and paralysis, and in most cases results in death within 1 year (Dix & Bredesen, 1988). Berger and Mucke (1988) reported prolonged survival (more than 30 months) after diagnosis in two individuals with AIDS and PML.

Clinical Presentation. Berger and colleagues (1987) found that initial manifestations of PML included extremity weakness, cognitive dysfunction, visual loss, gait disturbance, limb incoordination, headache, and speech or language disturbance. In addition, they found that the spectrum of neurologic illness most often included spastic hemiparesis, visual field loss, and altered mentation throughout the course of disease.

Symptoms attributable to cerebellar involvement include ataxia, limb dysmetria, and dysarthria. Cortical infection manifestations include aphasia, apraxia, Gerstmann's syndrome, prosopagnosia, left-sided neglect, and impaired spatial orientation. Berger and colleagues (1987) concluded that some of these symptoms may be attributable to coexisting HIV encephalitis, since PML is a disease of white matter.

Diagnosis. The physician is faced with a differential diagnosis including central nervous system toxoplasmosis, primary central nervous system lymphoma, PML, the AIDS-dementia complex, cryptococcal meningitis, and other central nervous system opportunistic infections and neoplasms. Although CT scanning, magnetic resonance imaging, angiography, and electroencephalography may contribute to diagnosis, a definitive diagnosis of PML requires microscopic examination of brain tissue usually obtained via stereotactic biopsy (CDC, 1987a; Dix & Bredesen, 1988).

Treatment. No form of therapy for PML has been efficacious. Attempted therapies have included prednisone, acyclovir, and adenine arabinoside administered both intravenously and intrathecally, cytosine arabinoside, human leukocyte antigen (HLA)-matched platelets, and HLA-matched lymphocytes (Berger et al., 1987; Dix & Bredesen, 1988).

Considerations for Nursing. PML requires intensive nursing care and places demands on the staff. Medicine has little to offer as far as treatment is concerned. Assessment and planning should take into account the psychologic trauma encountered by families, lovers, spouses, and significant others, as well as nursing staff, as they watch an ambulatory, communicative, social human being become bedbound, bowel and bladder incontinent, and devoid of interaction with surroundings. In the end-stages of disease, quadriparesis and coma often appear (Lehrich, 1990). With the support of significant others, many individuals can be safely cared for at home or in a hospice. In some cases the lack of these support systems or the burdens of care make a skilled nursing facility more appropriate for long-term care.

Related Nursing Care. See the discussions of weight loss, impaired vision, impaired mobility, and impaired cognition in Chapter 4.

KAPOSI'S SARCOMA

The noted physician Moriz Kaposi was born on Oct. 23, 1837, in Kaposvar, a regional trade center on the river Kapos in southern Hungary (Safai, 1985). Although his original studies at the University of Vienna led to degrees in medicine, surgery, and obstetrics, he eventually replaced his father-in-law as chairman of the department of dermatology at the university (Safai, 1985).

In 1872 Kaposi published a report titled "Idiopathic Multiple Pigmented Sarcoma of the Skin" (Friedman-Kien et al., 1989; Safai, 1985). Although Kaposi referred to the tumor as sarcoma idiopathicum multiplex hemorragicum, by 1881 it was designated Kaposi's sarcoma (KS) (Safai, 1985). The original disease described by Kaposi is referred to today as classic Kaposi's sarcoma, and many authors consider classic KS to have an indolent course of disease, confined to the lower extremities, and a survival of 10 to 15 years (Krigel & Friedman-Kien, 1988; Volberding, 1990).

Breimer (1984) reviewed the original paper by Kaposi and found remarkable similarities to the KS occurring in HIV-infected individuals today. According to Breimer, the original paper described the disease as incurable and rapidly lethal, with death occurring within 2 to 3 years after symptoms appear. Kaposi regarded the disorder as a generalized disease with the characteristic lesions not only on the lower limbs but also in the pharynx, larynx, trachea, stomach, liver, and both the small and large intestines. Breimer raised an intriguing question: did Moriz Kaposi describe AIDS in 1872 or did he describe KS?

Until 1981 KS was considered a rare and unusual neoplasm. Most cases occurred in North America among primarily elderly men of Mediterranean or Eastern European Jewish (Ashkenazic) descent and in equatorial Africa among young black adult males and prepubescent children. The disease was also found in organ transplant patients receiving immunosuppressive therapy (Friedman-Kien et al., 1989). By 1982 KS was seen in homosexual men in New York City and California and was identified as one of the most common manifestations of the newly identified disorder AIDS (CDC, 1981b, 1982b, 1982c).

Today variations in the epidemiologic patterns, clinical manifestations, and course of KS are classified as four types: (1) classic or non-HIV-related KS; (2) African or endemic KS; (3) KS associated with iatrogenic immunosuppression, sometimes referred to as renal transplant KS; and (4) epidemic or HIV-related KS (Friedman-Kien et al., 1989; Krigel & Friedman-Kien, 1988). The most notable characteristics distinguishing epidemic or HIV-related KS from the other three types are its fulminant, widely disseminated course and shorter survival. The histopathologic features of KS are essentially the same for all four variations (Friedman-Kien et al., 1989). The following discussion is limited to the HIV-related or epidemic form of KS.

Epidemiology. Although KS has been noted to occur in all risk categories of adults and in children, the predominant incidence has been in men who have sex with men. This has led to extensive investigation of possible cofactors that may predispose an HIV-infected individual to KS. Haverkos (1990) stated that sufficient evidence exists to consider nitrite inhalants ("poppers") as a KS cofactor and that individuals who use this as a recreational drug should avoid doing so until sufficient evidence is found to refute this drug-virus interaction hypothesis. Lifson and co-workers (1990), comparing men with AIDS-related KS to men with AIDs without KS, looked specifically at such cofactors as the number of sexual partners, history of certain recreational drugs including nitrite inhalants, or participation in certain specific sexual practices. They found no difference between the groups and could not support these activities as cofactors. Messiah and associates (1989) compared men who had AIDS and KS with men who had AIDS but not KS and found that the men with KS were less likely to have used nitrite inhalants, have engaged in anonymous sex with multiple partners, or have significant health histories of syphilis. Again the findings did not support the hypothesized association between nitrite inhalation and Kaposi's sarcoma. To date the evidence of nitrite inhalants as a cofactor to KS is not clear.

Another area of investigation has been the role of CMV in the development of KS in persons with HIV disease. However, some patients with AIDS and KS show no evidence of current or previous CMV infection, and CMV infection is common in many populations affected by AIDS in whom KS is infrequently seen (Heyer et al., 1990).

An earlier theory of the possibility of genetic factors in the development of KS was evaluated at New York University Medical Center. The presence of the genetic marker HLA-DR5 was studied, but no significant incidence of its presence in persons with AIDS-related KS was found when compared with control groups (Friedman-Kien et al., 1989).

Other supported theories regarding the origins of AIDS-related KS include (1) the immune surveillance theory, that the immune system is unable to detect and prevent a spontaneous neoplasm; (2) the HIV theory, that HIV has a direct oncogenic potential; and (3) the circulating endothelial growth factors theory, that KS is not a true malignancy but a stimulated response to HIV disease, in which lymphatic endothelial cells proliferate (Heyer et al., 1990).

Beral and associates (1990) proposed that KS in people with AIDS is caused by an unidentified sexually transmitted infection. These investigators provided several arguments in favor of this explanation: (1) the risk is greater among individuals who acquire HIV sexually than those who acquire it parenterally; (2) the risk of KS is greater among men who have sex with men, with the highest incidence occurring in California and New York City; (3) women who acquired HIV heterosexually from men who had sex with men had a fourfold higher incidence of KS than women who acquired HIV from other sexual partners; and (4) the incidence of KS is high among adults who acquire HIV heterosexually in Puerto Rico, Haiti, other Caribbean countries, Mexico, Central America, and Africa. The authors noted also that the steep decline in the occurrence of KS in men who have sex with men and are HIV infected might reflect different trends in exposure to the causal agent as a result of changes in sexual behavior that occurred during the first decade of the AIDS epidemic. During the early years of the AIDS epidemic in the United States, KS was reported in more than 30% of patients with AIDS (Safai, 1985). In 1989 AIDS-related KS reported to the CDC occurred in 11% of the adult cases and less than 1% of the pediatric cases (CDC, 1990a).

Friedman-Kien and associates (1990), in reporting six cases of KS in homosexual men without HIV disease, suggested that KS may be caused by another sexually transmitted infectious agent. In addition, Kumar and colleagues (1989) reported a fatal case of KS in a white heterosexual man without any serologic or immunologic evidence of HIV disease.

Pathogenesis. Although some studies suggest a vascular endothelial cell origin of KS, theories about lymphatic endothelial cell origin are consistent with the clinical distribution of KS lesions along cutaneous lymphatic drainage channels, as well as lymphedema frequently seen in persons with AIDS-related KS (Heyer et al., 1990). KS is a multicentric process that can occur in the lymphatic endothelium at any site, including internal organs; however, the first lesions often appear subtly on the face or head or in the oral cavity. In most cases KS progresses rapidly and is detected because of the appearance of new lesions on mucocutaneous surfaces and the viscera (Heyer et al., 1990).

Heyer and associates (1990) at the San Francisco General Hospital made the following observations regarding the prognosis of AIDS-related KS: (1) prognosis is best for individuals with only a few small nodular lesions, especially if they have been present for months before diagnosis; (2) prognosis is better for individuals with no previous opportunistic infection or recent fever, weight loss, or night sweats; (3) persons with lesions involving multiple anatomic regions or with previous opportunistic infections will probably not do well; (4) persons with AIDS and KS diagnosed before 1983 have a longer survival than those whose disease was diagnosed after 1983 (who probably have more severe immunologic impairment and the development of KS at a later stage of HIV disease); and (5) visceral KS implies a poor prognosis.

The development of KS, unlike the development of opportunistic infections seen in AIDS, is not directly linked to immunosuppression. KS can develop in an individual with HIV disease and a relatively normal T4 cell count. Conversely, a relationship exists between degree of immunosuppression and aggressive presentation and survival (Heyer et al., 1990; Mitsuyasu, 1988). The relationship between KS aggression and degree of immunosuppression is seen clearly in non-HIV-infected patients with KS who have iatrogenic immunosuppression because of immunosuppressive medications; once the medications are discontinued, the KS regresses in the majority of cases (Volberding, 1990).

Clinical Presentation. KS is manifested cutaneously as subcutaneous, painless, nonpruritic tumor nodules that are usually pigmented and violaceous (red to blue), nonblanching, and palpable (Heyer et al., 1990). Discrete patch-stage lesions appear early in some individuals and may be mistaken for bruises, purpura, or diffuse cutaneous hemorrhages (Friedman-Kien et al., 1989). The patches can then form into plaques and eventually coalesce and form nodular tumors. New multifocal lesions may appear at any time, and characteristic sites include the tip of the nose, eyelid, hard palate, posterior pharynx, glans penis, thigh, and sole of the foot (Heyer et al., 1990). Although rare, skin breakdown over the tumors can occur and can bleed, necrose, and become painful. Lymphedema can occur in the face, penis, scrotum, and lower extremities. The client is usually aware of its presence and points it out when being examined. The consistency of the fluid collection is usually firm and nonpitting (Heyer et al., 1990).

Gastrointestinal KS is often clinically inapparent, although signs and symptoms of obstruction may be present; in some cases enteropathies from small bowel involvement are noted and very rarely bleeding occurs (Friedman, 1988; Mitsuyasu, 1988). Pulmonary KS may be indistinguishable from pneumonia and may be manifested as fever, as well as cough, dyspnea, and wheezing if the tumors are causing airflow obstruction; hemoptysis has also been reported (Ognibene & Shelhamer, 1988). KS of the central nervous system is rare, and reported symptoms are transient hemiparesis and dizziness (So et al., 1988).

Diagnosis. Although many clinicians state that KS lesions are readily recognized, and the CDC revised definition of AIDS in 1987 included presumptive diagnosis of KS (based on the characteristic gross appearance of any erythematous or violaceous plaquelike lesion on skin or mucous membrane), numerous mucocutaneous lesions that are manifestations of other conditions can be easily confused with epidemic KS (Table 3–2).

The CDC (1987a) cautioned clinicians against making a presumptive diagnosis if they have seen only a few cases of epidemic KS. In addition, a presumptive diagnosis should be made only when laboratory evidence supports the diagnosis of HIV disease. Definitive diagnosis is by tissue biopsy to establish a histologic diagnosis.

TABLE 3–2. Mucocutaneous Lesions and Other Conditions Mimicking Kaposi's Sarcoma

Multiple lesions of purpura and variations thereof	Postinflammatory hyperpigmentation
	Dermatofibroma
Hemangioma	Pyogenic granulomas
Necrotizing vasculitis	Nevi
Angiokeratoma	Malignant melanoma
Venous lake	Basal cell carcinoma
Lesions of secondary syphilis	Pseudolymphoma
Condylomata lata	Cutaneous lymphoma
Pityriasis rosea	Mycosis fungoides
Erythema multiforme	Reticulum cell sarcoma
Granuloma annulare	Adenocarcinoma
Immune reaction to scabies	Eruptive xanthomata
Scabies	Glomus tumor
Urticaria pigmentosa	Leiomyoma
Lichen planus	Keloids
Prurigo nodularis	Sarcoidosis
Granulomatous dermatitis	

Data from Hennessey, N.P., and Friedman-Kien, A.E. (1989). Clinical simulators of the lesions of Kaposi's sarcoma. In A.E. Friedman-Kien (Ed.), *Color atlas of AIDS* (pp. 49-70). Philadelphia: W.B. Saunders.

Recently the Oncology Subcommittee of the AIDS Clinical Trials Group, sponsored by National Institutes of Health, proposed a new staging classification based on tumor bulk, immune function, and the presence of systemic illness (Krown et al., 1989). This system essentially predicts a favorable prognosis for individuals with tumors confined to skin or lymph nodes or with minimal oral disease; T4 cell counts of more than 200 cells/mm^3; no history of thrush, opportunistic infection, or constitutional symptoms; and a Karnofsky performance status score of 70 or better. Poor prognosis is associated with tumor-related edema or ulceration, extensive oral KS, gastrointestinal KS, or KS in other nonnodal viscera; a T4 cell count less than 200 cells/mm^3; history of thrush, opportunistic infections, or neurologic or constitutional disease; and a Karnofsky performance status score of less than 70.

Treatment. Mitsuyasu (1988) pointed out that treatment approaches for a person with KS and AIDS should include careful consideration of the degree of immunocompromise and the relative intolerance to myelosuppressive effects of the many chemotherapeutic agents. No difference in median survival rates has been found between groups of persons with AIDS-related KS treated with chemotherapy or alpha-interferon and those who received no treatment (Volberding et al., 1989).

Kaplan (1990a), noting that treatment is not indicated for all persons with AIDS-related KS, identified subgroups of patients for whom the goals of therapy are palliative and cosmetic. Indications for palliation include painful or uncomfortable intraoral or pharyngeal lesions that interfere with nutrition, respiratory tumors that may cause airway obstruction, lymphedema related to KS, plantar lesions that interfere with ambulation, and containment of rapidly progressive disease.

Treatment plans often include a variety of options for local and systemic therapies. Radiation therapy is commonly used for persons with single or locally symptomatic areas. Intralesional therapy with vinblastine may be used for cosmetic purposes on small cutaneous lesions, and laser therapy and cryotherapy have also been used on small isolated KS lesions (Kaplan, 1990a).

For individuals with rapidly progressive disease or advanced, widespread symptomatic disease, systemic therapy with antineoplastic agents may be appropriate. Single or combination agents used for systemic therapy include vincristine, vinblastine, etoposide, doxorubicin, and bleomycin. Kaplan (1990a) recommended the use of doxorubicin for advanced disease or for persons with previous unsuccessful therapy and the use of vincristine with or without bleomycin for persons with cytopenia. Intravenous chemotherapy with bleomycin and vincristine has been demonstrated to be safe and effective in persons taking zidovudine (Brunt et al., 1989).

Alpha-interferon is used for the treatment of epidemic KS because it possesses both antineoplastic and anti-HIV activity (Groopman & Scadden, 1989; Kaplan, 1990a; Lane et al., 1988). The success of alpha-interferon is related to the state of health of an HIV-infected person. Persons with higher T4 cell counts and no history of opportunistic infection have a greater response to therapy and a better prognosis than individuals with low T4 cell counts (fewer than 200 cells/mm³) (Kaplan, 1990a; Lane et al., 1988). Combination therapy with alpha-interferon and zidovudine has been found to be somewhat dose-limiting but effective therapy for epidemic KS (Kovacs et al., 1989).

Considerations for Nursing. Many clinical issues surrounding the development of epidemic KS may cause confusion, not only among clients and significant others, but also among nurses. First, KS can develop at any time during the course of HIV disease and does not necessarily result from immunosuppression. Therefore KS can develop in an HIV-infected client who is in a relatively good state of health as evidenced by lymphocyte subset studies. Second, clients and staff who have heard of long-term survivors of AIDS (most of whom have epidemic KS) may become complacent, believing the course of the disease to be indolent. All clients with KS must be monitored regularly for clinical progression, immunosuppression, and the development of opportunistic infections. Third, some nurses may think that not seeking active treatment is fatalistic and need assistance in understanding the indicators for therapy. Finally, some nurses, especially in areas with a low incidence of HIV disease, think that KS develops in all clients with AIDS and are not aware of the decreasing incidence of this AIDS-related malignancy.

Clients with external KS lesions usually have alterations in body image, as well as the potential for developing ineffective coping strategies. Every time clients with facial KS lesions look in a mirror, or at the facial expression of someone new, they see a reflection reminding them of their illness. Referrals to support groups, especially groups of persons with AIDS-related KS, can be invaluable in helping clients adjust to the diagnosis and develop positive coping strategies. Learning to cover lesions with makeup (best results are with theatrical makeup) can also contribute immensely to clients' self-esteem and sense of well-being.

Another insufficiently addressed problem is sexual dysfunction related to dermal KS lesions, especially on the abdomen, genitalia, or upper thighs. Clothing that the client and sexual partner find arousing and erotic helps to eliminate some of the related performance problems. Colored condoms may cover penile lesions and allow more normal sexual activities. This is an especially important consideration for clients with KS who are not severely immunocompromised or ill and are sexually active.

Related Nursing Care. See the discussions of dry skin and skin lesions, weight loss, pain, edema, dry and painful mouth, and sexual dysfunction in Chapter 4.

NON-HODGKIN'S LYMPHOMA

The lymphomas are cancers of the immune system. In all forms of lymphatic cancer, lymph tissue cells begin growing abnormally and spread to other organs. According to Kaplan (1990a), the non-Hodgkin's lymphomas (NHLs) are a heterogeneous group of malignancies that range from indolent to fulminant in their disease course. NHLs can originate as a malignancy of T cells, but the vast majority occur as B cell malignancies. NHLs are commonly classified according to pathologic and morphologic characteristics and are divided into three categories: low-grade, intermediate-grade, and high-grade lymphomas.

Reports of NHL in persons with AIDS began to appear in 1982 (Doll & List, 1982; Ziegler et al., 1982). Ziegler and associates (1984) published a report of the first large study indicating a relationship between NHL and AIDS. In June 1985 the CDC revised its case surveillance definition to include NHL in the list of AIDS-indicator diseases (CDC, 1985b).

Epidemiology. According to Doll and Ringenberg (1989), the exact incidence of malignant NHL in individuals with HIV disease is unknown, since the NHL is often diagnosed at postmortem examination. Levine (1987) estimated the incidence of NHL in persons with AIDS to be approximately 4% to 10%. The incidence of NHL in HIV-infected populations is highest in never married males, followed by intravenous drug users, hemophiliacs, transfusion recipients, and heterosexuals (Ahmed et al., 1987; Doll & Ringenberg, 1989; Egerter & Beckstead, 1988; Harnly et al., 1988; Knowles et al., 1988; Kristal et al., 1988; Lowenthal et al., 1988). NHL is also seen in women and children infected with HIV (Doll & Ringenberg, 1989; Knowles et al., 1988).

Pathogenesis. The etiology of NHL in persons with HIV disease remains unknown (Kaplan, 1990a). In the majority of patients with AIDS-related NHL, the malignancies are of B cell origin and are classified as either the intermediate- or the high-grade type. At the time of diagnosis the HIV-infected individual usually has widespread disease involving extranodal sites, most commonly in the gastrointestinal tract, central nervous system, bone marrow, and liver (Kaplan, 1990a). Original attempts to implicate Epstein-Barr virus in the lymphogenesis of NHL in persons with AIDS have not been supported (Kaplan et al., 1989; Subar et al., 1988).

To determine the incidence of NHL in AIDS, Pluda and associates (1990) studied symptomatic persons with HIV disease who had survived for up to 3 years with antiretroviral therapy. They concluded that prolonged survival in the presence of severe T4 cell depletion was associated with a relatively high probability of the development of NHL. The direct oncogenic potential of the antiretroviral therapy could not be discounted.

Clinical Presentation. Most persons with AIDS-related NHL have nonspecific constitutional symptoms such as unexplained fever, night sweats, or weight loss greater than 10% of their total body weight (Doll & Ringenberg, 1989). Many of the individuals with AIDS-related NHL have histories of persistent generalized lymphadenopathy and have follicular hyperplasia detected by lymph node biopsy (Kaplan, 1990a). Sites and symptoms vary with the extranodal site of the disease.

In up to 25% of persons with HIV disease and NHL, the lymphoma is confined to the central nervous system (Formenti et al., 1989; Rosenblum et al., 1988). The most common symptoms are confusion, lethargy, and memory loss. Other symptoms include hemiparesis, aphasia, seizures, cranial nerve palsies, and headache (Kaplan, 1990a).

Another common site of presentation for NHL (up to 25% of the cases) is the gastrointestinal tract (Doll & Ringenberg, 1989). Tumors may arise in the mouth, esophagus, stomach, duodenum, small bowel, mesentery, colon, and rectum, as well as the liver, gallbladder, and pancreas (Friedman, 1988). The clinical signs and symptoms of gastrointestinal NHL associated with AIDS depend on the site of occurrence but are generally associated with pain, obstruction, changes in bowel habits, bleeding, and in some cases fever.

Bone marrow involvement, which occurs in 26% to 46% of the cases, is often associated with meningeal invasion (Doll & Ringenberg, 1989). Although unusual, NHL involving the myocardium and pericardium has been reported and may be manifested as chest pain and dyspnea (Doll & Ringenberg, 1989; Kaplan, 1990a). Other unusual sites of presentation include the subcutaneous and soft tissue, epidural spaces, appendix, gingiva, parotid gland, and paranasal sinuses (Kaplan, 1990b).

Diagnosis. Because of the nonspecific nature of the clinical presentation and the possibility of various other opportunistic diseases and Kaposi's sarcoma, the diagnosis of NHL in a person with HIV disease can be difficult. Kaplan (1990b) recommended that biopsy be performed on HIV-infected individuals with generalized lymphadenopathy who have asymmetric node enlargement or rapidly enlarging bulky nodes. CT scanning and fine needle biopsy may assist in the diagnosis of abdominal and gastrointestinal involvement. Complaints of anorectal symptoms may indicate NHL. Perirectal abscess was an initial complaint of anorectal NHL in persons with AIDS treated at San Francisco General Hospital (Kaplan et al., 1989).

The diagnosis of central nervous system lymphoma is complicated. NHL cannot be differentiated from other central nervous system infections, such as toxoplasmosis, on the basis of CT scan or MRI (Kaplan, 1990b). To avoid brain biopsy, the patient may have to undergo empiric treatment for toxoplasmosis. Definitive diagnosis of NHL is by histologic tissue examination.

Treatment. Response and survival of persons with AIDS-related NHL have been poor, despite variations in intensive chemotherapy. Kaplan (1990b) pointed out that an HIV-infected person with a low total T4 cell count and poor performance status, who had a complicated history of AIDS before NHL developed, is unlikely to benefit from chemotherapy. Such an individual will probably have not only a shortened survival, but also a poorer quality of his or her remaining life because of the toxicity of cytotoxic agents. Patients with T4 cell counts above 100 cells/mm^3, a good performance status, and no other AIDS-indicator diseases may do well with combination chemotherapy (Kaplan, 1990b). Some patients with low-grade NHL have remained asymptomatic without therapy (Doll & Ringenberg, 1989).

Since no standard regimen for treating NHL associated with AIDS has been established, therapy must be individualized. Successful therapy has been associated with a modification of the combination of methotrexate, bleomycin, doxorubicin, cyclophosphamide, vincristine, and dexamethasone (m-BACOD regimen, modified) (Kaplan, 1990a). Survival time with various cytotoxic treatment regimens has been 4 to 7 months (Kaplan, 1990a). Brain irradiation for central nervous system lymphoma may be of benefit.

Considerations for Nursing. Persons with HIV disease and NHL may require the nurse's assistance in making decisions about therapy. Questions regarding risk versus benefit, survival, and adverse effects of chemotherapy and irradiation are common, especially if the client has been learning about HIV disease. A client's demands for concrete statistics and survival data can be frustrating for both the client and the nurse, since a standard treatment approach has not been established.

Related Nursing Care. See the discussions of weight loss, dry skin and skin lesions, fatigue, dry painful mouth, and pain in Chapter 4.

SUMMARY

A current definition of nursing is "the diagnosis and treatment of human responses to actual or potential health problems" (American Nurses' Association, 1980). Therefore nursing a client with a diagnosis of AIDS means the nurse must have full knowledge of the pathologic nature of HIV disease, as well as the common AIDS-related diseases (Ungvarski, 1988). Without this knowledge, identification of the client's biobehavioral responses becomes difficult, limiting the effectiveness of the nurse-client relationship and the nursing process. This chapter has focused on current information about the epidemiology, pathogenesis, clinical presentation, diagnosis, treatment, and considerations for nursing of the opportunistic infections and neoplasms associated with HIV disease. As the complexities of HIV disease and advances in its treatment continue to evolve, the nurse will be challenged to maintain an up-to-date knowledge base. See Appendix I for a summary of drugs commonly in use and their side effects.

References

Aaron, J.S., Wynter, C.D., Kirton, O.C., et al., (1988). Cytomegalovirus associated with acalculous cholecystitis in a patient with acquired immunodeficiency syndrome. *American Journal of Gastroenterology, 83*(8), 879–881.

Abd, A.G., Nierman, D.M., Ilowite, J.S., et al. (1988). Bilateral upper lobe *Pneumocystis carinii* pneumonia in a patient receiving inhaled pentamidine prophylaxis. *Chest, 94*(2), 329–331.

Abrams, J., Farhood, A.I. (1989). Infection associated vascular lesions in acquired immunodeficiency syndrome patients. *Human Pathology, 20*(10), 1025–1026.

Ahmed, T., Wormser, G.P., Stahl, R.E., et al. (1987). Malignant lymphomas in a population at risk for acquired immune deficiency syndrome. *Cancer, 60*(4), 719–723.

Almagro, P., Nava, J., Garau, J., et al. (1988). Herpetic bronchitis and case definition of AIDS [letter]. *Lancet, 2*(8618), 1024.

American Foundation for AIDS Research (1990). Treatment for opportunistic infections and neoplasms. *AIDS/HIV treatment directory, 4*(1), 65–76.

American Nurses' Association (1980). *Nursing: A social policy,* Kansas CIty, MO: The Association.

Ampel, N.M., Wieden, M.A., Galgiani, J.N. (1989). Coccidioidomycosis: Clinical update. *Review of Infectious Diseases, 11*(6), 897–911.

Anaissie, E., Fainstein, V., Samo, T., et al. (1988). Central nervous system histoplasmosis: An unappreciated complication of the acquired immunodeficiency syndrome. *American Journal of Medicine, 84*(2), 215–217.

Anderson, R., Boedicker, M., Ma, M., et al. (1986). Adverse reactions associated with pentamidine isethionate in AIDS. *Drug Intelligence and Clinical Pharmacy, 20*(11), 862–868.

Armstrong, D. (1989). Problems in management of opportunistic fungal diseases. *Review of Infectious Diseases, 11*(suppl 7), S1591–S1599.

Armstrong, M. (1987). Cryptosporidiosis, *Medical Laboratory Sciences, 44*(3), 280–284.

Balcarek, K.B., Bagley, R., Cloud, G., et al. (1990). Cytomegalovirus infection among employees of a children's hospital: No evidence for increased risk associated with patient care. *Journal of the American Medical Association, 263*(6), 840–844.

Balfour, C.L., Balfour, H.H. (1986). Cytomegalovirus is not an occupational risk for nurses in renal transplant and neonatal units: Results of a prospective study. *Journal of the American Medical Association, 256*(14), 1909–1914.

Barbaro, D.J., Orcutt, V.L., Coldiron, B.M. (1989). *Mycobacterium avium-Mycobacterium intracellulare* infection limited to the skin and lymph nodes in patients with AIDS. *Review of Infectious Diseases, 11*(4), 625–628.

Barone, R., Ficarra, G., Gaglioti, D., et al. (1990). Prevalence of oral lesions among HIV infected intravenous drug abusers and other risk groups. *Oral Surgery, Oral Medicine and Oral Pathology, 69*(2), 169–173.

Baskin, M.I., Abd, A.G., Ilowite, J.S. (1990). Regional deposition of aerosolized pentamidine: Effects of body position and breathing pattern. *Annals of Internal Medicine, 113*(9), 677–683.

Becker, M.H., Joseph, J.G., (1988). AIDS and behavioral change to reduce risk: A review. *American Journal of Public Health, 78*(4), 394–410.

Behar, R., Wiley, C., McCutchan, J.A. (1987). Cytomegalovirus polyradiculoneuropathy in acquired immune deficiency syndrome. *Neurology, 37*(4), 557–561.

Benson, M.C., Kaplan, M.S., O'Toole, K., et al. (1988). A report of cytomegalovirus cystitis and a review of other genitourinary manifestations of the acquired immune deficiency syndrome. *Journal of Urology, 140*(1), 153–154.

Beral, V., Peterman, T.A., Berkelman, R.L., et al. (1990). Kaposi's sarcoma among persons with AIDS: A sexually transmitted infection? *Lancet, 335*(8682), 123–128.

Berger, J.R., Kaszovitz, B., Post, M.J., et al. (1987). Progressive multifocal leukoencephalopathy associated with human immunodeficiency virus infection: A review of the literature with a report of sixteen cases. *Annals of Internal Medicine, 107*(1), 78–87.

Berger, J.R., Mucke, L. (1988). Prolonged survival and partial recovery in AIDS associated progressive multifocal leukoencephalopathy, *Neurology, 38*(7), 1060–1065.

Berger, T. (1990). Dermatologic manifestations of AIDS. In P.T. Cohen, M.A. Sande, & P.A. Volberding (Eds.), *The AIDS knowledge base* (pp. 531.1, 531.25). Waltham, MA: Medical Publishing Group.

Bevan, J.S., Doski, M., Grocutt, M., et al. (1989). Bilateral spontaneous pneumothoraces complicating AIDS-related *Pneumocystis carinii* pneumonia. *Respiratory Medicine, 83*(3), 245–246.

Bleweiss, I.J., Pervez, N.K., Hammer, G.S., et al. (1986). Cytomegalovirus induced adrenal insufficiency and associated renal cell carcinoma in AIDS. *Mount Sinai Journal of Medicine, 53*(8), 676–679.

Bloch, A.B., Rieder, H.L., Kelly, G.D., et al. (1989). The epidemiology of tuberculosis in the United States: Implications for diagnosis and treatment. *Clinical Chest Medicine, 10*(3), 297–313.

Bloom, J.N., Palestine, A.G. (1988). The diagnosis of cytomegalovirus retinitis. *Annals of Internal Medicine, 109*(12), 963–969.

Boccellari, A., Dilley, J.W., Shore, M.D. (1988). Neuropsychiatric aspects of AIDS dementia complex: A report on a clinical series. *Neurotoxicology, 9*(3), 381–389.

Borgstein, B.J., Koster, P.A., Portegies, P., et al. (1989). Myelography in patients with acquired immunodeficiency syndrome. *Neuroradiology, 31*(4), 326–330.

Bouchard, P., Sai, P., Reach, G., et al. (1982). Diabetes mellitus following pentamidine induced hypoglycemia in humans. *Diabetes, 31*(1), 40–45.

Bourn'erias, I., Boisnic, S., Patey, O., et al. (1989). Unusual cutaneous cytomegalovirus involvement in patients with acquired immunodeficiency syndrome. *Archives of Dermatology, 125*(9), 1243–1246.

Bozzette, S.A., Sattler, F.R., Chiu, J., et al. (1990). A controlled trial of early adjunctive treatment with corticosteroids for *Pneumocystis carinii* pneumonia in the acquired immunodeficiency syndrome. *New England Journal of Medicine, 323*(21), 1451–1457.

Braun, M.M., Truman, B.I., Marguire, B., et al. (1989). Increasing incidence of tuberculosis in a prison inmate population: Association with HIV infection. *Journal of the American Medical Association, 261*(3), 393–397.

Breimer, L.H. (1984). Did Moriz Kaposi describe AIDS in 1872? *Clio Media, 19*(1–2), 156–158.

Brodman, M., Deligdisch, L. (1986). Cytomegalovirus endometritis in a patient with AIDS. *Mount Sinai Journal of Medicine, 53*(8), 673–675.

Bronnimann, D.A., Adam, R.D., Galgiani, J.N., et al. (1987). Coccidioidomycosis in the acquired immunodeficiency syndrome. *Annals of Internal Medicine, 106*(3), 372–379.

Brown, H.H., Glasgow, B.J., Holland, G.N., et al. (1988). Cytomegalovirus infection of the conjunctiva in AIDS. *American Journal of Ophthalmology, 106*(1), 102–104.

Brown, S., Senekjian, E.K., Montag, A.G. (1988). Cytomegalovirus infection of the uterine cervix in a patient with acquired immunodeficiency syndrome. *Obstetrics and Gynecology, 71*(3, Pt. 2), 489–491.

Brunt, A.M., Goodman, A.G., Phillips, R.H., et al. (1989). The safety of intravenous chemotherapy and zidovudine when treating epidemic Kaposi's sarcoma. *AIDS, 3*(7), 457–460.

Burroughs-Wellcome Company (1990, April). *Product information monograph: Retrovir (zidovudine)*, Research Triangle Park, NC: The Company.

Byrne, W.R., Dietrich, R.A. (1989). Disseminated coccidioidomycosis with peritonitis in a patient with acquired immunodeficiency syndrome: Prolonged survival associated with positive skin test reactivity to coccidioidin. *Archives of Internal Medicine, 149*(4), 947–948.

Cannon, R.O., Hook, E.W., Nahmiss, A.J., et al. (1988). Association of herpes simplex virus type 2 infection in heterosexual patients attending sexually transmitted disease clinic [meeting abstract]. *Proceedings of the Fourth International Conference on AIDS*, Stockholm (Book II) (p. 201). Geneva, Switzerland: World Health Organization.

Cantrill, H.L., Henry, K., Melroe, N.H., et al. (1989). Treatment of cytomegalovirus retinitis with intravitreal ganciclovir: Long-term results. *Ophthalmology, 96*(3), 367–374.

Cello, J.P. (1988). Gastrointestinal manifestations of HIV infection. In M.A. Sande & P.A. Volberding (Eds.), *The medical management of AIDS* (pp. 141–152). Philadelphia: W.B. Saunders.

Cello, J.P., Wilcox, C.M. (1988). Evaluation and treatment of GI tract hemorhage. *Gastroenterology Clinics of North America, 17*(3), 639–648.

Centers for Disease Control (1981a). *Pneumocystis* pneumonia—Los Angeles. *Morbidity and Mortality Weekly Report, 30*(21), 250–252.

Centers for Disease Control (1981b). Kaposi's sarcoma and *Pneumocystis* pneumonia among homosexual men—New York City and California, *Morbidity and Mortality Weekly Report, 30*(25), 305–308.

Centers for Disease Control (1982a). Human cryptosporidiosis—Alabama. *Morbidity and Mortality Weekly Report, 31*(19), 251–254.

Centers for Disease Control (1982b). Update on Kaposi's sarcoma and opportunistic infections in previously healthy persons. *Morbidity and Mortality Weekly Report, 31*(21), 294–301.

Centers for Disease Control (1982c). A cluster of Kaposi's sarcoma and *Pneumocystis carinii* pneumonia among homosexual male residents of Los Angeles and Orange counties, California. *Morbidity and Mortality Weekly Report, 31*(23), 305–307.

Centers for Disease Control (1983). CDC guidelines for isolation precautions in hospitals. In J.S. Garner and B.P. Simmons (Eds.), *Guidelines for prevention and control of nosocomial infections* (pp. 47–78). Atlanta: CDC (U.S. Government Printing Office No. 747-459).

Centers for Disease Control (1984). Update: Treatment of cryptosporidiosis in patients with acquired immunodeficiency syndrome (AIDS). *Morbidity and Mortality Weekly Report, 33*(9), 117–119.

Centers for Disease Control (1985a). Disseminated *Mycobacterium bovis* infection from BCG vaccination of a patient with acquired immunodeficiency syndrome. *Morbidity and Mortality Weekly Report, 34*(16), 227–228.

Centers for Disease Control (1985b). Revision of case definition of acquired immunodeficiency syndrome for national reporting—United States. *Morbidity and Mortality Weekly Report, 34*(25), 373–375.

Centers for Disease Control (1986). Tuberculosis and acquired immunodeficiency syndrome. *Morbidity and Mortality Weekly Report, 35*(37), 587–590.

Centers for Disease Control (1987a). Revision of the CDC surveillance case definition for acquired immunodeficiency syndrome. *Morbidity and Mortality Weekly Report, 36*(1S), 3S–15S.

Centers for Disease Control (1987b). Tuberculosis and acquired immunodeficiency syndrome—New York City. *Morbidity and Mortality Weekly Report, 36*(48), 785–790, 795.

Centers for Disease Control (1988). Tuberculosis, final data—United States, 1986. *Morbidity and Mortality Weekly Report, 36*(50–51), 817–820.

Centers for Disease Control (1989a). Tuberculosis and human immunodeficiency virus infection: Recommendations of the advisory committee for the elimination of tuberculosis (ACET). *Morbidity and Mortality Weekly Report, 38*(14), 236–238, 243–250.

Centers for Disease Control (1989b). Prevention and control of tuberculosis in correctional institutions: Recommendations of the advisory committee for the elimination of tuberculosis. *Morbidity and Mortality Weekly Report, 38*(18), 313–320, 325.

Centers for Disease Control (1989c). *Mycobacterium tuberculosis* transmission in a health clinic—Florida, 1988. *Morbidity and Mortality Weekly Report, 38*(15), 256–258, 263–264.

Centers for Disease Control (1989d). Guidelines for prophylaxis against *Pneumocystis carinii* pneumonia for persons with human immunodeficiency virus. *Morbidity and Mortality Weekly Report, 38*(suppl 5), 1–9.

Centers for Disease Control (1990a, January). *HIV/AIDS Surveillance Report,* Vol. 3.

Centers for Disease Control (1990b). Update: *Salmonella enteritidis* infections and grade A shell eggs—United States, 1989. *Morbidity and Mortality Weekly Report, 38*(51–52), 877–882.

Centers for Disease Control (1990c). Herpes gladiatorum at a high school wrestling camp— Minnesota. *Morbidity and Mortality Weekly Report, 39*(5), 69–71.

Centers for Disease Control (1990d). Outbreak of multidrug resistant tuberculosis—Texas, California and Pennsylvania. *Morbidity and Mortality Weekly Report, 39*(22), 369–372.

Centers for Disease Control (1990e). Screening for tuberculosis and tuberculosis infection in high-risk populations and the use of preventative therapy for tuberculosis infection in the United States. *Morbidity and Mortality Weekly Report, 39*(RR-8), 1–12.

Chaisson, R.E., Griffin, D.E. (1990). Progressive multifocal leukoencephalopathy in AIDS. *Journal of the American Medical Association, 264*(1), 79–82.

Chaisson, R.E., Sande, M.A., Gerberding, J.L. (1990). Salmonella. In P.T. Cohen, M.A. Sande, & P.A. Volberding (Eds.), *The AIDS knowledge base* (pp. 611.1–611.6). Waltham, MA: Medical Publishing Group.

Chaisson, R.E., Schecter, G.F., Theuer, C.P., et al. (1987). Tuberculosis in patients with the acquired immunodeficiency syndrome: Clinical features, response to therapy, and survival. *American Review of Respiratory Diseases, 136*(3), 570–574.

Chaisson, R.E., Volberding, P.A. (1990). Clinical manifestations of HIV infection. In G.L. Mandell, R.G. Douglas, Jr., and J.E. Bennett (Eds.). *Principles and practice of infectious diseases* (3rd ed.) (pp. 1059–1092). New York: Churchill Livingstone.

Chandrasekar, P.H. (1987). "Cure" of chronic cryptosporidiosis during treatment with azidothymidine in a patient with the acquired immunodeficiency syndrome [letter]. *American Journal of Medicine, 83*(1), 187.

Cheng-Mayer, C., Weiss, C., Seto, D., et al., (1989). Isolates of human immunodeficiency virus type 1 from the brain may constitute a special group of the AIDS virus. *Proceedings of the National Academy of Sciences of the United States of America, 86*(21), 8575–8579.

Chernoff, D. (1990). Histoplasmosis. In P.T. Cohen, M.A. Sande, & P.A. Volberding (Eds.). *The AIDS knowledge base*, (pp. 634.1–634.4). Waltham, MA: Medical Publishing Group.

Chernoff, D., Sande, M.A. (1990a). Candidiasis. In P.T. Cohen, M.A. Sande, & P.A. Volberding (Eds.). *The AIDS knowledge base* (pp. 632.1–632.6). Waltham, MA: Medical Publishing Group.

Chernoff, D., Sande, M.A. (1990b). Cryptococcosis. In P.T. Cohen, M.A. Sande, & P.A. Volberding (Eds.). *The AIDS knowledge base* (pp. 633.1–633.8). Waltham, MA: Medical Publishing Group.

Chiodi, F., Valentin, A., Keys, B., et al. (1989). Biological characterization of paired human immunodeficiency virus type 1 isolates from blood and cerebrospinal fluid. *Virology, 173*(1), 178–187.

Chuck, S.L., Sande, M.A. (1989). Infections with *Cryptococcus neoformans* in the acquired immunodeficiency syndrome. *New England Journal of Medicine, 321*(12), 794–799.

Clark, R.A., Greer, D.L., Valainis, G.T., et al. (1990). *Cryptococcus neoformans* pulmonary infection in HIV-1-infected patients. *Journal of Acquired Immune Deficiency Syndromes, 3*(5), 480–484.

Clement, M. (1989). Patient care queries: Why does ketoconazole lose its effectiveness against *Candida? AIDS Clinical Care, 1*(8), 74.

Clement, M. (1990a). Patient care queries: What is the recommended therapy for *Mycobacterium avium* complex (MAC) infection? *AIDS Clinical Care, 2*(2), 14.

Clement, M. (1990b). Fluconazole: A promising new antifungal. *AIDS Clinical Care, 2*(6), 53–54.

Cohen, J.I., Saragas, S.J. (1990). Endophthalmitis due to *Mycobacterium avium intracellulare* in a patient with AIDS. *Annals of Ophthalmology, 22*(2), 47–51.

Cohn, J.A., McMeeking, A., Cohen, W., et al. (1989). Evaluation of the policy of empiric treatment of suspected *Toxoplasma* encephalitis in patients with the acquired immunodeficiency syndrome. *American Journal of Medicine, 86*(5), 521–527.

Collier, A.C., Meyers, J.D., Corey, L., et al. (1987). Cytomegalovirus infection in homosexual men: Relationship to sexual practices, antibody to human immunodeficiency virus, and cell-mediated immunity. *American Journal of Medicine, 82*(3), 593–601.

Conces, D.J., Jr., Kraft, J.L., Vix, V.A., et al. (1989). Apical *Pneumocystis carinii* pneumonia after inhaled pentamidine prophylaxis. *American Journal of Roentgenology, 152*(6), 1193–1194.

Concus, A.P., Helfand, R.F., Imber, M.J., et al. (1988). Cutaneous cryptococcosis mimicking molluscum contagiosum in a patient with AIDS [letter]. *Journal of Infectious Diseases, 158*(4), 897–898.

Connolly, G.M., Dryden, M.S., Shansin, D.C., et al. (1988). Cryptosporidial diarrhea in AIDS and its treatment. *Gut, 29*(5), 593–597.

Connolly, G.M., Shanson, D., Hawkins, D.A., et al. (1989). Non-cryptosporidial diarrhea in human immunodeficiency virus (HIV) infected patients. *Gut, 30*(2), 195–200.

Conover, B., Goldsmith, J.C., Buehler, B.A., et al. (1988). Aerosolized pentamidine and pregnancy [letter]. *Annals of Internal Medicine, 109*(11), 927.

Conte, J.E., Jr., Hollander, H., Golden, J.A. (1987). Inhaled or reduced dose intravenous pentamidine for *Pneumocystis carinii* pneumonia: A pilot study. *Annals of Internal Medicine, 107*(4), 495–498.

Corey, L., Spear, P.G. (1986). Infection with herpes simplex viruses. *New England Journal of Medicine, 314*(11), 686–691.

Corkery, K.J., Luce, J.M., Montgomery, A.B. (1988). Aerosolized pentamidine for treatment and prophylaxis of *Pneumocystis carinii* pneumonia: An update. *Respiratory Care, 33*(8), 676–685.

Cote, R.J., Rosenblum, M., Telzak, E.E., et al. (1990). Disseminated *Pneumocystis carinii* infection causing extra-pulmonary organ failure: Clinical, pathologic and immunohistochemical analysis. *Modern Pathology, 3*(1), 25–30.

Cotton, D.I. (1989). Improving survival in acquired immunodeficiency syndrome: Is experience everything? [editorial]. *Journal of the American Medical Association, 261*(20), 3016–3017.

Coulman, C.U., Greene, I., Archibald, R.W. (1987). Cutaneous pneumocystosis. *Annals of Internal Medicine, 106*(3), 396–398.

Crider, S.R., Horstman, W.G., Massey, G.S. (1988). *Toxoplasma* orchitis: Report of a case and a review of the literature. *American Journal of Medicine, 85*(3), 421–424.

Crocker, K.S. (1989). Gastrointestinal manifestations of the acquired immunodeficiency syndrome. *Nursing Clinics of North America, 24*(2), 395–406.

Cuzzell, J.Z. (1990). Clues: Itching and burning skin folds. *American Journal of Nursing, 90*(1), 23–24.

Daicker, B. (1988). Cytomegalovirus panuveitis with infection of corneotrabecular endothelium in AIDS. *Ophthalmologica, 197*(4), 169–175.

Dalakas, M., Wichman, A., Sever, J. (1989). AIDS and the nervous system. *Journal of the American Medical Association, 261*(16), 2396–2399.

Dannemann, B.R., Israelski, D.M., Remington, J.S. (1988). Treatment of toxoplasmic encephalitis with intravenous clindamycin. *Archives of Internal Medicine, 148*(11), 2477–2482.

Davis, C.E., (1986). Cryptococcus. In A.I. Braude (Ed.), *Infectious diseases and medical microbiology* (2nd ed.) (pp. 564–571). Philadelphia: W.B. Saunders.

DeHovitz, J.A., Pape, J.W., Boncy, M., et al. (1985). Clinical manifestations and therapy of *Isospora belli* infection in patients with the acquired immunodeficiency syndrome. *New England Journal of Medicine, 315*(2), 87–90.

DeRiso, A.J., Kemeny, M.M., Torres, R.A., et al. (1989). Multiple jejunal perforations secondary to cytomegalovirus in a patient with acquired immune deficiency syndrome: Case report and review. *Digestive Diseases and Sciences, 34*(4), 623–629.

Derouin, F., Sarfati, C., Beauvals, B., et al. (1989). Laboratory diagnosis of pulmonary toxoplasmosis in patients with AIDS. *Journal of Clinical Microbiology, 27*(7), 1661–1663.

D'Esopo, N.D. (1982). Clinical trials in pulmonary tuberculosis. *American Review of Respiratory Disease, 125*(3, Pt. 2), 85–93.

DesPrez, R.M., Heim, C.R. (1990). *Mycobacterium tuberculosis*. In G.L. Mandell, R.G. Douglas, Jr., & J.E. Bennett (Eds.), *Principles and practice of infectious diseases* (3rd ed.) (pp. 1877–1906). New York: Churchill Livingstone.

Diamond, R.D., (1990). *Cryptococcus neoformans*. In G.L. Mandell, R.G. Douglas, Jr., and J.E. Bennett (Eds.). *Principles and practice of infectious diseases*, (3rd ed.) (pp. 1980–1989). New York: Churchill Livingstone.

DiPerri, G., Cruciani, M., Danzi, M.C., et al. (1990). Nosocomial epidemic of active tuberculosis among HIV infected patients. *Lancet, 2*(8678–8679), 1502–1504.

Dismukes, W.E. (1988). Cryptococcal meningitis in patients with AIDS. *Journal of Infectious Disease, 157*(4), 624–628.

Dix, R.D., Bredesen, D.E. (1988). Opportunistic viral infections in acquired immunodeficiency syndrome. In M.L. Rosenblum, R.M. Levy, & D.E. Bredesen (Eds.), *AIDS and the nervous system* (pp. 221–261). New York: Raven Press.

Doll, D.C., List, A.F. (1982). Burkitt's lymphoma in a homosexual [letter]. *Lancet, 1*(8279), 1026–1027.

Doll, D.C., Ringenberg, O.S. (1989). Lymphomas associated with HIV infection. *Seminars in Oncology Nursing, 5*(4), 255–262.

Dressler, R., Peters, A.T., Lynn, R.I. (1989). Pseudomonal and candidal peritonitis as a complication of continuous ambulatory peritoneal dialysis in human immunodeficiency virus–infected patients. *American Journal of Medicine, 86*(6, Pt. 2), 787–790.

Drew, W.L., Erlich, K.S. (1990a). Cytomegalovirus epidemiology. In P.T. Cohen, M.A. Sande, & P.A. Volberding (Eds.), *The AIDS knowledge base* (pp. 643.1–643.4). Waltham, MA: Medical Publishing Group.

Drew, W.L., Erlich, K.S. (1990b). Cytomegalovirus as a cofactor in AIDS. In P.T. Cohen, M.A. Sande & P.A. Volberding (Eds.), *The AIDS knowledge base* (pp. 644.1–644.2). Waltham, MA: Medical Publishing Group.

Drew, W.L., Erlich, K.S. (1990c). Cytomegalovirus: Diagnosis. In P.T. Cohen, M.A. Sande, & P.A. Volberding (Eds.). *The AIDS knowledge base* (pp. 647.1–647.2). Waltham, MA: Medical Publishing Group.

Drew, W.L., Jacobson, M.A., Erlich, K.S. (1990). Cytomegalovirus: Clinical presentations. In P.T. Cohen, M.A. Sande, & P.A. Volberding (Eds.). *The AIDS knowledge base* (pp. 646.1–646.3). Waltham, MA: Medical Publishing Group.

Drew, W.L., Mills, J., Hauer, L.B., et al. (1988). Declining prevalence of Kaposi's sarcoma in homosexual AIDS patients paralleled by fall in cytomegalovirus transmission [letter]. *Lancet, 1*(8575–8576), 66.

duMoulin, G.C., Stotlmeier, K.D., Pelletier, P.A., et al. (1988). Concentration of *Mycobacterium avium* by hospital hot water systems. *Journal of the American Medical Association, 260*(11), 1599–1601.

Dunagan, W.C. (1990). Mycobacterial infection and HIV disease. *Modern Medicine, 87*(2), 79–81.

Edwards, J.E. (1990). *Candida* species. In G.L. Mandell, R.G. Douglas, Jr., & J.E. Bennett (Eds.), *Principles and practice of infectious diseases* (3rd ed.) (pp. 1943–1958). New York: Churchill Livingstone.

Efferen, L.S., Nadarajah, D., Palat, D.S. (1989). Survival following mechanical ventilation for *Pneumocystis carinii* pneumonia in patients with the acquired immunodeficiency syndrome: A different perspective. *American Journal of Medicine, 87*(4), 401–404.

Egerter, D.A., Beckstead, J.H. (1988). Malignant lymphomas in the acquired immunodeficiency syndrome: Additional evidence for a B-cell origin. *Archives of Pathology and Laboratory Medicine, 112*(6), 602–606.

Ehni, W.F., Ellison, R.T. (1987). Spontaneous *Candida albicans* meningitis in a patient with the acquired immune deficiency syndrome [letter]. *American Journal of Medicine, 83*(4), 806–807.

Engel, J.P., Englund, J.A., Fletcher, C.V., et al. (1990). Treatment of resistant herpes simplex virus with continuous infusion acyclovir. *Journal of the American Medical Association, 263*(12), 1662–1664.

Erice, A., Chou, S., Biron, K.K., et al. (1989). Progressive disease due to ganciclovir-resistant cytomegalovirus in immunocompromised patients. *New England Journal of Medicine, 320*(5), 289–293.

Erlich, K.S., Jacobson, M.A., Koehler, J.E., et al. (1989a). Foscarnet therapy for severe acyclovir-resistant herpes simplex virus type-2 infections in patients with the acquired immunodeficiency syndrome (AIDS). *Annals of Internal Medicine, 110*(9), 710–713.

Erlich, K.S., Mills, J. (1990). Herpes simplex virus. In P.T. Cohen, M.A. Sande, & P.A. Volberding (Eds.), *The AIDS knowledge base* (pp. 642.1–642.16). Waltham, MA: Medical Publishing Group.

Erlich, K.S., Mills, J., Chatis, P., et al. (1989b). Acyclovir-resistant herpes simplex virus infections in patients with acquired immunodeficiency syndrome. *New England Journal of Medicine, 320*(5), 293–296.

Etinger, N.A. (1990). *Pneumocystis carinii* pneumonia: Advances in diagnosis and therapy. *Missouri Medicine, 87*(1), 19–22.

Fanning, M.M., Read, S.E., Benson, M., et al. (1990). Foscarnet therapy of cytomegalovirus retinitis in AIDS. *Journal of Acquired Immune Deficiency Syndromes, 3*(5), 472–479.

Farr, B.M., Mandell, G.L. (1990). Rifamycins. In G.L. Mandell, R.G. Douglas, Jr., & J.E. Bennett (Eds.), *Principles and practice of infectious diseases* (3rd ed.) (pp. 295–303). New York: Churchill Livingstone.

Federation of American Societies for Experimental Biology (1990). Nutritional therapy and nutrition education in the care and management of AIDS patients (tentative report). Washington, DC: Center for Food Safety and Applied Nutrition, Food and Drug Administration, Department of Health and Human Services.

Fels, A.O. (1988). Bacterial and fungal pneumonias. *Clinics in Chest Medicine, 9*(3), 449–457.

Fernandez, F., Adams, F., Levy, J.K., et al. (1988). Cognitive impairment due to AIDS-related complex and its response to psychostimulants. *Psychosomatics, 29*(1), 38–46.

Ferreiro, J., Vinters, H.V. (1988). Pathology of the pituitary gland in patients with the acquired immunodeficiency syndrome (AIDS). *Pathology, 20*(3), 211–215.

Fertel, D., Pitchenik, A.E. (1989). Tuberculosis in acquired immunodeficiency syndrome. *Seminars in Respiratory Infections, 4*(3), 198–205.

Fitzgibbon, M.L., Cella, D.F., Humfleet, G., et al. (1989). Motor slowing in asymptomatic HIV infection. *Perceptual and Motor Skills, 68*(3, Pt. 2), 1331–1338.

Formenti, S.C., Gill, P.S., Lean, E., et al. (1989). Primary central nervous system lymphoma in AIDS: Results of radiation therapy. *Cancer, 15*(63), 1101–1107.

Francis, N.D., Boylston, A.W., Roberts, A.H., et al. (1989). Cytomegalovirus infection in gastrointestinal tracts of patients infected with HIV-1 or AIDS. *Journal of Clinical Pathology, 42*(10), 1055–1064.

Frank, T.S., LiVolsi, V.A., Conner, A.M. (1987). Cytomegalovirus infection of the thyroid in immunocompromised adults. *Yale Journal of Biology and Medicine, 60*(1), 1–8.

Freedberg, R.S., Gindea, A.J., Dieterich, D.T., et al. (1987). Herpes simplex pericarditis in AIDS. *New York State Journal of Medicine, 87*(5), 304–306.

Freeman, W.E., O'Quinn, J.L., Lesher, J.L., Jr. (1989). Fever and hyperpigmented papules in an intravenous drug user: Disseminated histoplasmosis in acquired immunodeficiency syndrome (AIDS). *Archives of Dermatology, 125*(5), 689, 692–693.

Friedman, S.L. (1988). Gastrointestinal and hepatobiliary neoplasms in AIDS. *Gastroenterology Clinics of North America, 17*(3), 465–486.

Friedman, S.L. (1990). Weight loss. In P.T. Cohen, M.A. Sande, & P.A. Volberding (Eds.), *The AIDS knowledge base* (5103.1–5103.4). Waltham, MA: Medical Publishing Group.

Friedman-Kien, A.E., Ostreicher, R., Saltzman, B. (1989). Clinical manifestations of classical, endemic African, and epidemic AIDS-associated Kaposi's sarcoma. In A.E. Friedman-Kien (Ed.), *Color atlas of AIDS* (pp. 11–48). Philadelphia: W.B. Saunders.

Friedman-Kien, A.E., Saltzman, B.R., Cos, Y.Z., et al. (1990). Kaposi's sarcoma in HIV-negative homosexual men [letter]. *Lancet, 335*(8682), 168–169.

Fuller, G.N., Guiloff, R.J., Scaravilli, F., et al. (1989a). Combined HIV-CMV encephalitis presenting with brainstem signs. *Journal of Neurology, Neurosurgery and Psychiatry, 52*(8), 975–979.

Fuller, G.N., Jacobs, J.M., Guiloff, R.J. (1989b). Association of painful peripheral neuropathy in AIDS with cytomegalovirus infection. *Lancet, 2*(8669), 937–941.

Gabuzda, D.H., Hirsch, M.S. (1987). Neurologic manifestations of infection with human immunodeficiency virus: Clinical features and pathogenesis. *Annals of Internal Medicine, 107*(3), 383–391.

Gagnon, S., Boota, A.M., Fischl, M.A., et al. (1990). Corticosteroids as adjunctive therapy for severe *Pneumocystis carinii* pneumonia in the acquired immunodeficiency syndrome—double-blind, placebo-controlled trial. *New England Journal of Medicine, 323*(21), 1444–1450.

Gallaher, M.M., Herndon, J.L., Nims, L.J., et al. (1989). Cryptosporidiosis and surface water. *American Journal of Public Health, 79*(1), 39–42.

Gallant, J.E., Enriquez, R.E., Cohen, K.L., et al. (1988). *Pneumocystis carinii* thyroiditis. *American Journal of Medicine, 84*(2), 303–306.

Gapen, P. (1982). Medical news: Neurological complications now characterizing many AIDS victims. *Journal of the American Medical Association, 248*(22), 2941–2942.

Gartner, S., Markovits, P., Markovitz, P., et al. (1986). Virus isolation from and identification of HTLV III/LAV producing cells in brain tissue from a patient with AIDS. *Journal of the American Medical Association, 256*(17), 2365–2371.

Gerberding, J.L. (1989). Risks to health care workers from occupational exposure to hepatitis B virus, human immunodeficiency virus, and cytomegalovirus, *Infectious Disease Clinics of North America, 3*(4), 735–745.

Gerberding, J.L., Bryant-LeBlanc, C.E., Nelson, K., et al. (1987). Risk of transmitting the human immunodeficiency virus, cytomegalovirus, and hepatitis B virus to health care workers exosed to patients with AIDS and AIDS-related conditions. *Journal of Infectious Diseases, 156*(1), 1–8.

Girard, P.M., Landman, R., Gaudebout, C., et al. (1989). Prevention of *Pneumocystis carinii* pneumonia relapse by pentamidine aerosol in zidovudine-treated AIDS patients. *Lancet, 1*(8651), 1348–1353.

Glass, R.M. (1988). AIDS and suicide [editorial]. *Journal of the American Medical Association, 259*(9), 1369–1370.

Glaser, J.B., Morton-Kute, L., Berger, S.R., et al. (1985). Recurrent *Salmonella typhimurium* bacteremia associated with the acquired immunodeficiency syndrome. *Annals of Internal Medicine, 102*(2), 189–193.

Glatt, A.E., Chirgwin, K. (1990). *Pneumocystis carinii* pneumonia in human immunodeficiency virus—infected patients. *Archives of Internal Medicine, 150*(2), 271–279.

Glatt, A.E., Chirgwin, K., Landesman, S.H. (1988). Treatment of infections with human immunodeficiency virus. *New England Journal of Medicine, 318*(22), 1439–1448.

Glick, M., Cohen, S.G., Cheney, R.T., et al. (1987). Oral manifestations of disseminated *Cryptococcus neoformans* in a patient with acquired immunodeficiency syndrome. *Oral Surgery, Oral Medicine, Oral Pathology, 64*(4), 454–459.

Glickel, A.Z., (1988). Hand infections in patients with acquired immunodeficiency syndrome. *Journal of Hand Surgery, 13*(5), 770–775.

Godfrey-Faussett, P., Miller, R.F., Semple, S.J. (1988). Nebulized pentamidine [letter]. *Lancet,1*(8586), 645–646.

Golden, J.A., Chernoff, D., Hollander, H., et al. (1989). Prevention of *Pneumocystis carinii* pneumonia by inhaled pentamidine. *Lancet, 1*(8639), 654–657.

Gould, E., Kory, W.P., Raskin, J.B., et al. (1988). Esophageal biopsy findings in the acquired immunodeficiency syndrome (AIDS): Clinicopathologic correlation in 20 patients. *Southern Medical Journal, 81*(11), 1392–1395.

Grant, I.H., Armstrong, D. (1988). Fungal infections in AIDS: Cryptococcosis. *Infectious Disease Clinics of North America, 2*(2), 457–464.

Gray, J.R., Rabeneck, L. (1989). Atypical mycobacterial infection of the gastrointestinal tract in AIDS patients. *American Journal of Gastroenterology, 84*(12), 1521–1524.

Gray, R.H. (1983). Similarities between AIDS and PCM [letter]. *American Journal of Public Health, 73*(10), 1332.

Greenberg, R.G., Berger, T.G. (1989). Progressive disseminated histoplasmosis in acquired immunodeficiency syndrome: Presentation as a steroid-responsive dermatosis. *Cutis, 43*(6), 535–538.

Greenberg, R.E., Mir, R., Bank, S., et al. (1989). Resolution of intestinal cryptosporidiosis after treatment of AIDS with AZT. *Gastroenterology, 97*(5), 1327–1330.

Greene, J.B. (1988). Clinical approach to weight loss in the patient with HIV infection. *Gastroenterology Clinics of North America, 17*(3), 573–586.

Greenspan, J.S., Greenspan, D., Winkler, J.R. (1988). Diagnosis and management of the oral manifestations of HIV infection and AIDS. *Infectious Disease Clinics of North America, 2*(2), 373–385.

Gregg, R.W., Friedman, B.C., Williams, J.F., et al. (1990). Continuous positive airway pressure by face mask in *Pneumocystis carinii* pneumonia. *Critical Care Medicine, 18*(1), 21–24.

Groopman, J.E., Scadden, D.T. (1989). Interferon therapy for Kaposi's sarcoma associated with the acquired immunodeficiency syndrome (AIDS). *Annals of Internal Medicine,* *110*(5), 335–337.

Guyer, D.R., Jabs, D.A., Brant, A.M., et al. (1989). Regression of cytomegalovirus retinitis with zidovudine. A clinicopathologic correlation. *Archives of Ophthalmology, 107*(6), 868–874.

Hagopian, W.A., Huseby, J.S. (1989). *Pneumocystis* hepatitis and choroiditis despite successful aerosolized pentamidine pulmonary prophylaxis. *Chest, 96*(4), 949–951.

Hamoudi, A.C., Qualman, S.J., Marcon, M.J., et al. (1988). Do regional variations in prevalence of cryptosporidiosis occur? The central Ohio experience. *American Journal of Public Health, 78*(3), 273–275.

Hanson, C.A., Reichman, L.B. (1989). Tuberculosis skin testing and preventative therapy. *Seminars in Respiratory Infection, 4*(3), 182–188.

Harnly, M.E., Swan, S.H., Holly, E.A., et al. (1988). Temporal trends in the incidence of non-Hodgkin's lymphoma and selected malignancies in a population with a high incidence of acquired immunodeficiency syndrome (AIDS). *American Journal of Epidemiology, 128*(2), 261–267.

Haskell, L., Fusco, M.J., Ares, L., et al. (1989). Disseminated toxoplasmosis presenting as symptomatic orchitis and nephrotic syndrome. *American Journal of the Medical Sciences, 298*(3), 185–190.

Haverkos, H.W. (1987). Assessment of therapy for *Toxoplasma* encephalitis: The TE study group. *American Journal of Medicine, 82*(5), 907–914.

Haverkos, H.W. (1990). The search for cofactors in AIDS, including an analysis of the association of nitrate inhalant abuse and Kaposi's sarcoma. *Progress in Clinical and Biological Research, 325,* 93–102.

Hayes, E.B., Matte, T.D., O'Brien, T.R., et al. (1989). Large community outbreak of cryptosporidiosis due to contamination of a filtered public water supply. *New England Journal of Medicine, 320*(21), 1372–1376.

Heinemann, M.H. (1989). Long-term intravitreal ganciclovir therapy for cytomegalovirus retinopathy. *Archives of Ophthalmology, 107*(12), 1767–1772.

Henderson, D.K., (1990). Nosocomial herpes virus infections. In G.L. Mandell, R.G. Douglas, Jr., & J.E. Bennett (Eds.), *Principles and practice of infectious diseases* (3rd ed.) (pp. 2236–2245). New York: Churchill Livingstone.

Hernandez, A.D. (1989). Cutaneous cryptococcosis. *Dermatology Clinics, 7*(2), 269–274.

Henry, K., Cantrill, H., Fletcher, C., et al. (1987). Use of intravitreal ganciclovir (dihydroxy propoxymethylguanine) for cytomegalovirus retinitis in a patient with AIDS. *American Journal of Ophthalmology, 103*(1), 17–23.

Henry, K., Thurn, J. (1990). The evolving challenge of *Pneumocystis carinii:* A deadly opportunist in AIDS. *Postgraduate Medicine, 87*(2), 45–50, 53, 56.

Herskovitz, S., Siegel, S.E., Schneider, A.T., et al. (1989). Spinal cord toxoplasmosis in AIDS. *Neurology, 39*(11), 1552–1553.

Heyer, D.M., Kahn, J.O., Volberding, P.A. (1990). HIV-related Kaposi's sarcoma. In P.T. Cohen, M.A. Sande, & P.A. Volberding (Eds.), *The AIDS knowledge base* (pp. 713.1–713.19). Waltham, MA: Medical Publishing Group.

Heyman, M.R., Rasmussen, P. (1987). *Pneumocystis carinii* involvement of the bone marrow in acquired immunodeficiency syndrome. *American Journal of Clinical Pathology, 87*(6), 780–783.

Hilton, C.W., Harrington, P.T., Prasad, C., et al. (1988). Adrenal insufficiency in the acquired immunodeficiency syndrome. *Southern Medical Journal, 81*(12), 1493–1495.

Hirsch, M.S., (1990). Herpes simplex virus. In G.L. Mandell, R.G. Douglas, Jr., & J.E. Bennett (Eds.), *Principles and practice of infectious diseases* (3rd ed.) (pp. 1144–1153). New York: Churchill Livingstone.

Hirschmann, J.V., Chu, A.C. (1988). Skin lesions with disseminated toxoplasmosis in a patient with the acquired immunodeficiency syndrome [letter]. *Archives of Dermatology, 124*(9), 1446–1447.

Ho, D.D., Bredesen, D.E., Vinters, H.V., et al. (1989). The acquired immunodeficiency syndrome (AIDS) dementia complex (clinical conference). *Annals of Internal Medicine, 111*(5), 400–410.

Ho, D.D., Rota, T.R., Schooley, R.T., et al. (1985). Isolation of HTLV-III from cerebrospinal fluid with neural tissues of patients with neurologic syndromes related to the acquired immunodeficiency syndrome. *New England Journal of Medicine, 313*(24), 1493–1497.

Ho, M. (1990). Cytomegalovirus. In G.L. Mandell, R.G. Douglas, Jr., & J.E. Bennett (Eds.), *Principles and practice of infectious disease* (3rd ed.) (pp. 1159–1172). New York: Churchill Livingstone.

Holland, G.N., Buhles, W.C., Jr., Mastre, B., et al., (1989). A controlled retrospective study of ganciclovir treatment for cytomegalovirus retinopathy: Use of a standardized system of disease outcome; UCLA CMV Retinopathy Study Group. *Archives of Ophthalmology, 107*(12), 1759–1766.

Holliman, R.E., (1988). Toxoplasmosis and the acquired immune deficiency syndrome. *Journal of Infection, 16*(2), 121–128.

Holmberg, S.D., Stewart, J.A., Gerber, A.R., et al. (1988). Prior herpes virus type 2 infection as a risk factor for HIV infection. *Journal of the American Medical Association, 259*(7), 1048–1050.

Hommes, M., Romijin, J.A., Godfried, M.H., et al. (1989). Increased resting energy expenditure in HIV-infected men [abstract]. In *Proceedings of the Fifth International Conference on AIDS*, Montreal (p. 218). Geneva, Switzerland: World Health Organization.

Hook, E.W. (1990). *Salmonella* species (including typhoid fever). In G.L. Mandell, R.G. Douglas, Jr., & J.E. Bennett (Eds.), *Principles and practice of infectious diseases* (3rd ed.) (pp. 1700–1716). New York: Churchill Livingstone.

Hopewell, P.C. (1989). Prevention of lung infection associated with human immunodeficiency virus infection. *Thorax, 44*(12) 1038–1044.

Hopewell, P.C. (1990). *Pneumocystis carinii* pneumonia. In M.A. Sande & P.A. Volberding (Eds.), *The medical management of AIDS* (2nd ed.) (pp. 209–240). Philadelphia: W.B. Saunders.

Houin, H.P., Gruenberg, J.C., Fisher, E.J., et al. (1987). Multiple small bowel perforations secondary to cytomegalovirus in a patient with acquired immunodeficiency syndrome. *Henry Ford Hospital Medical Journal, 35*(1), 17–19.

Hoy, J., Mijch, A., Sandland, M., et al. (1990). Quadruple drug therapy for *Mycobacterium avium-intracellulare* bacteremia in AIDS patients. *Journal of Infectious Diseases, 161*(4), 801–805.

Huber, M.A., Hall, E.H., Rathbun, W.A. (1989). The role of the dentist in diagnosing infection in the AIDS patient. *Military Medicine, 154*(6), 315–318.

Hughes, W.T. (1982). Natural mode of acquisition for de novo infection with *Pneumocystis carinii*. *The Journal of Infectious Diseases, 145*(6), 842–848.

Ibanez, H.E., Ibanez, M.A. (1989). A new presentation of disseminated histoplasmosis in a homosexual man with AIDS. *American Journal of Medical Science, 298*(6), 407–409.

Iseman, M.D. (1987). Is standard chemotherapy adequate in tuberculosis patients infected with the HIV? [editorial]. *American Review of Respiratory Disease, 436*(6), 1326.

Israel, H.L., Gottlieb, J.E., Schulman, E.S. (1987). Hypoxemia with normal chest roentgenogram due to *Pneumocystis carinii* pneumonia: Diagnostic errors due to low suspicion of AIDS. *Chest, 92*(5), 857–859.

Israelski, D.M., Dannemann, B.R., Remington, J.S. (1990). Toxoplasmosis in patients with AIDS. In M.A. Sande & P.A. Volberding (eds.), *The medical management of AIDS* (2nd ed.) (pp. 241–264). Philadelphia: W.B. Saunders.

Israelski, D.M., Remington, J.S. (1988). Toxoplasmosis encephalitis in patients with AIDS. In M.A. Sande & P.A. Volberding (Eds.), *The medical management of AIDS* (pp. 193–211). Philadelphia: W.B. Saunders.

Israelski, D.M., Skowron, G., Leventhal, J.P., et al. (1988). Toxoplasmosis peritonitis in a patient with acquired immunodeficiency syndrome. *Archives of Internal Medicine, 148*(7), 1655–1657.

Jabs, D.A., Enger, C., Bartlett, J.G. (1989). Cytomegalovirus retinitis and acquired immunodeficiency syndrome. *Archives of Ophthalmology, 107*(1), 75–80.

Jacobs, J.L., Gold, J.W., Murray, H.W., et al. (1985). *Salmonella* infections in patients with the acquired immunodeficiency syndrome. *Annals of Internal Medicine, 102*(2), 186–188.

Jacobson, E. (1990). New hospital hazards: How to protect yourself. *American Journal of Nursing. 90*(2), 36–41.

Jacobson, M.A. (1988). Mycobacterial diseases: Tuberculosis and *Mycobacterium avium* complex. In M.A. Sande & P.A. Volberding (Eds.), *The medical management of AIDS.* Philadelphia: W.B. Saunders.

Jacobson, M.A., Cello, J.P., Sande, M.A. (1988). Cholestasis and disseminated cytomegalovirus disease in patients with the acquired immunodeficiency syndrome. *American Journal of Medicine, 84*(2), 218–224.

Jacobson, M.A., Mills, J. (1988). Serious cytomegalovirus disease in the acquired immunodeficiency syndrome (AIDS): Clinical findings, diagnosis, and treatment. *Annals of Internal Medicine, 108*(4), 585–594.

Jacobson, M.A., Mills, J., Rush, J., et al. (1988). Failure of antiviral therapy for acquired immunodeficiency syndrome–related cytomegalovirus myelitis. *Archives of Neurology, 45*(10), 1090–1092.

Jacobson, M.A., O'Donnell, J.J. (1991). Approaches to treatment of cytomegalovirus retinitis: ganciclovir and foscarnet. *Journal of Acquired Immune Deficiency Syndromes, 4*(suppl 1), S11–S15.

Jacobson, M.A., O'Donnell, J.J., Mills, J. (1989). Foscarnet treatment of cytomegalovirus retinitis in patients with the acquired immunodeficiency syndrome. *Antimicrobial Agents and Chemotherapy, 33*(5), 736–741.

Janoff, E.N., Smith, P.D. (1988). Perspectives on gastrointestinal infections in AIDS. *Gastroenterology Clinics of North America, 17*(3), 451–463.

Janssen, R.S., Saykin, A.J., Cannon, L., et al. (1989). Neurological and neuropsychological manifestations of HIV-1 infection: Association with AIDS-related complex but not asymptomatic HIV-1 infection. *Annals of Neurology, 26*(5), 592–600.

Joe, L., Ansher, A.F., Gordin, F.M. (1989). Severe pancreatitis in an AIDS patients in association with cytomegalovirus infection. *Southern Medical Journal, 82*(11), 1444–1445.

Johnson, P.C., Hamill, R.J., Sarosi, G.A. (1989). Clinical review: Progressive disseminated histoplasmosis in the AIDS patient. *Seminars in Respiratory Infections, 4*(2), 139–146.

Johnson, P.C., Sarosi, G.A., Septimus, E.J., et al., (1986). Progressive disseminated histoplasmosis in patients with the acquired immune deficiency syndrome: A report of 12 cases and a literature review. *Seminars in Respiratory Infections, 1*(1), 1–8.

Jokipii, L., Jokipii, A.M.M. (1986). Timing of symptoms and oocyst excretion in human cryptosporidiosis. *New England Journal of Medicine, 315*(26), 1643–1647.

Jokipii, L., Pohjola, S., Jokipii, A.M.M. (1983). *Cryptosporidium:* A frequent finding in patients with gastrointestinal symptoms. *Lancet, 2*(8346), 358–361.

Jones, C., Orengo, I., Rosen, T., et al. (1990). Cutaneous cryptococcosis simulating Kaposi's sarcoma in the acquired immunodeficiency syndrome. *Cutis, 45*(3), 163–167.

Kales, C.P., Murren, J.R., Torres, R.A., et al. (1987). Early predictors of in-hospital mortality for *Pneumocystis carinii* pneumonia in the acquired immunodeficiency syndrome. *Archives of Internal Medicine, 147*(8), 1413–1417.

Källenius, G., Hoffner, S.E., Svenson, S.B. (1989). Does vaccination with bacille Calmette-Guerin protect against AIDS? *Review of Infectious Diseases, 11*(2), 349–351.

Kanas, R.J., Jensen, J.L., Abrams, A.M., et al. (1987). Oral mucosal cytomegalovirus as a manifestation of the acquired immune deficiency syndrome. *Oral Surgery, Oral Medicine, Oral Pathology, 64*(2), 183–189.

Kaplan, L.D. (1990a). The malignancies associated with AIDS. In M.A. Sande & P.A. Volberding (Eds.). *The medical management of AIDS* (2nd ed.) (pp. 339–364). Philadelphia: W.B. Saunders.

Kaplan, L.D. (1990b). HIV-associated non-Hodgkin's lymphoma. In P.T. Cohen, M.A. Sande, & P.A. Volberding (Eds.). *The AIDS knowledge base* (pp. 721.1–721.7). Waltham, MA: Medical Publishing Group.

Kaplan, L.D., Abrahms, D.I., Feigal, E., et al. (1989). AIDS-associated non-Hodgkin's lymphoma in San Francisco. *Journal of the American Medical Association, 261*(5), 719–724.

Katz, A.S., Niesenbaum, L., Mass, B. (1989). Pleural effusion as the initial manifestation of disseminated cryptococcosis in acquired immune deficiency syndrome: Diagnosis by pleural biopsy. *Chest, 96*(2), 440–441.

Kavesh, N.G., Holzman, R.S., Seidlin, M. (1989). The combined toxicity of azidothymidine and antimycobacterial agents: A retrospective study. *American Review of Respiratory Disease. 139*(50), 1094–1097.

Kida, M., Abramowsky, C.R., Santoscoy, C. (1989). Cryptococcosis of the placenta in a woman with acquired immunodeficiency syndrome. *Human Pathology, 20*(9), 920–921.

King, A.B. (1990). Malnutrition in HIV infection: Prevalence, etiology and management. *PAAC Notes, 2*(3), 122–129.

Kingsley, L.A., Armstrong, J., Rahman, A., et al. (1990). No association between herpes simplex virus type-2 seropositivity or anogenital lesions and HIV seroconversion among homosexual men. *Journal of Acquired Immune Deficiency Syndromes, 3*(8), 773–779.

Knowles, D.M., Chamulak, G.A., Subar, M., et al. (1988). Lymphoid neoplasia associated with the acquired immunodeficiency syndrome (AIDS): The New York University Medical Center experience with 105 patients (1981-1986). *Annals of Internal Medicine, 108*(5), 744–753.

Koralnik, I.J., Beaumanoir, A., Hausler, R. et al. (1990). A controlled study of early neurologic abnormalities in men with asymptomatic human immunodeficiency virus infection. *New England Journal of Medicine, 323*(13), 864–870.

Kotler, D. (1989). Clinical gastrointestinal (G.I.) diseases in AIDS [abstract]. In *Proceedings of the Fifth International Conference on AIDS*, Montreal (p. 208). Geneva, Switzerland: World Health Organization.

Kotler, D.P., Tierney, A.R., Altilio, D., et al. (1989). Body mass repletion during ganciclovir treatment of cytomegalovirus infections in patients with acquired immunodeficiency syndrome. *Archives of Internal Medicine, 149*(4), 901–905.

Kotler, D.P., Tierney, A.R., Brenner, S.K., et al. (1990). Presentation of short term energy balance in clinically stable patients with AIDS. *American Journal of Clinical Nutrition, 51*(1), 7–13.

Kotler, D.P., Tierney, A.R., Wang, J., et al. (1989). Magnitude of body-cell-mass depletion and the timing of death from wasting in AIDS. *American Journal of Clinical Nutrition, 50*(3), 444–447.

Kovacs, J.A., Deyton, L., Davey, R., et al. (1989). Combined zidovudine and interferon-alpha therapy in patients with Kaposi's sarcoma and the acquired immunodeficiency syndrome (AIDS). *Annals of Internal Medicine, 111*(4), 280–287.

Krigel, R., Friedman-Kien, A.E., (1988). Kaposi's sarcoma in AIDS: Diagnosis and treatment. In V.T. DeVita, Jr., S. Hellman, & S.A. Rosenberg (Eds.), *AIDS: Etiology, diagnosis, treatment and prevention* (pp. 245–261). Philadelphia: J.B. Lippincott.

Kristal, A.R., Nasca, P.C., Burnett, W.S., et al. (1988). Changes in the epidemiology of non-Hodgkin's lymphoma associated with epidemic human immunodeficiency virus (HIV) infection. *American Journal of Epidemiology, 128*(4), 711–718.

Krown, S.E., Metroka, C., Wernz, J.C. (1989). Kaposi's sarcoma in the acquired immunodeficiency syndrome: A proposal for uniform evaluation, response, and staging criteria. *Journal of Clinical Oncology, 7*(9), 1201–1207.

Kumar, S., Schade, R.R., Peel, R., et al. (1989). Kaposi's sarcoma with visceral involvement in a young heterosexual male without evidence of the acquired immune deficiency syndrome. *American Journal of Gastroenterology, 84*(3), 318–321.

Kurtin, P.J., McKinsey, D.S., Gupta, M.R., et al. (1990). Histoplasmosis in patients with acquired immunodeficiency syndrome: Hematologic and bone marrow manifestations. *American Journal of Clinical Pathology, 93*(3), 367–372.

Lafont, A., Wolff, M., Marche, C., et al. (1987). Overwhelming myocarditis due to *Cryptococcus neoformans* in an AIDS patient [letter]. *Lancet, 2*(8568), 1145–1146.

Lane, H.C., Kovacs, J.A., Feinberg, J., et al. (1988). Antiretroviral effects of interferon-alpha in AIDS-associated Kaposi's sarcoma. *Lancet, 2*(8622), 1218–1222.

Larsen, R.A., Bozzette, S., McCutchan, J.A., et al. (1989). Persistent *Cryptococcus neoformans* infection of the prostrate after successful treatment of meningitis: California Collaborative Treatment Group. *Annals of Internal Medicine, 111*(2), 125–128.

Laskin, O.L., Stahl-Bayliss, C.M., Morgello, S. (1987). Concomitant herpes simplex virus type 1 and cytomegalovirus ventriculoencephalitis in acquired immunodeficiency syndrome. *Archives of Neurology, 44*(8), 843–847.

Lee, J.Y., Peel, R. (1989). Concurrent cytomegalovirus and herpes simplex virus infections in skin biopsy specimens from two AIDS patients with fatal CMV infection. *American Journal of Dermatopathology*, 11(2), 136–143.

Lehrich, J.R. (1990). JC, BK, and other polyomaviruses (progressive multifocal leukoencephalopathy). In G.L. Mandell, R.G. Douglas, Jr., & J.E. Bennett (Eds.), *Principles and practice of infectious diseases* (3rd ed.) (pp. 1200–1203). New York: Churchill Livingstone.

Leoung, G.S., Feigal, D.W., Montgomery, A.B., et al. (1990). Aerosolized pentamidine for prophylaxis against *Pneumocystis carinii* pneumonia. *New England Journal of Medicine*, 323(12), 769–775.

Levine, A.M. (1987). Non-Hodgkin's lymphoma and other malignancies in the acquired immune deficiency syndrome. *Seminars in Oncology*, 14(2 suppl 3), 34–39.

Levine, S.J., White, D.A. (1988). *Pneumocystis carinii*. *Clinics in Chest Medicine*, 9(3), 395–423.

Levy, R.M., Bredesen, D.E. (1988). Central nervous system dysfunction in acquired immunodeficiency syndrome. In M.L. Rosenblum, R.M. Levy, & D.E. Bredesen (Eds.), *AIDS and the central nervous system* (pp. 29–63). New York: Raven Press.

Levy, R.M., Bredesen, D.E. (1989). Controversies in HIV-related central nervous system disease: Neuropsychological aspects of HIV-1 infection. In P.A. Volberding & M.A. Jacobson (Eds.) *AIDS clinical review 1989* (pp. 151–191). New York: Marcel Dekker.

Levy, R.M., Bredesen, D.E., Rosenblum, M.L. (1985). Neurological manifestations of the acquired immunodeficiency syndrome (AIDS): Experience at UCSF and a review of the literature. *Journal of Neurosurgery*, 62(4), 475–495.

Levy, R.M., Bredesen, D.E., Rosenblum, M.L. (1990). Neurologic complications of HIV infection. *American Family Physician*, 41(2), 517–536.

Levy, R.M., Bredesen, D.E., Rosenblum, M.L., Davis, R.L. (1988). Central nervous system disorders in AIDS. *Public Health Reports*, 103(3), 246–254.

Lifson, A.R., Darrow, W.W., Hessol, N.A., et al. (1990). Kaposi's sarcoma in a cohort of homosexual and bisexual men: Epidemiology and analysis for cofactors. *American Journal of Epidemiology*, 131(2), 221–231.

Lindley, D.A., Schleupner, C.J. (1988). Aerosolized pentamidine and conjunctivitis [letter]. *Annals of Internal Medicine*, 109(12), 988.

Lipson, B.K., Freeman, W.R., Beniz, J., et al. (1989). Optic neuropathy associated with cryptococcal arachnoiditis in AIDS patients. *American Journal of Ophthalmology*, 107(5), 523–527.

Lortholary, O., Deny, P., Boudes, P., et al. (1990). Bilateral adrenal hypertrophy in an AIDS patient with multivisceral human cytomegalovirus infection [letter]. *Journal of Infectious Diseases*, 161(3), 585–586.

Lowenthal, D.A., Straus, D.J., Campbell, S.W., et al. (1988). AIDS-related lymphoid neoplasia: The Memorial Hospital experience. *Cancer*, 61(11), 2325–2327.

Loyd, J.E., DesPrez, R.M., Goodwin, R.A., Jr. (1990). *Histoplasma capsulatum*. In G.L. Mandell, R.G. Douglas, Jr., J.E. Bennett (Eds.), *Principles and practice of infectious diseases* (3rd ed.) (pp. 1989–1998). New York: Churchill Livingstone.

Lubat, E., Megibow, A.J., Balthazar, E.J., et al. (1990). Extrapulmonary *Pneumocystis carinii* infection in AIDS: CT findings. *Radiology*, 174(1), 157–160.

Lucas, S.B., Parr, D.C., Wright, E., et al. (1989). AIDS presenting as cytomegalovirus cystitis. *British Journal of Urology*, 64(4), 429–430.

Lynch, D.P., Naftolin, L.Z. (1987). Oral *Cryptococcus neoformans* infection in AIDS. *Oral Surgery, Oral Medicine, Oral Pathology*, 64(4), 449–453.

Lynch, D.P., Naftolin, L.Z. (1990). Oral *Cryptococcus* in AIDS patients [letter]. *Journal of Oral and Maxillofacial Surgery*, 48(3), 329.

Lyphomed (1989). NebuPent (pentamidine isethionate): Product monograph. Rosemont, IL: Lyphomed.

Ma, P., Villanueva, T.G., Kaufman, D., et al. (1984). Respiratory cryptosporidiosis in acquired immune deficiency syndrome. *Journal of the American Medical Association*, 252(10), 1298–1301.

MacDonell, K.B., Glassroth, J. (1989). *Mycobacterium avium* complex and other nontuberculosis mycobacteria in patients with HIV infection. *Seminars in Respiratory Infections*, 4(2), 123–132.

Macher, A.M., Bardenstein, D.S., Zimmerman, L.E., et al. (1987). *Pneumocystis carinii* choroiditis in a male homosexual with AIDS and disseminated pulmonary and extrapulmonary *P. carinii* infection [letter]. *New England Journal of Medicine, 316*(17), 1092.

MacPhail, L.A., Greenspan, D., Schiodt, M., et al. (1989). Acyclovir-resistant, forcarnet-sensitive oral herpes simplex type 2 lesion in a patient with AIDS. *Oral Surgery, Oral Medicine, Oral Pathology, 67*(4), 427–432.

Mahieux, F., Gray, F., Fenelson, G., et al. (1989). Acute myeloradiculitis due to cytomegalovirus as the initial manifestation of AIDS. *Journal of Neurology, Neurosurgery and Psychiatry, 52*(2), 270–274.

Marks, G.L., Nolan, P.E., Erlich, K.S., et al. (1989). Mucocutaneous dissemination of acyclovir-resistant herpes simplex virus in a patient with AIDS. *Review of Infectious Diseases, 11*(3), 474–476.

Martin, J.L. (1987). The impact of AIDS on gay male sexual behavior patterns in New York City. *American Journal of Public Health, 77*(5), 578–581.

Martinez, C.M., Romanelli, A., Mullen, M.P., et al. (1988). Spontaneous pneumothoraces in AIDS patients receiving aerosolized pentamidine [letter]. *Chest, 94*(6), 1317–1318.

Masdeu, J.C., Small, C.B., Weiss, L., et al. (1988). Multifocal cytomegalovirus encephalitis in AIDS. *Annals of Neurology, 23*(1), 97–99.

Masur, H., Lane, H.C., Kovacs, J.A., et al. (1989). *Pneumocystis* pneumonia: From bench to clinic. *Annals of Internal Medicine, 111*(10), 813–826.

Masur, H., Pass, H.I., Travis, W.D. (1990). Thin-walled cavities, cysts, and pneumothorax in *Pneumocystis carinii* pneumonia: Further observations with histopathologic correlation. *Radiology, 174*(3), 697–702.

McArthur, J.C., Cohen, B.A., Selnes, O.A., et al. (1989). Low prevalence of neurological and neuropsychological abnormalities in otherwise healthy HIV-1 infected individuals: Results from the multicenter AIDS cohort study. *Annals of Neurology, 26*(5), 601–611.

McCabe, R.E., Remington, J.S. (1988). Toxoplasmosis: The time has come. *New England Journal of Medicine, 318*(5), 313–315.

McCabe, R.E., Remington, J.S. (1990). *Toxoplasma gondii.* In G.L. Mandell, R.G. Douglas, Jr., & J.E. Bennett (Eds.), *Principles and practice of infectious diseases* (pp. 2090–2103). New York: Churchill Livingstone.

Medlock, M.D., Tilleli, J.T., Pearl, G.S. (1990). Congenital cardiac toxoplasmosis in a newborn with acquired immunodeficiency syndrome. *Pediatric Infectious Diseases, 9*(2), 129–132.

Mehle, M.E., Adamo, J.P., Mehta, A.C., et al. (1989). Endobronchial *Mycobacterium avium-intracellulare* infection in a patient with AIDS. *Chest, 96*(1), 199–201.

Mendelson, M.H., Finkel, L.J., Meyers, B.R., et al. (1987). Pulmonary toxoplasmosis in AIDS. *Scandinavian Journal of Infectious Diseases, 19*(6), 703–706.

Merenich, J.A., McDermott, M.T., Asp, A.A., et al. (1990). Evidence of endocrine involvement early in the course of human immunodeficiency virus infection. *Journal of Clinical Endocrinology and Metabolism, 70*(3), 566–571.

Messiah, A., Rozenbaum, W., Vittecoq, D., et al. (1989). Possible correlation between exposure to AIDS risk factors, clinical presentation in AIDS, and subsequent prognosis. *European Journal of Epidemiology, 5*(3), 336–342.

Meyohas, M.C., Roullet, E., Rouzioux, C., et al. (1989). Cerebral venous thrombosis and dual primary infection with human immunodeficiency virus and cytomegalovirus. *Journal of Neurology, Neurosurgery, and Psychiatry, 52*(8), 1010–1011.

Miller, J.H. (1986). The protozoa. In A.I. Braude (Ed.), *Infectious diseases and medical microbiology* (2nd ed.) (pp. 610–625). Philadelphia: W.B. Saunders.

Miller, J.S. (1988). Cutaneous *Cryptococcus* resembling molluscum contagiosum in a patient with acquired immunodeficiency syndrome. *Cutis, 41*(6), 411–412.

Miller, R.F., Millar, A.B., Weller, I.V., et al. (1989). Empirical treatment without bronchoscopy for *Pneumocystis carinii* pneumonia in the acquired immunodeficiency syndrome. *Thorax, 44*(7), 559–564.

Minamoto, G., Armstrong, D. (1988). Fungal infections in AIDS: Histoplasmosis and coccidioidomycosis. In M.A. Sande & P.A. Volberding (Eds.), *The medical management of AIDS* (pp. 213–223). Philadelphia: W.B. Saunders.

Mitsuyasu, R.T. (1988). Kaposi's sarcoma in the acquired immunodeficiency syndrome. *Infectious Disease Clinics of North America, 2*(2), 511–523.

Modilevsky, T., Sattler, F.R., Barnes, P.F. (1989). Mycobacterial diseases in patients with human immunodeficiency virus infection. *Archives of Internal Medicine, 149*(10), 2201–2205.

Montaner, J.S., Russell, J.A., Lawson, L., et al. (1989). Acute respiratory failure secondary to *Pneumocystis carinii* pneumonia in the acquired immunodeficiency syndrome: A potential role for systemic corticosteroids. *Chest, 95*(4), 881–884.

Montgomery, A.B., Corkery, K.J., Brunette, E.R., et al. (1990). Occupational exposure to aerosolized pentamidine. *Chest, 98*(2), 386–388.

Montgomery, A.B., Luce, J.M., Turner, J., et al. (1987). Aerosolized pentamidine as sole therapy for *Pneumocystis carinii* pneumonia in patients with acquired immunodeficiency syndrome. *Lancet, 2*(8557), 480–483.

Moskovitz, B.L., Stanton, T.L., Kusmierek, J.J. (1988). Spiramycin therapy for cryptosporidial diarrhea in immunocompromised patients. *Journal of Antimicrobial Chemotherapy, 22*(suppl B), 189–191.

Murray, J.F., Felton, C.P., Garay, S.M., et al. (1984). Special report: Pulmonary complications of the acquired immunodeficiency syndrome. *New England Journal of Medicine, 310*(25), 1682–1688.

Murray, R.J., Becker, P., Furth, P., et al. (1988). Recovery from cryptococcemia and the adult respiratory distress syndrome in the acquired immunodeficiency syndrome. *Chest, 93*(6), 1304–1306.

Nadelman, R.B., Mathur-Wagh, U., Yancovitz, S.R., et al. (1985). *Salmonella* bacteremia associated with the acquired immunodeficiency syndrome (AIDS). *Archives of Internal Medicine, 145*(11), 1968–1971.

Nahmias, A.J., Muther, J., Lee, G. (1988). Herpes simplex virus type-2 (HSV-2)—a marker of behavioral and biological risk for the acquisition of HIV infection [meeting abstract]. In *Proceedings of the Fourth International Conference on AIDS* (Book II) (p. 198). Geneva, Switzerland: World Health Organization.

Nardell, E.A. (1989). Tuberculosis in homeless, residential care facilities, prisons, nursing homes, and other close communities. *Seminars in Respiratory Infections, 4*(3), 206–215.

National Institute of Allergy and Infectious Diseases (1990, May). HIV associated opportunistic infections: NIAID-supported clinical research. *OI Backgrounder*. Bethesda, MD: The Institute.

Newman, T.G., Soni, A., Acaron, S., et al. (1987). Pleural cryptococcosis in the acquired immune deficiency syndrome. *Chest, 91*(3), 459–461.

New York City Department of Health (1983). Cryptosporidiosis. *City Health Information, 2*(13), 1–3.

New York Statewide Professional Standards Review Council Inc. (1990). *Criteria manual for the treatment of AIDS* (2nd ed.). New York: New York State Department of Health.

Nistal, M., Regadera, J., Paniagua, R., Rodriguez, M.C. (1990). Nuclear bodies (sphaeridia) in Sertoli cells of a man with acquired immunodeficiency syndrome (AIDS) and testicular infection by cytomegalovirus. *Ultrastructural Pathology, 14*(1), 21–26.

Norris, S.A., Kessler, H.A., Fife, K.H. (1988). Severe progressive herpetic whitlow caused by an acyclovir-resistant virus in a patient with AIDS [letter]. *Journal of Infectious Diseases, 157*(1), 209–210.

O'Brien, J.J., Campoli-Richards, D.M. (1989). Acyclovir—an updated review of its antiviral activity, pharmacokinetic properties and therapeutic efficacy. *Drugs, 37*(3), 233–209.

O'Brien, R.J. (1989). The epidemiology of nontuberculosis mycobacterial disease. *Clinical Chest Medicine, 10*(3), 407–418.

Ognibene, F.P., Shelhamer, J.H. (1988). Kaposi's sarcoma. *Clinics in Chest Medicine, 9*(3), 459–465.

Ong, E.L., Ellis, M.E., Tweedle, D.E., et al. (1989). Cytomegalovirus cholecystitis and colitis associated with the acquired immunodeficiency syndrome. *Journal of Infections, 18*(1), 73–75.

Pagano, J.S., Lemon, S.M. (1986). The herpesviruses. In A.I. Braude (Ed.), *Infectious diseases and medical microbiology* (2nd ed.) (pp. 470–481). Philadelphia: W.B. Saunders.

Pape, J.W., Verdier, R.I., Johnson, W.D., Jr. (1989). Treatment and prophylaxis of *Isospora belli* infection in patients with the acquired immunodeficiency syndrome. *New England Journal of Medicine, 320*(16), 1044–1047.

Pape, J.W., Verdier, R.I., Johnson, W.D., Jr. (1990). *Isospora belli* and the acquired immunodeficiency syndrome [letter]. *New England Journal of Medicine, 322*(2), 131–132.

Peterson, P., Stahl-Bayliss, C.M. (1987). Cytomegalovirus thrombophlebitis after successful DHPG therapy [letter]. *Annals of Internal Medicine, 106*(4), 632–633.

Pilla, A.M., Rybak, M.J., Chandrasekar, P.M. (1987). Spiramycin in the treatment of cryptosporidiosis. *Pharmacotherapy, 7*(5), 188–190.

Pilon, V.A. (1990). Dissemination of *Pneumocystis. New York State Journal of Medicine, 90*(3), 121–122.

Pluda, J.M., Yarchoan, R., Jaffee, E.S., et al. (1990). Development of non-Hodgkin's lymphoma in a cohort of patients with severe human immunodeficiency virus (HIV) infection on long-term antiretroviral therapy. *Annals of Internal Medicine, 113*(4), 276–282.

Pomeroy, C., Englund, J.A. (1987). Cytomegalovirus: Epidemiology and infection control. *American Journal of Infection Control, 15*(3), 107–119.

Portegies, P., de Gans, J., Lange, J.M., et al. (1989). Declining incidence of AIDS dementia complex after introduction of zidovudine treatment. *British Medical Journal, 299*(6703), 819–821.

Price, R.W., Brew, B., Sidtis, J., et al. (1988). The brain in AIDS: Central nervous system HIV-1 infection and the AIDS dementia complex. *Science, 239*(4840), 586–592.

Price, R.W., Sidtis, J.J., Navia, B.A., et al. (1989). The AIDS dementia complex. In M.L. Rosenblum, R.M. Levy, & D.E. Bredesen (Eds.), *AIDS and the nervous system* (pp. 203–219). New York: Raven Press.

Price, R.W., Sidtis, J., Rosenblum, M. (1988). The AIDS dementia complex: Some current questions. *Annals of Neurology, 23*(suppl), S27–S33.

Quinn, T.C., Mann, J.M., Curran, J.W., et al. (1986). AIDS in Africa: An epidemiologic paradigm. *Science, 234*(4779), 955–963.

Rabinowitz, M., Bassan, I., Robinson, M.J. (1988). Sexually transmitted cytomegalovirus proctitis in a woman. *American Journal of Gastroenterology, 83*(8), 885–887.

Raufman, J.P. (1988). Odynophagia/dysphagia in AIDS. *Gastroenterology Clinics of North America, 17*(3), 599–614.

Ravalli, S., Garcia, R.L., Vincent, R.A., et al. (1990). Disseminated *Pneumocystis carinii* infection in the acquired immunodeficiency syndrome. *New York State Journal of Medicine, 90*(3), 155–157.

Reif, J.S., Wimmer, L., Smith, J.A., et al. (1989). Human cryptosporidiosis associated with an epizootic in calves. *American Journal of Public Health, 79*(11), 1528–1530.

Rein, M.F. (1990). Vulvovaginitis and cervicitis. In G.L. Mandell, R.G. Douglas, Jr., & J.E. Bennett (Eds.), *Principles and practice of infectious diseases* (3rd ed.) (pp. 953–964). New York: Churchill Livingstone.

Reinis-Lucey, C., Sande, M.A., Gerberding, J.L. (1990). Toxoplasmosis. In P.T. Cohen, M.A. Sande, & P.A. Volberding (Eds.), *The AIDS knowledge base* (pp. 656.1–656.15). Waltham, MA: Medical Publishing Group.

Remington, J.S., McLeod, R. (1986). Toxoplasmosis. In A.I. Braude (Ed.), *Infectious diseases and medical microbiology* (2nd ed.) (pp. 1521–1535). Philadelphia: W.B. Saunders.

Resnick, L., di Marzo-Veronese, F., Schupback, J., et al. (1985). Intra-blood-brain-barrier synthesis of HTLV-III specific IgG in patients with neurologic symptoms associated with AIDS or AIDS-related complex. *New England Journal of Medicine, 313*(24), 1498–1504.

Restrepo, C., Macher, A.M., Radany, E.H. (1987). Disseminated extra-intestinal isosporiasis in a patient with acquired immunodeficiency syndrome. *American Journal of Clinical Pathology, 87*(4), 536–542.

Rhoads, J.L., Wright, D.C., Redfield, R.R., et al. (1987). Chronic vaginal candidiasis in women with human immunodeficiency virus infection. *Journal of the American Medical Association, 257*(22), 3105–3107.

Richardson, E.P. (1988). Progressive multifocal leukoencephalopathy: 30 years later [editorial]. *New England Journal of Medicine, 318*(5), 315–317.

Rieder, H.L., Cauthen, G.M., Kelly, G.D., et al. (1989). Tuberculosis in the United States. *Journal of the American Medical Association, 262*(3), 385–389.

Riley, K.B., Antoniskis, D., Maris, R., et al. (1988). Rattlesnake capsule–associated *Salmonella arizona* infections. *Archives of Internal Medicine, 148*(5), 1207–1210.

Rolston, K.V. (1990). Cryptosporidiosis in patients with the acquired immunodeficiency syndrome. *AIDS Medical Report, 3*(2), 13–22.

Rolston, K.V., Fainstein, V., Bodey, G.P. (1989). Intestinal cryptosporidiosis treated with eflornithine: A prospective study among patients with AIDS. *Journal of Acquired Immune Deficiency Syndromes, 2*(5), 426–430.

Rooney, J.F., Felser, J.M., Ostrove, J.M., et al. (1986). Acquisition of genital herpes from an asymptomatic sexual partner. *New England Journal of Medicine, 314*(24), 1561–1564.

Rosenblum, M.L., Levy, R.M., Bredesen, D.E., et al. (1988). Primary central nervous system lymphomas in patients with AIDS. *Annals of Neurology, 23*(suppl), S13–S16.

Rossi, J.F., Eledjam, J.J., Delage, A., et al. (1990). *Pneumocystis carinii* infection of bone marrow in patients with malignant lymphoma and acquired immunodeficiency syndrome. *Archives of Internal Medicine, 150*(2), 450–452.

Ryan, C.A., Nickels, M.K., Hargrett-Bean, N.T., et al. (1987). Massive outbreak of antimicrobial-resistant salmonellosis traced to pasteurized milk. *Journal of the American Medical Association, 258*(22), 3269–3274.

Safai, B. (1985). Kaposi's sarcoma and other neoplasms in acquired immunodeficiency syndrome. In J.I. Gallin & A.S. Fauci (Eds.), *Advances in host mechanisms: Acquired immunodeficiency syndrome (AIDS)* (Vol. 5) (pp. 59–73). New York: Raven Press.

Saldana, M.J., Mones, J.M. (1989). Cavitation and other atypical manifestations of *Pneumocystis carinii* pneumonia. *Seminars in Diagnostic Pathology, 6*(3), 273–286.

Sall, R.K., Kauffman, C.L., Levy, C.S. (1989). Successful treatment of progressive acyclovir-resistant herpes simplex virus using intravenous foscarnet in a patient with the acquired immunodeficiency syndrome. *Archives of Dermatology, 125*(11), 1548–1550.

Salzman, S.H., Smith R.L., Aranda, C.P. (1988). Histoplasmosis in patients at risk for the acquired immunodeficiency syndrome in a nonendemic setting. *Chest, 93*(5), 916–921.

Sanders, W.E., Horowitz, E.A. (1990). Other *Mycobacterium* species. In G.L. Mandell, R.G. Douglas, Jr., & J.E. Bennett (Eds.), *Principles and practice of infectious diseases* (3rd ed.) (pp. 1914–1926). New York: Churchill Livingstone.

Sarti, G.M. (1989). Aerosolized pentamidine in HIV: Promising new treatment for *Pneumocystis carinii* pneumonia. *Postgraduate Medicine, 86*(2), 54–56, 59–60, 63.

Sattler, F.R., Cowan, R., Nielsen, D.M., et al. (1988). Trimethoprim-sulfamethoxazole compared with pentamidine for treatment of *Pneumocystis carinii* pneumonia in the acquired immunodeficiency syndrome: A prospective, noncrossover study. *Annals of Internal Medicine, 109*(4), 280–287.

Scalfano, F.P., Jr., Prichard, J.G., Lamki, N., et al. (1988). Abdominal cryptococcoma in AIDS: A case report. *Journal of Computerized Tomography, 12*(3), 237–239.

Scannell, K.A. (1990). Pneumothoraces and *Pneumocystis carinii* pneumonia in two AIDS patients receiving aerosolized pentamidine. *Chest, 92*(2), 479–480.

Scevola, D., Barbarini, G., Zambelli, A., et al. (1989). Nutritional status in AIDS patients [abstract]. In *Proceedings of the Fifth International Conference on AIDS*, Montreal (p. 465). Geneva, Switzerland: World Health Organization.

Schechter, G.F. (1990). *Mycobacterium tuberculosis*. In P.T. Cohen, M.A. Sande, & P.A. Volberding (Eds.), *The AIDS knowledge base* (pp. 622.1–622.4). Waltham, MA: Medical Publishing Group.

Schmitt, F.A., Bigley, J.W., McKinnis, R., et al. (The AZT Collaborative Working Group). (1988). Neuropsychological outcome of zidovudine (AZT) treatment of patients with AIDS and AIDS-related complex. *New England Journal of Medicine, 319*(24), 1573–1578.

Selwyn, P.A., Hartel, D., Lewis, V.A., et al. (1989). A prospective study of the risk of tuberculosis among intravenous drug users with human immunodeficiency virus infection. *New England Journal of Medicine, 320*(9), 545–550.

Similowski, T., Datry, A., Jais, P., et al. (1989). AIDS-associated cryptococcosis causing adult respiratory distress syndrome. *Respiratory Medicine, 83*(6), 513–515.

Skeels, M.R., Sokolow, R., Habbard, V., et al. (1990). *Cryptosporidium* infection in Oregon public health patients 1985-1988: The value of statewide surveillance. *American Journal of Public Health, 80*(3), 305–308.

Smaldone, G.C., Perry, R.J., Deutsch, D.G. (1988). Characteristics of nebulizers used in the treatment of AIDS-related *Pneumocystis carinii* pneumonia. *Journal of Aerosol Medicine, 1*(2), 113–126.

Small, P.M., Hopewell, P.C. (1990). *Mycobacterium avium* complex. In P.T. Cohen, M.A. Sande, & P.A. Volberding (Eds.), *The AIDS knowledge base* (pp. 621.1–621.4). Waltham, MA: Medical Publishing Group.

Small, P.M., McPhaul, L.W., Sooy, C.D., et al. (1989). Cytomegalovirus infection of the laryngeal nerve presenting as hoarseness in patients with acquired immunodeficiency syndrome. *American Journal of Medicine, 86*(1), 108–110.

Smart, P.E., Weinfeld, A., Thompson, N.E., et al. (1990). Toxoplasmosis of the stomach: A cause of antral narrowing. *Radiology, 174*(2), 369–370.

Smith, C.L. (1990). Nursing management of aerosolized pentamidine administration. *AIDS Patient Care, 4*(1), 13–17.

Smith, E., Franzmann, M., Mathiesen, L.R. (1989). Disseminated histoplasmosis in a Danish patient with AIDS. *Scandinavian Journal of Infectious Diseases, 21*(5), 573–575.

Smith, P.D., Janoff, E.N. (1988). Infectious diarrhea in human immunodeficiency virus infection. *Gastroenterology Clinics of North America, 17*(3), 587–598.

Smith, P.D., Macher, A.M., Bookman, M.A., et al. (1985). *Salmonella typhimurium* enteritis and bacteremia in the acquired immunodeficiency syndrome. *Annals of Internal Medicine. 102*(2), 207–209.

Snider, W.D., Simpson, D.M., Nielsen, S., et al. (1983). Neurological complications of acquired immune deficiency syndrome: Analysis of 50 patients. *Annals of Neurology, 14*(4), 403–418.

So, Y.T., Choucair, A., Davis, R.L., et al. (1988). Neoplasms of the central nervous system in acquired immunodeficiency syndrome. In M.L. Rosenblum, R.M. Levy, & D.E. Bredesen (Eds.), *AIDS and the nervous system* (pp. 285–300). New York: Raven Press.

Soave, R., Weikel, C.S. (1990). *Cryptosporidium* and other protozoa including *Ispospora, Sarcocystis, Balantidium coli,* and *Blastocystis.* In G.L. Mandell, R.G. Douglas Jr., & J.E. Bennett (Eds.), *Principles and practice of infectious diseases* (3rd ed.) (pp. 2122–2130). New York: Churchill Livingstone.

Sorvillo, F., Lieb, L., Iwakoshi, K., et al. (1990). *Isospora belli* and the acquired immune deficiency syndrome [letter]. *New England Journal of Medicine, 322*(2), 131.

Spika, J.S., Waterman, S.H., SooHoo, G.W., et al. (1987). Chloramphenicol-resistant *Salmonella newport* traced through hamburger to dairy farms. *New England Journal of Medicine, 316*(10), 565–570.

Spiller, R.C., Lovell, D., Silk, D.B. (1988). Adult acquired cytomegalovirus infection with gastric and duodenal ulceration. *Gut, 29*(8), 1109–1111.

Staib, F., Seibold, M., L'age, M., et al. (1989). *Cryptococcus neoformans* in the seminal fluid of an AIDS patient. *Mycoses, 32*(4), 171–180.

Stahl-Bayliss, C.M., Kalman, C.M., Laskin, O.L. (1986). Pentamidine-induced hypoglycemia in patients with the acquired immune deficiency syndrome. *Clinical Pharmacology and Therapeutics, 39*(3), 271–275.

Stevens, D.A. (1990). *Coccidioides immitis.* In G.L. Mandell, R.G. Douglas, Jr., & J.E. Bennett (Eds.), *Principles and practice of infectious diseases* (3rd ed.) (pp. 2008–2017). New York: Churchill Livingstone.

Stoler, M.H., Eskin, T.A., Benn, S., et al. (1986). Human T-cell lymphotropic virus type-III infection of the central nervous system: A preliminary in-situ analysis. *Journal of the American Medical Association, 256*(17), 2360–2364.

Straus, S.E. (1990). Introduction to herpesviridiae. In G.L. Mandell, R.G. Douglas, Jr., & J.E. Bennett (Eds.). *Principles and practice of infectious diseases* (3rd ed.) (pp. 1139–1144). New York: Churchill Livingstone.

Subar, M., Neri, A., Inghirami, G., et al. (1988). Frequent c-myc oncogene activation and infrequent presence of Epstein-Barr virus genome in AIDS-associated lymphoma. *Blood, 72*(2), 667–671.

Task Force on Nutrition Support in AIDS (1990). Guidelines for nutrition support in AIDS. *Nutrition, 5*(1), 39–46.

Tawney, S., Masci, J., Berger, H.W., et al. (1986). Pulmonary toxoplasmosis: An unusual nodular radiographic pattern. *Mount Sinai Journal of Medicine, 83*(3), 599–600.

Telzak, E.E., Budnik, L.D., Zweig-Greenberg, M.S., et al. (1990). A nosocomial outbreak of *Salmonella enteritidis* infection due to the consumption of raw eggs. *New England Journal of Medicine, 323*(6), 394–397.

Tenholder, M.F., Moser, R.J., Tellis, C.J. (1988). Mycobacteria other than tuberculosis: Pulmonary involvement in patients with acquired immunodeficiency syndrome. *Archives of Internal Medicine, 148*(4), 953–955.

Tindall, B., Hing, M., Edwards, P., et al. (1989). Severe clinical manifestations of primary HIV infection. *AIDS, 3*(11), 747–749.

Toma, E., Poisson, M., Claessens, M.R., et al. (1989). Herpes simplex type 2 pericarditis and bilateral facial palsy in a patient with AIDS [letter]. *Journal of Infectious Disease, 160*(3), 553–554.

Torres, R.A. (1987). Cryptococcal mediastinitis mimicking lymphoma in the acquired immune deficiency syndrome [letter]. *American Journal of Medicine, 83*(5), 1004–1005.

Tuazon, C.U. (1989). Toxoplasmosis in AIDS patients. *Journal of Antimicrobial Chemotherapy, 12*(5), 315–317.

Tucker, R.M., Swanson, S., Wenzel, R.P. (1989). Cytomegalovirus and appendiceal perforation in a patient with acquired immunodeficiency syndrome. *Southern Medical Journal, 82*(8), 1056–1057.

Tyler, K.L., Fields, B.N. (1990). Introduction to viruses and viral diseases. In G.L. Mandell, R.G. Douglas, Jr., J.E. Bennett (Eds.), *Principles and practice of infectious diseases* (3rd ed.) (pp. 1124–1134). New York: Churchill Livingstone.

Tzipori, S. (1988). Cryptosporidiosis in perspective. *Advances in Parasitology, 27*, 63–129.

Ungvarski, P.J. (1987). Demystifying AIDS: Educating nurses for care. *Nursing and Health Care, 8*(10), 570–573.

Ungvarski, P.J. (1988). Coping with infections that AIDS patients develop. *RN, 51*(11), 53–59.

Ungvarski, P.J. (1989). Nursing management of the adult client. In J.H. Flaskerud (Ed.), *AIDS/HIV infection: A reference guide for nursing professionals* (pp. 74–110). Philadelphia: W.B. Saunders.

Ungvarski, P.J. (1991). Administration of pentamidine aerosol therapy. *Journal of the Association of Nurses in AIDS Care, 2*(1), 12–14.

U.S. Pharmacopeial Convention, Inc. (1990). *USP DI: Vol. I. Drug information for the health care professional.* Rockville, MD: The Convention.

Van Calck, M., Motte, S., Rickaert, F., et al. (1988). Cryptococcal anal ulceration in a patient with AIDS. *American Journal of Gastroenterology, 83*(11), 1306–1308.

Vasudevan, V.P., Mascarenhas, D.A., Klapper, P., et al. (1990). Cytomegalovirus necrotizing bronchiolitis with HIV infection. *Chest, 25*(3), 311–312.

Villalona-Calero, M.A., Schrem, S.S., Phelps, K.R. (1989). Pneumomediastinum complicating *Pneumocystis carinii* pneumonia in a patient with AIDS. *American Journal of Medical Science, 297*(5), 328–330.

Vinters, H.V., Ferreiro, J.A. (1990). CMV: What is its effect on AIDS patients, and how do you treat it? *AIDS Medical Report, 3*(5), 43–56.

Vinters, H.V., Kwok, M.K., Ho, H.W., et al. (1989). Cytomegalovirus in the nervous system of patients with the acquired immune deficiency syndrome. *Brain, 112*(Pt. 1), 245–268.

Volberding, P.A. (1989). HIV infection as a disease: The medical indications for early diagnosis. *Journal of Acquired Immune Deficiency Syndrome, 2*(5), 421–426.

Volberding, P.A. (1990). Non-HIV Kaposi's sarcoma: Classic KS and KS associated with immunosuppression. In P.T. Cohen, M.A. Sande, & P.A. Volberding (Eds.), *The AIDS knowledge base* (pp. 712.1–712.2). Waltham, MA: Medical Publishing Group.

Volberding, P.A., Kusich, P., Feigal, D.W. (1989). Effect of chemotherapy for HIV-associated Kaposi's sarcoma on long-term survival [meeting abstract]. In *Proceedings of the Annual Meeting of the American Society of Clinical Oncology, 8*, A11.

von Roenn, J.H., Murphy, R.L., Weber, K.M., et al. (1988). Megestrol acetate for treatment of cachexia associated with human immunodeficiency virus (HIV) infection. *Annals of Internal Medicine, 109*(10), 840–841.

Wajsman, R., Cappell, M.S., Biempica, L., et al. (1989). Terminal ileitis associated with cytomegalovirus and the acquired immune deficiency syndrome. *American Journal of Gastroenterology, 84*(7), 790–793.

Wallace, J.M., Hannah, J. (1987). Cytomegalovirus pneumonitis in patients with AIDS: Findings in an autopsy series. *Chest, 92*(2), 198–203.

Wallace, J.M., Hannah, J.B. (1988). *Mycobacterium avium* complex infection in patients with acquired immunodeficiency syndrome: A clinicopathologic study. *Chest, 93*(5), 926–932.

Walzer, P.D. (1990). *Pneumocystis carinii.* In G.L. Mandell, R.G. Douglas, Jr., & J.E. Bennett (Eds.), *Principles and practice of infectious diseases* (3rd ed.) (pp. 2103–2110). New York: Churchill Livingstone.

Wasser, L., Talavera, W. (1987). Pulmonary cryptococcosis in AIDS. *Chest, 92*(4), 692–695.

Weiler, P.G. (1989). AIDS and dementia. *Generations: Journal of the American Society on Aging, 13*(4), 16–18.

Weiler, P.G., Mungas, D., Pomerantz, S. (1988). AIDS as a cause of dementia in the elderly. *Journal of the American Geriatric Society, 36*(2), 139–141.

Weisberg, L.A., Ross, W. (1989). AIDS dementia complex: Characteristics of a unique aspect of HIV infection. *Postgraduate Medicine, 86*(1), 213–220.

Wexner, S.D., Smithy, W.B., Trillo, C., et al. (1988). Emergency colectomy for cytomegalovirus ileocolitis in patients with the acquired immune deficiency syndrome. *Diseases of the Colon and Rectum, 31*(10), 755–761.

Wiley, C.A., Nelson, J.A. (1988). Role of human immunodeficiency virus and cytomegalovirus in AIDS encephalitis. *American Journal of Pathology, 133*(1), 73–81.

Wofsy, C.B. (1990a). Cryptosporidiosis. In P.T. Cohen, M.A. Sande, & P.A. Volberding (Eds.), *The AIDS knowledge base* (pp. 655.1–655.8). Waltham, MA: Medical Publishing Group.

Wofsy, C.B. (1990b). *Isospora belli.* In P.T. Cohen, M.A. Sande, & P.A. Volberding (Eds.), *The AIDS knowledge base* (pp. 657.1–657.4). Waltham, MA: Medical Publishing Group.

Woods, G.L., Goldsmith J.C. (1989). Fatal pericarditis due to *Mycobacterium avium-intracellulare* in acquired immunodeficiency syndrome. *Chest, 96*(6), 1355–1357.

Yarchoan, R., Thomas, R.V., Grafman, J., et al. (1988). Long-term administration of 3'-azido-2', 3'-dideoxythymidine to patients with AIDS-related neurological disease. *Annals of Neurology, 23*(suppl), S82–S87.

Youle, M.M., Hawkins, D.A., Collins, P., et al. (1988). Acyclovir-resistant herpes in AIDS treated with foscarnet [letter]. *Lancet, 2*(8606), 341–342.

Young, F.E., Nightengale, S.L., Cooper, E.C., et al. (1989). Aerosolized pentamidine: Approved for HIV-infected individuals at high risk for *Pneumocystis carinii* pneumonia. *Archives of Internal Medicine, 149*(11), 2412–2413.

Young, T.L., Robin, J.B., Holland, G.N., et al. (1989). Herpes simplex keratitis in patients with acquired immune deficiency syndrome. *Ophthalmology, 96*(10), 1476–1479.

Zakowski, P., Fligiel, S., Berlin, G.W., et al. (1986). Disseminated *Mycobacterium avium intracellulare* infection in homosexual men dying of acquired immunodeficiency. In H.M. Cole & G.D. Lundberg (Eds.), *AIDS from the beginning* (pp. 158–160). Chicago: American Medical Association.

Ziegler, J., Beckstead, J., Volberding, P.A., et al. (1984). Non-Hodgkin's lymphoma in 90 homosexual men: Relation to generalized lymphadenopathy and the acquired immunodeficiency syndrome. *New England Journal of Medicine, 311*(9), 565–570.

Ziegler, J.L., Drew, W.L., Miner, R.C., et al. (1982). Outbreak of Burkitt's-like lymphoma in homosexual men. *Lancet, 2*(8299), 631–632.

4

Nursing Management of the Adult Client

Peter J. Ungvarski

The major responsibility of the professional nurse with regard to HIV disease is health maintenance. This can be best described as nursing activities directed toward (1) concerns of individuals and groups about potential health problems and (2) reactions of individuals and groups to actual health problems (American Nurses Association, 1980).

When planning nursing care for a person with, or at risk for, HIV disease, the nurse should consider the entire spectrum of this illness and not simply focus on AIDS, which represents only the later stages of HIV disease. A three-tiered model can be used to clarify and facilitate communication about the responses of individuals with or at risk for HIV disease and to identify the appropriate nursing activities (Table 4–1).

TABLE 4–1. Levels of Health Maintenance Related to HIV Disease

Primary level:	Nursing activities directed toward the health appraisal of persons concerned about or with HIV disease
Secondary level:	Nursing activities directed toward health protection for persons with HIV disease
Tertiary level:	Nursing activities directed toward minimizing the residual disabilities related to advancing HIV disease or AIDS and maximizing the quality of life for persons with these illnesses

Data from Pender, N.J. (1987). Part I. The quest for health: Health-protecting (preventive) behavior. In *Health promotion in nursing practice* (pp. 37-56). Norwalk, CT: Appleton & Lange.

PRIMARY HEALTH MAINTENANCE

Primary health maintenance is the category of nursing care that focuses on an organized, systematic approach to health appraisal to (1) identify individuals with risk behaviors associated with HIV transmission, (2) detect signs and symptoms of HIV disease or of a related illness that is indicative of AIDS, (3) determine the need for health teaching to reduce the risk of acquiring HIV infection, or (4) determine the need for secondary or tertiary levels of health maintenance and nursing care.

Because the majority of persons with HIV infection are members of already stigmatized groups within our society (i.e., homosexual and bisexual men and intravenous drug users), the nurse taking the patient's history should be aware of his or her own feelings regarding these lifestyles. History taking should be performed, as much as possible, in a nonjudgmental manner (Ungvarski, 1988).

Making subjective assumptions about a client's risk potential for HIV disease can lead to an unnecessary delay in diagnosis. An example of this is a common assumption that HIV affects only younger people. The avoidance of taking sexual histories with elderly clients has caused HIV dementia to be misdiagnosed as Alzheimer's disease and has delayed diagnosis of *Pneumocystis carinii* pneumonia in HIV-infected elderly individuals (Fillit et al., 1990; Hargreaves et al., 1988; Weiler et al., 1988).

Health History. The health history should include a social history beginning with exploration of the person's sexual activities. The major error when taking a sexual history is to jump to conclusions based on a single answer to the simple question of sexual preference. If the client is homosexual and has been in a monogamous relationship with another man for the past 25 years, and neither has participated in sexual activities with other persons, they are no more at risk for HIV disease than a monogamous heterosexual couple about to celebrate their silver wedding anniversary. Sexual preferences and sexual behaviors are two different things. Sexual behaviors can be categorized as absolutely safe, very safe, probably safe, and risky with regard to the potential for HIV transmission (see Table 8–3). It is the specific sexual behaviors that increase the risk of HIV transmission between two individuals.

The question of condom use should be raised with both male and female clients. Questioning should also address the brand or type of condom, since research has demonstrated that latex condoms are the safest. The nurse should ascertain whether the client knows how to use condoms properly.

When asking about the use of drugs, the nurse should explore their relationship to sexual activities, since drugs such as alcohol or marijuana reduce inhibitions and may lead to high-risk activities during sex. The nurse should not ask, "Do you ever use drugs?" but rather "Have you ever used drugs?", since previous IV drug use or drug and sex behaviors may have placed the client at risk for HIV infection.

Questions about drug use will lead to questions about needle exposure. Although some exposures, such as those of an IV heroin addict, are obvious, other types of needle exposure may put people at risk, such as tattooing done on the streets or needle sharing among individuals who self-administer estrogens intramuscularly because they plan eventually to have transsexual surgery. In the early years of the AIDS epidemic, epidemiologic studies in Haiti traced HIV transmission to dirty needles used by untrained persons to give intramuscular injections (Pape & Johnson, 1989).

When the health history is used to identify persons at risk for HIV disease, questions should include occupational history and accidental exposure to blood, needles, or instruments (Soloway & Hecht, 1990). Attempting to sort out which occupations may be at risk might be difficult. In addition to the more obvious occupational groups, such as physicians, nurses, laboratory workers, and phlebotomists, others such as police officers, paramedics, and sanitation workers are at risk and should not be overlooked. To be as inclusive as possible, questioning should include all individuals.

When reviewing the medical history, the nurse should ask about illnesses that are likely to recur in an HIV-infected person as the immune system's ability to fight disease decreases. Most noteworthy are past infections with herpes simplex virus (HSV) and varicella zoster virus (VZV), both of which remain dormant in the body after the initial infection. Recurrent chronic HSV infection or the secondary appearance of VZV (commonly referred to as shingles) should be appropriately monitored.

The last part of the health history, the review of systems, is a detailed look for signs and symptoms of HIV disease and possibly of an associated AIDS-indicator disease. After the history is completed, it should be carefully reviewed with the client. The session should conclude with a question regarding the client's satisfaction with past behaviors and any other areas the client would like to change. This provides the basis for nursing care planning and health teaching. Table 4–2 presents a detailed outline for taking a health history.

Physical Examination. The physical examination findings are as diversified as the spectrum of HIV disease. Findings range from normal in an asymptomatic HIV-infected person to evidence of an opportunistic disease or infection that is associated with a diagnosis of AIDS. HIV-related conditions have demonstrated the ability to affect virtually every anatomic structure and organ system (Hernandez, 1990a). Therefore a complete physical examination should be performed and any deviations from normal findings should be considered significant if HIV infection is suspected.

Table 4–3 provides guidelines for conducting the physical exami-

TABLE 4–2. Primary Health Maintenance: Health History Specific for HIV Disease

A. Social history
  1. Sexual activities
     a. Absolutely safe behavior: abstinence or mutually monogamous with a noninfected partner
     b. Very safe behavior: noninsertive sexual practices
     c. Probably safe behavior: insertive sexual practices with the use of condoms and spermicide
     d. Risky behavior: everything else
     e. Use of condoms including application, removal, and use of lubricants
     f. Engaging in sex with multiple partners
     g. Use of mood-affecting drugs before sexual activities
     h. Whether AIDS has developed in anyone with whom client has had sex
  2. Use of mood-affecting drugs
     a. Drugs such as alcohol, marijuana, cocaine, crack, LSD, Quaalude, amphetamines, barbiturates, tranquilizers, amyl or butyl nitrate (called "poppers"), heroin
     b. Route of administration: oral, inhalation (including sniffing, snorting, and smoking), intravenous
     c. Any current or previous treatment for substance abuse
  3. Needle exposure
     a. Use of drugs via intravenous route, sharing of needles, syringes, and other drug paraphernalia
     b. Other needle-exposure activities such as tattoos, acupuncture, treatment by unlicensed individuals or "folk doctors," or sharing prescribed drugs between friends
     c. Whether AIDS has developed in anyone with whom client has shared needles
  4. Occupational history
     a. Client's occupation and responsibilities in relation to risk potential for HIV exposure
     b. Whether client has experienced any exposures
     c. What type of health care follow-up the client has pursued since exposure
     d. Client's knowledge level regarding the signs and symptoms or seroconversion and need for follow-up
  5. Travel
     a. Within the past 10 years
     b. Sexual activities when traveling in areas where the number of AIDS cases is high, such as New York, California, New Jersey, Texas, Florida, or countries such as Haiti or Zaire
B. Medication history: Current or previous use of medication that suppresses the immune system, such as steroids; current treatment for drug addiction if applicable
C. Medical history
  1. Major disease including (but not limited to) tuberculosis; hepatitis A or B or non A/B; mononucleosis; and hemophilia; receiving treatment with clotting replacements such as factor VIII
  2. Treatment for psychiatric or emotional disorders
  3. Transfusion donor or recipient
D. Surgical history
E. Childhood illnesses, including but not limited to varicella

Table continued on following page

TABLE 4–2. Primary Health Maintenance: Health History Specific for HIV Disease *Continued*

F. Sexually transmitted diseases (STDs), including (but not limited to) syphilis; gonorrhea; amebiasis; herpes simplex (oralis or genitalis); *Giardia lamblia* enteritis, and lymphogranuloma venereum

G. Review of systems
1. General: a comment from the client concerning a self-appraisal of current state of health should be elicited
2. Skin: eruptions, lesions, itching, dryness, redness, rashes, lumps, color changes, changes in hair or nails
3. Head: headaches, lightheadedness, or other sensations
4. Eyes: blurred vision or diploplia
5. Ears: impaired hearing or tinnitus
6. Nose and sinuses: obstruction, pain, discharges, or nosebleed
7. Mouth and throat: creamy white patches, lesions, bleeding gums, dysphagia, odynophagia, changes in taste, or sore throat
8. Respiratory: dyspnea with or without certain activities, coughing, wheezing, chest pain, "cold" or "flulike" symptoms, as well as the date of last chest x-ray examination and tuberculin test and results
9. Cardiovascular: chest pain, palpitations, edema, and known hypertension or hypotension
10. Gastrointestinal: changes in appetite, involuntary weight loss, abdominal pain or cramping, changes in bowel habits, diarrhea, blood in stool, rectal or perianal pain or itching
11. Genitourinary: dysuria, nocturia, pain, itching, discharges, or lesions
12. Gynecologic: changes in menstruation, dyspareunia, vaginal discharge, breast problems, obstetrical history, and contraception
13. Musculoskeletal: arthralgia or myalgia
14. Neurologic and emotional: problems with memory, nervousness, personality changes, confusional states, stiff neck, photophobia, tremors, paresthesias, seizures, or syncope
15. Endrocrine: polyuria, polyphagia, polydipsia, fevers, or night sweats
16. Hematopoietic: lymphadenopathy, bruising or bleeding, history of anemia

nation. Tables 4–2 and 4–3 identify the more common significant findings when the health appraisal is specific for HIV infection. These guidelines are not intended as a complete review and do not preclude the need for a more detailed history and physical examination based on the client's individual needs. Table 4–4 lists the common laboratory abnormalities associated with HIV disease (Burroughs Wellcome, 1990; Hernandez, 1990b; Hollander, 1990).

SECONDARY HEALTH MAINTENANCE

The secondary level of health maintenance should be implemented as soon as HIV infection is diagnosed. This category of nursing care focuses

TABLE 4-3. Primary Health Maintenance: Physical Examination Specific for HIV Disease

A. Neurologic examination
  1. Cerebral functions: impaired cognitive functions, decreased level of consciousness, anger, inattentiveness, depression, denial
  2. Cranial nerve (CN) examination
    a. CN II (optic nerve): papilledema, cotton-wool patches (exudate); visual field deficiencies, blurred vision
    b. CNs III, IV, VI (oculomotor, trochlear, abducens nerves): impaired extraocular movements, unequal pupils, diplopia, ptosis, nystagmus
    c. CN V (trigeminal nerve): photophobia
    d. CN VII (facial nerve): hemiparesis
    e. CN VIII (acoustic nerve): tinnitus, vertigo, impaired hearing
    f. CNs IX, X (glossopharyngeal and vagus nerves): dysphagia, dysarthria
  3. Motor examination: hemiparesis, paraparesis
  4. Sensory examination: dysesthesias, paresthesia, areas of anesthesia
  5. Cerebellar examination: ataxia, dysmetria, intention tremors
  6. Reflexes: abnormal reflexes, positive Babinski's sign
  7. Meningeal signs: nuchal rigidity, Brudzinski's sign, Kernig's sign
B. Mouth and throat examination: lesions, discoloration, exudates
C. Cardiovascular examination
  1. Heart: disturbances in cardiac rate rhythm and presence of pericardial friction rub
  2. Peripheral vascular: edema, decrease in peripheral pulse(s)
D. Respiratory examination: tachypnea, lag of excursion on palpation, dullness to percussion, presence of rales (crackles) or rhonchi (wheezes)
E. Lymphatic examination: lymphadenopathy
F. Abdominal examination: masses, tenderness, hepatomegaly, splenomegaly, hyperactive bowel sounds
G. Examination of genitalia and perianal region: lesions or discharges
H. Musculoskeletal examination: pain on range of motion
I. Skin examination
  1. Lesions or discolorations
  2. Dryness
  3. Thinning of hair or alopecia

TABLE 4-4. Common Laboratory Abnormalities Associated with HIV Disease

Anemia
Anergy to antigens
Decreased T4 lymphocytes
Decreased T4/T8 lymphocyte ratio
Decreased levels of anti-p24 antibody
Elevated erythrocyte sedimentation rate
Elevated serum beta$_2$-microglobulin
Elevated serum globulin (hypergammaglobulinemia)
Elevated serum lactate dehydrogenase (LDH)
Elevated serum neopterin
Elevated serum acid-labile interferon
Low serum cholesterol
Neutropenia
Positive serologic test for syphilis
Thrombocytopenia

on health protection for persons with HIV infection. Basic to planning is the nurse's knowledge that infection is the leading cause of morbidity in immunodeficient persons. The depressed activity of the T4 lymphocytes in persons with HIV infection leaves them vulnerable to a variety of infections. Therefore infection prevention should be considered a pragmatic necessity rather than an abstract concept. The vulnerability to opportunistic infections among persons with HIV infection is increased when they are treated with antimicrobial or antineoplastic agents, many of which induce leukopenia and cause cellular or mucosal damage. Critical to infection development in the person with HIV is an interaction of multiple predisposing factors, such as (1) local colonization of potentially pathogenic organisms from normal flora or the environment, (2) local damage to the integument or mucosa that allows entry of these organisms, and (3) a decrease in the number of T-helper cells, which results in rapid progression of the infectious process. Thus health protection on a secondary level focuses on maintaining or improving the individual's level of wellness through health teaching, as well as instructing the client about ways to avoid spreading HIV to others. Table 4–5 lists the key elements to be covered with the HIV-positive individual.

The nurse should include the client's lover, spouse, friends, or family (whomever the client designates as significant others) in health teaching and should provide printed materials they can use as a reference source. This is especially true when health teaching is implemented soon after the initial diagnosis of HIV infection. Weisman (1979) best describes this period as one of existential plight. The overwhelming impact of the initial diagnosis precipitates psychologic turmoil that can last for several weeks. Although clients are unlikely to retain much information given at this time, this may be the only contact the nurse will have with the client. Providing printed material and sharing information with the client and significant other will at least ensure that the information has been made available. It is also important at this time that the nurse provide a printed schedule and information for health care follow-up, as well as a list of community-based organizations for professional and peer support.

Follow-up for an individual whose HIV disease has just been diagnosed should be scheduled immediately rather than waiting until problems develop. Recommended intervals between follow-up visits vary from 3 to 6 months (Hecht & Soloway, 1991; Hollander, 1990). Since a repeat of the baseline history and physical examination is unnecessary, the assessment should focus on weight; vital signs; examination of skin, mouth, lymph nodes, and abdomen; neuropsychiatric examination; and funduscopic examination and testing of the visual fields (Hecht & Soloway, 1991; Hollander, 1990).

Women with HIV disease should be examined for vaginal candidiasis during each routine visit. Since a high prevalence of cervical cytologic abnormalities has been reported in HIV-infected women, they should be screened for cervical cancer at 6- to 12-month intervals (Hecht & Soloway, 1991).

TERTIARY HEALTH MAINTENANCE

The tertiary level of nursing activity is concerned with minimizing the disabilities that result from advancing HIV disease, including the clinical manifestations associated with AIDS-indicator diseases. It is also concerned with maintaining or improving the quality of life for clients in the later stages of illness. The focus is on nursing management, exclusive of medical orders.

NURSING CARE PLANNING

Planning and implementing the client's nursing care involves assessment, diagnosis, goal setting, interventions and health teaching, referrals, and evaluation. It is organized around the symptoms of impaired cognition (below), weight loss (p. 162), dry skin and skin lesions (p. 167), fatigue (p. 170), diarrhea (p. 172), shortness of breath (p. 175), cough (p. 177), edema (p. 178), impaired vision (p. 180), dry or painful mouth (p. 183), bleeding and bruising (p. 185), fever (p. 187), pain (p. 189), motor impairment (p. 191), and sexual dysfunction (p. 193) (Carpenito, 1989).

SYMPTOM: **Impaired Cognition**

Etiology:

A. HIV induced (primary infection) such as:
    1. AIDS dementia complex (subacute encephalitis)
    2. Aseptic meningitis
B. Opportunistic infections (secondary infection) caused by a:
    1. Bacterium
    2. Fungus
    3. Protozoan
    4. Virus
C. Cerebrovascular accidents resulting from:
    1. Infarction
    2. Hemorrhage
    3. Vasculitis
D. Complications of HIV therapy such as:
    1. Drug side effects
    2. Irradiation side effects

Text continued on page 158

TABLE 4-5. Secondary Health Maintenance: Health Protection for the Person with HIV Disease

CURRENT HEALTH ACTIVITIES	ENCOURAGE
Skin care	Showering daily Using mild soap Damp drying Using emollient cream such as petroleum jelly
Hair care	Washing hair infrequently Using mild shampoo Using conditioner Covering head while in bed Combing hair
Mouth care	Using soft toothbrush Using nonabrasive toothpaste (or baking soda) Brushing surface of teeth only Using Toothettes for mucosal surface cleaning Performing mouth care t.i.d.
Handwashing	Frequent washing after activities of daily living Using soap in a pump dispenser Rinsing well Applying emollient cream to protect the skin Wearing rubber or latex gloves when cleaning Demonstration of handwashing
Nutrition (Federation of American Societies for Experimental Biology, 1990)	Building up the client's current intake pattern High-protein, high-calorie diet Six small meals a day Cooking meat and eggs thoroughly Thawing frozen meats in refrigerator or microwave Serving hot foods while hot and cold foods while cold Washing fruits and vegetables thoroughly Using only pasteurized products Checking food labels for expiration date Using separate cutting boards for raw and cooked foods Washing hands before and after handling foods
Environmental cleaning and safety	Using household bleach (5.25% sodium hypochlorite) diluted 1:10 with water for cleaning Discarding solution daily and remixing when necessary Cleaning up blood or body fluids with this solution Using household bleach for laundry soiled with blood or body fluids

DISCOURAGE	INDIVIDUAL IS AT RISK FOR
Tub baths Drying, perfumed soap Creams and lotions that have a high alcohol content and are drying	Secondary skin infections or transfer of infections from one part of the body to another
Washing hair daily Drying, perfumed shampoo Brushing hair	Excessive hair loss related to chronic infection (HIV) and/or decreased nutritional intake
Using firm or hard toothbrush Using abrasive toothpaste Brushing mucosal surfaces Performing mouth care only q.d. or b.i.d.	Secondary oral infections, especially thrush
Using hot water Using bar soap Teaching handwashing without demonstrating correct method	Secondary infections related to poor handwashing practices
Introducing an entirely new menu or standardized menus that may be irrelevant to the client Diets low in protein and calories Three large meals or skipping meals Sushi, raw protein foods such as eggs, rare meat, cracked eggs should not be used Thawing meats at room temperature Allowing foods to stand at room temperature longer than 2 hours Eating foods with molds or expired freshness dates Using wooden cutting boards	Secondary infections related to inadequate protein and calorie intake or contaminated foods
Using expensive ineffective (for disinfection) household detergents Using cleaning solutions beyond 24 hours after mixing Discarding soiled disposable items without using double plastic bags Throwing used needles and sharps directly into household garbage	Secondary infections related to unclean environment; contamination of environment with HIV

Table continued on following page

CURRENT HEALTH ACTIVITIES	ENCOURAGE
	Using double plastic bags to discard disposable items contaminated with blood or body fluids
	Changing filters on air conditioners frequently
	Placing used needles and sharps in puncture-resistant containers
Pet care	Having pet care performed by someone other than person with HIV disease
	When necessary, wearing gloves and washing hands when finished
Health care follow-up	Establishing a pattern for health care follow-up (physician, nurse practicioner, visiting nurse, clinic, etc.)
	Establishing a relationship with health care professional knowledgeable about HIV disease
	Watching for signs and symptoms indicating secondary complications of HIV disease including but not limited to:
	1. Skin lesions, rashes, itching, lumps, or bruising
	2. Swollen lymph nodes
	3. Lesions or exudate in mouth
	4. Persistent fever, night sweats
	5. Extreme fatigue even when getting plenty of rest
	6. Weight loss
	7. Changes in digestion, difficulty swallowing, and diarrhea
	8. Shortness of breath, persistent coughing
	9. Headaches, visual changes, numbness in arms and legs, forgetfulness, dizziness
	10. Unusual bleeding, e.g., bleeding gums
Sexual practices	Safer sexual practices (see Table 8-3)
Procreation	Contraception
Intravenous drug use	Cessation of drug use and referral for treatment
	Not sharing drug paraphernalia with others
	Disinfecting drug paraphernalia before sharing equipment (if client persists in sharing)
	Open dialogue regarding continued drug use

Handling pet excreta or cleaning litter boxes, bird cages, or aquariums	Secondary infections related to microbes in pet excreta
Changing patterns of health care follow-up Seeking health care from health care professionals with knowledge deficits of HIV disease Ignoring warning signs	Delayed health care intervention when secondary complications develop
Risky sexual practices	Sexually transmitted disease and transfer of HIV to a noninfected person or transfer of secondary infection
Conception	Perinatal transmission of HIV
Sharing of contaminated drug paraphernalia Client and health care professional avoiding discussion of drug use	Secondary infections related to contaminated "works" and transmission of HIV to others

Table continued on following page

TABLE 4–5. Secondary Health Maintenance: Health Protection for the Person with HIV Disease *Continued*

CURRENT HEALTH ACTIVITIES	ENCOURAGE
Stress management, coping	Joining support groups from the community-based AIDS organizations or seeking professional guidance
	Meditation
	Use of visualization
	Relaxation techniques
	Use of therapeutic touch
	Getting factual answers to health concerns related to HIV infection from reliable sources such as health care professionals knowledgeable about HIV infection
	Review of financial status of client and health insurance, as well as Medicaid/Medicare eligibility
Additional considerations	Using own personal care items (e.g., razors, toothbrushes, makeup)
	Refraining from donating blood or organs
	Informing health care professionals responsible for primary care that the client has HIV disease
	Receiving influenza vaccination by December of each year (CDC, 1990)

Nursing Assessment (McArthur, 1990; Ungvarski, 1989):

A. Subjective data (obtained from client and significant other)
  1. History of symptoms
  2. Problems with memory, concentration, and conversation
  3. Problems with missing appointments or forgetting to do things
  4. Changes in leisure activities (e.g., loss of interest in reading printed materials or watching television)
  5. Withdrawal from social activity
  6. History of life-style, including occupation and recreation and leisure interests
  7. Coping patterns, including substance use
  8. Availability of support systems
  9. Ability and interest in performing activities of daily living
  10. History of a typical week of client's activities
  11. Self-assessment of cognitive activities
  12. Changes in upper motor function, such as signature change, or lower motor function, such as walking
  13. Behavior changes noticed by the significant other
  14. Medical and surgical history

DISCOURAGE	INDIVIDUAL IS AT RISK FOR
Continued use of recreational drugs as a method of coping Relying on friends, gossip, or the media for "latest" information about AIDS Delays in accessing required health care owing to lack of financial planning	Stress and continued use of recreational drugs such as alcohol and tobacco adversely affect the immune system and increase the potential for secondary infections and diseases Undue stress related to hysterical media reports Delays in obtaining health care related to inability to pay
Sharing of personal care items Donating blood or making plans to donate body organs Withholding information about HIV disease from health care professionals responsible for coordinating care	Transmitting HIV to others Delay in diagnosis of HIV-related problems and inappropriate care planning

    15. Psychiatric history
    16. Current drug therapy
B. Objective data
    1. General appearance, including grooming and dress
    2. Examination of cerebral functioning, including level of consciousness, orientation, and cognitive function testing including calculations
    3. Behavior (e.g., apathetic, withdrawn, irritable)
    4. Affect (e.g., appropriate or flat)
    5. Cranial nerve examination
    6. Motor examination
    7. Sensory examination
    8. Cerebellar examination
    9. Reflexes
    10. Meningeal signs

Nursing Diagnosis:

Sensory-perceptual alterations related to sensory overload and/or deprivation

Goals:

After discussing and validating the findings of assessment and the nursing diagnosis, the client, significant other, and nurse will select interventions to:
A. Promote independence
B. Identify factors that contribute to sensory-perceptual alteration
C. Provide meaningful and sufficient sensory input
D. Minimize disorientation
E. Provide for safety
F. Improve the individual's ability to cope with reality

Interventions and Health Teaching:

A. Assess for causative factors
　1. In the acute care setting
　　a. Sleep interruption because of hospital routines
　　b. Auditory overload because of staff talking at night, alarms going off, etc.
　　c. New, unfamiliar staff providing care
　　d. Social isolation because of infection control practices
　　e. Restricted movement
　　f. Lack of routine
　　g. Lack of familiar visitors
　　h. Fear, especially of loss of control
　　i. Medication side effects
　　j. Physiologic alterations
　2. In the community
　　a. Lack of supervision or motivation
　　b. Change in housing (e.g., being placed in a nursing home or AIDS shelter)
　　c. Lack of social support (e.g., visitors)
　　d. Lack of psychologic support (e.g., participation in peer support groups)
　　e. Lack of established routines
　　f. Changes in home care staff
　　g. Medication side effects
　　h. Continued substance use
　　i. Physiologic alterations
B. Reduce or eliminate causative factors
　1. Provide a written schedule of activities for client and encourage all involved in care to adhere to schedule as much as possible
　2. Provide a copy of the routines for client to follow
　3. Avoid staff assignment changes as much as possible

4. Decrease noise input, especially at night
5. Encourage regular visiting by friends
6. When friends visit, encourage them to take client out; in acute care settings, even take client for a walk to another area or for coffee
7. Encourage participation in weekly peer support groups
8. When barrier precautions are necessary, put them on in front of client, explaining the purpose
9. Discuss dangers of substance use with impaired cognition (especially to friends who may bring substances to client)
10. When external auditory stimuli cannot be controlled, consider use of personal radio with earplugs
11. Keep pictures of loved ones nearby

C. Promote cognitive stimulation and orientation
1. Address client by name
2. Identify self frequently (especially important with telephone conversations)
3. Explain all care activities
4. Engage client in areas of pleasure or interest such as board games, cards
5. Encourage friends to watch television and read newspapers with client
6. Keep calendar visible and cross off each day
7. Have client wear wristwatch, and check time with client periodically

D. Promote independence and self-esteem
1. Engage client in decision making
2. Keep important telephone numbers next to telephone for client's use
3. Pre-pour medications and supervise client's ability to self-medicate
4. Encourage client to do as much as possible in activities of daily living, including cleaning, shopping, and cooking
5. Have client dress and groom daily; do not allow client to sit around in bed clothes
6. Encourage client to verbalize fears and concerns

E. Promote exercise
1. Include exercise as a part of each day's routine
2. Plan purposeful exercise (e.g., shopping or visiting a friend)
3. If client was previously engaged in exercise (e.g., aerobics), continue within physical limitations of client's current capabilities

F. Provide for safety
1. Assist with potentially dangerous activities: cooking, using appliances, etc.

2. Assess with client, significant other, and physician the client's ability to continue to drive a motor vehicle
3. If client smokes, monitor safety and attempt to prohibit smoking in bed
4. Assess for hazards in the home and make necessary changes such as removing scatter rugs and breakable objects
5. Continually assess the need for assist devices such as a cane, walker, or bath bar

NOTE WELL: Because of the nature of cognitive impairment it is extremely important to include the client's designated care partner in all care planning and health teaching. Documentation on the client's record should reflect all instructions and concerns provided to both individuals.

Referrals:

A. Clinical nurse specialist (CNS) in HIV disease or neurologic disorders or mental health
B. Physical therapist
C. Occupational therapist
D. Community-based AIDS organization for participation in a volunteer visitor program
E. Day care program for cognitively impaired individuals (if available)

Evaluation:

The client or significant other will:
A. Identify causative factors contributing to sensory-perceptual alterations
B. Demonstrate the reduction or elimination of identified factors
C. Provide a safe home environment
The client will:
A. Participate in decision making
B. Maintain or improve appearance
C. Participate in plan of care
D. Verbalize fears and concerns
E. Be free from injury

SYMPTOM: **Weight Loss**

Etiology (King, 1990; Kotler et al., 1989):

A. Increased nutrient requirements resulting from primary systemic infection with HIV or secondary systemic (opportunistic) infection causing:

1. Hypermetabolism
2. Fever
3. Catabolism
B. Decreased food intake resulting from side effects of medication or systemic infection causing:
1. Anorexia
2. Nausea
3. Vomiting
4. Alterations in taste
C. Oral or esophageal infection causing:
1. Impaired chewing
2. Difficulty swallowing
D. Decreased assimilation of food because of primary intestinal infection with HIV or secondary (opportunistic) gastrointestinal infection causing:
1. Malabsorption
2. Diarrhea
E. Inability to obtain food because of:
1. Fatigue
2. Lack of money
3. Distance from shopping
4. Lack of utilities to store and prepare food
F. Lack of knowledge of the importance of nutrition in HIV infection and its impact on survival
G. Neuropsychiatric problems such as:
1. Depression
2. Impaired cognition
3. Paralysis

Nursing Assessment:

A. Subjective data
1. History of problem
2. Amount of weight loss
3. Present dietary patterns, likes, and dislikes (include 24-hour fluid intake)
4. Ability to pay for and obtain food
5. Living arrangement and ability and interest in preparing food
6. Mental status
7. Response to stress as related to eating (increase or decrease)
8. Basic knowledge of nutrition
9. Medical and surgical history
10. Current drug therapy

B. Objective data
 1. Height and weight
 2. Anthropometric measurements
 3. Examination of skin, hair, nails, and oral cavity
 4. Examination of cranial nerves I (olfactory); V (trigeminal); IX (glossopharyngeal); X (vagus)
 5. Evaluation of ability to feed self

Nursing Diagnosis:

Altered nutrition: less than body requirements related to anorexia, difficulty in chewing or swallowing, and/or inability to obtain or prepare food

Goals:

After discussing and validating the findings of assessment and the nursing diagnosis, the client and nurse will select interventions to:
A. Identify contributing factors associated with weight loss
B. Increase nutritional intake and reduce weight loss

Interventions and Health Teaching (Task Force on Nutrition Support in AIDS, 1989):

A. Minimize factors contributing to anorexia
 1. For alterations in the sense of smell
  a. Hyperosmia (increased sense of smell): avoid cooking odors by keeping windows open and the home well aerated; encourage meals that include cold foods
  b. Hyposmia (decreased sense of smell): use spices such as basil, oregano, rosemary, thyme, cloves, mint, cinnamon, or lemon juice to enhance smell
 2. For alterations in sense of taste (especially related to distaste for red meat)
  a. Marinate meat before cooking in commercial marinade, wine, or vinegar
  b. As substitutes for red meat use other protein sources such as eggs, peanut butter, tofu, cheeses, poultry, or fish
 3. For persons living alone or experiencing fatigue or depression:
  a. Explore the use of complete frozen dinners that can be prepared in oven or microwave
  b. Explore the use of easily prepared foods such as canned creamed soups and commercially prepared liquid nutritional supplements

      c. Explore the availability of community resources that provide meals and social gatherings for persons with AIDS

      d. Explore the availability of community volunteers to assist with meal preparation at home (e.g., Meals on Wheels)

      e. Plan for rest periods before meals

   4. For nausea and vomiting

      a. Avoid odors; keep home well aerated

      b. If possible have someone else prepare food

      c. Restrict liquids before, during, and immediately after meals

      d. Between meals sip liquids and ice chips

      e. Avoid lying down after meals; if immobilized and in bed, keep head of bed elevated

      f. Encourage taking antiemetic on a scheduled basis rather than p.r.n. (as needed)

      g. Explain that when the client feels good, food intake should increase to promote weight gain that will tide client over when periods of nausea and vomiting occur

B. Minimize factors related to difficulty chewing, dysphagia (difficulty swallowing), or odynophagia (painful swallowing)

   1. Avoid:

      a. Rough foods such as raw fruits and vegetables

      b. Spicy, acidic, or salty foods

      c. Alcohol and tobacco

      d. Excessively hot or cold foods

      e. Sticky food such as peanut butter and slippery foods such as gelatin, bologna, and elbow macaroni

   2. Encourage:

      a. Eating foods at room temperature

      b. Choosing mild foods and drinks, e.g., apple juice rather than orange juice

      c. Eating dry grain foods such as breads, crackers, and cookies after softening in milk, tea, etc.

      d. Eating nonabrasive, easy to swallow foods such as ice cream, pudding, well-cooked eggs, noodle dishes, baked fish, and soft cheese

      e. Eating popsicles to numb pain

      f. Using a straw when drinking

      g. Tilting the head back or moving it forward to make swallowing easier

C. Minimize factors related to inability to obtain food

   1. Evaluate financial resources and the need for referral for Medicaid, food stamps, etc.

   2. Evaluate the home and the client's ability to prepare and obtain food, looking for such factors as:

        a. Absence of cooking facilities, e.g., living in a shelter or hotel for the homeless

        b. Need for alternative housing arrangements

    3. Explore community resources that provide free meals

D. Discuss nutritional requirements for persons with HIV disease, including:

    1. High-protein sources and ways to increase protein intake by:

        a. Adding skim milk powder to regular whole milk

        b. Preparing canned creamed soups with heavy cream instead of water or milk

        c. Increasing intake of peanut butter and eating it on whole wheat bread

        d. Adding pasteurized processed cheeses to soups and vegetables

        e. Eating hard-boiled eggs for snacks

    2. Increasing caloric intake by:

        a. Using extra peanut butter, cream cheese, sugar, honey, sour cream, and mayonnaise

        b. Substituting heavy cream for milk in coffee, tea, soups, etc.

        c. Eating sweets for snacks

        d. Drinking commercially prepared liquid dietary supplements

        e. Making a liquid nutritional supplement at home by mixing:

            (1) A one-quart packet of powdered milk with

            (2) One quart of whole milk and

            (3) Four packets of a flavored instant breakfast mix

                NOTE: This powdered package recipe is significantly easier to travel with than ready-to-use canned preparations.

        f. Eating small frequent meals instead of a few large meals

    3. Reviewing a balanced diet selection for a 24-hour menu plan

E. Review essential elements of a low-microbial diet and food safety and preparation

F. See "Diarrhea"

NOTE WELL: The nutritional teaching should as much as possible follow the client's usual pattern of food intake rather than expecting the client to follow a totally new, unfamiliar prescription for meal planning.

Referrals:

A. Dietitian

B. Social worker

C. CNS in HIV disease

D. Visiting nurse

E. Community-based AIDS program that provides meals

Evaluation:

The client will:

A. Demonstrate weight maintenance or gain
B. Identify factors related to anorexia, difficulty chewing, dysphagia, or odynophagia
C. Identify sufficient resources to obtain and prepare food or social work intervention has been established to obtain food stamps or public assistance (welfare)
D. Identify means of increasing protein and calorie intake
E. Identify key concepts in planning a low-microbial diet
F. Select a balanced 24-hour menu

SYMPTOM: **Dry Skin and Skin Lesions**

Etiology:

A. Commonly seen skin conditions in HIV diseases (Berger, 1990)
 1. Herpes simplex
 2. Herpes zoster (shingles)
 3. *Candida albicans* infection
 4. *Mycobacterium avium-intracellulare* infection
 5. Staphylococcal folliculitis
 6. Bacillary angiomatosis
 7. Molluscum contagiosum
 8. Insect bite reactions
 9. Photosensitivity
 10. Eosinophilic folliculitis
 11. Seborrheic dermatitis
 12. Psoriasis or Reiter's syndrome
B. Dry skin secondary to diaphoresis and febrile states associated with HIV disease
C. Anemia
D. Cutaneous invasion by Kaposi's sarcoma
E. Immobility
F. Malnutrition
G. Cutaneous reactions to drug therapy

Nursing Assessment:

A. Subjective data
 1. History of symptoms
 2. Usual patterns of bathing and skin care
 3. Bathing facilities in home
 4. Current nutritional history

5. Past medical and surgical history
6. Exercise and rest patterns
7. Current drug therapy
B. Objective data
   1. Examination of skin, paying particular attention to:
      a. Areas under skin folds
      b. Pressure points
      c. Sites of invasive procedures (e.g., incisions, biopsy sites, venipuncture sites)
      d. Genital, perineal, and perianal regions
   2. Palpate skin for temperature, texture, pain, turgor, moisture, circulation, and edema

Nursing Diagnoses:

A. *Impaired skin integrity related to dryness, immobility, malnutrition, or skin lesions*
B. *Pain related to pruritus*

Goals:

After discussing and validating the findings of assessment and the nursing diagnosis, the client and nurse will select interventions to:
A. Maintain the integrity of healthy skin
B. Reduce the potential for secondary infections of the skin
C. Reduce or relieve symptoms of inflammatory process

Interventions and Health Teaching:

A. Keep skin clean and well moisturized
   1. Have shower or bed bath daily
   2. Use mild soap in pump dispenser
   3. Damp dry
   4. Apply emollient cream
   5. Apply cool, moist compresses for pruritus
B. Prevent dissemination of infection or development of secondary infection
   1. Avoid tub baths or sitz baths
   2. Avoid bar soap
   3. Use separate washcloth to bathe areas with infectious lesions
   4. Explain dangers of scratching and extension of infection and lesions
C. Maintain skin integrity for immobile persons
   1. Turn and position frequently

2. Massage bony prominences frequently
3. Institute a schedule of both active and passive range of motion exercises
4. Use pressure-relieving devices such as egg crate mattress, sheepskin, foam protectors, and alternating-pressure devices
5. Use a "pull-sheet" for turning and positioning
6. Apply skin barriers such as Skin-prep to bony prominences and before applying tape to skin
7. Use a foot board to prevent sliding
8. When the client is out of bed, use a reclining chair that supports legs and alternate the chair positions frequently
9. For comatose persons, use pillows and blanket to support normal body alignment

D. Provide adequate nutrition and hydration
1. Hydrate with 2.5 to 3 liters of fluid per day
2. Provide high-calorie, high-protein diet; see also "Weight Loss"

E. Provide incontinent care
1. For confused clients
   a. Observe incontinent periods to determine a pattern of occurrence
   b. Establish a schedule of toileting to prevent incontinence
   c. When client is ambulatory, use protective pads or adult diaper
2. When client is incontinent, wash with soap and water, rinse well, and apply protective cream
3. Consider use of external catheter and fecal incontinence collecting bags when situation cannot be controlled

F. Implement specific skin care regimens in collaboration with physician's orders

NOTE WELL: "Occlusive dressings such as Stomahesive, Op-site, and Duo Derm are contraindicated for immunocompromised patients" (McDonnell & Sevedge, 1986, p. 572). For safe use of this type of dressing, the body's host defenses should be intact (Hotter, 1990). In vitro studies have shown that in persons with AIDS the body's chemotactic response to bacterial substances are altered, interfering with monocyte-macrophage-mediated organisms (Crowe et al., 1990). In addition, *Candida albicans* flourishes under occlusive dressings (Cuzzel, 1990).

Referrals:

A. Physical therapist
B. CNS in HIV disease or dermatologic disorders
C. Visiting nurse

Evaluation:

The client will:

A. Describe factors that contribute to dry skin and secondary skin infections
B. Demonstrate the ability to provide special skin care
C. Change position frequently when immobilized
D. Plan a diet high in protein and calories for a 24-hour period
E. Retain intact mucocutaneous surfaces without evidence of redness, dryness, or secondary infection
F. Verbalize a decrease in pruritus

SYMPTOM: **Fatigue**

Etiology:

A. Chronic HIV infection
B. Secondary opportunistic infection(s) or malignancies
C. Anemia
D. Malnutrition
E. Diarrhea
F. Prolonged immobility

Nursing Assessment:

A. Subjective data
    1. History of symptoms
    2. Associated symptoms
    3. Current ability to perform activities of daily living
    4. Medical and surgical history
    5. Current drug therapy
    6. Nutrition history
B. Objective data
    1. Assess activity tolerance by taking vital signs before and immediately after the performance of an activity such as bathing, dressing, or ambulating
    2. Assess for associated symptoms such as pallor, diaphoresis, or complaints of dyspnea or dizziness

Nursing Diagnosis:

Activity intolerance related to insufficient oxygen transport, nutritional deficiencies, diarrhea and fluid loss, prolonged immobility, and / or knowledge deficit regarding need for rest and pacing activities of daily living

Goals:

After discussing and validating the findings of assessment and nursing diagnosis, the client and nurse will select interventions to:
A. Identify contributing factors associated with fatigue
B. Identify methods that will increase activity tolerance and promote independence in activities of daily living

Intervention and Health Teaching:

A. Minimize factors contributing to fatigue
   1. See "Shortness of Breath"
   2. See "Weight Loss"
   3. See "Diarrhea"
   4. For prolonged immobility or the potential for prolonged immobility
      a. Plan a schedule of turning, positioning, and active and passive range of motion exercises
      b. Plan a schedule of getting out of bed daily and sitting in a recliner if possible or necessary (even if intubated while in hospital)
      c. Increase activities gradually when recovering from an acute episode of immobilization
   5. Encourage the use of assist devices when necessary to mobilize client and promote independence; teach safe use of:
      a. Trapeze bar while in bed
      b. Wheelchair
      c. Walker or crutches
      d. Cane
      e. Bath-shower chair, tub bars, hand-held shower, etc.
B. Assist by planning to pace activities of daily living
   1. Plan a 24-hour schedule for activities of daily living that alternates short activities with rest periods
   2. Assist in identifying activity priorities such as eating breakfast and then resting before bathing in the morning as opposed to the reverse
   3. Evaluate the individual's needs and point out ways to conserve energy, such as:
      a. Sitting down while dressing, shaving or preparing food
      b. Sitting in a shower chair while bathing
      c. Using disposable items for eating so no clean-up is needed

Referrals:

A. Physical therapist
B. Occupational therapist
C. CNS in HIV disease or rehabilitation

D. Visiting nurse

E. Community-based AIDS program that provides visitors or "buddies"

Evaluation:

The client will:

A. Identify causative factors that increase fatigue

B. Demonstrate the ability to plan a schedule of paced activity for a 24-hour period

C. Demonstrate the ability to use assist devices safely

D. Verbalize a decrease in the fatigue experienced over a 24-hour period

SYMPTOM: **Diarrhea**

Etiology:

A. Gastrointestinal infection caused by:
   1. HIV
   2. *Giardia lamblia*
   3. *Entamoeba histolytica*
   4. *Salmonella*
   5. *Shigella*
   6. *Campylobacter*
   7. *Isospora belli*
   8. *Cryptosporidium*
   9. *Mycobacterium avium-intracellulare*
   10. Cytomegalovirus
   11. Herpes simplex
B. Kaposi's sarcoma in the gastrointestinal tract
C. Gastrointestinal reaction to medications
D. Lactose intolerance
E. Inappropriate dietary intake
F. Intolerance to dietary supplements with a high osmolarity

Nursing Assessment:

A. Subjective data
   1. Usual pattern of elimination
   2. Usual pattern of nutrition
   3. Food intolerance
   4. History of diarrhea
   5. Associated symptoms
   6. Current drug therapy
   7. Sexual activities involving anal intercourse or oral-anal contact
   8. Current and past medical and surgical history

B. Objective data
 1. Observation of fecal material
 2. Assessment of mucocutaneous surfaces (hydration status)
 3. Assessment of blood pressure for orthostatic hypotension
 4. Auscultation and palpation of abdomen
 5. Examination of perianal region

Nursing Diagnoses:

A. *Diarrhea related to lack of knowledge regarding dietary control of symptom*
B. *Fluid volume deficit related to abnormal fluid loss*

Goals:

After discussing and validating the findings of assessment and the nursing diagnosis, the client and the nurse will select interventions to:
A. Reduce symptoms and facilitate the restoration of usual bowel patterns
B. Prevent associated complications such as dehydration and skin break-down

Interventions and Health Teaching:

A. Low-residue, high-protein, high-calorie diet (Culhane, 1984; Task Force on Nutrition Support in AIDS, 1989)
 1. Diet includes:
    a. Cottage cheese, cream cheese, and mild processed cheeses
    b. Cooked eggs
    c. Boiled low-fat milk, yogurt, and buttermilk
    d. Clear broth and bouillon
    e. Baked, broiled, or roasted fish, poultry, or lean ground beef
    f. Gelatin, pudding, custard
    g. Cooked Cream of Wheat or Cream of Rice cereal
    h. Bananas, applesauce, peeled apples, apple juice, grape juice, or avocados
    i. White bread, toast, or crackers made from refined flour
    j. Noodles, pasta, or white rice, cooked vegetables such as baked potatoes, carrots, squash, peas, green or wax beans
    k. Cream soups
 2. Diet excludes:
    a. Whole grain bread, cereals, or brown rice
    b. Nuts, seeds, popcorn, pretzels, potato chips, and similar snacks
    c. Fried foods
    d. Fresh fruits (except those listed previously), dried fruits
    e. Raw vegetables and fresh salads

    f. Rich pastries

    g. Strong spices such as chili powder or curry

    h. Foods that increase flatus such as cabbage, broccoli, and onions

    i. Coffee, tea, colas, chocolate

    j. Carbonated beverages

    k. Alcoholic beverages

    l. Tobacco

B. Hydrate with at least 2.5 to 3 liters of fluid per day including:

    1. Water

    2. Gatorade

    3. Noncarbonated drinks or soda that has been opened and is relatively "flat" (with minimum carbonation left)

    4. Caffeine-free drinks

    5. Diluted fruit juices

C. Provide small frequent meals and dietary supplements

D. Avoid foods that are very hot, very cold, or spicy

E. In the presence of lactose intolerance use lactose-free dairy products such as Lactaid

F. Provide skin care by washing perianal region with soap and water, damp drying, and applying creams or ointments

G. For ambulatory persons

    1. Use plastic squeeze bottle filled with warm water and use soap to wash perianal area while sitting on toilet after each bowel movement

    2. Carry Tucks to cleanse perianal area when not at home

    3. Wear "panty-liners" (sanitary napkins) to protect clothing and prevent embarrassment from incontinence or staining of fecal liquid, or from creams applied to perianal region; if incontinence is severe, adult diapers may be used.

    4. Assess for orthostatic hypotension and teach gradual assumption of upright position

H. Avoid anal intercourse or oral-anal sexual activities

I. Encourage the use of antidiarrheal agents on a scheduled basis, not p.r.n.

Referrals:

A. Dietitian

B. CNS in HIV disease or ostomy care

C. Visiting nurse

Evaluation:

The client will:

A. Identify factors that contribute to diarrhea

B. Plan a 24-hour menu of low-residue, high-protein, high-calorie foods
C. Demonstrate the ability to provide proper skin care after each bowel movement
D. Verbalize the need to avoid anal sexual practices
E. Verbalize a decrease in the number of bowel movements over a 24-hour period

SYMPTOM: **Shortness of Breath**

Etiology

A. Infections of the respiratory system caused by:
  1. *Pneumocystis carinii*
  2. Cytomegalovirus
  3. *Cryptococcus neoformans*
  4. *Mycobacterium avium-intracellulare*
  5. *Mycobacterium tuberculosis*
  6. *Histoplasma capsulatum*
  7. *Candida albicans*
  8. *Cryptosporidium*
B. Respiratory tract invasion by:
  1. Kaposi's sarcoma
  2. Lymphomas
C. Autoimmune manifestation of HIV infection
  1. Lymphocytic interstitial pneumonitis
  2. Diffuse infiltrative lymphocytosis syndrome (Itescu et al., 1990)
D. Anemia
E. Exercise intolerance

Nursing Assessment:

A. Subjective data
  1. History of problem
  2. Associated symptoms
  3. Presence of associated contributing factors such as smoking, drug use, and pain
  4. Medical and surgical history
  5. Current drug therapy
  6. Self-evaluation by client of ability to dress, bathe, toilet, ambulate, etc.
B. Objective data
  1. Detailed respiratory assessment including observation, palpation, and auscultation

2. Cardiovascular assessment including blood pressure, pulse, and skin color
3. Evaluation of cardiovascular and respiratory system in relation to client's response to simple activities of daily living
4. Situational assessment including living arrangements, presence of significant other(s), and community and social support

Nursing Diagnosis:

Impaired gas exchange related to shortness of breath and/or fatigue

Goals:

After discussing and validating the findings of assessment and the nursing diagnosis the client and the nurse will select interventions to:
A. Identify causative factors related to the perception of breathlessness.
B. Develop and implement a plan of care that will allow maximum independence through pacing activities of daily living to conserve energy.

Interventions and Health Teaching:

A. Minimize factors contributing to the client's perception of shortness of breath.
   1. For smoking:
      a. If client has a need to continue, discourage smoking before eating and before, during, and immediately after performing activities of daily living
      b. Discuss a daily reduction schedule of cigarettes smoked
      c. Consider use of commercial filters to reduce the amount of tar, nicotine, and carbon monoxide inhaled (especially if client uses marijuana)
   2. For inadequate pulmonary hygiene or immobility:
      a. Change position frequently
      b. For immobilized client develop a regimen of frequent coughing and deep breathing exercises
      c. If necessary and not contraindicated, consider use of incentive spirometer and chest physical therapy
      d. Provide adequate hydration: 2.5 to 3 liters of fluid per day: monitor fluid intake and output
      e. If client has productive cough or copious secretions, see "Cough"
B. Develop a plan of care that will minimize client's perception of breathlessness
   1. See "Fatigue"

Referrals:

A. Physical therapist
B. Occupational therapist
C. CNS in HIV disease or respiratory disorders
D. Visiting nurse

Evaluation:

The client will:
A. Identify the contributing factors related to breathlessness
B. Develop a plan of self-care by pacing activities of daily living
C. Verbalize a decrease in the number of times per day breathlessness is experienced

SYMPTOM: **Cough**

Etiology:

A. See "Shortness of Breath"
B. After bronchoscopic procedures

Nursing Assessment:

A. See "Shortness of Breath"
B. Observation of client with chronic coughing

Nursing Diagnosis:

Ineffective airway clearance related to chronic, nonrelieved cough, pain or fear of pain, viscous secretions, or sore throat

Goals:

After discussing and validating the findings of assessment and the nursing diagnosis, the client and nurse will select interventions to:
A. Promote optimum respiratory function
B. Minimize the discomfort associated with chronic cough

Interventions and Health Teaching:

A. Minimize discomfort associated with chronic nonrelieved cough
   1. Encourage client to take cough medications on a scheduled basis rather than p.r.n. and to schedule doses appropriately between, not with, meals
   2. Encourage use of cough drops and tea with lemon and honey

    3. Consider warm saline gargle frequently to soothe sore throat

    4. Avoid oxygen administration without adequate humidification

B. Minimize factors that contribute to cough suppression

    1. If chest pain from chronic, nonrelieved cough is present, medicate on a scheduled basis and not p.r.n.

    2. Demonstrate splinting techniques to minimize pain associated with coughing

C. Minimize cough related to viscous secretions

    1. Hydrate with 2.5 to 3 liters of fluid per day

    2. Assist client in controlled coughing exercise schedule

Referrals:

A. CNS in HIV disease or respiratory disorders

B. Visiting nurse

Evaluation:

The client will:

A. Identify effective cough remedies

B. Demonstrate the ability to cough effectively

C. Verbalize a decrease in the amount of cough experienced daily

SYMPTOM: **Edema**

Etiology:

A. Lymphatic occlusion caused by:

    1. HIV

    2. Kaposi's sarcoma

    3. *Mycobacterium avium-intracellulare*

    4. *Cryptococcus*

    5. *Histoplasma capsulatum*

    6. Epstein-Barr virus

    7. Cytomegalovirus

    8. *Toxoplasma gondii*

B. Vascular invasion by Kaposi's sarcoma

C. Medication side effects

Nursing Assessment:

A. Subjective data

    1. History of edema

    2. Contributing or causative factors

    3. Current drug therapy

4. Dietary intake
5. Limitations of activities of daily living related to immobility
B. Objective data
   1. Observation of edematous areas
   2. Palpation of:
      a. Lymph nodes
      b. Skin for edema
      c. Arterial pulses
   3. Condition of skin over edematous areas
   4. Weighing patient routinely

Nursing Diagnosis:

Fluid volume excess: edema related to excess sodium intake, inadequate lymphatic drainage, and/or venostasis

Goals:

After discussing and validating the findings of assessment and the nursing diagnosis, the client and the nurse will select interventions to:
A. Identify causative factors and methods of reducing the edema
B. Develop a plan of care to protect the skin over edematous areas

Interventions and Health Teaching:

A. Avoid excessive sodium intake
   1. Read labels; look for low-sodium canned products
   2. Avoid convenience snack foods and frozen foods
   3. Substitute other spices for salt
B. Avoid dependent venous pooling
   1. Keep edematous areas above level of heart
      a. Extremities should be extended, not flexed
      b. Affected arm(s) should be in abduction
      c. Affected leg(s) should be completely supported, avoiding pillow placement at pressure points, especially behind the knees
      d. If the face is edematous, the head should be kept elevated while in bed
   2. Reduce potential impediments to venous return
      a. Discourage leg or ankle crossing
      b. Avoid constrictive garments such as girdles, garters, and knee-length socks or stockings
   3. Consider the use of elastic bandages and support hose applied in the morning before getting out of bed

C. Protect the affected area from injury
   1. Examine the skin over edema regularly for circulation and skin discolorations or breakdown
   2. See symptom "Dry Skin"

Referrals:

A. Physical therapist
B. CNS in HIV disease or cardiovascular disorders
C. Visiting nurse

Evaluation:

The client will:
A. Identify factors that increase edema
B. Plan a low-sodium menu for a 24-hour period
C. Demonstrate the ability to provide special skin care to edematous areas
D. Exhibit a decrease in edema

SYMPTOM: **Impaired Vision**

Etiology:

A. Chorioretinitis caused by:
   1. Cytomegalovirus
   2. *Toxoplasma gondii*
   3. *Pneumocystis carinii*
   4. Herpes zoster
   5. *Histoplasma capsulatum*
B. Central nervous system malignancy such as:
   1. Kaposi's sarcoma
   2. Lymphoma
C. Central nervous system infection such as progressive multifocal leukoencephalopathy
D. Side effects of medications

Nursing Assessment:

A. Subjective data
   1. Previous health history related to vision
   2. History of visual impairment
   3. Description of visual impairment limitations on activities of daily living, especially noting:
      a. Housing

  b. Egress from home
  c. Assistance needed
  d. Ability to summon assistance
  e. Ability to feed, bathe, dress, toilet, and medicate self
 4. Current drug therapy
B. Objective data
 1. Examination of cranial nerves II (optic); III, IV, and VI (oculomotor, trochlear, and abducens); V (trigeminal)
 2. Evaluation of ability to:
  a. Negotiate immediate surroundings
  b. Feed self
  c. Bathe self
  d. Dress self
  e. Toilet self
  f. Medicate self

Nursing Diagnoses:

A. *High risk for injury related to sensory (visual) deficit*
B. *Self-care deficit related to inability to feed, bathe, dress, toilet, and medicate self*

Goals:

After discussing and validating the findings of assessment and the nursing diagnosis, the client and the nurse will select interventions to:
A. Identify potential hazards in the environment and methods to avoid injury
B. Maintain maximum independence in activities of daily living

Interventions and Health Teaching:

A. Provide for safety
 1. Orient to unfamiliar surroundings
  a. Explain call system and assess client's ability to use it
  b. Keep bed in lowest position
  c. Assess frequently at night and keep a night light on at all times
  d. Encourage client to ask for assistance at night, especially when first adjusting to impaired vision
 2. Discuss general safety measures for the home
  a. Avoid changing furniture arrangements
  b. Remove hazards such as small, unsecured area rugs, and exposed sharp objects
  c. Avoid smoking when alone or unsupervised

B. Accommodate client with unilateral visual loss by:
   1. Assigning client to a bed in which client's intact visual field is toward the door
   2. Placing overbed table, telephone, call light, etc. on appropriate side of person's bed
C. Minimize sensitivity to light by:
   1. Encouraging the use of sunglasses
   2. Keeping environment dimly lit
   3. Encouraging client to wear brimmed hat when out of doors
   4. Keeping television at low level of brightness
D. Promote independence and assist in relearning activities of daily living
   1. Feeding self
      a. Describe location of utensils when serving food
      b. Describe location of food on a plate referring to clock (e.g., the potatoes are at 12 o'clock, meat at 6 o'clock)
      c. Use "finger foods" for snacks
      d. Use cups or mugs for liquids such as soups
   2. Bathing and grooming self
      a. Arrange equipment according to client's preference and replace in same location when finished with toileting
      b. Consider use of assist devices such as bath bar or shower chair
      c. Provide supervision until client is comfortable performing alone
      d. Encourage short hair styles that require a minimum of care and grooming
      e. Encourage use of electric shaver
   3. Dressing self
      a. Assist client in planning location of clothing
      b. Place matching clothing on same hanger
   4. Toileting self
      a. If bedpan or urinal is necessary, keep accessible at all times
      b. If diarrhea is present, evaluate usefulness of bedside commode
      c. If confusion is present, consider use of external catheter with drainage bag on leg or use of adult diapers
   5. Medicating self
      a. Develop a plan for medication
      b. Frequently review side effects of drugs, such as narcotic analgesics, that may further increase the potential for injury and the need to restrict activities

Referrals:

A. Occupational therapist
B. CNS in HIV disease or neurological disorders

C. Visiting nurse
D. Local organization for the blind

Evaluation:

The client will:
A. Identify potential hazards in the environment
B. Demonstrate the ability to move about the environment safely
C. Demonstrate the ability to feed, bathe, dress, and toilet self
D. Describe a plan for assistance with medication administration and other activities of daily living

SYMPTOM: **Dry and Painful Mouth**

Etiology:

A. Primary infection of HIV
   1. Diffuse infiltrative lymphocytosis syndrome (Itescu et al., 1990)
B. Secondary infections caused by:
   1. *Candida albicans*
   2. Herpes simplex
   3. *Histoplasma capsulatum*
   4. *Mycobacterium avium-intracellulare*
   5. *Cryptococcus neoformans*
   6. Herpes zoster
   7. Papillomavirus
   8. Epstein-Barr virus (causing oral hairy leukoplakia)
C. Malnutrition
D. Dehydration
E. Reaction to drug therapy or local radiation therapy
F. Dentures that fit poorly because of weight loss
G. Mouth breathing
H. Inadequate oral hygiene
I. Continued alcohol and tobacco use
J. Periodontal disease

Nursing Assessment:

A. Subjective data
   1. History of symptoms
   2. Associated symptoms
   3. History of recent nutritional intake
   4. History of oral hygiene habits
   5. Use of alcohol and tobacco

6. Medical and surgical history
7. Current drug therapy
B. Objective data
1. Examination of the lips, tongue, buccal mucosal surfaces, teeth, and dental appliances
2. Assessment for pain

Nursing Diagnosis:

Altered oral mucous membrane related to inadequate oral hygiene and/or stomatitis

Goals:

After discussing the findings of assessment and the nursing diagnosis, the client and the nurse will select interventions to:
A. Establish a routine oral hygiene regimen
B. Minimize the potential for or severity of stomatitis

Interventions and Health Teaching:

A. Implement an oral hygiene regimen
1. Perform oral hygiene with a mirror over sink or with an emesis basin if in bed
2. Remove dental appliances
3. Examine oral cavity with adequate lighting
4. Brush teeth using a soft toothbrush; avoid brushing mucosal surfaces
5. Use sodium bicarbonate made into paste with water in place of toothpaste
6. Use a sponge on a stick (Toothette) or small, soft toothbrush
7. Rinse thoroughly with cool water
8. Floss between teeth
9. Establish this routine after meals and before sleep at night
10. Consider use of denture adhesive for poorly fitting dentures
B. For profound fatigue, or for client who is not interested in changing habits:
1. Consider saline mouth rinses after meals and at bedtime
2. Consult with the physician about ordering an oral pharmacologic rinse such as chlorhexidine (National Institutes of Health, 1990)
C. For oral pain:
1. Provide straws
2. Popsicles and ice can temporarily numb painful lesions
3. Avoid very hot or spicy foods

4. Apply topical agents to control pain before meals
5. Evaluate the need for systemic analgesia

D. For dry mouth:
1. Suggest artificial saliva solutions
2. Keep water near client at all times and encourage client to take sips frequently

E. Provide adequate nutrition and hydration; see "Weight Loss"

Referrals:

A. CNS in HIV disease
B. Dental hygienist
C. Visiting nurse

Evaluation:

The client will:
A. Demonstrate the ability to assess oral cavity before and after hygiene
B. Demonstrate the ability to perform an oral hygiene routine
C. Demonstrate moist, pink, intact mucosal surfaces
D. Verbalize a decrease in perceived symptoms

SYMPTOM: **Bleeding and Bruising**

Etiology:

A. Autoimmune responses to HIV disease
1. Immune thrombocytopenic purpura
2. Lupuslike anticoagulants
B. Vascular invasion by Kaposi's sarcoma
C. Bone marrow suppression resulting from drug therapy

Nursing Assessment:

A. Subjective data
1. History of symptoms
2. Associated symptoms
3. History of skin care and oral hygiene
4. Medical and surgical history
5. Current drug therapy
B. Objective data
1. Examination of mucocutaneous surfaces for bleeding, bruises, and petechiae

Nursing Diagnosis:

Altered health maintenance related to the lack of knowledge of the potential for bleeding

Goals:

After discussing the findings of assessment and the nursing diagnosis, the client and the nurse will select interventions to:
A. Minimize the potential for injury that may result in bleeding
B. Prevent environmental contamination by HIV related to bleeding

Interventions and Health Teaching:

A. Maintain skin integrity; see "Dry Skin and Skin Lesions"
    1. Wear loose clothing
    2. Avoid heavy objects, especially those that may rest and bump against the body (e.g., over-the-shoulder bags)
B. Maintain good oral hygiene
    1. Clients with bleeding gums should not use a toothbrush; they should use nonwaxed dental floss and Toothettes only
    2. See "Dry and Painful Mouth"
C. Maintain nutrition and hydration; see "Weight Loss"
D. Avoid medications that increase the potential for bleeding, such as aspirin products, anticoagulants, phenothiazines, indomethacin, and alcohol (Gannon, 1984)

NOTE: Clients with Hickman and Broviac catheters who require low-dose anticoagulant therapy need additional observation and teaching for bleeding.

E. Prevent environmental contamination with HIV
    1. For clients with continuously bleeding gums an oxygen face tent, lined with several layers of gauze, can be used to prevent blood splash when ambulating and when talking
    2. For rectal bleeding suggest panty-liners to contain bleeding
    3. Clean up splashes and spills with 1:10 dilution of household bleach (5.25% sodium hypochlorite)

Referrals:

A. CNS in HIV disease
B. Visiting nurse

Evaluation:

The client will:
A. Identify factors that increase the potential for bleeding

B. Identify appropriate interventions to decrease bleeding potential
C. Identify the methods for minimizing environmental contamination and the correct method for cleaning up splashes and spills

SYMPTOM: **Fever**

Etiology:

A. Chronic HIV infection
B. Secondary opportunistic infection(s)
C. Diarrhea
D. Dehydration

Nursing Assessment:

A. Subjective data
  1. History of symptom
  2. Associated symptoms
  3. 24-hour dietary history
  4. Medical and surgical history
  5. Current drug therapy
B. Objective data
  1. Vital signs, including temperature, pulse, respiration, and blood pressure
  2. Mental status, including alertness, cognition, and orientation
  3. Skin assessment, including integrity, temperature, turgor, appearance, and signs of injury or infection
  4. Assessment for dehydration including the preceding plus fluid intake and output estimates and urine color, quantity, and consistency

Nursing Diagnoses:

A. *Potential altered body temperature related to infection*
B. *Fluid volume deficit related to abnormal fluid loss*

Goals:

After discussing the finding of assessment and the nursing diagnosis, the client and the nurse will select interventions to:
A. Control fever
B. Replace fluid loss and maintain electrolyte balance

Interventions and Health Teaching:

A. Maintain near normal body temperature
  1. Predetermine with physician the antipyretic of choice
  2. Provide tepid water sponge bath

3. Eliminate excessive clothing and bed covers
4. Maintain bed rest when fever occurs
5. Keep room well aerated and cool
6. Provide plenty of cool liquids to drink (2.5 to 3 liters per day); monitor fluid intake and output
7. Assess client's ability to take and record temperature

B. Increase caloric intake
1. Provide a plan for six feedings distributed over a 24-hour period
2. Provide high-protein, high-calorie nutritional supplements, especially in the presence of anorexia
3. Record food intake on a 24-hour basis

C. Maintain comfort and skin integrity
1. Provide dry clothes and bed linens; use cotton materials rather than synthetics
2. Use lotions and emollient creams for dry skin
3. Provide frequent sponge baths

D. Maintain safety
1. Monitor mental status frequently, especially when client is febrile
2. Evaluate client safety for independent ambulation

E. For chronic recurrent night fever and night sweats:
1. Suggest client take the antipyretic of choice before going to sleep
2. Have a change of bed clothes nearby in case a change is necessary
3. Keep a plastic cover on pillow
4. Place a towel over pillow in case of profuse diaphoresis

Referrals:

A. CNS in HIV disease
B. Dietitian
C. Visiting nurse

Evaluation:

The client will:
A. Identify appropriate measures to be taken in the presence of fever
B. Demonstrate the ability to initiate and maintain adequate hydration and nutrition
C. Demonstrate the ability to take and record the temperature accurately

NOTE WELL: Aspirin is contraindicated in the presence of low platelet counts (a common finding in many HIV-infected persons). Although concern has been expressed about concomitant administration of zidovudine and acetaminophen, Steffe and colleagues (1990) found no significant interaction between the two drugs when given together.

SYMPTOM: **Pain**

Etiology:

A. Localized pain in bone, nerve, and viscera caused by:
1. Tumor invasion
2. Opportunistic infection(s)
B. Generalized arthralgia and myalgia associated with chronic HIV disease
C. Autoimmune response to HIV disease resulting in:
1. Vasculitis
2. Chronic demyelinating neuropathy
3. Inflammatory myopathy

Nursing Assessment:

A. Subjective data
1. History of symptom
2. Associated symptoms
3. Nondrug remedies
4. Limitations of activities
5. Medical and surgical history
6. Current drug therapy
B. Objective data
1. Assess vital signs
2. Assess effect
3. Observe ability and willingness to participate in activities of daily living

Nursing Diagnosis:

Pain related to knowledge deficit of pain control measures

Goals:

After discussing the findings of assessment and the nursing diagnosis, the client and the nurse will select interventions to:
A. Identify factors that increased the perception of pain
B. Reduce the pain experience and improve mobility

Interventions and Health Teaching:

A. Identify aggravating factors
1. Ask client to identify activities of daily living that appear to increase the type and amount of pain perceived

    2. Use a visual analogue scale to rate and record the perception of pain (on a scale of 0 to 10) relating to activities identified in No. 1

B. Maximize comfort and pain control by:

    1. Explaining the need for the client controlling the pain versus the pain controlling the client and give medications on a scheduled basis rather than p.r.n.

    2. Exploring the use of nonmedicinal techniques such as relaxation, visualization, and distraction

    3. Encouraging client to plan activities of daily living in relation to therapeutic schedule (e.g., bathing after taking analgesic or performing relaxation techniques)

    4. Institute comfort measures such as:

        a. Using egg crate mattress, air mattress, etc.

        b. Frequent massage and back rubs

        c. Warm soaks to painful muscles and joints

        d. Ice bag or cold washcloth for headaches

        e. Positioning and supporting limbs comfortably when in bed or sitting up in a chair

        f. Using "pull-sheet" to move patient and change position

    5. Encourage the family or significant other to bring in familiar objects such as:

        a. Pillows and blankets

        b. Pictures

        c. Religious articles

        d. Clothing

        e. Colognes, makeup, powders, etc.

Referrals:

A. Occupational therapist

B. Physical therapist

C. CNS in HIV disease or mental health

D. Visiting nurse

Evaluation:

The client will:

A. Identify aggravating or precipitatory factors related to the pain experienced

B. Identify measures to control pain

C. Verbalize a decrease in the amount and type of pain experienced over a 24-hour period

SYMPTOM: **Motor Impairment**

Etiology:

A. Primary infection of HIV
B. Secondary opportunistic infection
   1. Toxoplasma
   2. JC virus
C. Reiter's syndrome (Winchester et al., 1987)

Nursing Assessment:

A. Subjective data
   1. History of problem
   2. Associated symptoms
   3. Medical and surgical history
   4. Current drug therapy
B. Objective data
   1. Examination of musculoskeletal system
   2. Evaluation of ability to:
      a. Sit
      b. Stand
      c. Transfer
      d. Ambulate
      e. Turn self
      f. Feed self
      g. Bathe self
      h. Dress
      i. Toilet
      j. Self-medicate
   3. Evaluate endurance
   4. Evaluate motivation

Nursing Diagnosis:

Impaired physical mobility related to limited use of upper and/or lower extremities

Goals:

After discussing and validating the findings of assessment and the nursing diagnosis, the client and nurse will select interventions to:
A. Identify potential hazards and the need for appropriate assist devices
B. Maintain maximum independence in activities of daily living

Interventions and Health Teaching:

A. Provide for safety
  1. Identify potential hazards in the home such as:
     a. Area rugs
     b. Sharp objects
     c. Hot objects and liquids
     d. Smoking unattended
  2. Protect areas of decreased or absent sensation with emphasis on avoidance of:
     a. Tight-fitting clothing and shoes
     b. Sitting near radiators or stoves
     c. Using devices such as a heating pad
  3. Assess the need for assist devices, including:
     a. Cane
     b. Walker
     c. Crutches
     d. Wheelchair
     e. Siderails
     f. Bath bar
     g. Shower stool
     h. Hand-held shower
  4. Demonstrate correct use of assist devices
  5. Teach client how to handle urgent situations such as:
     a. Falling
     b. Calling for help
B. Maintain and if possible increase limb mobility
  1. Provide range of motion exercises
     a. Establish a daily schedule for exercise, giving consideration to the individual need for rest periods between activities of daily living
     b. Allow client to perform exercises actively to the extent possible
     c. If pain is present, medicate before exercises
  2. Assess the need for items that promote independence such as:
     a. Shoes and clothing that fasten with Velcro closures
     b. Builtup eating utensils
     c. Speaker telephone
  3. Explain importance of promoting independence to significant other(s), who may wish to do everything for client

Referrals:

A. CNS in HIV disease or rehabilitation
B. Physical therapist

C. Occupational therapist
D. Visiting nurse

Evaluation:

The client will:
A. Identify potential hazards in the environment
B. Describe safety measures to be observed and how to manage urgent situations
C. Demonstrate safe use of assist devices
D. Demonstrate activities to increase mobility

SYMPTOM: **Sexual Dysfunction**

Etiology:

A. Chronic genital lesions (e.g., herpes simplex or Kaposi's sarcoma)
B. Chronic *Candida* vaginitis
C. Physical limitations (e.g., fatigue, shortness of breath, paralysis)
D. Medications
E. Partner unwilling, uninformed, or unavailable
F. Religious conflict
G. Lack of knowledge
H. Pain
I. Substance use
J. Fear of failure
K. Fear of transmitting or acquiring infection
L. Depression

Nursing Assessment (Fogel et al., 1990):

A. Subjective data
   1. History of problem
   2. Desire for sexual experience
      a. Changing patterns: increase or decrease or fluctuations
      b. Concern about adequacy
   3. Concerns about body image and desire to have sex
   4. Current sexual interaction with partner
   5. Initiation of sexual activity
      a. Communication, both verbal and nonverbal
      b. Use of substances (drugs and alcohol)
      c. Use of enhancements (e.g., clothing, sexual devices, videotapes)
   6. Use of fantasy during sexual activities

    7. Sexual dislikes

    8. Sexual experiences with multiple or different partners

    9. Male-specific questions

       a. Erections, quality, failure, and satisfaction with size of penis

       b. Orgasms, frequency, how achieved (by penetration, oral sex, masturbation) and concern over partner reaching climax

       c. Sexual experiences, degree of experimentation

   10. Female-specific question

       a. Facility for vaginal lubrication, sufficient time for lubrication, vaginal pain with penile penetration

       b. Orgasms, frequency and method (masturbation, manual and oral manipulation by partners)

       c. Situations that inhibit orgasms

   11. Presence, absence, or fear of pain

   12. Knowledge of safer sexual practices

   13. Fear of infection

   14. Comfort level with sexual orientation

   15. Sexually related fears (e.g., conflict with religious belief, concern about disease transmission)

   16. Medical and surgical history

   17. Current drug therapy

B. Objective data

   1. Unwillingness to acknowledge problem

   2. Avoidance behaviors when topic is mentioned

   3. Presence of physical limitations (e.g., dyspnea, paralysis)

Nursing Diagnoses:

A. *Altered sexuality patterns related to ineffective coping, change in body part, or fear of disease transmission*

B. *Sexual dysfunction related to physiologic limitations*

Goals:

After discussing and validating the findings of assessment and nursing diagnosis, the client and nurse will select interventions to:

A. Encourage free expression of concerns about sexual activities

B. Minimize fear of sexual experience in the presence of HIV disease

Interventions and Health Teaching (Annon, 1976):

A. Permission: provide a milieu in which client and significant other can freely discuss their sexual feelings and concerns

   1. Assure client that sexuality is an expression of an individual's identity

2. Assess for areas of concern and contributing factors of sexual problems, both psychologic and physical
3. Particularly note any knowledge deficits about sexual practices that may place the client at risk for disease transmission (e.g., exchange of body fluids)
4. Assess for presence of conflicts between sexual practices and client's spiritual beliefs

B. Limited information: provide information relevant to client's concerns; explain effects of HIV disease and client's symptoms, as well as medication effects, on sexual desires and performance

C. Specific suggestions: offer suggestions that can facilitate sexual functioning
1. Concern over having sex when one partner has HIV disease
   a. Explain prevention of harm to client and others during sexual activity through discussion of specific sexual behaviors
   b. Provide resource information on local AIDS support groups and events sponsored for HIV-positive persons
   c. If having sex with a partner is unacceptable to client, consider masturbation
2. Concern over genital lesions or infection
   a. For men, using colored condoms
   b. For women, using a vaginal pouch (sometimes referred to as a female condom)
3. Concern over sexual appeal related to weight loss or to lesions on legs, torso, or arms
   a. Wear garments that may stimulate sexual arousal in both client and partner (allow client and significant other to identify garments that stimulate sexual arousal)
   b. Consider reducing lighting in room when engaging in sexual activities
4. Promote stimulation of all senses and perceptions
   a. Use oils for body rubs and colognes
   b. Consider use of sexually explicit and appealing videotapes
   c. Consider use of sexual devices such as vibrators and dildoes
5. Shortness of breath
   a. Client should remain passive in relation to position changes during sexual activities
   b. Client should avoid lying flat
   c. Use oxygen during sex if needed
   d. Avoid sexual practices (e.g., fellatio) that may interfere with breathing
6. Fatigue
   a. Plan rest before sexual activity
   b. Client should remain passive in relation to positional changes

7. Pain
   a. Assist client in determining best time for medication in relation to sexual activities (e.g., 30 to 60 minutes before)
   b. Use a water-soluble lubricant for intercourse
   c. For localized painful lesions use anesthetic creams or ointments before sexual activity
D. Intensive therapy: when indicated, assist client with referral for counseling and therapy

Referrals:

A. CNS in HIV disease or human sexuality
B. Psychologist or psychiatrist
C. Support groups for persons with HIV disease

Evaluation:

The client will:
A. Discuss sexual concerns and feelings
B. Identify sexual activities that prevent transmission of body fluids during sex
C. Express concerns over changes in body image and identify strategies to cope with the changes
D. Discuss physiological limitations to having sex and strategies to minimize their interference with sex
E. When appropriate, identify the need for further counseling and seek out assistance with referral

SUMMARY

Planning nursing care for clients with or at risk for HIV disease begins with a knowledge of behaviors and activities that place individuals at risk. The findings of this risk assessment are then nonjudgmentally incorporated into all client care. For HIV-positive individuals nursing care focuses on providing information and options to change behavior in order to maintain and improve health. Since HIV disease has no cure, emphasis is placed on reducing symptoms through nursing interventions throughout the spectrum of illness (McMahon & Coyne, 1989).

References

American Nurses Association (1980). Nursing—a social policy statement (Report No. NP-63 22M 11/84R). Kansas City, MO: American Nurses Association.

Annon, J.S. (1976). The PLISS + model: A proposed conceptual scheme for the behavioral treatment of sexual problems. *Journal of Sex Education and Therapy*, 2(1), 211–215.

Berger, T.G. (1990). Dermatologic care in the AIDS patient. In M.A. Sande & P.A. Volberding (Eds.), *The medical management of AIDS* (2nd Ed.) (pp. 114–130). Philadelphia: W.B. Saunders.

Burroughs Wellcome (1990, September). *Changing issues in the management of HIV infection*. New York: World Health Communications.

Carpenito, L.J. (1989). *Nursing diagnosis: application to clinical practice* (3rd Ed.). Philadelphia: J.B. Lippincott.

Centers for Disease Control (1990). Prevention and control of influenza. *Morbidity and Mortality Weekly Report*, 39(RR-7), 1–15.

Crowe, S., Mills, J., McGrath, M.S. (1990). Monocyte/macrophages. In P.T. Cohen, M.A. Sande, & P.A. Volberding (Eds.), *The AIDS knowledge base* (pp. 324.1–324.2). Waltham, MA: Medical Publishing Group.

Culhane, B. (1984). Diarrhea. In J.M. Yasko (Ed.), *Nursing management of symptoms associated with chemotherapy* (pp. 41–47). Reston, VA: Reston Publishing.

Cuzzel, J.Z. (1990). Clues: Itching, burning in skin folds. *American Journal of Nursing*, 90(1), 23–24.

Federation of American Societies for Experimental Biology (1990). *Nutritional therapy and nutritional education in the care and management of AIDS patients* (tentative report). Washington, DC: Center for Food Safety and Applied Nutrition, Food and Drug Administration, Department of Health and Human Services.

Fillit, H., Fruchtman, M.D., Sell, L., et al. (1990). AIDS in the elderly: A case and its implications. *AIDS Patient Care*, 4(1), 8–12.

Fogel, C.I., Forker, J., Welch, M.B. (1990). Sexual health care. In C.I. Fogel & D. Lauver (Eds.), *Sexual health promotion* (pp. 19–38). Philadelphia: W.B. Saunders.

Gannon, C.T. (1984). Bleeding due to thrombocytopenia. In J.M. Yasko (Ed.), *Nursing management of symptoms associated with chemotherapy* (pp. 77–83). Reston, VA: Reston Publishing.

Hargreaves, M.R., Fuller, G.N., Gazzard, B.G. (1988). Occult AIDS: *Pneumocystis carinii* pneumonia in elderly people. *British Medical Journal*, 297(6650), 721–722.

Hecht, F., Soloway, B. (1991). The physical exam in HIV infection. *AIDS Clinical Care*, 3(1), 4–5.

Hernandez, S.R. (1990a). History and physical exam of HIV infected patients. In P.T. Cohen, M.A. Sande, & P.A. Volberding (Eds.), *The AIDS knowledge base* (pp. 421.1–421.7). Waltham, MA: Medical Publishing Group.

Hernandez, S.R. (1990b). Laboratory testing and management of HIV infected patients. In P.T. Cohen, M.A. Sande, & P.A. Volberding (Eds.), *The AIDS knowledge base* (pp. 422.1–422.11). Waltham, MA: Medical Publishing Group.

Hollander, H. (1990). Care of the individual with early HIV infection: Unanswered questions, including the syphilis dilemma. In M.A. Sande & P.A. Volberding (Eds.), *The medical management of AIDS* (2nd Ed.) (pp. 93–102). Philadelphia: W.B. Saunders.

Hotter, A.N. (1990).Wound healing and immunocompromise. *Nursing Clinics of North America*, 25(1), 193–203.

Itescu, S., Brancato, L.J., Buxbaum, J., et al. (1990). A diffuse infiltrative CD_8 lymphocytosis syndrome in human immunodeficiency virus (HIV) infection: A host immune response associated with HLA-DR5. *Annals of Internal Medicine*, 112(1), 3–10.

King, A.B. (1990). Malnutrition in HIV infection: Prevalence, etiology and management. *PACCNOTES*, 2(3), 122–129.

Kotler, D.P., Tierney, A.R., Wang, J., Pierson, R.N., Jr. (1989). Magnitude of body-cell-mass depletion and the timing of death from wasting in AIDS. *American Journal of Clinical Nutrition*, 50(3), 444–447.

McArthur, J. (1990). AIDS dementia: Your assessment can make all the difference. *RN*, 53(3), 36–42.

McDonnell, M., Sevedge, K. (1986). Acquired immune deficiency syndrome (AIDS). In M.H. Brown, M.E. Kiss, E.M. Outlaw, & C.M. Viamontes (Eds.), *Standards of oncology practice* (pp. 565–594). New York: John Wiley & Sons.

McMahon, K.M., Coyne, N. (1989). Symptom management in patients with AIDS. *Seminars in Oncology Nursing, 5*(4), 288–301.

National Institutes of Health (1990). Oral complications of cancer therapies: Diagnosis, prevention, and treatment. *Clinical Courier, 8*(3), 1-8.

Pape, J.W., Johnson, W.D. (1989). HIV-1 infection and AIDS in Haiti. In R.A. Kaslow & D.P. Francis (Eds.), *The epidemiology of AIDS* (pp. 194–221). New York: Oxford University Press.

Soloway, B., Hecht, F. (1990). Identifying patients at risk for HIV infection. *AIDS Clinical Care, 2*(10), 85, 87–88.

Steffe, E.M., King, J.H., Inciardi, J.F., et al. (1990). The effect of acetaminophen on zidovudine metabolism in HIV infected patients. *Journal of Acquired Immunodeficiency Syndromes, 3*(7), 691–694.

Task Force on Nutrition Support in AIDS (1989). Guidelines for nutrition support in AIDS. *Nutrition, 5*(1), 39–46.

Ungvarski, P.J. (1988). Assessment: The key to nursing an AIDS patient. *RN, 51*(9), 28–34.

Ungvarski, P.J. (1989). AIDS dementia complex: Considerations for nursing care. *Journal of the Association of Nurses in AIDS Care, 1*(1), 10–12.

Weiler, P.G., Mungas, D., Pomerantz, S. (1988). AIDS as a cause of dementia in the elderly. *Journal of the American Geriatric Society, 36*(2), 139–141.

Weisman, A.D. (1979). A model for psychological phasing in cancer. *General Hospital Psychiatry, 1,* 187–195.

Winchester, R., Bernstein, D.H., Fischer, H.D., et al. (1987). The co-occurrence of Reiter's syndrome and acquired immunodeficiency. *Annals of Internal Medicine, 106*(1), 19–26.

5

Nursing Care of the Child

Mary G. Boland and Richard Conviser

OVERVIEW

As the decade of the 1990s began, the HIV epidemic was spreading with particular rapidity among infants and children. In the United States the Centers for Disease Control (CDC) recorded its 2500th case of pediatric AIDS during 1990, and experts predict as many as 2.5 million HIV-infected infants and children in the world by the end of the decade (Chin, 1990). Although in the mid-1980s cases of pediatric AIDS in the United States were concentrated in urban centers in New York, New Jersey, and Florida, by 1990 the pediatric HIV epidemic had begun to reach into rural areas and the country's heartland (Arpadi & Caspe, 1990). In one of the urban areas where the epidemic was most advanced, blinded seroprevalence studies conducted by the CDC between 1988 and 1990 showed 0.5% of newborn infants testing positive for HIV antibodies and infection rates approaching 8% in one group of women of childbearing age. In the country as a whole, through 1989, the risk of AIDS in black women was more than 13 times as high as that in white women, and the risk for Hispanic women was more than 8 times as high (Lambert, 1990).

Transmission

Many of the earliest cases of pediatric AIDS in the United States resulted from the use of infected blood in transfusions and in blood products administered to people with hemophilia. Since the screening of blood

199

and treatment of blood products began in 1985, however, the vast majority of pediatric HIV infection in the United States has been a result of perinatal transmission. This is most often related to the use of intravenous drugs by the infant's mother or heterosexual transmission of HIV to the mother from a sexual partner who has injected illicit drugs. Several cases of HIV infection have also been traced to transmission through breast feeding. In addition, a very small proportion of the cases of HIV infection among children has resulted from sexual abuse.

In Europe the vectors of transmission for pediatric HIV infection have been similar to those in the United States. Through mid-1990, the World Health Organization (WHO) had reported more than 1500 cases of AIDS among children under 13 years of age in 32 European countries, representing more than 4% of all reported AIDS cases in these countries (World Health Organization, 1990). In other parts of the world, heterosexual transmission of HIV among adults (unrelated to drug use) has been a chief contributor to the pediatric HIV epidemic. Public health authorities have estimated that in some African countries 5% to 10% of women of child-bearing age are HIV infected (Eckholm & Tierney, 1990). The spread of the epidemic in Third World and Eastern European countries has been quickened by the reuse of unsterilized needles and syringes. (Despite the apparently small risk of pediatric HIV infection from breast milk, breast feeding is still advised where children face more serious health risks from the use of infant formula made with unsafe water supplies.) In short, health care and social service professionals the world over will be called on to care for HIV-infected infants and children as long as the epidemic continues.

Prognosis

Until recently the prognosis for infected children was generally poor: without medical intervention, most perinatally infected children had symptoms of HIV infection within a year, and most with HIV-related conditions survived for less than 3 years (Pollock & Boland, 1990). In a far smaller proportion of children, disease manifestations did not become evident for as long as 9 years (Auger et al., 1988). The speed with which HIV-related illnesses develop may be related to the mode of transmission of the disease, with symptoms developing most quickly in perinatally infected children (Rogers et al., 1987). That symptoms of HIV infection generally develop so much more rapidly in infants than in adults may be attributed to the infants' immature immune systems. However, there are growing indications that early intervention and prophylaxis for infected infants and children can allow their more normal development, forestalling the onset and lessening the effects of life-threatening conditions (Pizzo, 1989). The antiretroviral drug zidovudine (azidothymidine, AZT) has been approved for use with children, and children have also become increasingly involved in clinical trials of other drugs with immunomodulating and prophylactic effects. Clinical care and research have become more closely intertwined as the medical community searches for a definitive treatment for HIV.

Diagnosis

The identification of HIV-infected infants is complicated by the fact that infants receive maternal antibodies to HIV transplacentally and retain them for up to 15 months. Because current tests for HIV infection detect HIV antibodies rather than the virus itself, virtually all infants born to infected mothers initially test positive for HIV. However, evidence suggests that HIV infection will develop in only about 20% to 50% of these infants (Semprini et al., 1987; Gonik & Hammill, 1990). The remainder will seroconvert, eventually showing no signs of HIV antibody or—in the vast majority of cases—of HIV infection. The stages of pregnancy or delivery at which infants can become infected are not yet known, although signs of infection have been detected in fetal tissues as early as 13 weeks after conception (Falloon et al., 1989).

There are several ways to obtain information about which infants are infected and would benefit from early intervention to slow the progression of HIV disease. Knowledge of the HIV status of all pregnant women would help health care professionals know which infants are at risk for HIV. For this reason many public health officials have recommended that testing be offered routinely, particularly for women whose histories indicate a risk of exposure to HIV. For other women of childbearing age, knowledge of their serostatus could have an important influence on their decisions whether to bear children. In general, HIV symptoms in infants and children are different from those in adults. Among the HIV-related symptoms often seen in children are recurrent fever, serious bacterial infections, failure to thrive, developmental delay, and loss of developmental milestones. Health care workers who know how HIV infection manifests itself among children can conduct regular medical checkups to look for those manifestations. Such checkups also allow health professionals to monitor growth and development, provide appropriate immunizations, and perform laboratory evaluations of immune function. Children born to drug-addicted mothers may also show symptoms of developmental delay resulting from addiction or withdrawal. In children as in adults, HIV infection leaves all organ systems susceptible to illness. Several specialized tests, described later in the chapter, can provide direct evidence of HIV infection, in contrast to the evidence of antibody formation provided by the standard enzyme-linked immunosorbent assay (ELISA) and Western blot test.

Care Delivery

Infected children have a better quality of life when as much of their care as possible is administered at home and in community-based settings. As noted previously, however, a majority of infected children in the United States are from families in which one or both parents are infected. As both a cause and a consequence of injected drug use, these families are often disorganized and have poor access to health care (including prenatal care), substandard housing, inadequate nutrition, and little money. Moreover, one or both parents may already have HIV-related illnesses in addition to their drug addictions, rendering them psychologically unwilling or physically unable to care for their children. In such cases foster care may be necessary; it is often available from members of the extended family. In contrast, some infected mothers dedicate themselves to the care of their ailing children and neglect their own need for services (Abrams & Nicholas, 1990). All of these factors complicate the delivery of care to HIV-infected children. The development of comprehensive networks of community-based, family-centered, multidisciplinary services can help deliver care to both infected children and their mothers.

Role of Nurses

Nurses have played a central role in building and staffing networks for HIV-infected infants, children, and their families. The range of services needed by infected families is broad and may include home care, hospice care, counseling, nutrition, housing, transportation, financial and legal assistance, many forms of outpatient care and therapy, and inpatient care. Hospital- and community-based nurses can contribute to the success of patient outcomes by functioning as case managers who quickly link children and their families with the services they need. (Pollock & Boland, 1990). Nurses can also provide the support and educational services that help make adult family members (whether natural, foster, or extended) part of the child's primary caregiving team, promoting the normal growth and development of both infected children and their siblings.

Progress in the development of antiretroviral and prophylactic drugs for infected children will increase their life spans substantially. Longer survival will create a demand for health and social services over an extended period and in an increasing variety of settings, including long-term care facilities, day care centers, and schools. To protect infected children against prejudice and discrimination, and to protect themselves against infection, workers in these settings will need accurate information about HIV transmission and must be comfortable working with infected children. Nurses can play an important role in providing authoritative information and reshaping the attitudes of others who work with infected children. In addition, nurses will continue to be a key source of support in providing critical services and comfort to this newest population of chronically ill children.

NATURAL HISTORY OF HIV INFECTION IN CHILDREN

Most of the studies of perinatal HIV transmission rates, which report the development of HIV disease in 20% to 50% of infants born to infected mothers, have been based on small, retrospectively obtained samples (Blanche et al., 1989; Johnson et al., 1989; Ryder et al., 1989; Gonik & Hammill, 1990; Prieto & Hansen, 1990). Recent prospective studies suggest that the overall figure is likely to be 30% or less (Andiman et al., 1990). Why some children of infected mothers become infected and others do not is not yet known. Possibly children of symptomatic mothers are more likely to be infected than those of asymptomatic mothers (Lambert, 1990). However, the chance that a child will be infected appears to be independent of whether the mother has previously given birth to an infected child (Boland & Klug, 1986). Delivery by cesarean section also appears to make no difference in the perinatal infection rate (Semprini et al., 1987; Falloon et al., 1989). Scientists are attempting to discover how and when infants are infected during the course of pregnancy and delivery. Such a discovery might allow the timely administration of drugs to pregnant women to prevent prepartum or intrapartum transmission of HIV.

Initially HIV-infected infants were thought to have a visible dysmorphism, but more recent studies have shown no significant physical differences between infected and noninfected infants at birth; dysmorphism appears to be related instead to maternal intravenous drug use (Johnson et al., 1989; Lambert, 1990). Because HIV suppresses the immune system, the range of symptoms in children is broad. Many of the opportunistic infections that affect immunosuppressed adults—for example, *Pneumocystis carinii* pneumonia (PCP), toxoplasmosis, tuberculosis, cryptococcosis, and histoplasmosis—are reactivations of conditions that had been held in check by healthy immune systems before the onset of HIV disease. Such opportunistic infections are less common in children, but when they do occur, they typically represent initial infection rather than reactivation of latent infection (Falloon et al., 1989).

HIV-Related Abnormalities

In children as in adults, HIV affects all of the organ systems. Generalized lymphadenopathy is a common abnormality in HIV-infected children, and many children with this condition also have splenomegaly. Hepatomegaly commonly occurs late in the child's first year. Skin conditions are also common, especially candidiasis and seborrheic rash (from either unidentifiable chronic infection or circulating immune complexes) (Johnson et al., 1989). *Candida* esophagitis occurs frequently, interfering with nutrition by making swallowing painful. Failure to thrive (Rogers, 1985) may be related to anemia, recurrent diarrhea, and gastrointestinal problems. Children with HIV may have infections caused by unusual enteric pathogens, including *Cryptosporidium*, persistent adenovirus infection, and cytomegalovirus (CMV) enteritis (Johnson et al., 1989).

HIV-infected children have a high incidence of lower respiratory tract infections, especially PCP and bacterial pneumonia. Lymphoid interstitial pneumonitis (LIP) affects as many as half of HIV-infected children (Falloon et al., 1989). Sinusitis and chronic otitis media are also found. Neurologic disorders are often subtle in their initial manifestations, but one study identified such problems by 6 months of age in half of HIV-infected infants, several of whom had no other evidence of associated immunodeficiency disease at the time (Johnson et al., 1989). Infants with HIV infection appear to be particularly susceptible to encephalopathy, which is manifested in developmental delays, a deterioration of motor skills and intellectual abilities, and abnormal behaviors (Falloon et al., 1989; Pizzo, 1989). Malignancies and susceptibility to unusual bacterial infections are also typical manifestations of HIV in children. Serious infections such as sepsis, pneumonia, meningitis, abscesses, and cellulitis are often among the early symptoms of pediatric HIV infection (Falloon et al., 1989).

Classification of Pediatric HIV

The CDC has issued several classification schemes for pediatric HIV infection. The system currently in use, issued in 1987, was developed for epidemiologic purposes. It classifies pediatric infection according to the presentation of symptoms, and it does not necessarily correlate with stage of illness (Arpadi & Caspe, 1990; Boland, 1990). Shown in Table 5–1, the system identifies three broad classes of infection—indeterminate, asymptomatic, and symptomatic—and divides the latter two into subclasses. Although class P-2 does not explicitly distinguish CDC-defined AIDS from other symptomatic conditions, the CDC defines pediatric AIDS to include opportunistic infection and wasting syndrome, LIP, progressive enceph-

TABLE 5–1. Summary of Classification of HIV Infection in Children Under 13 Years of Age

Class P-0	Indeterminate infection
Class P-1	Asymptomatic infection
Subclass A	Normal immune function
Subclass B	Abnormal immune function
Subclass C	Immune function not tested
Class P-2	Symptomatic infection
Subclass A	Nonspecific findings
Subclass B	Progressive neurologic disease
Subclass C	Lymphoid interstitial pneumonitis
Subclass D	Secondary infectious diseases
Category D-1	Specified secondary infectious disease listed in the CDC surveillance definition for AIDS
Category D-2	Recurrent serious bacterial infections
Category D-3	Other specified secondary infectious diseases
Subclass E	Secondary cancers
Category E-1	Specified secondary cancers listed in the CDC surveillance definition for AIDS
Category E-2	Other cancers possibly secondary to HIV infection
Subclass F	Other diseases possibly due to HIV infection such as hepatitis, cardiopathy, nephropathy, hematologic (anemia, thrombocytopenia), dermatologic diseases

From Centers for Disease Control (1987). Classification system for human immunodeficiency virus (HIV) infection in children under 13 years of age. *Morbidity and Mortality Weekly Report, 36,* 225–230.

alopathy, and malignancy. These AIDS-defining conditions correspond to P-2 subclasses D, C, B, and E-1, respectively.

Disease Course

Several studies that have traced the natural history of HIV infection in groups of children show that the disease does not follow any single course (Mok et al., 1987; Rogers et al., 1987; Krasinski et al., 1989; Scott et al., 1989). The most complete published natural history data come from two studies, each of which analyzed infected children treated at a single institution. A more accurate picture of the natural history of HIV infection in children awaits the publication of large longitudinal studies with data pooled from many hospitals (Krasinski et al., 1989). However, the two published studies are worth exploring; they show that both age at diagnosis of HIV infection and presenting diagnosis of opportunistic infections or neoplasms affect the course of HIV disease in infected children.

One of the studies examined 172 children treated at a Miami hospital between 1979 and 1987 (Scott et al., 1989). All of these children were infected perinatally; 69% of their mothers were infected heterosexually, and of these, 74% were Haitian born. The ages of children at diagnosis ranged from 1 to 100 months, with a median age of 8 months. In more than half (57%) HIV infection was diagnosed in the first year of life, and in 79% it was diagnosed before the second birthday. Fifteen percent of the children died in their first year; in subsequent years the mortality rate was lower. The median age at death was 77 months, and the median survival time from diagnosis was 38 months. The latter contrasts with an earlier, more pessimistic estimate of 9 months' survival from early CDC epidemiologic data (Falloon et al., 1989).

The other study, at a New York hospital, examined records for 111 children and adolescents whose HIV infection was diagnosed between 1980 and 1988; 86% were perinatally infected (Krasinski et al., 1989). Among those with perinatal infections, survival times ranged from 2.5 to 124 months, with a median age at death of 23 months. The mean survival time for perinatally infected children was 67 months, in contrast to a mean survival time of 90 months for children who were infected by transfusion when they were over 2 years of age. These findings complement those from an earlier CDC study showing that the interval between infection and evidence of disease was shorter for children infected perinatally than for children infected by transfusion (Rogers et al., 1987; Falloon et al., 1989).

The Miami study examined the diagnosis and survival times of children whose initial diagnosis was one or more of seven patterns of disease: PCP, encephalopathy, recurrent bacterial infections (RBIs), *Candida* esophagitis, cardiomyopathy, renal disease, or LIP. Sixty percent of the children had at least one of these conditions; 5% had other conditions leading to an AIDS diagnosis, such as disseminated CMV, disseminated herpes simplex, or cerebral toxoplasmosis; and the remaining 35% had less specific findings, including failure to thrive. The condition most likely to occur first was LIP, which affected 30% of the sample; in children with LIP the median survival time was 72 months and PCP was unlikely to develop. Yet another study showed a median survival time from birth of 91 months for children with LIP, making it one of the less immediately life-threatening conditions (Thomas et al., 1987).

PCP was most often an initial disease presentation in the Miami study, and it was associated with a median survival time from diagnosis of just 1 month. (Unpublished data from other institutions show a marginally higher median survival time for children with PCP but confirm the relatively poor prognosis of these children.) Encephalopathy, renal disease, and *Candida* esophagitis all had median survival times from diagnosis of less than 1 year, and the median survival time from a diagnosis of RBI was 50 months. (The survival time for encephalopathy may be underestimated because this condition is sometimes difficult to detect initially.) Cardiomyopathy never appeared in the Miami sample as the initial pattern of illness, and renal disease seldom did. These data show a considerable diagnosis-related variation in the survival times of HIV-infected children. Moreover, even in the absence of antiretroviral and prophylactic therapy, half of the children in each study lived to more than 5 years of age. The findings from these studies underscore the need to develop health care delivery systems that manage pediatric HIV as a chronic illness.

MANAGEMENT OF CLINICAL MANIFESTATIONS OF HIV IN CHILDREN

Diagnosis of HIV in Infants

HIV-exposed infants can be identified at birth if pregnant women are tested. For this reason public health officials increasingly recommend voluntary confidential testing for all pregnant women and those contemplating pregnancy, particularly if they have a history of risk activity. Such testing should always be accompanied by culturally sensitive counseling, both before tests are conducted and when the results are given. At a minimum, pretest counseling should clarify that the test is for HIV infection, how HIV infection is related to AIDS, why the test is desirable, and what its possible outcomes and consequences are. Techniques to prevent HIV transmission can also be discussed at counseling sessions. Before an infant is tested the consent of a parent or guardian (or a child protective agency, when appropriate) should be obtained. Test results should be given only in person to the test subject (in the case of infants, the caregiver), and their implications should be carefully explored. Chapter 6 discusses HIV antibody test counseling, risks, and benefits in detail.

Because infants retain maternal HIV antibodies for as long as 15 months after birth, the standard ELISA and Western blot test used to diagnose HIV infection in older children and adults yield indeterminate results for infants. Consequently, a variety of other diagnostic tools are used to detect HIV infection in infants. These are often employed in combination and with clinical and nonspecific laboratory parameters. Among the diagnostic tools currently in use or development are detection of HIV antigen, viral culture, serial antibody determinations, and polymerase chain reaction (PCR) (Husson et al., 1990). Although some of these tools do not provide definitive diagnoses, their use is important. Because of the toxicities associated with antiviral and prophylactic treatments, these should be given only to truly infected infants and children, not to all children in whom infection is suspected. Early intervention can be of substantial benefit to children in whom the tests detect HIV infection.

Antigen Testing. One approach to diagnosing HIV infection in infants is to look for the presence of a specific HIV antigen (p24) in blood or tissue specimens. The level of this antigen, however, varies with the amount of virus in the subject, making it particularly difficult to detect in the early, asymptomatic phase of HIV infection. Many infants and children with indeterminate infection status fit into this category. Despite this, a positive antigen test may be indicative of HIV infection, especially when there are other positive tests or clinical signs of immunocompromise.

Viral Culture. Another approach to testing infants is coculturing of peripheral blood mononuclear cells with uninfected mononuclear cells that can support HIV growth. HIV presence in such samples can be determined through measurement of p24 antigen or reverse transcriptase activity. Viral cultures have yielded positive results in more than 90% of infected adults regardless of their stage of infection. However, because this method has failed to detect infection in close to 10% of infected adult subjects, cultures negative for HIV in infants do not definitively rule out HIV infection.

Antibody Detection. Maternal immunoglobulin HIV antibody of class G (IgG) is present in infants of infected mothers. However, class M and A antibodies (IgM and IgA) are not passed transplacentally; thus any IgM and IgA antibodies found in infants can be taken as signs of HIV infection. These antibodies can be detected through modifications of ELISA and immunoblot antibody testing techniques. However, IgM and IgA antibodies are often transient and are present only in low concentrations. Therefore serial testing should be done for these antibodies, and their absence cannot rule out HIV infection in infants (Husson et al., 1990). An alternative approach to antibody testing currently under development differentiates between IgG antibodies of maternal and infant origins by means of isoelectric focusing or titer differences. Also being developed is a way of detecting HIV antibody produced in vitro by the infant's lymphocytes.

Polymerase Chain Reaction. PCR amplifies specific nucleic acid sequences, such as HIV proviral DNA, facilitating their detection. This technique's sensitivity in diagnosing HIV has been greater in adults than in infants, especially those in whom AIDS does not develop in the first year of life. Also, viral levels in the months immediately following birth are often below the current limits of detection of the PCR assay. Moreover, the PCR technique sometimes yields false-negative results and discordant results are sometimes obtained from the same sample (Bremer & Hollinger, 1990; Husson et al., 1990). Therefore this technology still cannot diagnose HIV infection definitively.

CD4 Counts. Combinations of these experimental tests, along with nonspecific laboratory tests for immunoglobulin levels and T cells, are often used to detect HIV infection in infants. The nonspecific tests can be ordered by pediatricians and performed at many local laboratories; experimental tests may be available only at referral centers. Although HIV-infected children often have hypergammaglobulemia, they show poor humoral responses (Bye & Bernstein, 1989). In T4 (CD4 +) tests, counts less than 500 cells/mm³ are generally taken to indicate serious immunocompromise in HIV-infected adults (contrasting with normal counts in the 600 to 1200 range); the onset of opportunistic illnesses (such as PCP) in adults typically occurs among those with counts below 200 cells/mm³. PCP also occurs frequently in adults whose CD4 + cells account for less than 20% of their circulating lymphocytes (Leibovitz et al., 1990). However, adult CD4 + count standards appear to be far too low to signify immunocompromise in infants and young children. In one study of perinatally infected young children with definitively diagnosed PCP, CD4 + counts were found to be between 200 and 1700 (Connor et al., 1991). CD4 + counts in uninfected newborn infants may be as high as 3500 and decrease to 1500 to 2000 within 2 years (Leibovitz et al., 1990). This has led investigators to suggest that CD4 + counts less than 1500 be taken to indicate immunocompromise in children under 1 year of age and that counts less than 1000 be considered evidence of HIV infection in at-risk children aged 1 to 2 years. In a healthy individual the ratio of T4 (helper) to T8 (suppressor) cells is generally about 2:1. A T4/T8 ratio below 1 is another indicator of immune dysfunction.

Other Indicators. In addition to depressed CD4 + levels, nonspecific clinical findings that suggest an HIV diagnosis include hepatomegaly, splenomegaly, or lymphadenopathy; hypergammaglobulinemia; nonspecific pulmonary infiltrates; and opportunistic infections in the absence of other causes of immunodeficiency (Husson et al., 1990). Table 5–2 lists

TABLE 5–2. Possible Indicators of Pediatric HIV Infection

MEDICAL HISTORY	PHYSICAL EXAMINATION	LABORATORY RESULTS
Recurrent fever	Failure to maintain percentiles or gain weight	Anemia
Serious bacterial infections	Failure to grow in length or head circumference	Liver function elevations
Recurrent otitis media	Diaper dermatitis or condyloma	Hypergammaglobulinemia Hyperproteinemia
Recurrent or chronic oral thrush	Candida or seborrhea	Leukopenia
Recurrent or chronic diarrhea	Otitis media, rhinitis, parotitis	Thrombocytopenia
Monilial diaper rash	Generalized lymphadenopathy (>0.5 cm significant)—cervical, axillary, or inguinal	Evidence of p24 antigen, IgM or IgA antibodies, viral culture, other positive experimental test results, or low CD4 count
Lymphadenopathy	Hepatomegaly	
Parotitis	Splenomegaly	
Failure to thrive	Loss of developmental milestones	
Poor feeding	Clubbing	
Microcephaly		
Developmental delay		

conditions suggestive of HIV infection that can be detected through medical histories, physical examinations, and laboratory tests. Many of these conditions may have causes other than HIV, but their presence should raise the index of suspicion that a young child is infected, especially when other indicators of infection are present. The prolonged indeterminate HIV status of an infant is a source of stress for the family and caregivers, even when the infant eventually becomes seronegative. Nurses should thus be aware of the need for strong medical and social support systems to help families cope with the immediate and the long-term implications of an HIV diagnosis.

Immunization and Care of Children with Indeterminate HIV Status or No Symptoms

Immunization. Infants whose mothers tested positive prenatally and those who test positive for HIV antibody by ELISA and Western blot test in the newborn period should be watched closely for the signs of immunocompromise listed in Table 5–2. If an infant is well and presents no physical symptoms or laboratory findings associated with HIV infection, it is impossible to know whether infection is present. Viral cultures and other immunologic studies should be performed during the first few months of their lives, and depending on the results, ELISA and the immunoblot test, as well as experimental tests, should be performed every 3 to 6 months until they are 2 years old. Because HIV-infected children are particularly susceptible to disease, all at-risk children should be immunized against childhood diseases, following the schedule of the American Academy of Pediatrics (AAP) with inactivated polio vaccine (Salk) substituted for oral vaccine (Sabin). AAP recommendations for the immunization of HIV-infected children are shown in Table 5–3.

TABLE 5–3. Recommended Routine Immunizations for HIV-Infected Children in the United States

VACCINE	RECOMMENDATION
Diphtheria, tetanus toxoids, pertussis	Yes
Oral poliovirus vaccine	No
Inactivated poliovirus vaccine	Yes
Live virus measles, mumps, and rubella	Yes
Haemophilus diphtheria toxoid conjugate vaccine	Yes
Pneumococcal	Yes
Influenza	Yes if symptomatic; considered if asymptomatic

From Peters G. (Ed.) (1988). Reprinted with permission from Report of the Committee on Infectious Diseases. Copyright © 1991 American Academy of Pediatrics.

HIV-infected children who have been exposed to such diseases as measles should be immunized within 72 hours of exposure, even if they have not yet reached the normal age for immunization. Parents should report varicella (chickenpox) exposure immediately, and HIV-infected children should receive varicella zoster immune globulin (VZIG) within 96 hours of exposure to prevent or modify infection. Nurses must be aware that VZIG prolongs the incubation period to 10 to 28 days. Normally varicella virus is controlled by cell-mediated immune mechanisms. In children with immune impairment, however, it can cause prolonged and disseminated morbidity, with complications including neurologic encephalitis and pneumonia. Its symptoms include pruritic vesicular rash on the face, scalp, and trunk; these may be preceded by systemic symptoms including fever, chills, myalgia, and arthralgia. Treatment is by intravenous acyclovir, 10 mg/kg administered every 8 hours for 5 to 7 days until lesions dry. This decreases pain and hastens healing. Side effects of acyclovir include renal toxicity and an increase in serum creatinine level. Immunocompromised children who have had varicella are at risk for its reactivation as herpes zoster (shingles), which can be severe and disseminated. Zoster in children is treated with intravenous acyclovir, 10 mg/kg every 8 hours for 5 to 7 days or until lesions dry.

For most at-risk children, immunization recommendations for healthy children should be followed. For those less than 3 years old, doses are sometimes divided and given in several administrations. In immunocompromised children, immunization may not produce functioning antibody but may result in symptoms of infection (Borkowsky et al., 1987). (This result may be a further indication of immunocompromise.) For children with documented humoral or antibody deficiencies, many physicians recommend intravenous immune globulin infusions every 3 to 4 weeks to provide antibodies. The study of this practice is ongoing, and no data are available yet to document its effectiveness; practitioners have varying opinions about its appropriateness.

Home Care. Illnesses contracted by children with indeterminate HIV status and those with asymptomatic HIV infection (CDC classes P-0 and P-1, respectively) rarely require hospitalization; most of their care can be given on an outpatient basis. The major goal of care for children with asymptomatic HIV infection is to prevent infections and opportunistic illnesses, through both supportive care and prophylaxis. Educating parents or other caregivers about supportive care is basic and important. Topics covered should include handwashing; bathing children regularly (daily or every other day); keeping their skin clean and dry, especially in the diaper area; moisturizing skin in other areas to prevent it from cracking and itching, thus preventing fungal infections and impetigo; changing diapers; and cleaning bottles. Nurses can be instrumental in providing this education and can also sensitize caregivers to the signs and symptoms of infection that should lead them to seek medical attention (Table 5–2).

Prophylaxis. Prophylaxis is intended to prevent primary or recurrent infection in children known to be HIV infected. Although studies of prophylaxis for PCP have not yet been conducted on children, results in adults have shown aerosolized pentamidine and trimethoprim-sulfamethoxazole (TMP-SMX; Bactrim, Septra) to be effective in both preventing the onset of PCP and reducing its morbidity and mortality. TMP-SMX can also prevent recurrent otitis media and other infections in children. Other prophylactic and antiviral therapies for children are discussed later in the chapter.

Care and Disease Prevention in Symptomatic Children

Immune Function, Nutrition, and Infection. A child's immune function interacts with his or her nutrition and infection status: if one of them is impaired, the others tend to worsen as well. For example, malnutrition impairs immune function (even in a healthy child), and an immune deficiency (an inability to produce functioning antibody) increases the risk of infection. Infections in immunocompromised children have more rapid onset and greater severity than in normal children; they also typically involve more than one infectious agent.

Age and Symptoms. Symptoms and their presentation vary by age among HIV-infected children. Infants frequently have recurrent infections of bacterial, fungal, or protozoal origins. In early childhood most infections are bacterial and not life threatening; they should generally be handled the way they are for young children who are not immunocompromised. Few adolescents have thus far shown symptoms of HIV infection, so its modes of presentation in this population are still largely unknown. Early experience with adolescents suggests that opportunistic infections are often the first symptoms of HIV disease. As in adults, these often involve reactivations of infectious agents already carried, such as PCP, sexually transmitted diseases, tuberculosis, toxoplasmosis, and *Mycobacterium avium-intracellulare* (MAI) infection. In female adolescents, as in older women, gynecologic symptoms—including sexually transmitted diseases—may be the first signs of HIV infection, but health care workers have often overlooked their significance (New Jersey Women and AIDS Network, 1990).

Hospitalization. When infected children are hospitalized, the risk for nosocomially transmitted infections should be recognized. Following universal precautions in the handling of blood and body fluids from these patients is critical. Handwashing between patients is the single most effective way of preventing the spread of disease. An HIV-infected child admitted with a diagnosis of possible infection should be given a private room for 24 to 48 hours or until a definitive etiology or agent has been ruled out. HIV-infected children who are hospitalized with a noninfectious process or are completing treatment for an infectious disease do not need a private room. However, most institutions still place such children by themselves or in a room with other HIV-infected children.

Acute Treatment. For acute treatment of children thought to have infectious conditions, diagnosis is often the most challenging problem. Many times such children run a fever but no infectious agent can be identified. It is appropriate to treat these children with empiric therapy and broad-spectrum coverage for 3 to 5 days. Generally one sees a result in such cases because a viral agent simply has run its course. However, infectious organisms can rarely be eradicated in an immunocompromised child; once treatment is halted, the organism reappears. Pending diagnosis, treatment should cover organisms associated with B cell defects, such as *Staphylococcus aureus*, *Streptococcus pneumoniae*, and *Haemophilus influenzae*. If an agent is identified for which there is no definitive treatment, supportive or symptomatic treatment can be given.

Need for Ongoing Treatment. Once an agent of opportunistic infection has been identified, lifelong treatment will be required. For some opportunistic infections no treatment is currently available; for others, existing experimental treatments often have side effects. Decisions about what course to follow should be discussed between the physician and the parents or other caregivers. Factors to be taken into account include the child's overall medical condition, the accessibility of treatment, the ability of parents or caregivers to administer necessary treatment, the stage of illness of the child, the family's ability to obtain needed services, the financial impact of treatment decisions on the family, and the impact of these decisions on the quality of the child's life. The nurse can play an important role in working with the family to provide information and validate the impact of treatment. Because nurses often understand better than physicians how treatment will affect the lives of the child and the family, they should be actively involved in decision making.

As a child's degree of immunocompromise increases, more frequent hospitalizations will be required. Among children with less severe symptoms, most conditions can be treated on an outpatient basis. However, once AIDS has developed, it is not unusual for a child to be hospitalized as many as three times in a year for the treatment of acute illnesses. Each hospitalization forces families to confront anew the uncertain outcome of the illness (Boland & Klug, 1986).

SPECIFIC INFECTIONS AND MALIGNANCIES IN SYMPTOMATIC CHILDREN

Bacterial Infections

Bacterial and fungal skin infections have been noted at many sites in HIV-infected children. The most recent (1987) CDC definition of AIDS-related conditions among children less than 13 years of age includes at least two multiple or recurrent bacterial infections within 2 years, excluding skin and otitis media. Because of secondary impaired humoral response, HIV-infected children are susceptible to both gram-positive and gram-negative bacterial infections, and these can become acute if treatment is absent or incomplete. Bacterial infections affect a variety of organ systems, including the skin, respiratory system, gastrointestinal tract, and blood.

Common skin infections include cellulitis and abscess caused by *Staphylococcus* and *Streptococcus*; the latter is the bacterial pathogen most frequently identified in children with HIV disease and is often implicated in pneumonia and bacteremia (Hauger & Powell, 1990). Skin infections may follow bites, eczema, or the insertion of catheters. Sinopulmonary complications include chronic otitis media, sinusitis, and pneumonia; chronic recurrent pneumonia predisposes some children to chronic lung diseases such as bronchiectasis. In the gastrointestinal tract, diarrhea is the most common symptom, and infectious agents are usually opportunistic, including CMV, *Salmonella*, *Cryptosporidium*, MAI, and *Giardia*. In the blood, any bacterial agent (e.g., *Haemophilus influenzae*) can cause sepsis. Blood infections often occur secondarily in children hospitalized for acute infections. Like other bacterial infections, they are appropriately treated with antibiotics administered for the maximum "normal" time with follow-up to ensure that the infection has been resolved. When care is given at home, nurses can teach parents or other caregivers to administer medication.

Opportunistic Infections

Infectious agents that present no threat to people with healthy immune systems can cause serious damage in immunocompromised individuals. Table 5–4 lists some of the common sources of opportunistic infection in infants and children with HIV disease and typical therapeutic responses. A more detailed discussion of several of these infections follows.

***Pneumocystis carinii* Pneumonia.** The protozoan that causes PCP is commonly found in air, water, and soil (although some geographic vari-

TABLE 5–4. Opportunistic Infections in Infants and Children with HIV Disease

OPPORTUNISTIC INFECTION	THERAPY	COMMENTS
Pneumocystis carinii pneumonia (PCP)	Trimethoprim-sulfamethoxazole (TMP-SMX) Pentamidine Dapsone	Prophylaxis indicated in children with immunocompromise Post-infection prophylaxis indicated Diagnosis established by bronchoalveolar lavage or open lung biopsy
Candida esophagitis (thrush)	Nystatin Clotrimazole troches Ketoconazole Fluconazole Amphotericin B	Recalcitrant oral thrush may require treatment for esophagitis Appropriate prophylaxis regimen not established, but prolonged use of nystatin relatively safe
Cytomegalovirus (CMV)	Ganciclovir Foscarnet*	No established treatment HIV-infected infants who are CMV antibody negative should receive CMV-negative blood
Mycobacterium avium intracellulare (MAI)	No therapy effective Amikacin sulfate*	*M. tuberculosis hominis* (MTB) may become more prevalent in pediatric HIV infection, with unusual manifestations
Cryptococcus meningitis (and other systemic infections)	Amphotericin B 5-Fluorocytosine	After initial daily treatment for 4-6 weeks, lifelong weekly treatment with amphotericin B; CSF and serum cryptococcal antigen should be serially measured
CNS toxoplasmosis	Sulfadiazine and Pyrimethamine Folic acid Clindamycin*	Biopsy of CNS lesion may be needed to differentiate from CNS lymphoma Lifelong treatment necessary
Cryptosporidiosis	No therapy effective	MAI of GI tract and cryptosporidiosis potentiate malnutrition, intermittent ileus

From Boland, M. (1991). The child with HIV infection. In Durham, J., Cohen, F. (Eds.), *The person with AIDS: Nursing perspectives* (2nd Ed.) (pp. 324–326). © 1991 Springer Publishing Company, Inc., New York 10012. Used by permission.
*Denotes investigational use.

ation exists) and is carried by many domestic animals and people. Most children are exposed to the protozoan by the age of 4 years and form specific antibodies to it. However, illness from PCP has occurred in more than 70% of the pediatric AIDS cases reported to the CDC. Before the use of prophylaxis, both adults and children had a high mortality rate from PCP, with about half of the deaths among children occurring during the first episode and a large proportion of the rest occurring during the second. With prophylaxis the prognosis has improved substantially, although PCP remains the most serious opportunistic infection in children and is often observed in conjunction with a failure to thrive, encephalopathy, and renal disease. Its onset is quicker and its progression is more fulminant than in adults (Hauger & Powell, 1990). Correlates of death from PCP in children include young age, depleted CD4 + counts, and associated clinical manifestations, including failure to thrive, oral or esophageal candidiasis, and encephalopathy. Survival times for children with PCP are shorter than those in adults. Lymphocyte proliferative responses to phytohemagglutinin are useful as a predictor of pediatric survival (Connor et al., 1991).

The primary site of PCP infection is the lungs, although disseminated infection is also found in the spleen, lymphatic system, and blood. Clinical symptoms of disease include acute tachypnea, dyspnea, fever, dry cough, hypoxemia, and bilateral pulmonary infiltrates. Definitive diagnosis can be made through lung biopsy or flexible bronchoscopy performed with bronchoalveolar lavage. The most prominent laboratory finding is a large alveolar/arterial oxygen gradient denoting hypoxemia. The roentgenographic pattern is similar to that seen in diffuse interstitial lung disease; PCP should be suspected when hypoxemia is out of proportion (Hauger & Powell, 1990). Isomorphic elevation of lactic dehydrogenase (LDH) levels is sensitive to PCP but not specific. However, given the high mortality rates associated with untreated PCP, a presumptive diagnosis based on clinical symptoms is preferabe to waiting for a definitive diagnosis.

Treatment is generally with TMP-SMX. The recommended dosages are intravenous TMP 20 mg/kg and SMX 100 mg/kg daily, divided into four doses, for 21 days (Hauger & Powell, 1990). TMP-SMX appears to be better tolerated in children than in adults. Adverse reactions to TMP-SMX include rash, fever, leukopenia, acute hypoglycemia, and a drop in blood pressure. For children who fail to improve within a few days or cannot tolerate TMP-SMX, an alternative treatment is intravenous pentamidine, 4 mg/kg, given for 21 days, although this has been associated with a high incidence of side effects, including renal insufficiency. Coadministration of corticosteroids in adults with PCP has helped to improve outcomes, but no information about their effectiveness in children is available. Aerosolized pentamidine, used for prophylaxis, is an ineffective treatment for acute PCP, and in children its use has still not been standardized. Side effects of aerosol treatment include bronchospasm and hypoglycemia as well as a strong metallic taste. These can be offset by preceding treatment with a bronchodilator, ventilating the room well, and offering hard candy or mints.

PCP is generally recurrent, necessitating prophylactic use of TMP-SMX, pentamidine, or dapsone. Recommended drugs used in the past among children with leukemia are TMP, 75 mg/m^2 and SMX, 375 mg/m^2, respectively, administered orally every 12 hours on three consecutive days a week (Connor et al., 1991).

Because PCP may be the initial illness associated with AIDS, HIV-exposed and HIV-infected infants must be identified as early as possible so that primary prophylaxis to prevent PCP can begin. Prophylaxis is recommended for infants under 1 year born to infected mothers with CD4 + counts less than 1500 cells/mm^3; for seropositive children between 1 and 2 years old with CD4 + counts less than 750 cells/mm^3, and for infected children more than 2 years with CD4 + counts less than 500 cells/mm^3 (Connor et al., 1991). Some observers recommend prophylaxis for all seropositive infants more than 2 months old, regardless of their ultimate serostatus (Leibovitz et al., 1990). Dapsone is recommended as the oral drug alternative to TMP-SMX at any age. The recommended dose is 1 mg/kg given orally once daily (not to exceed 100 mg/dose) to minimize toxicity. As with TMP-SMX, monthly complete blood counts with differential and platelet counts should be done to monitor for hematologic toxicity. TMP-SMX, dapsone, and other sulfa drugs may be more likely to cause hematologic anemia in patients with glucose-6-phosphate dehydrogenase (G6PD) deficiency.

Candidiasis (Thrush). Candidiasis is a fungal (yeast) infection often encountered in children. Before the HIV epidemic, *Candida* infection was seen in infants under 2 months of age, particularly in the mouth and diaper area. In all children this organism also inhabits the oropharynx, vagina, large intestine, and skin but rarely causes disease unless the child is immunocompromised. *Candida* infection is most commonly localized but can be disseminated. Its symptoms vary with the site. Along with herpes simplex virus and CMV, it is among the causes of dysphagia (difficulty in swallowing) and odynophagia (pain in swallowing), both of which adversely affect infant feeding behaviors.

Treatment for *Candida* infection is site specific. When it occurs on the skin, mucous membranes, or diaper area, it calls for an antifungal cream; parents need to be instructed about cleaning bottles. Oral thrush is generally treated with an antifungal agent such as nystatin or chlotrimazole (Mycolex) troches. If no improvement occurs, short courses of ketoconazole can be given. *Candida* infection in the esophagus or trachea (diagnosed through a barium swallow) is treated with systemic doses of amphotericin B. As in adults, amphotericin B can produce severe reactions. Thus the child must be monitored closely and may require premedication with Benadryl or corticosteroids or both. Complaints such as fever and abdominal pain must be reported promptly to a physician. Disseminated *Candida* has recently been treated with fluconazole administered daily. Since fungal infection in children tends to be a recurrent problem, prophylactic treatment may be indicated. For oral thrush, nystatin can be administered prophylactically once or twice daily; in the diaper area, antifungal cream should be used.

Mycobacterium avium-intracellulare **Infection.** Before AIDS, MAI was rarely seen and then only in people with chronic lung disease; disseminated MAI was rare. It is still uncommon in adults with AIDS, occurring in 3% to 4% of AIDS cases, and is usually extrapulmonary, most often affecting the gastrointestinal tract. Because MAI is resistant to many antimicrobial agents, the outcome is generally poor. However, MAI seldom causes death in children. It generally becomes evident only as a late complication but is more common than was previously recognized, being found in 25% to 30% of HIV-infected children at autopsy. In addition to the gastrointestinal tract, sites include the blood, bone marrow, liver, spleen, adrenal glands, lungs, brain, and skin. The clinical presentation is often nonspecific, involving recurrent fever, chills, abdominal pain, failure to gain or maintain weight, hepatosplenomegaly, anemia, and diarrhea. Definitive diagnosis can be made by cultures of blood, sputum, bone marrow, or stool or through tissue biopsy. No curative therapy is available, and treatment decisions should be based on the child's condition; comfort and nutrition are the main issues to consider (Hauger & Powell, 1990). Although MAI is not communicable, enteric precautions should be followed.

Cryptosporidiosis. *Cryptosporidium* is an enteric protozoan that causes acute, self-limited disease in immunocompetent children but severe and persistent enteritis in those with AIDS. Because it is communicable, only toilet-trained symptomatic children should be permitted in group settings. Symptoms of cryptosporidiosis include fever, frequent and voluminous watery diarrhea, cramps and abdominal pain, weight loss and dehydration, and lactose intolerance. This is not a life-threatening condition, but early manifestations should be treated symptomatically. Total parenteral hyperalimentation is beneficial and may be decreased or terminated once the child is able to eat. Definitive diagnosis can be made from stool samples. No definitive treatment is available.

Malignancies

Kaposi's Sarcoma. Malignancies occur less frequently in HIV-infected children than in infected adults, although this discrepancy will not necessarily continue as survival times for children with HIV increase. Kaposi's sarcoma (KS), which is far more common in homosexual men than in other adults with HIV, is relatively rare in children, with 11 cases among the first 500 children with AIDS reported to the CDC (McClain & Rosenblatt, 1990). KS has occurred mostly among children with Haitian-born parents from the Miami area (Falloon et al., 1989). A variety of chemotherapeutic agents in combination—vincristine with bleomycin or methotrexate—have yielded response rates from 40% to 80% as in adults with KS. However, the biologic response modifier alpha-interferon has been effective in 20% to 50% of adults treated early and does not have the immunosuppressive effects of chemotherapy. For this reason it may prove more appropriate than chemotherapy for children with KS.

Lymphomas. Some evidence of B and T cell lymphomas in children has been found; these were present in 7 of 300 HIV-infected children in one study and 3% to 4% in a larger sample (Wiznia & Nicholas, 1990; McClain & Rosenblatt, 1990). HIV-associated lymphomas are uncommon in childhood, however, and B cell lymphomas in HIV-infected children may be hard to recognize as HIV related because they are similar to those found in about 25% of all children with lymphomas (Falloon et al., 1989; McClain & Rosenblatt, 1990). Symptoms of lymphoma in children include fever, weight loss, diffuse adenopathy, jaundice, hepatomegaly, abdominal distention, and pain. Early institution of intravenous chemotherapy with combinations of cyclophosphamide, vincristine, doxorubicin, methotrexate, cytosine arabinoside, and prednisone may extend life for these children (McClain & Rosenblatt, 1990). However, the course of lymphomas in some children is so rapid and severe that chemotherapy and radiation therapy may be precluded.

ORGAN SYSTEM INVOLVEMENT FROM HIV INFECTION

Respiratory Tract Disease

Pulmonary examinations of HIV-infected children should include a complete blood cell count, chest roentogenography, quantification of blood oxygenation (arterial blood gas or transcutaneous pulse oximetry), and blood culture if a fever is present. LIP is the most frequently occurring pulmonary disease among HIV-infected children (Wiznia & Nicholas, 1990). Other pulmonary complications include bacterial pneumonia, lower respiratory tract viral infection, herpes simplex viremia, and PCP.

Lymphoid Interstitial Pneumonitis. LIP is sometimes associated with hyperplasia of bronchus-associated lymphoid tissue (pulmonary lymphoid hyperplasia [PLH]). A slowly progressive disease, LIP-PLH causes chronic nonproductive cough and exertional dyspnea, leading to dyspnea and finally hypoxemia at rest. Chronic hypoxemia causes digital clubbing, mild lactate dehydrogenase (LDH) elevation, and a widened alveolar/arterial oxygen gradient. Chest roentgenograms may be helpful in diagnosis, although definitive diagnosis is based on lung biopsy. Signs of infection include worsening cough, increased respiratory rate, dyspnea, color changes, distress in feeding, and fatigue (Boland & Klug, 1986). LIP is often accompanied by wheezing, marked lymphadenopathy and hepatosplenomegaly, sharply elevated serum gammaglobulin levels, and occasonal parotitis (Wiznia & Nicholas, 1990). The progression of LIP is insidious with fever usually absent, and its short-term effects are far less serious than those of PCP. Associated viral or bacterial problems can be treated with a broad-spectrum antibiotic but not with TMP-SMX. LIP-PLH responds to corticosteroid therapy, but this should be withheld until there is evidence of significant hypoxemia. Then treatment should begin with prednisone, 2 mg/kg per day for 2 to 4 weeks, tapering to 0.5 to 0.75 mg/kg on alternate days; intravenous immune globulin is also used (Bye & Bernstein, 1989).

Other Respiratory Infections. In HIV-infected children bacterial pneumonia is generally manifested as an acute febrile illness with fever, malaise, and cough; most often the infectious agent is *Streptococcus, H. influenzae,* or *Staphylococcus.* Lower respiratory tract viral infection also occurs frequently, often as a result of respiratory syncytial virus (RSV). This is treated with aerosolized ribavirin, 6 g in 300 ml sterile water nebulized over 12 hours for a maximum of 5 days. Intermittent adenovirus infection occurs also, with a course similar to that in immunocompetent infants. Although it frequently occurs in HIV-infected adults and adolescents, tuberculosis (TB) is rare in young HIV-infected children. Since the latter are often anergic, however, negative test results do not eliminate the possibility of TB infection (Bye & Bernstein, 1989).

Gastrointestinal Tract Disorders

Diarrhea in HIV-infected children has both common and uncommon causes. When it is preceded by vomiting but the stool does not contain blood or mucus, viral (e.g., rotavirus) gastroenteritis should be the presumptive diagnosis. Diarrhea along with fever and abdominal pain may result from CMV; this can be diagnosed by endoscopic biopsy. No standard therapy for CMV has been established, although ganciclovir is believed to be effective in the treatment of adult enterocolitis. *Escherichia coli,* another cause of enterocolitis, responds to antibiotic therapy. *Yersinia enterocolitis* is also seen and responds to TMP-SMX and other broad-spectrum antibiotics. *Salmonella, Shigella,* and *Campylobacter* can also cause acute bacterial gastroenteritis (Hauger & Powell, 1990).

Central Nervous System Disorders

Encephalitis is the central nervous system (CNS) infection of greatest concern in HIV-infected children. It can result from many viruses (CMV, herpes simplex, varicella zoster, Epstein-Barr), as can meningitis or retinitis. *Toxoplasma gondii* infection is relatively uncommon in young HIV-infected children, although it does occur in adolescents. However, congenital syphilis has been on the rise; among its clinical manifestations are prolonged fever, rash, failure to thrive, and CNS involvement in the early or late stages of disease. Syphilis can be treated with parenteral penicillin G for 10 days (Hauger & Powell, 1990).

Developmental delay is a key symptom of HIV infection, and it may be compounded in children born to mothers who used intravenous drugs during pregnancy. Other signs of CNS involvement include acquired microcephaly, cognitive impairment, loss of milestones, seizures, ataxia, abnormal tonicity, and spasticity. Cerebrospinal fluid may be normal or may reveal mild pleocytosis and elevated protein levels. Corticospinal tract degeneration is frequently seen in HIV-infected children. Therefore children with HIV infection require regular neurodevelopmental evaluations. Encephalopathy can be static or progressive. Intervention can be of benefit for mild delays. Children with severe neurologic involvement require therapy to maximize ability and manage abnormal tone and spasticity; their parents must be taught how to care for them. Intravenously administered zidovudine has been shown to reverse developmental delay, with improvements in the performance of activities of daily living, socialization skills, and adaptive behavior (Pizzo, 1989). Orally administered zidovudine does not have this effect in children (Wiznia & Nicholas, 1990).

Hematologic Disease

Hematologic disease may result directly from HIV or appear as a secondary consequence of immune system dysfunction. Moderate anemia is present in nearly all perinatally infected infants by their fifth month, and severe anemia requiring aggressive evaluation occurs in some children. Anemia is a side effect of zidovudine, and some children require repeated blood transfusions while receiving zidovudine therapy. Thrombocytopenia occurs in 10% to 15% of HIV-infected children, in whom it is often the initial symptom of HIV infection. Most hematologic disease in infected children results from an increased rate of platelet destruction; drug therapy should be considered if the platelet count is consistently fewer than 40,000/mm^3. The count may rise spontaneously; intravenous immune globulin (1 g/kg for 3 days, with additional infusions every 2 to 4 weeks) frequently results in a significant but transient increase in the platelet count. The use of corticosteroids is also beneficial but may result in further immunosuppression. Splenectomy has had limited success in older infected children but carries the risk of sepsis. Some believe that neutropenia is best treated with intravenous gammaglobulin (Wiznia & Nicholas, 1990).

Renal Complications

HIV-infected adults commonly have nephropathy, with clinical signs of proteinuria and renal failure and histologic evidence of focal glomerulosclerosis. Perinatally infected children in a recent study had mesangial hyperplasia as often as focal glomerulosclerosis; severe renal failure developed in only half of the patients with nephropathy but in all patients with focal glomerulosclerosis (Strauss et al., 1990). The clinical course of the latter was not as rapid in children as in adults, and in no case was renal failure the cause of death. Other renal signs of HIV infection include parenchymal disease, B and T cell lymphomas infiltrating the kidney, electrolyte abnormalities (often secondary to other organ system involvement), hyponatremia, hypokalemia and hyperkalemia, and metabolic acidosis. Especially if nephrotoxic drugs such as pentamidine are used, renal function tests should be performed regularly on HIV-infected children (Wiznia & Nicholas, 1990).

Cardiomyopathy

Autopsy reveals evidence of cardiomyopathy in a majority of children with HIV, but whether this is primarily or secondarily related to HIV infection is unknown. Decreased left ventricular contractility and dilation develop in some children and result in congestive heart failure with pulmonary edema, tachycardia, tachypnea, hepatomegaly, and decreased peripheral pulses. The optimal management of cardiac disease in HIV-infected children is unclear (Wiznia & Nicholas, 1990).

Disorders of Other Organs

Children with HIV infection are thought to have other end-organ system dysfunctions. Although symptoms have been noted, etiology and management are not clear. Typically treatment is directed toward the symptoms.

PROPHYLACTIC, INVESTIGATIONAL, AND ANTIVIRAL THERAPIES

Strategies to prevent serious illness in HIV-infected children include attempts to block the action of specific infectious agents, to block replication of HIV, and to strengthen the immune system.

Prophylaxis

Drugs commonly used in both treatment and prophylaxis for pediatric HIV infection are summarized in Table 5–5. As already noted, since many HIV-related illnesses in children are recurrent, treatment for those illnesses may have to be lifelong. Only anecdotal evidence has been presented for the efficacy of intravenous gammaglobulin in decreasing bacterial and viral infections, but a controlled study is in progress (Rosenblatt et al., 1990). Otherwise, prophylaxis has been used in children primarily for PCP; recommended dosages of TMP-SMX were discussed previously and are shown in Table 5–5. Pentamidine is used prophylactically against PCP when treatment with TMP-SMX is ineffective or has serious side effects; it can be administered either intravenously or in aerosolized form. For aerosol administration a nebulizer is required to deliver the drug effectively. The patient must be old enough to cooperate with the nebulization procedures, must have lungs able to absorb the drug, and must be able to hold his or her breath for 3 to 5 seconds. Care must be taken during treatment to prevent aerosolizing pentamidine into the room. Prophylactic regimens for other illnesses such as MAI infection and toxoplasmosis are under development. Children with a history of chronic recurring infections such as otitis media and herpes may receive regular administration of the agent used for treatment, but at a less than treatment dose.

Investigational Therapies

For many of the conditions affecting HIV-infected children, investigational therapies offer the only hope for curative treatment. HIV damages many body systems. Therapy must reach multiple sites, and because proviral sequences are integrated into target cells, treatment may have to continue for the life of the child (Pizzo & Wilfert, 1991). Probably no one drug will be effective over the long term. Therapy will require multiple agents used in combination to minimize side effects or toxic effects while providing benefit. For this reason, children must have increased access to

TABLE 5-5. Drugs Commonly Used in Pediatric HIV Infection

MEDICATION	USE	COMMENTS/SIDE EFFECTS
AZT (zidovudine)	Treatment of proven HIV infection Dose: <12 yr 180 mg/m² q 6 hr >12 yr 100 mg/m² q 4 hr	Side effects: *neutropenia*, anemia, GI upset Follow patient with complete blood cell count plus differential Regular use increases mean corpuscular volume *Does not prevent infections*
Trimethoprim-sulfamethoxazole (TMP-SMX; Bactrim)	*Pneumocystis carinii* pneumonia Treatment: TMP 5 mg/kg q 6 hr IV or PO Prophylaxis: 75 mg/m² PO b.i.d. q Mon., Tues., Wed. only	Diagnosis by bronchoalveolar lavage, endotracheal suction (silver stain for *Pneumocystis*), lung biopsy Side effects: hypersensitivity, skin rash, fever, *neutropenia*, anemia, increased white blood cells, increased platelets (usual indication to stop drug), increased liver function studies, increased blood urea nitrogen (BUN), increased creatinine, nausea, vomiting sometimes Must get rash evaluated; desensitization may be successful *Alternative drug is pentamidine*
Pentamidine (Isethionate)	*Pneumocystis carinii* pneumonia Treatment: 4 mg/kg IV q 24 hr (in D5W run over 1 hr) Prophylaxis: 4 mg/kg as above q 4 wk (aerosolized used in older children 300 mg q 4 wk)	Alternative to Bactrim if hypersensitive or with depressed bone marrow or treatment failure Side effects: hypoglycemia, hypotension, *interstitial nephritis* (stop drug for severe kidney disease), possible nausea and vomiting, taste changes, hypocalcemia
Nystatin (Mycostatin)	Oral candidiasis (thrush) Treatment: 1-6 ml (depends on age); swish in cheeks t.i.d. or q 6-8 hr	Prolonged use of nystatin relatively safe May not work against recalcitrant thrush
Monostat vaginal cream Clortrimazole troches	Apply PO b.i.d. to q.i.d.	For small children, coat oral membranes
Ketoconazole	Severe oral candidiasis, esophagitis Treatment: 3.3-6.6 mg/kg/day	Side effects: potential liver toxicity, rash, pruritus *Evaluate liver function before starting*
Fluconazole	Systemic fungal infection, esophagitis Dose: 3-6 mg/kg PO or IV q day	Skin rash and allergic reaction well tolerated in adults Safety and efficacy in children not fully established

TABLE 5–5. Drugs Commonly Used in Pediatric HIV Infection *Continued*

MEDICATION	USE	COMMENTS/SIDE EFFECTS
Amphotericin B	Disseminated candidiasis, cryptococcal disease Dose: 0.25-1 mg/kg IV q 24 hr, run over 4-8 hr	*Severe side effects:* renal toxicity, electrolyte imbalance, fever chills, bone marrow depression, venous thrombosis, arrhythmia
Acyclovir (Zovirax)	Herpes simplex, herpes zoster Dose: 10 mg/kg q 8 hr IV (also used PO for prophylaxis)	Because of possible progression of mucocutaneous/skin lesions to systemic disease, IV administration is recommended *Side effects:* nephrotoxic (adequate hydration needed), nausea, vomiting
5-Fluorocytosine (Flucytosine)	Cryptococcal disease, disseminated candidiasis Dose: 50-150 mg/kg PO q 6 hr	Usually used with amphotericin B Lifelong weekly treatment for cryptococcal meningitis Side effects: nausea, vomiting, diarrhea, *possibly severe enterocolitis,* hepatotoxicity
Steroids (prednisone, others)	Lymphoid interstitial pneumonitis, hypoxemia (PaO$_2$ <65 mm Hg) Dose: varies	May mask signs of infection Side effects: weight gain, fluid retention Induces sense of well-being

Adapted from Children's Hospital AIDS Program (CHAP), Children's Hospital of New Jersey, Newark, N.J.

these therapies, many of which have been made available only to adults. Most clinical trials with adults have yielded no data about the effects of investigational therapies on children. Participation in a clinical trial is discussed in depth in Chapter 7.

Antiviral Therapies

The Food and Drug Administration (FDA) approved use of the antiviral drug zidovudine for children in the late spring of 1990, more than 3 years after its use in adults had become widespread. Zidovudine is now officially recommended for use in children in the advanced stages of HIV illness as indicated by CD4 + counts less than 400 cells/mm^3. As noted previously, its use may be indicated in all children under 15 months of age with definitively diagnosed HIV infection and in children with CD4 + counts less than 1500 cells/mm^3 in their first year of life or below 1000 cells/mm^3 in their second. As in adults, early studies of zidovudine in children showed improvements such as weight gain, improved neurologic function, and decreased levels of serum immunoglobulins. However, the effects did not reverse disease progression. Also, as in adults, zidovudine has bone marrow toxicity, necessitating a modified dose or transfusion. The recommended dosage for children to the age of 12 years is 180 mg/m^2 every 6 hours. Because this was the dosage used in the initial studies in children, clinicians have been reluctant to decrease the recommended dosage to adult levels. Adolescents are prescribed the adult dose of 100 mg/m^2 every 4 hours.

Certain second-generation antiretroviral drugs whose use is under investigation in adults, such as dideoxycytidine and dideoxyinosine, are also being given to children in clinical trials (Falloon et al., 1989). Their future availability to children depends on the outcome of the clinical trials. Studies are planned to investigate whether perinatal transmission of HIV to fetuses can be blocked by administering therapy to infected pregnant women. The FDA has given approval to the National Institutes of Health (NIH) for a phase II study to evaluate whether transmission from mother to infant can be interrupted with AZT (Prober & Gershon, 1991). For more information on clinical trials and phase II studies, see Chapter 7.

CHRONICITY OF DISEASE AND DELIVERY OF CARE

Organization of Care in the Clinic and the Home Setting

Challenges of Home Care. The ideal locus for the management of chronic childhood illnesses is the home. Often the parents of a chronically ill child are the only consistent link in the care system; they know the most about the child's symptoms, treatments, and responses (Boland & Czarniecki, 1991). Even in the best of circumstances, however, managing a chronic illness introduces stresses into the family (Jessop & Stein, 1989): it must reorient its existence around the child's constant need for care with the concomitant financial, social, and emotional strains. In the case of HIV-infected children, however, family stability may already have been compromised by drug addiction and a host of other social problems, such as poverty, substandard housing, inadequate support networks, and poor access to community resources, including medical care. Moreover, parents frequently discover that they are HIV infected only when HIV symptoms are diagnosed in their newborn child. This discovery, which may be the first concrete evidence of one partner's drug use or bisexuality, invariably transforms the relationship, often further destabilizing family life. The first reaction may be a denial of the child's diagnosis.

Importance of Early Diagnosis. Both psychosocial issues (discussed in more detail later in the chapter) and the progressive nature of HIV disease complicate the management of HIV as a chronic childhood illness. Nevertheless, it is critical for the child that the process begin early: if the signs and symptoms of HIV infection are recognized at the outset, the effects of the illness can be minimized through supportive and antiretroviral therapies. More widespread HIV testing and greater awareness of early signs of pediatric HIV infection by health care workers will result in more diagnoses being made before the appearance of symptoms. Early diagnosis will require that pediatric health professionals deal with issues not typically encountered in pediatric practice in the past, including substance abuse, sexuality, reproductive rights, early death, and bereavement.

Shifting Focus of Chronic Care. In general, those who provide care for chronically ill children should strive to minimize the disruption made by the disease process and treatment regimen on the family unit and the development of the children (Pollock & Boland, 1990). In recent years the focus of pediatrics has shifted from an exclusive concern with medical care toward psychosocial problem solving with an awareness of the contributions other disciplines can make to long-term care (Eaton et al., 1989). This shift has contributed to the development of care models that promote a normal life for the chronically ill child. In the case of HIV-infected children, health care and psychosocial needs are particularly complex and demand coordination. Most of these needs can be met by community-based providers, but regional tertiary care centers should be available to treat the children for severe infection or illness and to provide periodic evaluation and antiviral treatment (Boland et al., 1989). Acute care hospitalization is seldom needed before symptomatic AIDS develops.

Coordinating Care. HIV-infected children and their families require services from many helping professions. In addition to nurses, these may include physicians, social workers, psychologists, dietitians, teachers, clergy, and occupational, physical, and recreational therapists (Falloon et al., 1989). Care from these many sources can be coordinated through case management, which can prevent the two extremes of a failure to meet needs and the duplication of services. Indeed, families of HIV-infected children have testified that the constant availability of a single identified person to link them with services is the key factor that has enabled them to care for their children at home (McGonigel, 1988). Outpatient care can be made particularly accessible and effective if it is offered in special clinics that provide comprehensive care for both children and adults. In all care settings the special needs of children—such as the need to play—should be acknowledged and accommodated. In addition, health professionals must be culturally sensitive and nonjudgmental. By adopting positive attitudes, these professionals can promote such attitudes in families, which bear the brunt of care. A detailed explanation of the case management model is included in Chapter 7.

Family Assessment. A formal assessment of the family is important to determine their willingness and ability to provide care for the HIV-infected child (Boland & Harris, in press). Home care workers need to know how the family regards the diagnosis and who in the family is aware of it (Boland et al., 1989). The limited capacity of the medical profession to provide help for HIV-infected children may have shattered trust in the profession, and this trust will have to be rebuilt (Thorne & Robinson, 1989). Trust may be an issue particularly when the source of infection was blood products provided by medical authorities for a family member with hemophilia (Tiblier et al., 1989). Families may also have a general suspicion of authorities if illicit drug use was the route of infection. Even without these complicating factors, caretakers often do not understand the meaning of HIV testing or the complexities of immune system functioning. They may be overwhelmed with the amount of information provided them and many have difficulty remembering what was said. Education for parents or guardians should be provided at the many occasions on which they encounter health professionals, and it should be reinforced with printed materials. Parents of infected children have requested particular assistance in getting information about HIV disease and its treatment and in disclosing the diagnosis to family and friends (Falloon et al., 1989). Some parental concerns can be addressed in the context of support groups. Although many parents of infected children shy away from formal support group meetings, organized group social activities often spawn informal support systems.

Planning Care. The caregiving team should meet regularly to plan and coordinate patient and family care and to make referrals concerning such issues as child care, foster care, child custody, school arrangements, home health care, finances, and substance use (Falloon et al., 1989). Initial assessments of seropositive infants should include information about maternal drug withdrawal and sexually transmitted diseases, for which infants should be given appropriate treatment (Mendez, 1990). Ongoing outpatient care of the seropositive infant should include HIV antibody testing at regular intervals until the infant is 2 years of age. Growth (height, weight, head circumference) and development should be monitored at regular intervals with a growth chart and the Denver Developmental Screening Test or the Bayley or McCarthy scales. Regular immunizations such as measles-mumps-rubella, influenza, and pneumococcus vaccines should be administered. (Polio vaccination should be by injection of killed vaccine rather than oral administration of live vaccine.)

The need for preventive therapy should be reviewed early in the course of a child's illness and should include consideration of prophylaxis against PCP, the potential benefits of intravenous gammaglobulin, and the timing of zidovudine (Mendez, 1990). For school-age children the development of treatment protocols and drug regimens should take into account school schedules; late afternoon or evening clinic visits and adjusted medication schedules best accommodate the needs of these children (Abrams & Nicholas, 1990). As noted previously, ongoing information and education should be provided for parents or guardians. Infected parents should be encouraged to obtain regular health care, and health care workers should look for signs of parental compromise that could affect the care of the child, such as fatigue, weight loss, forgetfulness, or an inability to follow through with treatment.

Role of the Home Care Nurse. The home care nurse can act as a liaison between the family and the child's medical team and can serve as an advocate for the family in dealing with other providers. Because of the impairment in humoral and cell-mediated immunity, HIV-infected children are susceptible to bacterial, viral, and fungal infections. The nurse must have a good working knowledge of HIV disease processes, how they affect children at various stages of infection, and appropriate pharmacologic and nonpharmacologic interventions. The home care nurse should also know how well the child and caregivers understand diagnosis and treatment, sites of infection, respiratory status, growth and development, thought processes, physical mobility, nutritional status, skin integrity, level of comfort, and compliance with medical regimens. The most common diagnoses in immunocompromised children include increased susceptibility to infection, fever, increased pain, opportunistic infection, alteration in gas exchange, alteration in cognitive and motor function, alteration in nutrition, potential for bleeding, alteration in fluid/electrolyte balance, potential impairment of skin integrity, and potential fatigue and exhaustion of caregivers (Boland et al., 1989).

Outpatient Care. Even with well-coordinated home care, infected children are likely to make periodic visits to the hospital emergency room. Parents or guardians should be instructed to tell staff there about the child's HIV serostatus (Mendez, 1990). As symptoms develop, the frequency of outpatient visits will increase and hospitalizations will begin. This will make denial of the diagnosis more difficult, and parents will often ask for detailed information as they experience a loss of control and as treatment regimens become more complicated. These regimens may include intravenous and high-technology therapies that can be safely administered in the home. Nurses should be aware, however, that when denial does not interfere with medical care, it serves as a protective measure, decreasing stress and allowing caregivers to function (Boland & Klug, 1986).

AIDS Diagnosis and Family Stress. Once AIDS is diagnosed, the prognosis is generally poor. Most children die within 2 years of diagnosis. Most often the AIDS diagnosis results from a progression of existing symptoms such as failure to thrive, encephalopathy, or untreatable opportunistic infection. High levels of service and intervention are required, and these greatly increase the potential for parent-provider conflict as the involved parties grapple with the risks and benefits of aggressive, intrusive, and investigational therapies. An AIDS diagnosis is often accompanied by an immediate family crisis, manifested in guilt, shock, shame, and confusion (Pollock & Boland, 1990). Families often need assistance in clarifying issues and getting support for decision making. Disadvantaged families especially may assume that the physician is always right and may not realize how actively they can participate in making decisions. The family should be encouraged to discuss feelings about the child's prognosis, including the desire for pain management, use of life support mechanisms, and confidentiality. Often at a time when the medical staff has come to accept the child's impending death, parents favor heroic lifesaving measures. Conversely, some parents perceive and accept impending death before the medical team does. The different expectations of parent and provider must be recognized and addressed. The nurse can initiate discussion and facilitate recognition of differing perceptions.

Terminal Stage. In the terminal stage of illness, home care focuses on the comfort, care, and optimal quality of each day in the child's life. The hospice philosophy involves a partnership among child, family, and providers. Rather than recovery, the goal of hospitalization becomes achievement of a dignified and comfortable death. In contrast to previous hospitalizations, invasive procedures and aggressive management are not needed. The child should be kept pain free through a variety of therapeutic interventions. When death occurs, parents and other family members need adequate time to say good-bye, which may involve bathing the child or fixing the child's hair. Although such time is seldom provided in busy hospital settings, these hours are invaluable to parents. The family cannot be rushed; nurses who provide such support can assist the family in beginning the mourning process.

Financial constraints on home care and safety of personnel if the home is in a high-crime area are often provider concerns in the terminal stage of illness. Parents who have provided excellent home care may wish to place a child in the hospital as death approaches; some may refuse home-based hospice care because they do not want new people introduced into their lives. Rehospitalization should remain an option for terminally ill children.

Management of Chronic Illness by Family

Conditions Compromising Family Care. It was noted earlier that a majority of HIV-infected children in the United States have one or both parents infected and that the parents' infections are frequently a consequence of intravenous drug use. A mother's illness or addiction may interfere with her ability to care for an infected child, both physically and psychologically. She may be fearful of sharing her diagnosis with her significant other because of the possibility of rejection, abandonment, withdrawal of economic support, or even physical violence. Similar fears may isolate her and her partner from the network of friends or family to whom they would normally turn for support. The diagnosis may also precipitate arguments between a couple about who is to blame or it may reactivate previously buried family issues. In addition to the disruption of her relationship, an infected mother may be burdened by guilt over her child's condition. Moreover, although a diagnosis of HIV infection should be the occasion for adopting safer sexual behaviors, cultural or religious beliefs often make it difficult for a woman to initiate changes in sexual behaviors with her partner.

The mother's responses to HIV infection are further complicated when she has a history of substance use. She may continue to use drugs as an escape, and this may prevent her from coping with the child's infection or providing needed care and treatment (Boland et al., 1989). Addicted parents may be skilled at manipulating medical staff members and turning them against one another. There is also the risk that addicted parents may inappropriately use pain medications prescribed for their children; health care workers should monitor this. Health professionals can be helpful in making parents with substance use problems aware of the benefit of seeking treatment for these problems. When treatment is not an option and the parents' actions are disruptive, professionals experienced in dealing with substance use must be consulted. The nursing and medical staff must be consistent and clear about their expectations of parents and the plan of care. A concrete plan and frequent communication among care providers can minimize staff splitting and manipulation by family members. Health care workers can help parents overcome guilt for their past actions by refocusing them on the good they can do for their infected children in the present.

Surrogate Caregivers. In some circumstances surrogate caregivers for infected children are needed. Often they can be found within the extended family; in many black or Hispanic families the pattern of care involves extended family members such as grandmothers or aunts (Boyd-Franklin & Aleman, 1990). However, these caregivers may be impeded by struggles related to the life-styles, illnesses, or deaths of their own children. If they are advanced in age, they may lack the physical strength and stamina to provide care for young children at a time in their lives at which they might reasonably expect to be taken care of themselves. Although extended family members in some places are reimbursed for the foster care of a relative, services available to other caregivers—such as respite care—may not be available to them.

Early in the pediatric HIV epidemic there were periodic horror stories in the press about infected children who lived their entire lives as "boarder babies" in acute care hospitals. By 1990 the situation had changed markedly. Most states had improved their resources for recruiting and training foster care families; transitional care facilities for children awaiting foster care placements had been developed in many localities (Abrams & Nicholas, 1990). Foster parents of HIV-infected children have some of the same fears of rejection and isolation as do natural parents, but they face some additional challenges. They may lack the legal authority to participate in decision making about a child's medical treatment. In addition, they may be unrealistic in their expectations about what will be involved in caregiving. Their involvement may grow out of spiritual beliefs, a sense of higher calling, a strong sense of advocacy, or a belief that love will heal. Proper training for foster parents, conducted in hospitals and transitional care facilities, will help prepare them for the realities of caring for chronically ill children.

Dealing with Stress. The manner in which a biologic, extended, or foster family copes with an HIV diagnosis in a child is related to its previously established ways of dealing with crises and stresses. A diagnosis of HIV can magnify feelings of hopelessness and precipitate suicidal ideation in adults; in some cultural contexts adults may view illnesses as a moral judgment or punishment for past behavior. Similar feelings are involved when a child has HIV infection. A parent's guilt may manifest itself in overprotective or permissive behavior toward the child, possibly interfering with the child's development (Jessop & Stein, 1989). If the family fears the stigma often attached to an HIV diagnosis, they may be secretive and isolate themselves. This may confuse older siblings, who frequently become involved in caring for an ailing child and parents. These children may face the prospect of requiring a new home without understanding the illness that is the cause of their relocation (Abrams & Nicholas, 1990). Families often need assistance in dealing with issues of confidentiality and disclosure, that is, thinking through whom to tell, when, and how (Pollock & Boland, 1990). Because of difficulty in adjusting to the diagnosis, the family may have only intermittent contact with clinics at crisis or decision points and disappear in between. This intermittent contact may also be an outgrowth of a family's perception of outside agencies as intrusive, which may be more common in minority families with multiple socioeconomic problems who are most in need of help (Boland et al., 1989; Boyd-Franklin & Aleman, 1990).

Families with HIV-infected children may have to deal with the illness for many years and are likely to encounter practical problems that have no easy solutions. Most families with infected children are totally dependent on public health care programs, such as Medicaid, that are often inadequately funded. Even adequately insured families may have difficulty in getting complete coverage for HIV-related conditions in children: health care financing in the United States is typically geared to acute illnesses with policy limits for each condition. Other financial stressors include the loss of work time when a child must be supervised constantly, lost opportunities for career advancement, and the expenses involved in transporting the child to the clinic and other social service appointments (Jessop & Stein, 1989). Chronic illnesses such as HIV can also be more draining emotionally than acute illnesses. Parents of chronically ill children often fluctuate among a variety of reactions—shock, denial, sadness, anger—between periods of relative acceptance and equilibrium. Their feelings of guilt or inadequacy are brought to the fore repeatedly as they are confronted by the child's difference from healthy peers, especially at critical developmental stages such as starting day care or school (Jessop & Stein, 1989). Most of the literature on chronic illness has focused on children in middle-class families, so there is little understanding of how deprived and chaotic families may deal with a chronic illness such as HIV over the long run. In addition, families with an HIV-infected child typically have more than one chronically ill member.

Maintaining Family Autonomy. As noted earlier, health care professionals treating a chronic childhood illness should try to prevent both the illness and the treatment regimen from disrupting the child's development and the family unit. Typically the medical establishment reinforces the role of passive, dependent parents. This is particularly inappropriate in the management of a chronic illness such as HIV. Furthermore, forcing parents into a dependent role is counterproductive in families that are determined to maintain control over the child; this type of enforced dependence makes the lives of the adults feel out of control as well as that of the child. Health care workers should attempt to establish a partnership with the family (Boland et al., 1989). This may be challenging in the case of families unaccustomed to dealing with the health care system. To them, monthly appointments may appear time consuming, cost prohibitive, and unnecessary if they result in no prescription, procedure, or treatment. In addition, where case management and coordinated care systems have not been developed, the variety of sources and providers with whom the family must deal may include medical subspecialists with conflicting demands. This situation sets the stage for clashes between the values of middle-class professionals who provide services and those of poor families struggling to survive. Because responsibility for day-to-day supervision falls to family members, respecting their autonomy and providing a flexible system of care are important. The family of the HIV-infected child should be able to maintain its independence, autonomy, and self-determination without undue supervision and paternalism (Jessop & Stein, 1989). Health care workers must convince families that the services they offer are necessary if they expect parents to make use of these services. In addition, they sometimes have to deal with their own feelings of anger and blame toward parents if they are to avoid fantasies of rescuing children from evil parents.

Changing Needs. A complex interaction occurs among chronic illness, the family's response, and the child's developmental status. Changes in all three occur simultaneously: the child develops, the chronic condition changes as it follows its course, and the family changes through its life cycle and as its adaptation to the child's condition unfolds (Jessop & Stein, 1989). Care for most HIV-infected children requires lifelong treatment involving multiple drug regimens with oral and intravenous treatments and complex medical interventions (Abrams & Nicholas, 1990). As care proceeds, both medical professionals and caregivers need to be sensitive to changes in the child, the child's medical condition, and the family situation.

Psychosocial Issues

Disclosure of the Diagnosis. Infected children are children first, with typical wishes for acceptance and understanding. HIV compromises their development, and societal reactions to the illness—such as fear and rejection—impede their struggles for normal life experiences (Pollock & Boland, 1990). These children may have lived with several caretakers and lacked a consistent parental figure; this lack of a consistent family structure may inhibit their ability to deal with the diagnosis. Medical care is also stressful for them; they can expect to undergo repeated anxiety-producing, painful, and intrusive procedures throughout their treatment. Their ability to assimilate information is limited, and they may misunderstand what is told them. Young children often believe that their chronic illness is a result of magic or of their own action or inaction. As they grow older and more aware of their peers, they may worry about their differences from others, and these differences could become a primary mode of identification. Concealing their condition from others—however warranted it may be—may lead them to believe that their illness is something to be ashamed of (Perrin & Gerrity, 1984). For such reasons as these, children with chronic conditions appear to have a greater incidence of psychosocial problems than others (Pless, 1984).

Parents and caregivers of chronically ill older children and adolescents often struggle over whether to tell them the nature of their illness, what to tell them, when is the best time, and who should do the telling. The truth is less threatening to children than fear of the unknown. But the information given a child has to be geared to the child's developmental level. Psychologists can figure critically in the decision-making process, helping to frame the information given the child and helping the child to survive the aftermath of the disclosure. Before a disclosure is made the child's and parents' understanding of illness causality should be assessed. Awareness of the family's level of health knowledge and their beliefs about health and illness is also important in determining how to help them integrate the necessary medical information. Often families need assistance in finding words they can say comfortably and the child will understand (Pollock & Boland, 1990). Because HIV-infected children with neurologic involvement may not be functioning at normal chronologic levels, developmental evaluation may be helpful in determining how to communicate with them. It may be necessary to relate the information more than once. Developmentally appropriate language is needed when medical procedures and treatments are explained to children; play therapy and discussion may be helpful. The stigma and shame that often accompany an HIV diagnosis must be addressed therapeutically as well.

Overcoming Isolation. Some families of infected children isolate themselves in an attempt to maintain control over the child and the situation; their isolation may be a result of disapproval or fear of contagion by family members and friends. Caregivers may feel that they and their children are contaminated, and they may be angry with the medical profession and depressed over the many losses and potential losses they face (Boland et al., 1989). Counseling and psychologic support may be indicated to help caregivers—including mothers, grandmothers, and foster parents—and siblings deal with denial and feelings of shame or fear (Steiner, 1990). Families that have dealt with racism, poverty, and the intrusive scrutiny of entitlement programs may have strict rules about the privacy of family-related matters that have to be overcome (Boyd-Franklin & Aleman, 1990). Still, it is important for children to have contact with their peers, particularly in school settings (Boland & Klug, 1986).

Mental Health Needs. Often the mental health needs of HIV-infected children are neglected (Pollock & Boland, 1990). The death of friends from the clinic may heighten children's fears of death; a variety of approaches, including behavior therapy, play therapy, and medication, may be salutary. Therapy can be offered at the clinic, during hospitalizations, or at home. Offering children access to one another in play or support groups may also help them grieve. Children who survive the death of a parent— whether the children are infected or not—may need emotional support that is not available from their caregivers. Signs of their distress may include disruptive behavior at home and in school, increased aggression, and substance use (Boyd-Franklin & Aleman, 1990). Again, these cases require therapeutic intervention.

Grieving Process. The stigma associated with HIV disease and the resultant secrecy complicate the grieving process. Health and social service professionals should respect the family's need to maintain secrecy about the diagnosis. People vary greatly in the ways they handle their grief—what they feel, how deeply and intensely they feel, how they respond, and what coping mechanisms produce relief. Options for support include counseling, support groups, phone calls, contact with other bereaved families, home visits, and the use of volunteers or others who have established a close relationship with the family (Boland et al., 1989). Spiritual beliefs and connections with others in church communities may also be important coping mechanisms. A postdeath conference scheduled with the medical care providers can give parents an opportunity to ask about the events leading to the death and can help provide closure for both the providers and the parents.

SUMMARY

As the techniques for identifying HIV infection in infants and treating infected children with antiretroviral and prophylactic therapies improve, so does the prognosis for HIV-infected children. Already the management of HIV illness has shifted to a chronic illness model. As the life expectancy for infected children increases, the quality of their lives assumes greater importance. Many infected children will be able to participate in the normal growth processes and activities of childhood. Thoughtfully designed systems of care delivery and competently administered care will assist HIV-infected children to live for many years.

References

Abrams, E.J., Nicholas, S.W. (1990) Pediatric HIV infection. *Pediatric Annals, 19,* 482–487.

Andiman, W.A., Simpson, B.J., Olson, B., et al. (1990). Rate of transmission of human immunodeficiency virus type 1 infection from mother to child and short-term outcome of neonatal function. *American Journal of Disease in Children, 144,* 758–768.

Arpadi, S., Caspe, W.B. (1990). Diagnosis and classification of HIV infection in children, *Pediatric Annals, 19,* 409–420.

Auger, I., Thomas, P., DeGruttola, V., et al. (1988). Incubation periods for paediatric AIDS patients. *Nature, 336*(8), 575–577.

Blanche, S., Rouzioux, C., Moscato, M.L.G., et al. (1989). A prospective study of infants born to women seropositive for human immunodeficiency virus type 1. *New England Journal of Medicine, 320,* 1643–1648.

Boland, M.G. (1990). HIV infection in children. *NAACOG's Clinical Issues in Perinatal and Women's Health Nursing, 1,* 53–59.

Boland, M., Czarniecki, L. (1991). Starting life with HIV. *RN 54*(1), 54–58.

Boland, M., Harris, D. (in press). Living with HIV infection. In Connor, E., Yoger, R. (eds.) *The child with HIV infection.* Chicago: Yearbook Medical Publishers.

Boland, M.G., Klug, R.M. (1986). AIDS: The implications for home care. *MCN—The American Journal of Maternal and Child Nursing, 11*, 404–411.

Boland, M.G., Mahan-Rudolph, P., Evans, P. (1989) Special issues in the care of the child with HIV infection/AIDS. In Martin, B. (ed.), *Pediatric hospice care: What helps* (pp. 116–144). Los Angeles: Los Angeles Children's Hospital.

Boyd-Franklin, N., Aleman, J. (1990). Black, inner-city families and multigenerational issues: the impact of AIDS. *Psychologist, 40*(3), 14–17.

Borkowsky, W., Steele, C.J., Grubman, S., et al. (1987). Antibody responses to bacterial toxoids in children infected with human immunodeficiency virus. *Journal of Pediatrics, 110*(4), 563–566.

Bremer, J.W., Hollinger, F.B. (1990). Pediatric HIV infection and AIDS: Diagnostic tests. *Seminars in Pediatric Infectious Diseases, 1*(1), 27–30.

Bye, M.R., Bernstein, L.J. (1989). Identifying pulmonary sequelae in children with AIDS. *Journal of Respiratory Diseases, 10*(12), 27–39.

Centers for Disease Control (1987). Classification system for human immunodeficiency virus (HIV) infection in children under 13 years of age. *Morbidity and Mortality Weekly Report, 36*, 225–230.

Chin, J. (1990). Current and future dimensions of the HIV/AIDS pandemic in women and children. *Lancet, 336*, 221–224.

Connor, E., Bagarzzi, M., McSherry, G., Holland, B., Boland, M., Denny, T., Oliske, J. (1991). Clinical and laboratory correlates of *Pneumocystis carinii* pneumonia in children infected with HIV. *JAMA 265*, 1693–1697.

Eaton, A.P., Coury, D.L., Kern, R.A. (1989). The roles of professionals and institutions. In Stein, R. (Ed.), *Caring for children with chronic illness* (pp. 75–86). New York: Springer.

Eckholm, E., Tierney, J. (1990). Africa writhes with growing agony of AIDS. *The Sunday Oregonian*, September 23, A1, A24–25.

Falloon, J., Eddy, J., Wiener, L., Pizzo, P.A. (1989). Human immunodeficiency virus infection in children. *Journal of Pediatrics, 114*, 1–30.

Gonik, B., Hammill, H.A. (1990) AIDS in pregnancy. *Seminars in Pediatric Infectious Diseases, 1*(1), 82–88.

Hauger, S.B., Powell, K.R. (1990). Infectious complications in children with HIV infection. *Pediatric Annals, 19*, 421–436.

Husson, R.N., Corneau, A.M., Hoff, R. (1990). Diagnosis of human immunodeficiency virus infection in infants and children. *Pediatrics 86*(1), 1–10.

Jessop, D.J., Stein, R.E.K. (1989). Meeting the needs of individuals and families. In Stein, R. (Ed.), *Caring for children with chronic illness* (pp. 63–74). New York: Springer.

Johnson, J.P., Nair, P., Hines, S.E., et al. (1989). Natural history and serologic diagnosis of infants born to human immunodeficiency virus–infected women. *American Journal of Diseases in Children, 143*, 1147–1153.

Krasinski, K., Borkowsky, W., Holzman, R.S. (1989). Prognosis of human immunodeficiency virus infection in children and adolescents. *Pediatric Infectious Diseases Journal, 8*, 216–220.

Lambert, J.S. (1990). Maternal and perinatal issues regarding HIV infection. *Pediatric Annals, 19*, 468–472.

Leibovitz, E., Rigaud, M., Pollack, H., et al. (1990). *Pneumocystis carinii* pneumonia in infants infected with the human immunodeficiency virus with more than 450 CD4 lymphocytes per cubic millimeter. *New England Journal of Medicine, 323*(8), 531–533.

McClain, K.L., Rosenblatt, H. (1990). Pediatric HIV infection and AIDS: Clinical expression of malignancy. *Seminars in Pediatric Infectious Diseases, 1*(1), 124–129.

McGonigel, M. (1988). Family meeting on pediatric AIDS. Washington, DC: Association for the Care of Children's Health.

Mendez, H. (1990). Ambulatory care of infants and children born to HIV-infected mothers. *Pediatric Annals, 17*, 439–447.

Mok, J.Q., Gianquinto, C., DeRossi, A., et al. (1987). Infants born to mothers seropositive for human immunodeficiency virus: Preliminary findings from a multicentre European study. *Lancet, 1*, 1164–1168.

New Jersey Women and AIDS Network (1990). *Me first! Medical manifestations of HIV in women*. New Brunswick, NJ: The Network.

Perrin, E.C., Gerrity, P.S. (1984). Development of children with a chronic illness. *Pediatric Clinics of North America, 31,* 19–31.

Pizzo, P.A. (1989). Emerging concepts in the treatment of HIV infection in children. *Journal of the American Medical Association, 262,* 1989-1992.

Pizzo, P.A., Wilfert, C. (1991). Treatment considerations for children with HIV infection. In Pizzo, P., Wilfert, C. (Eds.), *Pediatric AIDS: The challenge of HIV infection in infants, children, and adolescents* (pp. 478–494). Baltimore: Williams & Wilkins.

Pless, I.B. (1984). Clinical assessment: Physical and psychological functioning. *Pediatric Clinics of North America, 31,* 33–45.

Pollock, S.W., Boland, M.G. (1990). Children and HIV infection. *Psychologist, 40*(3),17–21.

Prieto, C., Hansen, T.N. (1990). Pediatric HIV infection and AIDS: Neonatal AIDS. *Seminars in Pediatric Infectious Diseases, 1*(1), 89–93.

Prober, C., Gershon, A. (1991). Medical management of newborns and infants to seropositive mothers. In Pizzo, P., Wilfert, C. (Eds.), *Pediatric AIDS: The challenge of HIV infection in infants, children, and adolescents* (pp. 516–530). Baltimore: Williams & Wilkins.

Rogers, M.F. (1985). AIDS in children: A review of the clinical, epidemiologic and public health aspects. *Pediatric Infectious Diseases, 4*(3), 230–236.

Rogers, M.F., Thomas, P.A., Starcher, E.T., et al. (1987). Acquired immunodeficiency syndrome in children: Report of the Centers for Disease Control national surveillance, 1982 to 1985. *Pediatrics, 79,* 1008–1014.

Rosenblatt, H.M., Englund, J.A., Shearer, W.T. (1990). Immunotherapeutic approaches to pediatric HIV infection. *Seminars in Pediatric Infectious Diseases, 1*(1), 140–149.

Ryder, R.W., Nsa, W., Hassig, S.E., et al. (1989). Perinatal transmission of the human immunodeficiency virus type 1 to infants of seropositive women in Zaire. *New England Journal of Medicine, 320,* 1637–1642.

Scott, G.B., Hutto, C., Makuch, R.W., et al. (1989). Survival in children with perinatally acquired human immunodeficiency virus type 1 infection. *New England Journal of Medicine, 221,* 1791–1796.

Semprini, D.E., Vucetich, A., Pardi, R. (1987). HIV infection and AIDS in newborn babies of mothers positive for HIV antibody. *British Medical Journal, 194,* 610.

Steiner, G.L. (1990). Children, families and AIDS: Psychosocial and psychotherapeutic aspects. *Psychologist, 40*(3), 11–14.

Strauss, J., Abitbol, C., Zilleruelo, G., et al. (1990). Renal disease in children with the acquired immunodeficiency syndrome. *New England Journal of Medicine, 321*(10), 625–630.

Thomas, P.A., O'Donnell, R.E., Lessner, L. (1987). Survival analysis of children reported with AIDS in New York City, 1982–1986. Proceedings of the Third International Conference on AIDS. Washington, D.C.:WHO.

Thorne, S.E., Robinson, C.A. (1989) Guarded alliance: Health care relationships in chronic illness. *Image: Journal of Nursing Scholarship, 21,* 153–157.

Tiblier, K.B., Walker, G., Rolland, J.S. (1989). Therapeutic issues when working with families of persons with AIDS. In Macklin, J. (Ed.), *AIDS and families* (pp. 81–128). New York: Harrington Park Press.

Wiznia, A.A., Nicholas, S.W. (1990), Organ system involvement in HIV-infected children. *Pediatric Annals, 19*(8), 475–481.

World Health Organization (1990). WHO Collaborating Centre on AIDS, *AIDS Surveillance in Europe, Quarterly Report No. 26,* 30 June 1990. Paris: Institut de Médecine et d'Epidémiologie Africaines et Tropicales.

6

Psychosocial Aspects

Jacquelyn Haak Flaskerud

HIV disease generates a unique series of stresses for infected persons, sexual partners, family members, and health care professionals. It creates serious problems for everyone with whom the infected person has close contacts, including friends and employers. It causes stress in HIV-positive healthy people, in those with clinical disease, in the worried well, and in the general public.

UNIQUE FEATURES OF THE AIDS EPIDEMIC

HIV infection, AIDS, and its related conditions have a constellation of unique characteristics that make them public health problems without contemporary counterpart. AIDS is a relatively new, communicable, sexually transmitted, fatal disease. It was first identified and occurs most frequently in socially stigmatized groups: homosexual men, intravenous drug users (IVDUs), and ethnic and racial minorities. The diagnosis of AIDS is a traumatic event because the disease is known to have a progressive course, no curative treatment, and an extremely poor prognosis. The complexity and multiplicity of problems confronting people with HIV infection and the psychologic fear it engenders affect every aspect of a person's life. Specific features of the AIDS epidemic contribute to the unique psychologic, social, and medical aspects of the disease (Becker & Joseph, 1988; Christ et al., 1988; Fullilove, 1989; Govoni, 1988; Tross & Hirsch, 1988; Wolcott, 1986):

1. Persons diagnosed with HIV disease are generally young. About 21% are in their twenties, 47% in their thirties, and 21% in their forties (CDC, 1991).

2. HIV disease is incurable, requires lifelong changes in behavior, and threatens a person's most intimate relationships.

3. The diagnosis of HIV infection may force the person's identification as a likely member of a stigmatized minority.

4. The social stigma and fear associated with the contagious aspect of the disease can cause others, even family members, to avoid social and physical contact with the infected person.

5. Because of moral disapproval and negative societal attitudes, there is a tendency to blame the infected person for the disease if he or she is in one of the two largest transmission groups.

6. The entire continuum of HIV disease, from exposure through infection to diagnosis, is characterized by extreme uncertainty resulting in marked psychologic distress.

7. Persons with HIV disease are vulnerable to feelings of guilt, self-hatred, rejection, and ostracism, as well as to the commonly recognized feelings of fear, anxiety, depression, and anger that accompany life-threatening illnesses.

8. AIDS is associated with the highest incidence of neurologic and neuropsychiatric morbidity of any serious common illness not primary to the nervous system.

9. AIDS is associated with severe chronic physical disability that leaves persons debilitated and disfigured.

10. Health care professionals and the current patient treatment system for persons with AIDS (PWAs) are severely taxed and often overwhelmed by the complexity and multiplicity of problems associated with AIDS. This situation is likely to worsen as the numbers of patients increase. In addition, fear and a lack of knowledge and sensitivity among health care workers are detrimental to patient care.

11. AIDS has had a highly visible social and political impact. The disease has attracted a barrage of media attention that is not always accurate, is often stressful to PWAs, aggravates public fears, and leads to attempts at repressive measures such as quarantines.

Because of these characteristics of the disease and the epidemic, the care of PWAs requires special attention to the psychologic and social aspects of their disease. Also of concern to health professionals are the stresses experienced by the worried well, by asymptomatic seropositive persons, and by the sexual partners and families of PWAs. The stresses that health care professionals themselves experience in giving care to PWAs are a further consideration.

PSYCHOSOCIAL STRESSES ON ASYMPTOMATIC PERSONS

AIDS is occurring in a society that disapproves of homosexuality, drug use, and sexual promiscuity. This disapproval is accompanied by fear of contagion, prejudice, discrimination, stigmatization, and in extreme cases hatred and violence. It is within this social context that psychologic responses to HIV infection occur (Christ et al., 1988; Fullilove, 1989; Govoni, 1988).

Among asymptomatic persons are those who are not infected. They may be classified as the unworried well and the worried well. The major psychologic responses of the unworried well are denial and dissociation. Heterosexuals practice denial by underestimating their vulnerability to infection. Although they are very aware of AIDS, they do not consider it a threat to themselves. This underestimation of vulnerability is evidenced in the lack of behavioral change among heterosexual adolescents and young adults; in these groups use of condoms and number of sexual partners do not appear to have changed despite reported use of condoms. Risk reduction practices among urban minorities also appear to be limited (Becker & Joseph, 1988). Although a study of drugstore condom sales in the year following the Surgeon General's report on AIDS showed a 20% increase in sales over the previous year, syphilis rates increased 25% in that year, with urban areas having the highest rates (Moran et al., 1990).

Dissociation occurs among heterosexuals both by a physical separation of themselves from the so-called risk groups and by a psychologic dissociation with sexually transmitted diseases (STDs) and drug use. Many people think of both these conditions as so morally reprehensible that they would consider it an extreme insult to question a sexual partner about a history of STDs and drug use. Because of these two psychologic responses, dissociation and denial, to HIV infection, heterosexuals might be characterized as unworried, but also as not careful and therefore vulnerable. These persons rarely seek psychologic or social support related to their affective responses to AIDS.

Several studies on both the East and West coasts have reported that homosexual men have significantly changed their sexual behavior in response to the threat of AIDS (Becker & Joseph, 1988). However, Bauman and Siegel (1987) found that some asymptomatic gay men in New York City had only a weak perception of their vulnerability to HIV disease. Gay men in this study were engaging in risky behaviors but underestimated the risks associated with these behaviors because they knew their sexual partners. They believed the risk to be associated only with anonymous partners. This group might also be characterized as the unworried well.

Their psychologic responses are also those of denial and dissociation with any personal perception of vulnerability.

In addition to these psychologic responses, certain cognitive and affective responses among gay men and IV drug users may be influencing their willingness to change their behavior (Christ et al., 1988). The values gay men place on freedom of sexual expression may conflict with the sexual behavior change demanded by the AIDS epidemic. In the same way, among IVDUs the values placed on sharing, closeness, and interaction may conflict with required changes in needle-sharing behaviors. Persons with these beliefs may choose not to change their risk behaviors.

Another group of asymptomatic persons who are not infected are the worried well. This group includes both those who are not involved in risk behaviors and those whose life-styles have put them at risk for HIV infection (IVDUs or their sexual partners, bisexual and homosexual men, and heterosexuals with multiple sexual partners).The psychologic responses of the worried well are anxiety based (Fullilove, 1989). These responses include generalized anxiety and panic attacks, obsessive-compulsive behavior, hypochondriasis, and anxiety-based physical symptoms.

In some cases, anxieties of the worried well may be relieved by appropriate reassurance and negative HIV antibody tests. However, some persons in this group are not persuaded by laboratory evidence and are convinced that they are experiencing symptoms of HIV disease. These persons are in need of psychotherapy that relates their perception of symptoms to anxiety. However, the subject of HIV antibody testing raises a series of psychologic risks and benefits that must be carefully considered both in recommending and in implementing an HIV testing program.

HIV TESTING AND COUNSELING

HIV antibody testing and counseling usually involve asymptomatic persons concerned about their serostatus. A program of HIV testing and counseling must be concerned with complex ethical, legal, and psychologic issues. Testing has both benefits and harms, and pretest and posttest counseling guidelines must be followed to ensure a safe and beneficial program (Christ et al., 1988; Killian, 1990; Lo et al., 1989; McMahon, 1988).

Ethical and Legal Issues

The assurance of confidentiality is of the highest importance among the issues associated with testing. Disclosure of confidential information can result in discrimination in housing, insurance, health care, and employment. In addition, the impact on interpersonal relationships can be devastating. Some states, California and New York for example, permit physicians or public health officials to notify sexual partners that they are at risk without the consent of the seropositive person. In these cases ethical principles are in conflict: confidentiality and autonomy versus the responsibility to prevent harm.

To protect themselves and their clients, agencies must have clearly written and enforced policies regarding disclosure of test results and maintenance of confidentiality throughout the system. Lawsuits have occurred because confidential information was disclosed. In states where partner notification is permitted, persons considering HIV antibody testing must be notified of this statute before they are tested. In states where such a law does not exist, health providers should try to persuade the infected person to notify partners. If this fails, public health authorities should be notified and asked for their assistance in counseling the infected person and implementing voluntary notification of sexual partners.

A second ethical and legal concern is the presence of a comprehensive standard of care or teaching program within which HIV antibody testing is conducted. Severe psychologic trauma to individuals being tested has occurred because of the way in which seropositive test results were revealed to them. This trauma is compounded by lack of counseling, failure to make referrals, disclosure of inaccurate test results, or institution of inappropriate procedures (e.g., isolation) based on test results. The standard of care for HIV testing and counseling is mandated by law in some states and is recommended in guidelines by the Centers for Disease Control (CDC). The standard of care involves pretest and posttest counseling and may be characterized by its emphasis on completeness and consistency. All relevant information must be provided to persons considering testing. The information provided must be consistent from one person to the next and in accord with standards of practice (CDC guidelines) and the current understanding of HIV disease. Problems arise when different persons are provided with more or less information or conflicting information. In such a situation a person who suffers psychologic or physical harm or injury may be able to establish that a standard of practice was not followed. Improper or negligent counseling may result in liability of the agency. Finally, as part of any comprehensive standard of care, appropriate referral sources for continued counseling, education, medical care, and psychiatric emergencies must be in place before HIV testing begins.

A final ethical and legal issue is the predictive value of HIV antibody testing. Like all laboratory tests, HIV antibody tests are imperfect. Both false-positive and false-negative results can occur. Because false-positive results may have tragic psychologic and legal consequences, repeat testing on a second specimen using the Western blot test should be required before test results are communicated. In persons with no high-risk behaviors, positive results should be repeated on two new serum specimens in a reference laboratory. False-negative antibody results may also occur. A negative result may be misleading and falsely reassuring to a tested person. Seroconversion may take up to 3 months or in rare cases longer. Continued high-risk behaviors may lead to infection of the person and of his or her sexual or needle-sharing partners. Before HIV testing is conducted, persons considering testing must be carefully instructed about the occurrence of false-positive and false-negative test results. They must also be informed in detail what an HIV antibody test result does and does not mean.

Psychologic Issues

The previous section, on ethical and legal issues, referred frequently to the psychologic responses to HIV test results. For asymptomatic persons who are seropositive, significant adverse reactions in the form of depression, anxiety, and preoccupation with AIDS are reported commonly (Tross & Hirsch, 1988). Suicide risk is reported also to be high in persons recently found to be HIV positive (Hall et al., 1989). The devastating effects of seropositive test results include feelings of panic, depression, and hopelessness.

Interpersonal and social responses can also be devastating. Many individuals lose their sexual partners because of disclosure of seropositive results. In addition, discrimination in employment and housing, loss of insurance benefits, and social ostracism, can occur. Persons receiving HIV-positive test results may require prolonged counseling; they also need a variety of social, medical, and psychiatric support services.

Persons who test seronegative may have a false sense of security that could foster continued high-risk behavior. Some persons experience a feeling that they are immune to the virus. Other seronegative persons involved in high-risk behaviors experience ongoing anxiety related to the uncertainty of knowing their HIV antibody status. Still others vacillate between periods of hope and despair regarding their HIV status. Persons who are HIV negative but are engaged in high-risk behaviors may require ongoing counseling and repeated HIV testing. These interventions should include education and behavior change strategies.

Benefits and Risks of Testing

More than most clinical laboratory tests, HIV antibody testing has benefits and risks that must be weighed before a program of testing is instituted (Christ et al., 1988; Lo et al., 1989; McMahon, 1988). The benefits to individuals and society follow. For persons who test seronegative, the benefits include the following:

- Reassurance and reduction of anxiety
- Motivation for behavior change to prevent infection
- Information on which to base decisions about marriage, sexual relationships, childbearing, breast feeding, and immunizations for infants
- Support for an alternative medical diagnosis for unexplained symptoms when HIV disease is under consideration

Asymptomatic persons who test seropositive have these benefits:

- Closer medical follow-up
- Laboratory measurement of disease prognostic markers
- Opportunity for involvement in experimental protocols, early intervention programs, and alternative therapies
- Treatment or prophylaxis for other infectious diseases
- Protection of sexual partners
- Information as a basis for decisions about marriage, sexual relationships, childbearing, breast feeding, and immunizations for infants
- Information for use in future plans for employment, insurance, housing, legal affairs, and so forth

Society receives these benefits from testing:

- Preventing new HIV infections through sexual transmission, IV transmission, the blood supply and organ donations, and perinatal transmission
- Assisting scientists and researchers through enrollment in experimental protocols, through tracking the natural history of HIV infection and disease, and through establishing the incidence and prevalence of infection
- Assisting health providers and planners in designing programs to meet the HIV-related needs of the community and to provide services

There are also risks and harm associated with HIV antibody testing programs (Christ et al., 1988; Lo et al., 1989; McMahon, 1988; Tross & Hirsch, 1988). Persons who test seronegative may have had a false-negative result, resulting in a false sense of security, high-risk behaviors, and infection of others. Asymptomatic persons who test seropositive may experience these problems:

- Possibility of false-positive test results accompanied by psychologic trauma
- Discrimination and ostracism by health care professionals, resulting in medically inappropriate procedures
- Severe psychologic reactions, including anxiety, depression, sleep disturbances, and suicidal behavior
- Disrupted interpersonal relationships
- Sexual dysfunction
- Preoccupation with physical symptoms
- Stigmatization and ostracism by society
- Discrimination in housing and employment
- Loss of insurance
- Exposure to hatred and violence

The potential harm of HIV testing far exceeds that of other laboratory clinical tests. Therefore in any HIV antibody testing program every effort must be made to maximize the benefits and minimize the harm to persons tested. This can be achieved best through a comprehensive pretest and posttest counseling program.

Pretest Counseling

A comprehensive pretest counseling program that meets standards of care in both completeness and consistency has several essential elements (Christ et al., 1988; Killian, 1990; Lo et al., 1989; McMahon, 1988). The pretest counseling program should be extremely comprehensive both to maximize its benefits and because posttest counseling often occurs in a situation of such relief or anxiety that concentration is compromised. The essential elements of a comprehensive pretest counseling program include the following:

- Analysis of reasons for seeking testing and assessment of risk behaviors
- Review of what both positive and negative tests mean and do not mean
- Review of test procedures
- Review of possibility of false-negative and false-positive results

- Review of agency's policy for protecting confidentiality
- General information on the virus and AIDS
- Information on reducing the risk of transmission
- Advice on safer sexual practices, abstinence, and safer drug use
- Information on drug treatment programs
- Provision of condoms and bleach
- General health information on diet, rest, exercise, alcohol and tobacco use, avoiding infections (e.g., STDs and soft tissue infections)
- Information on pregnancy, breast feeding, and immunizations for infants
- Review of potential psychologic and emotional reactions to test results
- Review of potential interpersonal and societal reactions to test results
- Information on alternative testing sites for partners
- Information on medical, social, and psychiatric resources and follow-up counseling
- Review of the risks and benefits of testing

When the pretest counseling session is completed, the counselor should obtain a written informed consent for testing.

Posttest Counseling

As noted earlier, often when the HIV antibody test results are disclosed, the person may be distracted by feelings of relief or anxiety. Therefore a comprehensive approach should be taken during pretest counseling. However, some elements of posttest counseling are essential. These should be both discussed with the person and given in a written format so that he or she can review them later. For persons who test seronegative, posttest counseling includes:

- Interpretation of the test results
- Advice on HIV retesting after 3 months if the person engages in high-risk behaviors
- Information on safer sex and drug use practices
- Provision of condoms and bleach if desired
- Information on needle exchange programs where available

- Information on how to maintain a negative status
- General information on healthy life-style practices
- Information on alternative test sites for partners
- Referral for psychologic, social, medical, and psychiatric services and drug rehabilitation programs as needed
- Follow-up for retesting of persons engaging in high-risk behaviors

For asymptomatic persons who test seropositive, posttest counseling includes the following:

- Reconfirmation of test results on a second serum specimen in a reference laboratory
- Interpretation of the results (includes the information that the person does not have AIDS)
- Evaluation for suicide potential
- Crisis intervention counseling as needed
- Information on whom to tell: partners, health care providers, blood and organ donation centers
- Information on alternative test sites for partners
- Discussion of follow-up for partners and children
- Referral to a partner notification program if needed
- Information on transmission, safer sex and drug use practices, and reinfection
- Information on pregnancy and perinatal transmission
- Information on symptoms associated with the spectrum of HIV disease
- Referral to an early intervention program that includes attention to life-style practices that may suppress the immune system and activate the disease
- Referral to an HIV-positive persons' support group
- Referral for medical follow-up
- Referral for drug rehabilitation program
- Information on entering experimental protocols
- Referral for psychologic, social, and psychiatric services as needed
- Discussion of potential discrimination and effects on housing, employment, insurance, and so forth

Asymptomatic infected persons will benefit from the full range of medical and human services noted previously during the course of their HIV disease. At the time of immediate posttest counseling they may be extremely anxious and unable to absorb the information presented. They should be given written information as well and encouraged to return for additional counseling. Such persons need continual reassurance and support and access to consistent health care. That health care should promote clients' concern for their condition and encourage monitoring and prevention, but avoid an excessive approach that can lead to undue anxiety. One of the most useful forms of support is an ongoing involvement with groups or individuals who share the person's situation and concerns. The overall goals of a comprehensive program for HIV-infected asymptomatic persons are to assist them to (1) cope with psychologic reactions, (2) manage information and resources, and (3) develop a personal health and medical care plan.

PSYCHOSOCIAL STRESSES ON PERSONS WITH AIDS

When HIV-infected people begin having symptoms of disease, they experience all the psychologic and social stresses associated with AIDS. Knowledge of the psychosocial problems associated with other life-threatening illnesses can be applied to understanding the psychosocial consequences of AIDS and designing strategies to meet patients' needs. At this point in the epidemic the medical problems of PWAs, although complex, are somewhat more predictable. Between acute episodes HIV disease may be managed by a structured medical and psychosocial regimen that helps PWAs cope with the fear of the progressive effects of their disease. However, infections must be treated as they occur and often constitute crises. As noted earlier, the stresses associated with AIDS are compounded by the youth of the population affected; the high mortality rate and accompanying anxiety and depression; the social stigma, fear, ostracism, and discrimination associated with the diagnosis of the disease; the debilitation, disfigurement, and symptoms of the disease; and its contagious nature.

Psychosocial Assessment

Concepts important to the care of other persons with life-threatening illnesses have relevance to the care of PWAs (Christ et al., 1988; Govoni, 1988; Saunders, 1989; Tross & Hirsch, 1988; Volberding, 1988; Wolcott, 1986; Wolcott et al., 1986). Information about persons with HIV infection in various categories of assessment can assist the health care professional in anticipating reactions, needs, and vulnerability to psychologic dysfunction and in designing an appropriate psychosocial intervention model (Table 6–1).

Past Psychosocial History. The person's history of interpersonal relationships, education, and career can provide insight into vulnerability to psychologic dysfunction. Use of nonprescribed drugs and alcohol and prior psychiatric care are other indicators of psychologic dysfunction. Psychologically healthy individuals usually have stable jobs and stable interpersonal relationships. Psychologically vulnerable HIV-infected persons may have preillness behaviors that include drug use and multiple sexual contacts. Presence of a personality disorder, as in IVDUs, or of a previous psychiatric disorder is more apt to result in severe psychologic symptoms and a maladaptive response to the stresses of illness.

Current Distress and Crisis. What specific threats and losses is the person experiencing currently? What aspect of the illness is the most distressing and bothersome to the individual at the present time? The person's level of anxiety, fear, and behavioral disorganization will change from one time to the next and will be related to the duration, intensity, and precipitants of the current crisis.

Coping. The person will call into action previous patterns of understanding problems and methods of resolving them when facing HIV disease. Knowing which approaches have been successful for this person in the past and which approaches are currently being tried will give an indication of how he or she will attempt to cope with the illness and how successful that attempt might be. It will also give direction for providing support to the person's coping mechanisms.

Social Support. What sources of support are available to the person: family? spouse? lover? friends? social groups? What is the person's social identity? To which cultural or subcultural groups does he or she belong? What are the possibilities for support within that social identity? Gender, race and ethnicity, and transmission group all affect the amount and kind of social support available and needed by PWAs. Fewer organized resources are available for women, blacks and Hispanics, and IV drug users. Furthermore, the needs of these groups differ from one another and from those of gay white men. The following questions should be asked: What types of support and assistance does the PWA need: practical assistance?

TABLE 6–1. Psychosocial Assessment

1. Past psychosocial history	5. Life cycle phase
2. Current distress and crisis	6. Illness phase
3. Past and current coping	7. Individual identity
4. Social support needed and available	8. Experience with loss and grief

social interaction? emotional support? How can that assistance be provided?

Life Cycle Phase. People have different goals, resources, skills, and social roles depending on their age. The majority of persons with HIV infection are in their twenties, thirties, and forties. These young adults are not developmentally prepared to confront their mortality. Those in their twenties have fewer resources and skills than those in their forties. The former are involved in the psychosocial tasks of establishing independence, autonomy, and adult identity. At times of illness this age group typically becomes intensely reinvolved with the family of origin, emotionally and financially. Older persons (those in their thirties and forties) have more resources (money, housing, insurance) and have established independent adult roles. At times of illness they are more likely to depend on a spouse or lover and friends for support.

Illness Phase. People's needs for psychosocial support differ according to their phase of illness. Stresses on the person are different in the diagnosis, treatment, and after-treatment phases. They also differ depending on the clinical syndrome the person is experiencing: an opportunistic infection, a neoplasm, or a central nervous system (CNS) disease. PWAs fear CNS disease more than other clinical syndromes; the associated memory loss and mood changes result in depression, anger, and strain on their social network (Getzel & Mahony, 1990). Emotional reactions and methods of coping differ in response to the illness phase and clinical syndrome experienced.

Individual Identity. An individual's personal identity also affects his or her reaction to a life-threatening illness. The person's sources of self-esteem, valued achievements, and future goals make up that person's identity. These and the individual's orientation to living and search for meaning all play a role in how the person perceives and combats the illness.

Loss and Grief. The losses the individual has experienced, is experiencing currently, and anticipates experiencing as a result of the illness affect the kind of psychosocial support the person needs. Persons may be currently grieving a loss and going through the grief process. They may have previous experiences with loss and grief and feel some recognition and equanimity toward the process, or they may have no previous experience and be anxious and fearful about anticipated losses and the grieving process.

● ● ●

An assessment of the person with HIV disease in these various areas will provide the health care professional with the information needed to design a psychosocial intervention plan. This plan can be individualized to meet the specific needs of individuals as they move through the various phases of the disease and the phases of their emotional and social responses to the illness. The common psychosocial crises that occur in PWAs have been identified, and intervention strategies have been designed to support them during these crises.

Psychologic Stresses

The major psychologic stress on PWAs is the knowledge that they have a fatal disease with the potential for a rapid decline to death. Most symptoms are of fear, anxiety, and depression, which are compounded by the uncertainty of the course of the disease. Social stresses on PWAs include exposure, stigma, rejection, abandonment, and isolation. Common reactions are guilt, fear, anger, and suspicion (Baum & Nesselhof, 1988; Bennett, 1988, 1990; Christ et al., 1988; Frierson & Lippmann, 1988; Fullilove, 1989; Gambe & Getzel, 1989; Getzel & Mahony, 1990; Govoni, 1988; Hall et al., 1989; Saunders, 1989; Tross & Hirsch, 1988; Wolcott, 1986; Wolcott et al., 1986).

Certain crisis points in the course of the disease precipitate intense anxiety, fear, and depression (Table 6–2). The initial crisis is at diagnosis. The same existential issues that accompany a diagnosis of other life-threatening illnesses occur with AIDS. The normal response is charac-

TABLE 6–2. Crisis Points and Emotional Response

CRISIS POINT	EMOTIONS AND BEHAVIORS	INTERVENTIONS
Diagnosis	Intense anxiety; fear; anger; guilt; impulsive behavior; suicidal ideation	Suicide assessment Crisis intervention Pharmacotherapy
Treatment	Depression; weakness, alienation; dysphoria; fear of disfigurement, disability, pain	Individual therapy Education Resource provison Stress reduction techniques
Treatment termination	Anxiety; fear	Support groups
New symptoms	Hypochondriasis; demanding and dependent behavior; anxiety	Support assistance Clergy; attorney
Recurrence and relapse	Depression; dependence; apathy; isolation; suicidal ideation; dysphoria; fear of abandonment	
Terminal illness	Deterioration; decline; ambivalence; dependence; disinterest; resolution	

terized by disbelief, numbness, feeling already dead, and denial, followed by anger, turmoil, disruptive anxiety, and depressive symptoms. High levels of anxiety can exist for 2 to 3 months after diagnosis and can take the form of panic attacks, agitation, tachycardia, impulsive behaviors such as sexual acting-out, and suicidal ideation.

The treatment phase is often accompanied by weakness, depression, alienation, and dysphoria. Patients fear disfigurement, debilitation, and pain. Treatment often includes isolation procedures that make patients feel alienated and socially abandoned. The termination of treatment often brings on increased anxiety and fears of renewed disease progression. Hypervigilance with body functions and the appearance of new symptoms can result in hypochondriacal concerns, demanding behavior toward medical personnel, and excessive dependence on health care givers.

Recurrence or relapse of disease is often accompanied by feelings of hopelessness, helplessness, sadness, low self-esteem, discouragement, loss of control, dependence, isolation, and suicidal ideation. Patients fear being abandoned by health care givers who might decide that continued treatment is futile. This stage may be accompanied by cognitive impairment because of CNS disease. The terminal phase of illness is marked by deterioration and decline and can be accompanied by ambivalence, dependence, disinterest, or resolution.

The potential for suicide has been recognized at several crisis points in HIV infection and disease. Increased risk of suicide is associated with HIV antibody testing and learning of a seropositive status, with a diagnosis of AIDS, and with later stages of illness that may be characterized by pain and dementia (Glass, 1988; Perry et al., 1990). The suicide rate of men aged 20 to 59 years with AIDS in New York City in 1985 was 36 times that of men of the same age without this diagnosis and 66 times that of the general population (Marzuk et al., 1988). Persons with AIDS who are more likely to kill themselves are those with previous depressive episodes, high levels of environmental stress, inadequate counseling before and after the HIV antibody test, and poor support networks (Frierson & Lippmann, 1988). Several groups whose behavior puts them at risk for HIV infection are also those who are more at risk for suicide. IVDUs frequently have preexisting affective disorders. Gay men and lesbians attempt suicide twice as often as their heterosexual counterparts, and racial stigma has been linked with suicide (Hall & Stevens, 1988).

Assessment of suicide risk should accompany any of the crisis points in HIV infection and disease. Assessment should include a history of affective disorder and drug use; an investigation of a plan and method for suicide; an evaluation of the extent, availability, and supportiveness of the person's social network; whether significant others have committed suicide; whether the person is suffering grief and loss; socioeconomic status (housing, employment, insurance); and spirituality. Persons with

AIDS contemplating suicide may have made suicide pacts with friends and loved ones, and they may be grieving the loss of friends who died of AIDS. They may be experiencing the loss of independent functioning accompanied by a loss of self-esteem. They may be facing also an existential crisis in which life has ceased to have meaning. Any or all of these factors may be motivation for suicide.

During crisis points PWAs need a full range of psychosocial interventions. These include immediate crisis intervention or individual therapy, or both, to deal with feelings of extreme anxiety, fear, and anger and with impulsive behavior and suicidal thoughts and behaviors. Persons with HIV disease should be encouraged to express their anxiety, fear, sadness, and anger and to grieve with the understanding that grief is a healing process. Pharmacotherapy should be used for intense anxiety, depression, hopelessness, and insomnia. Whenever possible, health care givers should support and enhance the person's coping mechanisms and defenses and not work in opposition to these unless they are dangerous or destructive. Patients also need ongoing psychosocial support in the form of support groups to dispel self-blame and guilt, provide reassurance, share information and experiences, and reduce feelings of isolation and loneliness. Experience with persons with HIV disease in support groups and research on levels of distress in persons with AIDS, AIDS-related complex (ARC), and lymphadenopathy syndrome (LAS) suggest that separate support groups be developed for persons with clinical disease: one for persons with LAS and ARC, one for persons with Kaposi's sarcoma, and one for other PWAs. These suggestions are based on the differing levels of anxiety and areas of concern of these people (Ragsdale & Morrow, 1990).

Infected people need education regarding the disease and its treatment, liaison with community resources to help them resolve practical problems, instruction in stress and anxiety reduction tehniques such as relaxation, and suportive intervention from a social network that includes family, friends, health professionals, volunteers, attorney, and clergy, who can offer encouragement, comfort, concern, compassion, affection, and legal and spiritual assistance.

All of these interventions play a role in the treatment of PWAs during crisis stages. Which will take priority at any given time depends on individual response and can be determined by psychosocial assessments of the patient at crisis points. If possible, the patient should be assigned a primary caregiver, primary care nurse, or case manager to coordinate service needs and provide a central and familiar person the patient can see to ensure continuity of care throughout the course of the illness, hospitalizations, community care, and referrals.

People with HIV disease are subjected to an unusual number of psychologic or internal conflicts (Table 6–3). Some of these revolve around

TABLE 6–3. Internal Conflicts and Emotional Responses

PSYCHOLOGIC CONFLICT	EMOTIONS AND BEHAVIORS	INTERVENTIONS
Transmission	Anxiety; depression, fear; anger	Education
		Resource provision
Protection from infection	Suspicion; guilt	Support groups
Previous life-style	Internalized homophobia or societal prejudices; bargaining to go straight; preexisting affective symptoms	Stress reduction techniques
Personal relationships	Loneliness; frustration; rejection; abandonment	

transmission of the disease: who the person got it from or to whom he or she might have passed it. Emotional responses to these internal conflicts can be directed toward self and others and involve anxiety, depression, fear, anger, suspicion, and guilt.

Similar concerns and conflicts are evident in the person's efforts to protect himself or herself from the risk of infection. Fear of associating with others, anger at and suspicion of others who might transmit infection, and guilt and loneliness from abandoning friends for self-protection are all involved in this conflict. People may also experience guilt over their previous life-styles, especially if they have had a number of anonymous sexual partners or have used IV or recreational drugs. Getzel and Mahony (1990) report bargaining to go straight or denying a homosexual identity as part of a search for a magical cure among PWAs in group therapy in New York City. For IVDUs, the presence of preexisting affective disorders compounds the psychologic problems of HIV disease. Considerable feelings of guilt and self-blame among PWAs can cause them to internalize society's prejudicial attitudes toward the group(s) to which they belong and lead them, in turn, to stigmatize others. Among homosexuals this is called internalized homophobia, but it can happen in any group toward which society expresses disapproval, such as drug users, prostitutes, and persons with multiple sexual partners.

Finally, many conflicts occur over continuing personal relationships, especially if these have a sexual focus. Fears of social abandonment, isolation, and loneliness accompany giving up intimate sexual relationships. This is especially true if sexual relationships were used to provide interpersonal contacts.

Certain sexual practices (e.g., anal intercourse) among gay men and ritual needle sharing among IVDUs may have functioned to integrate the person into the homosexual or drug-using community. Giving up these practices and making major life-style changes may become an emotional crisis in itself. Restraints on sexual or drug use behavior may demand new social skills for negotiation, limit setting, or partner rejection, as well as new psychologic skills for tolerating frustration, managing anxiety, self-reassurance, and self-control.

Some of these psychologic conflicts can be resolved through education groups that focus on transmission and protection from infection. Others can be resolved through support groups and finding reassurance and shared experiences among other persons with the same concerns. These concerns include sharing unacceptable feelings, providing positive reinforcement, and exploring options to enhance the quality of daily life. Support groups can also help prevent loneliness and isolation and can identify ways for members to reach out to family and friends. Community resources can help people build social networks and develop sustained relationships that are not predicated on sex or drug use and sharing. The use of stress reduction techniques, such as relaxation or other behavioral techniques, can assist individuals in dealing with their fears and anxieties.

Social Stresses

Persons with HIV disease are subject to an unusual number of social conflicts and stresses (Table 6–4). The first of these may involve public identification as a member of a highly stigmatized group. Social stigmatization is attached to both of the largest transmission groups for HIV infection: male homosexuals and IVDUs. Persons who have considered their sexuality or drug use to be private matters are now subject to exposure and possible rejection by family and friends. Because the diagnosis is AIDS, they may be abandoned by friends who accept their sexual preference or drug use but are afraid of the disease. At a time when people most need social support, comfort, compassion, and closeness, they might be left alone and isolated. Confiding the diagnosis to family and friends

TABLE 6–4. Social Stress and Emotional Responses

SOCIAL CONFLICT	EMOTIONS AND BEHAVIORS	INTERVENTIONS
Disclosure and exposure	Fear of abandonment, isolation, and rejection	Support groups
		Stress reduction techniques
Stigma	Guilt; anger; suspicion	Resource provision
Employment and insurance	Insecurity because of loss of job and health benefits	Financial counseling
Social support limitations	Loneliness; alienation	
Distance from family		

is often not a matter of personal choice. A diagnosis of AIDS is difficult to hide because of the obvious physical signs, such as frequent illness, disfigurement, and debilitation.

Persons with ARC and LAS and asymptomatic persons who are seropositive are faced with a dilemma as to whether to confide in friends, family, and health care workers, since stigmatization and social rejection are likely to result from receipt of this information. Levels of psychologic distress in persons with ARC or asymptomatic seropositive persons are often high. Some studies have found that persons with ARC scored higher than persons with AIDS on several self-report measures of distress (King, 1989; Ragsdale & Morrow, 1990; Tross & Hirsch, 1988). In addition, among PWAs, one third had not discussed their health problems or sexual orientation with their families or employers; but among persons with ARC two thirds had not done so. Among those who had disclosed information one fourth experienced negative reactions: condemnation or outright rejection. These reactions occurred most commonly among confidants but were also found among employers and health care workers. Limandri (1989) reported that what persons seek from disclosure is compassion, understanding, and information. Participating in a support group can provide the opportunity to practice telling others in an environment that is least likely to be rejecting.

PWAs have been confronted with a variety of problems involving employment and insurance. Some individuals have been fired from their jobs because employers and coworkers feared they would contract AIDS. In some cases this discrimination has extended to the families of PWAs. Others have had to leave jobs because of physical disability. In many instances health insurance is lost when the job is lost. PWAs are often young and have limited experience with medical insurance policies. Many are, in fact, new in the work force and employed by small companies with no insurance coverage. In addition, some insurance companies have tried to avoid covering PWAs because of the high costs of care. Many PWAs are without financial security, resources, and insurance. Community resources they might need include Social Security Disability Insurance, Supplemental Security Income, and Medicaid. These should be applied for immediately and arrangements should be made also for legal assistance and personal assistance in the home, such as visiting nurse services and "buddies" to assist with chores and shopping.

Finally, many PWAs have limited social support networks. Many times families are not involved with the person, or they live in distant and separate places. This could be due to alienation from the family because of life-style or to relocation in a large urban area, such as New York, San Francisco, or Los Angeles, that is far from where the family lives. Some families abandon a relative with AIDS when they learn of the diagnosis. This action could be the result of a desire to avoid social stigma, an incorrect belief that homosexuality or drug use itself causes AIDS and that the disease is a just retribution, or fear of contagion. Such a situation leaves the person at a crucial time without a family to assist with basic physical needs and to provide emotional support and forces a greater dependence on spouses, lovers, and friends. Community resources can help to meet basic physical needs of PWAs at home through practical services such as shopping and housekeeping. Some clergy and churches assist visiting parents and siblings in finding places to stay when they come from out of town. The gay community and gay service agencies in large cities have organized a variety of supportive services for persons with limited or distant social support networks. These services include case management, which provides social service, nursing service, insurance, counseling, client advocacy, and emotional and physical support through a "buddy" system (Katoff & Dunne, 1988; Sonsel, 1989).

Political and social organizations that offer specialized services are less commonly available to drug users who have AIDS, women and children with AIDS, and hemophiliacs and blood transfusion recipients with AIDS (Christ et al., 1988; Tiblier et al., 1989). The social network and support resources of drug users usually consist of other drug users and family; they have no organized community for support. Close liaison with drug rehabilitation programs and self-help groups of former addicts may provide some supportive service for IVDUs with AIDS. Women with AIDS are often IVDUs or the sexual partners of IVDUs. Specialized AIDS services for women are extremely limited, but supportive services are sometimes provided through other women's organizations that focus on domestic violence, rape, and homelessness. Children with AIDS most frequently have parents with AIDS and a very limited support network. A few hospitals have begun support groups for children who have siblings or parents with AIDS. Nonspecific children's services might be useful also. Persons with hemophilia have supportive medical and social resources to deal with their hemophilia that might be mobilized to assist with problems associated with AIDS, but few specialized AIDS services. Blood transfusion recipients have extremely limited AIDS support services. In addition, both persons with hemophilia and blood transfusion recipients may feel betrayed by the medical system because of the means of their infection with HIV.

As can be noted from the foregoing discussion, the psychosocial stresses on persons with AIDS are overwhelming. They call for a range of psychologic, social, economic, and legal interventions, and at any given time in the course of a person's disease they may call for all the interventions and services discussed in this section. Added to the picture of psychosocial stresses and need for appropriate psychologic and social services to PWAs are the psychosocial stresses on lovers, spouses, and friends of the PWA and their needs for services and support.

PSYCHOSOCIAL STRESSES ON THE LOVER, SPOUSE, OR SEXUAL PARTNER

A diagnosis of AIDS has widespread consequences that affect the person's entire social support network. Affected most immediately and extensively is the lover, spouse, or sexual partner of the PWA. This person experiences both psychologic and social effects of having a partner with AIDS (Christ et al., 1988; Dean et al., 1988; Frierson & Lippmann, 1988; Greif & Porembski, 1989; Schoen & Schindelman, 1989; Tiblier et al., 1989; Wolcott, 1986; Wolcott et al., 1986) (Table 6–5). One psychologic stress experienced by the lover or spouse of a PWA might be guilt about possibly having transmitted the disease. Another is fear of being infected through sexual contact with the PWA. These issues can be discussed in support groups for the spouse, lover, or sexual partner of the PWA or in support groups for couples in which one partner has AIDS. Through sharing experiences, support groups help members avoid self-blame and guilt. They also provide information on contagion and transmission, as well as a safe setting in which members can frankly discuss needed changes in sexual practices.

The psychologic stresses related to a diagnosis of a life-theatening illness and the premature death of a young adult can cause the same existential crisis, anxiety, and depression in the lover or spouse as it does in the PWA. Among gay men especially, losses of loved ones can occur frequently, sometimes without any time to recuperate from previous losses and sometimes unrelentingly over a long period. Some social networks have been decimated by AIDS, leading to chronic bereavement in survivors. Often bereavement is accompanied by significant physical and psychologic symptoms. Despair over a loved one's death from AIDS can reach suicidal proportions. Lovers and spouses should seek individual counseling to assist them in dealing with their crisis, as well as with the ongoing sadness, fear, and anxiety that can accompany impending death in a young

TABLE 6–5. Psychosocial Stresses on Lover or Spouse

STRESS	INTERVENTIONS
Guilt over transmission	Lover-spouse support groups or couples
Fear of contagion	groups
Anxiety, fear, depression over life-threatening illness	Individual therapy
	Community resources
Disrupted relationship equilibrium	Attorney, clergy, liaison psychiatry
Decisions regarding treatment	Bereavement groups
Conflicts with family and hospital staff	
Anticipatory and postmortem grief	

partner. Support groups can also provide emotional support to spouses and lovers.

Various social stresses affect the spouse or lover of a PWA. Major stresses occur because the equilibrium of the relationship is disrupted. A relationship based on interdependence, mutual support, autonomy, and egalitarianism may be severely threatened when one partner becomes emotionally and physically dependent, unable to contribute financially, limited in the ability to provide support, and impaired in cognitive functions. Spouses and lovers can find themselves involved in activities that drain them physically, emotionally, and financially. Caring for the partner with AIDS can require losing time from work, constantly supervising the PWA, assisting with all aspects of daily living, and providing emotional support, comfort, compassion, and affection. The diagnosis of AIDS also requires a change in sexual activities, both to prevent transmission of infection and in response to decreased sexual desires because of illness. All of these changes in the relationship can be intensely stressful and demoralizing to the spouse or lover. Again, support groups for lovers and spouses or for couples can help resolve some of these issues through sharing of experiences. They also provide information on community resources to assist lovers and spouses in the care of the partner.

Stresses associated with frequent and prolonged hospitalization of the partner can range from the logistics of visiting, to making sure that the partner's financial and insurance resources remain adequate, to making decisions about the partner's medical treatment. The lover or spouse is often called on to make decisions when the partner's mental status is compromised or when the partner is extremely ill. Decisions about life support and the disposition of property often fall to the spouse or lover. Early in the illness the partner with AIDS and the lover or spouse should discuss the partner's wishes regarding treatment, life support, funeral, burial, and disposition of property. Lovers must obtain a durable power of attorney to carry out these decisions.

Decisions made by the PWA and his or her partner can create conflicts with hospital staff and with family and can cause additional stress on the lover or spouse. Decisions regarding treatment and life support may conflict with the course of action the hospital staff believes is necessary or indicated. These conflicts can often be resolved with the assistance of the psychiatric consultation-liaison team, hospital chaplain, and hospital attorney. These same persons can assist in mediating conflicts between the spouse or lover and the patient's family. Sometimes the partner of the PWA is blamed for the disease. Conflicts are more common when families are emotionally distant from the patient and do not realize the extent and depth of the relationship between the patient and lover in a gay relationship. Disputes can arise over treatment issues, burial, and disposition of property. In addition to helping resolve conflicts, hospital liaison psychiatry, clergy, and attorneys can assist the lover or spouse and patient in preparing for these situations and taking the necessary steps to implement their decisions.

Finally, lovers and spouses of PWAs must face anticipatory grief over the loss of a partner and postmortem grief when the partner dies. Sometimes a bereaved gay partner is denied a rightful place in funerals and memorial services. There may be disputes over wills and life insurance. AIDS support groups in large cities focus specifically on bereavement and the grief process. These groups encourage persons to grieve—to express sadness, fear, loneliness, anger, and guilt—with the understanding that grief is a healing process that is important to the recovery of the bereaved.

PSYCHOSOCIAL STRESSES ON FAMILY AND FRIENDS

The families and friends of PWAs often need supportive care themselves (Table 6–6). For gay men, friends may represent a reconstituted family. All of the emotional and social reactions that occur with PWAs, lovers, and spouses also occur with families and friends: shock, denial, anxiety, anger, fear, guilt, and depression (Britton & Zarski, 1989; Christ et al., 1988; Frierson & Lippmann, 1988; Greif & Porembski, 1989; Kelly & Sykes, 1989; Pheifer & Houseman, 1988; Rinella & Dublin, 1988; Schoen & Schindelman, 1989; Solomon, 1990; Tibesar, 1986; Tiblier et al., 1989). Families experience conflict under the best of circumstances; a chronic, eventually terminal illness strains family relationships and requires nurturing of a sick member at a time when families might least expect or be equipped to do so. Furthermore, preexisting conflicts between the family and the PWA regarding life-style or sexual preference may have resulted in the family's emotional and geographic distance from the patient. In other cases the distance is only geographic and results from the person's having relocated in a major metropolitan area. Either situation makes the

TABLE 6–6. Psychosocial Stresses on Families

STRESS	INTERVENTIONS
Preexisting conflicts	Supportive interventions of consultation-liaison
Revelation of life-style	team, clergy, attorney
Guilt over life-style	Support groups
Fear of social stigma	Community resources
Conflict with PWA's lover	
Physical, emotional, and financial drain	
Loss and grief	

family's relationship with the PWA difficult and imposes stress on the family. Families who are emotionally distant by choice may feel ambivalent about the PWA or may reject him or her, leading to psychologic turmoil that includes anger, bitterness, anxiety, embarrassment, and despair. Anger at the PWA may be generated by the thought that the person's behavior (i.e., sexuality or IV drug use) is killing him or her; however, often families are unwilling to express anger toward a family member with a terminal illness. Families who are geographically distant experience severe situational stresses in attempting to visit with no place to stay and being unable to provide emotional and physical assistance because of distance. Families should know that most large cities that are AIDS epicenters have local services available to family members even if they are from out of town.

Some families experience other stresses. The diagnosis of AIDS may be their first knowledge that their relative is homosexual, is a drug user, or has had multiple sexual partners. This news is greeted with shock, anger, bewilderment, rejection, and sometimes guilt. In this case families experience double grieving: for their relative's behavior or identity and for his or her terminal illness. Parents may feel guilty because they believe that they are responsible for their child's life-style. This is especially true of mothers, who traditionally have been blamed by society for their children's actions. Knowledge of a relative's homosexuality, drug use, or promiscuity may cause conflict and divided loyalties within a family. Sometimes certain family members, usually siblings, have known of the person's life-style but have kept it secret from parents. As a result they have felt isolated from their own support system. Sometimes a mother has kept such information secret from a father. Family members kept in the dark might feel hurt because they were not informed earlier. In other families no one has preexisting knowledge, but when the person's life-style is revealed some in the family decide to accept it and others to reject it. Fears and suspicions are aroused, and loyalties are threatened.

When the PWA is an IV drug user, other kinds of family conflicts occur. Some families serve as enablers of the person's drug use by providing support, housing, and money. Such families may feel guilty that they are responsible for the person's disease. In other cases the diagnosis of AIDS reveals to the family that a person is still using drugs. Under these circumstances families feel hurt, anger, and betrayal.

When the PWA is a young child, other stresses and conflicts occur within the family. In many such families parents are also infected. In these cases siblings may feel fear and insecurity about who will care for them. They may also feel resentment and anger toward the PWA because of the lack of attention given them by the family during the PWA's illness.

In all these situations, families need compassionate, supportive, constructive assistance from clergy, health care givers, and the psychiatric consultation-liaison team to deal with their feelings, work together, help the PWA cope, and assist in the PWA's care. They can also use assistance with such practical needs as housing and transportation and can benefit from sharing feelings and experiences in a support group for families. Support groups for children and younger siblings of PWAs can assist them in coping with their special issues.

As mentioned in the previous section, families sometimes perceive the PWA's lover as having too much control in treatment decisions. Families have to adjust to the lover's role as equivalent to that of a spouse. This is especially difficult if they have not met or known each other before. Since the lover's role and responsibilities are socially ambiguous, they often must be clarified before families and lovers can work together for the well-being of the PWA.

Another social stress that families face is whether to disclose the diagnosis of AIDS to friends and then which friends to tell. Having a child or sibling with AIDS subjects the family to the powerful threat of social stigma and rejection by friends, neighbors, co-workers, and schoolmates. Children and adolescents are often kept in the dark about a parent's or sibling's HIV disease in an effort to protect them from social stigma and rejection. They may be confused and distessed about being excluded from a family problem. On the other hand, rejection and taunting by schoolmates and neighbors are real possibilities if the family member's disease becomes known. In addition, adolescents may suffer embarrassment because they are in the process of confronting their own sexuality.

The consequence of social rejection and stigma is that families lack the social support they would normally receive when a family member has a life-threatening illness. In addition, during their bereavement some of the emotional support that usually accompanies mourning may not be available to them. When the diagnosis is not disclosed to others, often pain becomes intensified and sorrow is prolonged. Whether to tell friends can present a major conflict. Because of this situation, support groups become an important part of a family's social network. In addition, clergy can take the lead in establishing an atmosphere of compassion and concern among their parishioners so that the traditional social support of religion is available.

The prolonged pain and debility of the PWA is another stress to families. In some instances the PWA pressures the family to help him or her commit suicide. Prolonged debility brings with it great need for physical, emotional, and financial assistance. It can deplete family resources and drain family members emotionally and physically. Often families must make difficult decisions about life support or whether to continue to provide food and fluids. The provision of emotional support, physical assistance, financial assistance, and community resources is essential to supportive care of the family.

Families and friends also face fears of contagion and transmission and will benefit from education regarding the disease. Friends who have been involved in behaviors or circumstances similar to those of the PWA may feel vulnerable because they identify with the ill person. In addition, they might want to be supportive but not know how. For many the diagnosis of AIDS in a friend leads to difficult reappraisals and evaluations of their own life-styles and behaviors. As noted earlier, some gay social networks have been decimated by AIDS. In these instances bereavement is chronic, and some individuals wonder whether anyone will be left in the network to care for them.

Issues of bereavement affect both family and friends. Since PWAs are usually young, lovers, spouses, family, and friends are dealing with loss and grief in the context of an untimely, undeserved, and unjust illness and death. John Kennedy said at the death of his infant son that "it is an unnatural thing for parents to bury a child." These issues, as well as sadness, anger, anxiety, guilt, and loss, must be dealt with as part of the grief process. For many survivors of PWAs the grief and healing process is long. Sadness, hurt, anger, and guilt can go on for a significant period after the death. Families must deal with the ambivalence of grief and anger, as well as the confusion and pain caused by social rejection. In some survivors suicide is a concern; in others guilt over transmission or over survival is an issue. Ongoing involvement in family support groups for as long as 2 years has been found especially beneficial. The services of mental health counselors and clergy can greatly facilitate the grief process.

SPIRITUAL NEEDS

Throughout the discussion of psychosocial stresses on PWAs, their partners, families, and friends, references have been made to the need for the services of clergy. The spiritual needs of PWAs, their loved ones, and caregivers involve existential concerns about self-identity; the meaning of life, adversity, and individual destiny; the need for love and acceptance; and sometimes the need for reconciliation and forgiveness (Table 6–7). Spiritual needs of PWAs present a special challenge to nursing care, particularly in the face of organized religion's condemnation and rejection of homosexuals, drug users, and sexually promiscuous persons (Bellemare, 1988; Bennett, 1988; Dunphy, 1987; Govoni, 1988; Graydon, 1988; Hall & Stevens, 1988; Saynor, 1988; Tibesar, 1986; Tiblier et al., 1989).

Spirituality or the spiritual dimension of an individual's life involves questions about the meaning of life, hope, self-identity, and self-worth. It can also embody forgiveness and reconciliation. In contrast to religious practice and organized religion (although these are meant to serve the spiritual needs of their members), spirituality does not involve a particular

TABLE 6–7. Spiritual Needs and Care of Persons with AIDS

SPIRITUAL NEED	SPIRITUAL CARE
Meaning, value, hope, purpose, direction	Know spiritual concerns and issues
	Strengthen person's sense of worth, identity, and dignity
Love, acceptance	Provide compassionate, accepting care
Reconciliation with family, church	Listen
Rituals and practices of organized religion	Provide assistance in locating clergy, a religious community

creed, liturgy, or theism. The spiritual needs of PWAs and their significant others include a profound need for meaning and hope. Most people create a self-identity and a sense of self-worth from their professional and personal relationships and the consequent productivity and satisfaction engendered. These relationships give their lives meaning, a sense of purpose, direction, and value. AIDS threatens an individual's meaning and hope with physical debilitation, anxiety, loss of personal relationships, social alienation, rejection, and loss of job and productivity. PWAs often must reestablish the sense that their life has value, direction, and purpose. The significant others of PWAs also experience anxiety, personal and social isolation and alienation, and an unacceptable and abrupt death of a young loved one from a controversial disease.

Traditionally people turn to the clergy, religion, and pastoral care to help them meet their spiritual needs. Many PWAs, however, view organized religion and its value system as oppressive and irrelevant. Their experiences with organized religion often have been negative, and they are alienated from the religious community. Many have lived without spiritual comfort or support. When they feel spiritual needs, they may not recognize them as such or they may repress or deny them.

The ultimate spiritual concerns of PWAs include questions of self-identity (Who am I now?), questions about the meaning of life (Is there any value or purpose to this suffering? Is there a reason to go on living?), questions about adversity (Is life essentially cruel and unfair?), questions about destiny (Why did this happen to me?), and questions about being or existence (Has my life made a difference? Have I made a contribution to the world? Will I be remembered?). PWAs also ask other questions that relate directly to AIDS, its stigma, and social ostracism. Questions about AIDS being a punishment for homosexuality, for using drugs, or for enjoying life can leave PWAs guilt ridden.

To deal with all of these questions, both PWAs and their loved ones have a need for spiritual care. Often that care comes from clergy and is known as pastoral care. However, health care workers can also provide spiritual care. Knowing the spiritual concerns of the PWA is the first step.

Approaching the PWA with compassion, nurturance, and support is the second. Spiritual care for PWAs must respect their conscience and integrity, accept and affirm their lives and their relationships, and break through the perception that spirituality is the preserve of the religious. Spiritual care involves strengthening the person's sense of meaning, purpose, worth, dignity, and identity. A sense of meaning and hope is life affirming and nourishing, whereas the collapse of a person's meaning system is a primary motivation for suicide.

In addition to meaning and hope, PWAs need love and acceptance. Fulfilling this need is sometimes hard for significant others and health care workers because sick or dying people are often irascible, demanding, hostile, and unreasonable. The assistance of clergy and the religious community with these needs can be invaluable. Not only can they provide PWAs with the love and acceptance needed, but also they can support health care givers and significant others in meeting these spiritual needs on a consistent basis.

A third step in providing spiritual care is being available to listen. Health care workers can be open to discussions about faith, belief, meaning in life, and mortality. They can help PWAs review their lives, identify what has given them meaning and hope in the past, and plan experiences that will provide purpose and identity in the present and future. Sometimes PWAs request help in reconnecting with traditional faith and organized religion. Some ask for the ritual and practices of a particular religion. These practices provide comfort and give the person a sense of continuity with his or her past. They can decrease feelings of anxiety, isolation, and alienation by offering an experience of community. The health care worker can find clergy who are willing to work with PWAs and their families in approaching the spiritual dimension of the illness. Clergy can assist PWAs in reconciling with their families and their church. They can encourage PWAs, their families, and their congregations to forgive one another. Members of a congregation or religious community can be an important support system, providing spiritual, emotional, physical, and financial assistance. Furthermore, acceptance by a religious congregation can help PWAs and their families and loved ones counter the feelings of guilt and sin that have been associated with the disease.

An understanding and supportive response to the spiritual needs of the PWA can benefit the person's overall health and well-being. Responding to clients' spiritual needs will help them to live a life of meaning and purpose and to die with dignity and a sense of completion. Health care workers can provide spiritual care or can facilitate the provision of spiritual care to their clients. In addition, health care workers must be aware of their own spiritual and psychosocial needs in caring for PWAs.

PSYCHOSOCIAL STRESSES ON NURSES AND OTHER HEALTH CARE GIVERS

Caring for persons with HIV disease puts enormous stress on health care workers (Table 6–8). This is especially true of nurses and interns because they spend the most time with patients and have the closest contact with them through performing supportive care and procedures. Nurses and other health care workers are subject to a wide range of emotional, social, and work-related stresses, some of which are also experienced by patients, lovers, spouses, families, and friends of PWAs and some of which are unique to health care givers. In general, their reactions can be characterized as pertaining to disease and death, sexuality and intimacy, and the burdens and rewards of caretaking (Abbing, 1988; Bolle, 1988; Christ et al., 1988; Frierson & Lippmann, 1988; Gambe & Getzel, 1989; Getzel & Mahony, 1990; Govoni, 1988; Hall et al., 1989; Kelly et al., 1987; McKusick, 1988; Minkin, 1989; Pasacreta & Jacobsen, 1989; Rinella & Dublin, 1988; Tiblier et al., 1989; Volberding, 1988; Wolcott, 1986; Wolcott et al., 1986).

Initially nurses and other health care workers have anxiety and concerns about contagion and transmission. They are in contact with the patient's body fluids, administer medications and IV fluids, change beds, bathe patients, and provide toilet care. Their concerns include fears of personal exposure (e.g., needlesticks) and exposure of other staff members. In addition, they have concerns about appropriate infection control procedures. This extends to fears of introducing infection to the AIDS patient, of cross-infection of other patients, and of adequately teaching infection control procedures to families, friends, lovers, and spouses of patients. Since the introduction, through in-service education, of adequate and accurate information concerning AIDS and infection control procedures, anxiety has decreased somewhat. Willingness to work with patients with

TABLE 6–8. Psychosocial Stresses on Nurses and Other Health Care Workers

STRESS	INTERVENTIONS
Contagion and transmission	Education
Discomfort with homosexuality and drug use	Adequate staff and resources
Intensive complicated care	Psychosocial support groups
Facing own mortality	Crisis intervention and individual support
Repetitive grief	port
Conflicts over goals of treatment	Clear institutional policies and goals on treatment
	Personal stress reduction

AIDS and appropriate precautions and behavior toward PWAs have improved. The fear of transmission has had social consequences for health care workers, some of whose spouses or lovers have urged them to quit their jobs to avoid infection of themselves and their families. Others have experienced social stigma and avoidance by friends because they work with PWAs.

Stresses on nurses also result from the uncertainty and discomfort they feel in relating to drug users, prostitutes, sexually promiscuous persons, homosexuals, and the lover of the gay PWA. Personal values, cultural background, and religious ideals are challenged by the different backgrounds of these patients. Again, through education and with the assistance of the consultation-liaison psychiatric team or mental health consultants, nurses have become more comfortable discussing sexuality openly. This includes knowing enough about bisexuality and homosexuality to understand the issues and problems related to HIV transmission and being able to discuss sexual precautions and answer questions of lovers and family. Several studies have measured health care workers' attitudes toward homosexuals and AIDS. Both physicians and registered nurses have demonstrated homophobic and AIDS-phobic attitudes and behaviors (Kelly et al., 1987, 1988).

The intense physical care and emotional needs of hospitalized PWAs can cause health care workers to become overtaxed, stressed, fatigued, and fearful of being overwhelmed by the burden of the intensive complicated care. Enormous demands are made on their energies by the frequent necessity to meet immediate acute needs and by serious time pressures and overwork. In addition, they feel stressed because inattention to other responsibilities and other patients is necessitated by the seemingly all-encompassing needs of the AIDS population. These stresses increase each day because of the mushrooming incidence of the disease and tax institutional resources to the limit. In some institutions the quality and comprehensiveness of training programs have been questioned because students are taking care of only PWAs and have no experience with patients who have other problems.

Nurses have become overwhelmed by caring for PWAs day after day. Infection control procedures often leave them feeling isolated, and they are emotionally and physically drained by the intensive physical and psychologic needs of the patients. AIDS brings to the nurse's attention the constant responsibility for intense, complex monitoring of the sights, sounds, smells, and suffering of life and death struggles. Nursing care problems of the patient with AIDS can include concurrent needs for attention to respiratory distress, pain, nausea, vomiting, diarrhea, bleeding, fatigue, motor weakness, breakdown of skin, breakdown of oral mucous membranes, nutritional deficits, fluid volume deficit, alteration in mental status, and acute psychologic distress. Nurses have found it especially difficult to deal with patients' anger and seemingly unreasonable demands in complex nursing care situations. Interns are often fatigued and over-taxed by the immediate demands of acute situations. Interns are called on to manage acute crises in the illness; they perform such procedures as arterial blood gas measurements, blood cultures, lumbar punctures, and bone marrow biopsies. They also feel isolated from the rest of the staff and resentful that residents and attending physicians avoid discussing life-sustaining treatment with patients and families and leave do-not-re-suscitate orders up to them.

Dealing with patients with AIDS has a special impact on health care workers because they and the patients are usually about the same age. Identification and a sense of personal vulnerability to disease and death are elicited when patients are young, hitherto healthy persons who face rapid physical deterioration and death. Health care workers are forced to recognize the fact of their own death and dying and are faced with the need to reexamine the meaning and quality of their lives. Some handle these feelings with denial and distancing tactics; others identify with their patients. Physicians have expressed the level of distress they feel when diagnosing Pneumocystis pneumonia as "pronouncing a death sentence." The age of the patients has evoked the feeling that "it's like telling your brother that he's going to die." An especially difficult situation is dis-cussing life-sustaining treatments with a patient whom the health care worker has just met and who may need immediate intubation. These situations take their toll on health care workers in cumulative stress, depression, and psychic fatigue.

Nurses often become intensely involved with PWAs because of the time and closeness of the nursing care demanded. To some degree they become a family to the patient, and some nurses have been asked to hold the durable power of attorney for the patients and make decisions re-garding treatment, disposition of property, and burial. This relationship is highly stressful when the patient dies, and nurses and physicians react much more strongly than they would with patients who have relied more on family and friends for support. Repetitive grief and demoralization occur because of the high mortality of AIDS.

The traditional goals of nursing and medical care impose additional stresses on health care givers. In general these goals are to cure, to prolong life, and to improve the quality of remaining life when its duration is beyond control. Patients with AIDS fall into the second and often the third category. Prolonging life and improving quality of life become the prime focuses of service. However, even these goals cannot be carried out without personal conflict, ambiguity, and disagreements among staff. Many of the treatments for AIDS produce debilitating and distressing side effects, so that prolonging life and improving quality of life can be at odds. Often treatment fails. Health care workers become involved in questions about whether the treatment regimen is justified; they become pessimistic and wonder, "What's the use?" Their professional identity as persons who improve patients' lives is called into question, resulting in a feeling of professional impotence. Sometimes health care workers feel anger at colleagues for what they consider lack of involvement with or support for the patient. On the other hand, some staff members may empathize with a PWA's desire for suicide; they may even support medically assisted euthanasia on request. These conflicts can result in anxiety, depression, and anger among staff.

The care of the PWA presents a challenge to the nurse's competence, to professional and personal values, and to ethical convictions. To meet the psychosocial needs of health personnel caring for AIDS patients, a multifaceted program of institutional support is required:

1. All staff members should receive regularly scheduled educational and informational updates on HIV and its treatment. These educational programs must be repeated at intervals to reinforce and update information. Especially important is instruction on (a) transmission and contagion; (b) bisexuality and homosexuality; (c) drug use, drugs in use, and needle sharing; (d) assessment of mental status and recognition of delirium; (e) monitoring cognitive dysfunction and adjusting expectations for the patient's independent adherence to procedures and treatment; and (f) hospital and community resources to assist patients and families.

2. Clear, consistent policies and procedures should be developed about infection control, the ethical and professional responsibility to care for PWAs, and guidelines for testing. Such policies, adhered to by all staff, will decrease anxiety about transmission and ensure correct and appropriate behavior toward patients. Professionals most likely to experience occupational exposure (e.g., nurses and surgeons) should be involved in developing these policies.

3. Clear, consistent, and explicitly stated agreement among all hospital staff on the goals of treatment for PWAs will ensure a common approach and feelings of support for other staff members. This agreement on goals might address the issues of prolonging life through the use of available treatment; enhancing the quality of life for both patient and family through excellence in symptom control and attention to psychologic, social, spiritual, legal, and financial needs; and providing supportive care until death.

4. Regular and as-needed small group meetings to provide emotional support for staff specifically related to the care of PWAs and their families will promote a sense of shared experience and social and professional group support to health care workers. Nurses and physicians should be encouraged to discuss issues of grief and loss in this safe environment.

5. Easy access to mental health consultants who can provide emo-

tional support for patients and staff members can be helpful in crisis situations. Referrals can be made for staff desiring more long-term psychologic support.

6. Adequate institutional resources and support to provide the level of nursing and medical care needed will prevent staff from becoming overwhelmed, fatigued, and overtaxed by the care of PWAs.

On a personal level, nurses and other health care workers can implement several measures that can reduce their stress at work and away from work. At work they can:

- Work regular (consistent) hours or shifts
- Take lunch and coffee breaks
- Take brief respite breaks (look out the window, wash hands and face, massage face, isometric exercises)
- Acknowledge and reward work well done by one another

Away from work they can:

- Exercise, eat, and drink in moderation
- Create meaningful relationships and commit time to maintain them
- Develop an absorbing hobby or diversional activity
- Not bring work home
- Take regular vacations

Several psychosocial issues that usually arise separately are combined in the treatment of patients with AIDS, creating unusually difficult problems. These include fears of contagion, disease, and death in young persons; negative social attitudes and personal prejudices; overworked, fatigued, and overwhelmed health care workers; and overtaxed institutional resources. Such difficult problems require institutions to provide a set of supportive guidelines for nurses and other health care professionals in the care of patients with AIDS.

PSYCHOSOCIAL TASKS OF HEALTH CARE WORKERS TREATING PERSONS WITH AIDS

In caring for persons with AIDS, nurses and other health care workers engage in a variety of psychologic, social, and educational tasks to ensure that patient needs are met. Nursing models that emphasize care of the whole person are most useful. These provide guidelines for the nurse in meeting the physiologic, psychosocial, and educational needs of the patient (Bennett, 1988; Govoni, 1988; Hall et al., 1989; Katoff & Dunne, 1988; Mount, 1986; Pheifer & Houseman, 1988; Wolcott, 1986; Wolcott, et al., 1986):

- Accept, value, and provide longitudinal psychosocial and physical nursing care and medical care to the patient.
- Support the patient's capacity for hope, self-determination, autonomy, independence, and control.
- Provide accurate medical information concerning treatment alternatives, benefits, and risks and the rationale for suggested intervention.
- Provide accurate information regarding health-enhancing behavioral options (e.g., diet, rest, exercise, preventing infection) in a sensitive, nonjudgmental manner.
- Understand common psychosocial issues surrounding AIDS and provide assistance or referral for problems.
- Familiarize herself or himself with community psychologic, social, educational, political, and financial resources and make appropriate referrals for patients, lovers, spouses, families, and friends.
- Recognize and ensure treatment of neuropsychiatric syndromes common to AIDS.
- Control symptoms, reassure patients that this will be done, and provide supportive care or comfort measures.
- Carry out patients' decisions concerning life-sustaining treatment and reassure them that they will not be abandoned.
- Recognize the stress that co-workers experience in caring for patients with AIDS and work to minimize it.
- Assist survivors with bereavement support and grief counseling.

SUMMARY

The diagnosis of AIDS presents psychologic and social dilemmas, conflicts, and stresses for everyone intimately involved with the PWA, for less intimately involved acquaintances, and ultimately for society. An awareness of these stresses for the people involved, of the psychosocial supports needed and available, and of new developments in the treatment of HIV disease and care of patients will assist the nurse in giving optimal nursing care. In addition, nurses should care for themselves and request from their institutions and one another the support they need to battle HIV infection and AIDS.

References

Abbing, H.D.C. (1988). Dying with dignity, and euthanasia: A view from the Netherlands. *Journal of Palliative Care, 4*(4), 70–74.

Baum, A., & Nesselhof, S.E.A. (1988). Psychological research and the prevention, etiology, and treatment of AIDS. *American Psychologist, 43*(11), 900–906.

Bauman, L.J., & Siegel, K. (1987). Misperceptions among gay men of the risk for AIDS associated with their sexual behavior. *Applied Social Psychology, 17*, 329.

Becker, M.H., & Joseph, J.G. (1988). AIDS and behavioral change to reduce risk: A review. *American Journal of Public Health, 78*(4), 394–410.

Bellemare, D. (1988). AIDS: The challenge to pastoral care. *Journal of Palliative Care, 4*(4), 58–60.

Bennett, J. (1988). Helping people with AIDS live well at home. *Nursing Clinics of North America, 23*(4), 731–748.

Bennett, M.J. (1990). Stigmatization: Experiences of persons with acquired immune deficiency syndrome. *Issues in Mental Health Nursing, 11*, 141–154.

Bolle, J.L. (1988). Supporting the deliverers of care: Strategies to support nurses and prevent burnout. *Nursing Clinics of North America, 23*(4), 843–850.

Britton, P.J., & Zarski, J.J. (1989). HIV spectrum disorders and the family: Selected interventions based on stylistic dimensions. *AIDS Care, 1*(1), 85–92.

Centers for Disease Control (1991, April). *AIDS Weekly Surveillance Report*, Atlanta: AIDS Program.

Christ, G.H., Siegel, K., & Moynihan, R.T. (1988). Psychosocial issues: Prevention and treatment. In V.T. Devita, S. Hellman, & S. Rosenberg, (Eds.), *AIDS: Etiology, diagnosis, treatment, and prevention* (pp. 321-337). Philadelphia: J.B. Lippincott.

Dean, L., Hall, W.E., & Martin, J.L. (1988). Chronic and intermittent AIDS-related bereavement in a panel of homosexual men in New York City. *Journal of Palliative Care, 4*(4), 54–57.

Dunphy, R. (1987). Helping persons with AIDS find meaning and hope. *Health Progress, 68*, 58–63.

Frierson, R.L., & Lippmann, S.B. (1988). Suicide and AIDS. *Psychosomatics, 29*(2), 226–231.

Fullilove, M. (1989). Anxiety and stigmatizing aspects of HIV infection. *Journal of Clinical Psychiatry, 50*(suppl 11), 5–8.

Gambe, R., & Getzel, G.S. (1989). Group work with gay men with AIDS. *Journal of Contemporary Social Work*, 172–179.

Getzel, G.S., & Mahony, K.F. (1990). Confronting human finitude: Group work with people with AIDS (PWAs). *Journal of Gay and Lesbian Psychotherapy, 1*(3), 105–120.

Glass, R.M. (1988). AIDS and suicide. *Journal of the American Medical Association, 259*(9), 1369–1370.

Govoni, L.A. (1988). Psychosocial issues of AIDS in the nursing care of homosexual men and their significant others. *Nursing Clinics of North America, 23*(4), 749–765.

Graydon, D.N. (1988). AIDS: Observations of a hospital chaplain. *Journal of Palliative Care, 4*(4), 66-69.

Greif, G.L., & Porembski, E. (1989). Implications for therapy with significant others of persons with AIDS. *Journal of Gay and Lesbian Psychotherapy, 1*(1), 79–86.

Hall, J.M., Koehler, S.L., & Lewis, A. (1989). HIV-related mental health nursing issues. *Seminars in Oncology Nursing, 5*(4), 276-283.

Hall, J.M., & Stevens, P.E. (1988). AIDS: A guide to suicide assessment. *Archives of Psychiatric Nursing, 1*(2), 115–120.

Katoff, L., & Dunne, R. (1988). Supporting people with AIDS: The gay men's health crisis model. *Journal of Palliative Care, 4*(4), 88-95.

Kelly, J.A., St. Lawrence, J.S., Hood, H.V., et al. (1988). Nurses' attitudes toward AIDS. *The Journal of Continuing Education in Nursing, 19*, 78–83.

Kelly, J.A., St. Lawrence, J.S., Smith, S., et al. (1987). Stigmatization of AIDS patients by physicians. *American Journal of Public Health, 77*(7), 789–791.

Kelly, J., & Sykes, P. (1989). Helping the helpers: A support group for family members of persons with AIDS. *Social Work, 34*(3), 239–242.

Killian, W.H. (1990, September). HIV counseling—know the risks. *The American Nurse, 22*(8), 28.

King, M.B. (1989). Psychosocial status of 192 out-patients with HIV infection and AIDS. *British Journal of Psychiatry, 154*, 237-242.

Limandri, B.J. (1989). Disclosure of stigmatizing conditions: The discloser's perspective. *Archives of Psychiatric Nursing, 3*(3), 69–78.

Lo, B., Steinbrook, R.L., Cooke, M., et al. (1989). Voluntary screening for human immuno-deficiency virus (HIV) infection. *Annals of Internal Medicine, 110*(9), 727–733.

Marzuk, P.M., Tierney, H., Tardiff, K., et al. (1988). Increased risk of suicide in persons with AIDS. *Journal of the American Medical Association, 259*(9), 1333–1337.

McKusick, L. (1988). The impact of AIDS on practitioner and client. *American Psychologist, 43*(11), 935–940.

McMahon, K.M. (1988). The integration of HIV testing and counseling into nursing practice. *Nursing Clinics of North America, 23*(4), 803–821.

Minkin, T. (1989, November/December). On the front lines of caring, the newest enemy is compassion-fatigue. *Bostonia*, 43-45, 71.

Moran, J.S., Janes, H.R., Peterman, T.A., & Stone, K.M. (1990). Increase in condom sales following AIDS education and publicity, United States. *American Journal of Public Health, 80*(5), 607-608.

Mount, B.M. (1986). Dealing with our losses. *Journal of Clinical Oncology, 4*(7), 1127-1134.

Pasacreta, J.V., & Jacobsen, P.B. (1989). Addressing the need for staff support among nurses caring for the AIDS population. *Oncology Nursing Forum, 16*(5), 659-663.

Perry, S., Jacobsberg, L., & Fishman, B. (1990). Suicidal ideation and HIV testing. *Journal of the American Medical Association, 263*(5), 679–682.

Pheifer, W.G., & Houseman, C. (1988). Bereavement and AIDS: A framework for intervention. *Journal of Psychosocial Nursing, 26*(10), 21–26.

Ragsdale, D., & Morrow, J.R. (1990). Quality of life as a function of HIV classification. *Nursing Research, 39*(6), 355–359.

Rinella, V.J., & Dublin, W.R. (1988). The hidden victims of AIDS: Healthcare workers and families. *The Psychiatric Hospital, 19*(3), 115–20.

Saunders, J.M. (1989). Psychosocial and cultural issues in HIV infection. *Seminars in Oncology Nursing, 5*(4), 284-288.

Saynor, J.K. (1988). Existential and spiritual concerns of people with AIDS. *Journal of Palliative Care, 4*(4), 61-65.

Schoen, K., & Schindelman, E. (1989). AIDS and bereavement. *Journal of Gay and Lesbian Psychotherapy, 1*(2), 117-120.

Solomon, K. (1990). Facing AIDS with my mother. *The Body Positive*, 22–25.

Sonsel, G.E. (1989). Case management in a community-based AIDS agency. *Quality Review Bulletin, 15*(1), 31-36.

Tibesar, L.J. (1986). Pastoral care: Helping patients on an inward journey. *Health Progress, 67*, 41–47.

Tiblier, K.B., Walker, G., & Rolland, J.S. (1989). Therapeutic issues when working with families of persons with AIDS. In Macklin, E.D. (Ed.), *AIDS and Families* (pp. 81–128). New York: Harrington Park Press.

Tross, S., & Hirsch, D.A. (1988). Psychological distress and neuropsychological complications of HIV infection and AIDS. *American Psychologist, 43*(11), 929–934.

Volberding, P.A. (1988). Caring for the patient with AIDS: An integrated approach. *Infectious Disease Clinics of North America, 2*(2), 543–550.

Wolcott, D.L. (1986). Psychosocial aspects of acquired immune deficiency syndrome and the primary care physician. *Annals of Allergy, 57*(8), 95-102.

Wolcott, D.L., Fawzy, F.I., Landsverk, J., et al. (1986). AIDS patients' needs of psychosocial services and their use of community service organizations. *Journal of Psychosocial Oncology, 4*(1), 135-146.

7

Community-Based and Long-Term Care

Peter J. Ungvarski and Kathleen M. Nokes

When planning for the health care needs and social services of persons with HIV disease, nurses must look at the full range of services that may be required throughout the course of illness. In June 1988 the Presidential Commission on the HIV Epidemic pointed out in their final report that continued focus on AIDS, rather than the entire spectrum of the HIV epidemic, has left the United States unable to deal effectively with the epidemic (Presidential Commission, 1988). Most important, the report looked at health care delivery "through the lens of the HIV epidemic and found gaping holes, huge problems" (Gebbie, 1989, p. 869). In essence the HIV epidemic has vividly exposed the many weaknesses inherent in health care in the United States.

Gebbie (1989) noted that the HIV epidemic has revealed major deficits, such as (1) failure to offer each child born a comprehensive health and health education program, which would provide a basis for a healthy adult life; (2) failure to construct a coherent system of delivering illness care services and a method of paying for such services; and (3) failure to understand the dangers of creating a permanent underclass, a drug-linked culture that does not participate in the ordinary obligations and benefits of our social service system. In fact, the HIV epidemic has shown that there is no such thing as a "health care system" in the United States (Ungvarski, 1989). The definition of the word "system" implies an interdependence and interrelationship between elements, which forms a collective entity. In the United States we have the antithesis to this definition:

a fragmented array of health services provided by federal, state, local, nonprofit, voluntary, and proprietary agencies. The United States and the Republic of South Africa are the only developed industrialized countries that do not ensure that all citizens have access to basic health care (Lundberg, 1991).

In many respects the phrase "health care system" is a misnomer. What is actually provided in the United States is a system of acute care, not health care. Essentially, an individual who becomes seriously ill is provided a bed in a hospital. The emphasis is on hospitals, with limited focus on long-term care and virtually no investment in primary care or prevention. Primary care and prevention are available to those who can afford it and who seek it out.

Realizing and acknowledging these issues, the nurse can appreciate that planning care for an HIV-infected person from the time of diagnosis through the course of illness, can be not only difficult but also frustrating. What is needed in the early stages of HIV infection is clinical monitoring through primary care and psychosocial services, and in the later stages acute care, home care, long-term residential care, and hospice care are required. Many individuals have limited access to primary care and support services; they may be refused access to long-term residential care because they are HIV infected. Lack of entitlement and inability to pay, unfortunately, are barriers to care shared by most HIV-positive persons. This chapter not only discusses the various aspects of planning care in a nonacute setting, but also attempts to describe the realities.

CASE MANAGEMENT

Because the United States has no system of health care, and because the average consumer has great difficulty understanding and negotiating the complexities of entitlements such as private insurance policies, Medicaid, and Medicare, case management has become a necessity. Case management is not new. At the turn of the century, public health programs provided community service coordination that was the forerunner of case management (American Nurses Association [ANA], 1988). Coordination of services has always been the focus of public health nursing (ANA, 1980).

After World War II the term "case management" was used to describe the community services necessary for the care of discharged psychiatric patients (Grau, 1984). The term first appeared in social welfare literature in the early 1970s, followed closely by mentions in the nursing literature (ANA, 1988). In more recent years the U.S. government policy on health care has moved toward programs that offer a comprehensive, coordinated continuum of care at the community level. In 1981 the Omnibus Budget

Reconciliation Act and Medicare prospective reimbursement program encouraged case management to provide community-based alternatives to institutional placement.

The ANA (1988) defined case management as a system of elements including (1) health assessment, (2) planning, (3) procurement of services, and (4) monitoring to ensure that the multiple service needs of the client are met. Ideally case management should not only optimize the client's self-care capability through the efficient use of resources but also stimulate the creation of new services. The goals of case management are to provide high-quality care, minimize fragmentation of care across many settings, enhance the quality of the client's life, and contain costs (ANA, 1988; Morrison, 1990a). The best situation is to have a single designated case manager. However, because of the complex needs of clients with HIV disease and the numerous players involved with care, what actually takes place is multiagency case management (Table 7–1). To achieve the client's goals, the various health care professionals managing the case must be aware of one another's capabilities and limitations and develop a milieu of cooperation. Synonymous terms for case management include case coordination, service management, care management, and managed care. Case management can provide facilitating functions, gatekeeping functions, or a combination. Facilitating functions include assisting the client and significant others in obtaining the needed services in a maze of complex rules and regulations. The gatekeeping role of case management ensures that the client and significant others receive appropriate and cost-effective health care.

Less clearly defined is who should actually provide case management. Case management models vary and include a single designated case manager, an interdisciplinary team, or a multiagency team. In reality, the ubiquitous, monolithic case manager, does not exist.

TABLE 7–1. Team Members Who May Be Involved in Case Management of a Person with HIV Infection

1. Client and significant other(s)
2. Primary physician
3. Consulting physicians (e.g., ophthalmologist managing cytomegalovirus retinitis)
4. Hospital-based staff, including resident physicians, nurses, nutritionists, pharmacists, and discharge planners
5. Home care staff, including visiting nurse, homemakers, home attendants, home health aides, continuous care nurses in the home, and special teams providing in-home infusion therapy
6. Case workers and managers from AIDS organizations, Medicaid programs, child welfare agencies, drug treatment programs, and health clinics
7. Mental health professionals
8. Clergy

The ANA (1988) defined the component parts of case management in the framework of the nursing process. In this model, interaction with the client, family and significant others, and various providers is followed by assessment, planning, implementation, and evaluation. Professional nurses are uniquely qualified to be case managers because of their theoretical background in the biologic and social sciences and the humanities; their knowledge of health maintenance, disease processes, and medications; and their experience in collaboration as part of the health care team (ANA, 1988).

Regardless of the professional discipline of persons hired to perform case management, they should be provided the necessary education, reference tools, and resource persons to understand the complex biobehavioral and psychobehavioral responses individuals experience during the course of HIV disease. They should be good listeners and not individuals who make quick value judgments without a total picture of the situation. As part of their role preparation they should be taught the etiquette and value of telephone case management; they should be told that the telephone is an invaluable asset and should not be viewed as an interruption. Above all, case managers should keep in mind that they are not the client's only advocates. Advocacy based on a collaborative process, with mutual respect, will do more to obtain the needed services than will an adversarial approach.

Assessment

The collection of baseline data provides the framework on which the case manager structures the plan of care. Assessment is an interaction with the client, significant others, family members, and service providers. It is a time to introduce the role of the case manager and to establish a relationship between the case manager and the other parties. It is wise to remember that first impressions are lasting.

Comprehensive evaluation includes, but is not limited to, collection of data that describe (1) demographic and personal characteristics; (2) support persons; (3) functional status of the client; (4) clinical needs of the client; (5) family information; (6) legal issues; (7) social data; (8) financial data; and (9) summary of service providers, both individuals and agencies, that are involved in the case (see Appendix III for a detailed assessment outline). The primary purpose of the assessment are to identify the client's care needs and problems, to evaluate what needs are being met, and to determine what should be improved.

Ideally the initial interview should take place with the client and significant others in the client's home. The presence of a significant other is especially important when there is a potential for discrete or undiagnosed cognitive impairment of the client. For the initial interview the home setting provides the case manager with an opportunity to assess the home environment and community resources. Although at the initial assessment the client may be relatively healthy and independent, this information provides a basis for future evaluation of the feasibility for in-home service should the need arise. If the initial assessment is performed at the hospital or in an office, the case manager should arrange an in-home visit at a later date for assessment purposes.

Planning

The cardinal rule for the development of a service plan is that the client and significant others actively participate in developing the plan. This includes mutually agreed on goals. Involvement of the client in setting goals is probably the rule that health care professionals most frequently ignore. Unilaterally setting goals by the case manager will eventually lead to labeling the client as noncompliant. In this case the true statement would be "this client was noncompliant with the case manager's wishes"! For example, if the case manager decides that home attendant services are indicated, but the client views it as intrusive and can still manage on his or her own, a good deal of time and effort is wasted when the client refuses service the day the home attendant shows up. It is important to keep in mind that the plan of care belongs to the client, not the case manager.

The plan of care should also include measurable objectives, the steps to be taken to meet these objectives, and a timeframe. Documentation throughout the process is important, and constraints to achieving goals or meeting timeframes should be recorded. The case manager should realize that problems with the care plan are inevitable and should not view them as personal failure. Internalization of problems can lead to frustration and anger and impede the process.

The final requirement of the planning process is selecting the services needed. In the case of the HIV-infected person this may be limited, since access to institutional long-term care has been limited throughout the HIV-AIDS epidemic. Nursing homes and psychiatric facilities that will accept an HIV-infected person are scarce. Gaining access to addiction treatment services may be even more difficult. Day care is virtually nonexistent. Home care and hospice care, although available in most areas, may not be adequate or safe for the client's needs. The case manager, from time to time, may reach a dead end when other service providers reject the referral.

Implementation

In the implementation phase of the care plan, access to services is accomplished by completion of applications and contact with providers. Advocacy for entitlements will require providing all necessary information and educating the client and significant others to prevent future denial of services, or denial of financing services.

The case manager should anticipate problems and conflicts during the process of implementation: checks don't arrive on time, transportation is delayed, home care workers don't show up, clients miss appointments, and so forth. A backup plan is needed for such situations: petty cash for food until checks can be traced, alternative transportation or appointment rescheduling, and someone to stay with the client until a replacement home care worker is available. The more service providers involved with a case, the greater the likelihood of problems.

The case manager should watch for and avoid duplications in service. As the number of AIDS service organizations increases, so does the number of duplicative services provided. For example, if a client moves into supportive housing for persons with AIDS (PWAs) that provides health care monitoring, psychosocial support services, and food and shelter, there is little need to provide for medical appointments, counseling, friendly visitors, or volunteer "buddies" that were previously required.

Evaluation

Evaluation should be ongoing and planned; it should not be left to chance or wait for a crisis to occur. Planned visits to the client at specified intervals, or at least telephone audits to verify services and identify problems, can be invaluable tools in preventing a major crisis. Educating the client and significant others about the importance of self-care is essential in the provision of services and cost containment.

Unneeded services should not be continued for the sake of convenience. Likewise, the case manager should not provide services as "gifts" in an attempt to be liked by the client. Overservicing a client and significant others is antithetical to their achieving and maintaining independence.

Family members or significant others providing care may experience role fatigue. Plans of care that specify intervals of respite to prevent psychologic or physical fatigue are quite successful. Plans for respite care vary from a few hours a week to taking off for long weekends every few months. Redefining goals and modifying the care plan will be based on the ongoing assessment of the needs of the client and significant others. Table 7–2 lists constraints to case management.

TABLE 7–2. Constraints to Case Management

1. Case management usually is limited to the provision of services to persons with diagnosed AIDS, thus excluding persons who are HIV seropositive and in the earlier stages of disease.
2. Usually health care facilities and organizations are not reimbursed for case management.
3. Communication channels between case managers and other service providers are not always well established.
4. Power struggles can emerge between case managers from different agencies.
5. There is a lack of specialized training and resource materials that prepare case managers to interpret and understand the complex clinical problems of their clients, such as clinical needs related to opportunistic infections, research protocols, drugs, and alternative therapies.
6. Many case managers do not adequately involve the client in the plan of care.
7. Many case managers are unprepared to deal with an HIV-seropositive person who chooses to continue to engage in unsafe sexual activity or to continue to use drugs or wishes to get pregnant and have a baby.
8. Undiagnosed HIV-related cognitive impairment can complicate the decision-making process.
9. Confidentiality laws may leave case managers reluctant to provide adequate information to other service providers involved in the case.
10. Hospitals are not experienced in outpatient case management and are not familiar with solutions to problems that face persons with HIV infection or AIDS when they are at home in the community.
11. Emphasis on cost saving may result in conflict over supplies and medications prescribed by case managers and denied by third party payors.

HOME CARE

In 1981 the only option for care of PWAs was acute care hospitalization. Nursing responded to the need, however, and in 1984 the first program of home care services for PWAs was organized and implemented by the Visiting Nurse Association and Hospice of San Francisco. This was followed 1 year later by the development of a formal program of home care services at the Visiting Nurse Service of New York (VNSNY). Today VNSNY operates the largest home care program of its kind in the world for PWAs, with an average daily census of more than 900 clients.

Home care providers have responded to the growing health care needs of PWAs by designing special programs and adapting current ones to meet their needs. Home care is especially appropriate and effective for PWAs. It enables them to remain in familiar surroundings, thus providing maximum emotional support for them and their significant others. It provides maximum independence and control over decision making in the least restrictive setting. Home care can improve the quality of life significantly and can give PWAs the greatest use of their remaining time (Ungvarski, 1988). It promotes the participation of significant others in the plan of care. Finally, it provides an opportunity for case finding and health teaching in the community (Ungvarski, 1987). Health teaching is especially important in preventing transmission of both HIV and tuberculosis, which is rapidly becoming a major HIV-related illness.

One misconception about home care is that it consistently costs substantially less than institutional care. Costs for service in the home (excluding supplies such as medications, dressings, and intravenous [IV] infusion equipment) can range from about $140 per day to $1000 per day (New York City Department of Health, 1989). In addition, estimates comparing home care costs with institutional care rarely include total costs of care and may fail to include the average daily cost for rent, food, and utilities.

Another misconception is that home care is intended to take over or take away care and responsibility for the PWAs from the significant others. Nothing could be further from the truth. Home care is specifically designed to support the client and significant others and is not a system of care to take over custody of the client. In this respect, home care may be inappropriate for individuals who require continuous care in an institutional setting.

Many health care professionals throughout the United States place undue pressure on home care agencies to accept all PWAs who are referred, since there are virtually no other options for long-term care ouside the hospital. Therefore it is important for all health care professionals to understand the purposes of home care, as well as its limits and constraints.

As previously stated, home care is a supportive system of care for the client and significant others. Therefore, in addition to education of the client in self-care, the significant other, often referred to as the informal caregiver, must be educated, since he or she is the most important provider of care. Formal caregivers include professional and paraprofessional health care workers who participate in the plan of care (Table 7–3). The informal and formal caregivers should work together to develop a plan of care that is mutually agreeable, is designed to meet the needs of the client and significant others, and is realistic about the care that can be safely provided by the home care agency.

Case Management Issues and Home Care

Evidence suggests a failure to diagnose alcohol and drug dependencies when clients are referred for home care services. With the initiation of services, the problem becomes evident and directly affects the client's ability to comply with prescribed medical and nursing regimens, as well as the willingness of paraprofessional workers to go into the home to provide service. Even when the HIV-infected individual is alcohol or drug

TABLE 7–3. Formal Caregivers Providing Home Care Services

CATEGORY OF STAFF	FUNCTIONS
Professional staff	
Physician	Provides for medical care (usually through periodic office or clinic visits and telephone contact with the visiting nurse)
Visiting nurse (usually the case manager)	Provides orders for nursing care and coordinates all professional and paraprofessional services needed; promotes and teaches self-care to client and significant others
Medical social worker	Provides for necessary concrete social services as well as counseling
Therapists (occupational, physical, speech)	Provide maintenance or restorative therapies and teach self-care to client and significant other
Specialists	Provide specific services (e.g., respiratory therapists for aerosolized pentamidine or clinical nurse specialist for problems in case management)
Paraprofessional staff	
Housekeeper	Provides chore services such as shopping, cleaning, laundry, meal preparation (no personal care)
Personal care assistants (also referred to as home attendants or personal care attendants)	In addition to chore services, provide assistance with bathing, dressing, toileting, ambulating, and traveling to and from appointments
Home health aides	In addition to the above, assist with many nursing tasks such as taking temperatures, providing special exercises, taking care and providing safety with oxygen therapy
Homemakers	Usually provide chore services and child care services; may provide child care in the presence of an ill parent or may act as surrogate parent staying 24 hours when parent is hospitalized

These definitions and functions often vary from state to state.

free, the significant other(s) may be overtly using substances, which again leads to reluctance of paraprofessionals to enter the home or may result in abusive behavior toward home care workers. When the problem of drug or alcohol use is diagnosed by professional home care staff, treatment options for referral are limited. Alcohol and drug treatment programs that meet the needs of homebound clients are almost nonexistent. In the absence of a treatment plan for the chemical dependency, home care may not be feasible.

Because of the paucity of long-term care options for HIV-ill persons with psychiatric disorders, acute care facilities may withhold psychiatric diagnoses when making home care referrals. Once the client is at home, paraprofessional home care workers, as well as families and significant others, are often reluctant or unable to cope with combative, assaultive, or self-destructive behaviors. Again, home care may not be possible, and in some cases the only available plan of care will be to return the client to the hospital.

Cognitive impairment resulting from the neurotropic effects of HIV or an opportunistic central nervous system infection is a grossly under-diagnosed problem in the HIV-ill population. Once the client is home, the visiting nurse or paraprofessional home care worker is often the first to detect cognitive and motor impairment. In the case of clients who live alone, forgetting to take medications or miscalculating doses can lead to disastrous problems such as overmedication or the worsening or recurrence of an opportunistic infection because of inability to comply with suppressive therapy medication. In addition, the home is not the best milieu for the cognitive stimulation therapy necessary to keep the client at an optimal level of functioning. Home care in conjunction with a program of day care is most desirable.

In the absence of previous experience, it is not uncommon while the client is in the hospital for the significant others to agree to participate in the home-based plan of care. However, once faced with the harsh realities of intense levels of physical care and emotional support needed in the home, significant others or family members may withdraw active participation. Some family members or significant others insist that a client be returned home with home care services but may themselves be unable to participate in care because they live far away. The participation of family and significant others is the foundation of safe home care. Reimbursement for services varies with payor source, that is, private insurance, Medicaid, Medicare and so forth, and from state to state in the case of Medicaid. Capitations on the amount of service often require that significant others participate. If they do not, modifications of the original plan and referral to an institution for long-term care may be necessary.

Family cases referred for home care services provide a unique challenge. Among the situations that may be present are (1) husband and wife who are both infected, (2) infected parents and children, (3) uninfected children in the same household with infected parents and siblings, and (4) gay couples who are both infected and severely ill. Legal assistance is often required for planning wills and guardianship. Referrals will be necessary to assist survivors (e.g., grandparents, aunts, uncles) in caring for HIV-ill children whose parents have died or are in prison. In the absence of planned guardianship or relatives willing to provide child care, referrals to foster care agencies will be necessary.

The growing population of HIV-ill IV drug users who need home care services presents situations that will challenge not only the agency's resources but also the staff's ability to cope with the problems encountered. Home care staff will have to rely on the assistance of other community agencies when they encounter child neglect or abuse, incest, or truancy. A parent who repeatedly succumbs to the need to spend all available money on drugs and is unable to provide food for the children may require intervention from agencies that provide protective services for children. Such services are usually more readily available than are treatment resources for the parent's drug addiction.

Situations of abuse are not restricted to situations involving substance use. Client abuse by family members or lovers also occurs and may necessitate referral to community-based agencies that provide protective services for adults.

When home care service is provided to persons covered by Medicaid, their hospital-based medical care is often provided by house staff (residents in training). At the time of home care referral, the resident providing the initial medical orders is usually not assuming the role of primary care physician. Once the client is at home, the visiting nurse may find no physician willing to modify and provide orders for the medical portion of the plan of care. Visiting nurses spend an inordinate amount of time attempting to arrange ongoing medical care for Medicaid recipients receiving home care. In the absence of medical supervision, the visiting nurse may have to return a client to the acute care facility for simple matters that otherwise could be addressed by a telephone call and a primary care physician. This usually results in an unnecessary rehospitalization just so medical orders and prescriptions can be obtained. Many states regulating home care require physician's orders at specified intervals, but there is no legislation requiring physicians to provide a continuum of medical care to persons receiving home care. Ironically, the burden of ensuring adequate medical care for the person receiving home care is left to the professional nurse.

Home care cannot be provided in inadequate or unsuitable housing. Examples of HIV-ill persons with unsuitable housing include (1) persons with diarrhea who are housed in single-room occupancy hotels (often referred to as welfare hotels), have no bathroom or sink in the room, and are required to use distant, shared bathroom facilities; (2) those with significant weight loss who live in places without facilities for cooking and food storage and are too weak to go out for meals; (3) those who require IV therapy but have neither a telephone to use in case of a medical emergency nor a refrigerator for storing the solutions and drugs; and (4) clients who can no longer walk and live in buildings with broken or no elevators. The provision of home care services may require that the client be relocated to more suitable housing or that home care be delayed until necessary services are provided.

Home care cannot be provided in unsafe housing. Examples of unsafe housing include (1) buildings in which previous home care staff have been accosted or mugged; (2) buildings where entrances and hallways are used as "shooting galleries" for IV drug users or where crack and cocaine are sold; (3) buildings designated by local police departments as high-crime areas; and (4) homes in which overt drug using and trafficking takes place. Although most home care agencies in large urban areas provide an escort service for visiting nurses, this service is expensive and therefore extremely limited, since it is not directly reimbursable. Escort service is not usually provided for paraprofessionals, so they may refuse to provide service to clients in unsafe environments. This should not be misconstrued as refusal to care for a PWA, a commonly encountered misinterpretation. In some cases home care workers can arrange to be met by the family or significant others and escorted to and from the home.

Planning for Clinical Nursing Needs at Home

Managing client care at home and planning for care are directly related to the individual client's problems, which result from the numerous AIDS-indicator diseases that may develop in a PWA. Chapters 4 and 5 detail specific individual responses to HIV disease and the related nursing care. However, it is possible to make certain assumptions about a PWA's home care needs based on the medical diagnosis.

The following information is designed to provide the case manager, discharge planner, and visiting nurse with a brief explanation of what to anticipate for in-home service. The reader should refer to Chapter 3 for the overall clinical picture of a particular disease. Client-centered nursing care for specific physical problems can be found in Chapter 4, psychologic problems in Chapter 6, and medications and pentamidine aerosol therapy in the Appendix.

HIV Wasting. Clients with HIV wasting usually exhibit profound fatigue and therefore require help with chores (laundry, house cleaning, shopping, and meal preparation). Depending on the severity of fatigue, they may require assistance with personal care and getting to and from appointments. If the wasting is related to fat malabsorption, the nurse should pay particular attention to the fat content in any nutritional supplements ordered. Ideally the weight should be monitored, but this is often unrealistic because many clients cannot afford a scale. Evaluation may have to be based on the client's and nurse's subjective assessment using such measures as how clothes fit. In addition to monitoring weight, the visiting nurse should evaluate and document the presence or absence of factors contributing to weight loss. These include (1) thrush, (2) painful oral lesions such as herpes simplex and Kaposi's sarcoma, (3) dysphagia and odynophagia, (4) dysgeusia, (5) steatorrhea, (6) continued alcohol or drug use, (7) depression, (8) side effects of drugs, and (9) development of another opportunistic disease.

HIV Encephalopathy. Cognitive dysfunction associated with HIV encephalopathy or AIDS dementia complex (ADC) results in problems with memory. Consequently the client pays less attention to grooming and appearance and to the environment. Most important, the client may have problems complying with prescribed medication regimens such as taking medications on schedule and calculating dosages. Motor slowing, weakness, and ataxia may also be noticeable. Paraprofessional care for a client with HIV encephalopathy should focus on setting schedules for activities of daily living and reminding and assisting the client. Caregivers should avoid doing everything for the client; the goal is independence, cognitive stimulation, and exercise to assist in motor control.

From time to time the visiting nurse should count remaining medication to ensure that the client is taking the prescribed amounts. The client will need constant assistance with financial matters. Measures to avoid false accusations over being shortchanged when others shop for the client should be established. In addition to monitoring the client's neurologic status, the nurse should assess the presence of (1) depression (since most of these individuals are aware of the impaired cognition); (2) suicide ideation; (3) increasing need for assistive devices such as a cane, tub rail, or bath seat; (4) development of incontinence; and (5) development of another opportunistic disease. The designated significant other(s) should participate in developing the plan of care and later changes, since the client has poor memory.

Tuberculosis. A client with tuberculosis (TB) exhibits profound fatigue and weight loss and requires assistance with chores and personal care. When the client is refered to the home care agency, the nurse should establish whether the client has pulmonary TB or extrapulmonary TB or both and the client's response to chemotherapy. The nurse should monitor compliance with the medication regimen during each visit and should follow local health department regulations for reporting individuals who have problems taking medication. Case finding for contacts, especially those living in the same household, should be performed early in the case management process. In addition to monitoring the clinical progress of the TB, the visiting nurse should evalute (1) the need for acid-fast bacillus (AFB) precautions; (2) the need for medical evaluation of household members; (3) weight loss and nutritional status; and (4) the development of another opportunistic disease. For clients with extrapulmonary TB, drainage and secretion precautions should be followed during wound care (CDC, 1983).

***Mycobacterium avium* Complex.** *Mycobacterium avium* complex (MAC) disease results in profound fatigue and weight loss with or without abdominal pain and diarrhea. Clients with MAC need assistance with chores, personal care, and travel to and from appointments. If the client is not receiving medication to treat MAC, the visiting nurse should be alert for increases in symptom severity and report them to the physician, since this may be an indication for treatment. With clients receiving medication to treat MAC, in addition to monitoring for drug side effects the nurse should be alert for depression related to a lack of progress or clinical improvement despite medications. In addition to evaluating the client regularly for the development of another opportunistic disease, the visiting nurse should be alert for excessive self-medication with acetaminophen or aspirin to relieve the constitutional symptoms. Drainage and secretion precautions should be followed for wound care (CDC, 1983).

Salmonellosis. An important responsibility of the visiting nurse whose client has HIV illness is the prevention of salmonellosis through health teaching and focusing on a low-microbial diet (see Chapter 4). The primary problems associated with salmonellosis are fatigue, diarrhea, and weight loss. The client will need assistance with chores and personal care. Leaving the home and having immediate access to a toilet as needed are anxiety provoking, to say the least. Adult diapers offer protection against soiling clothing. The client should be instructed to take along extra diapers in case a change is needed and small plastic bags in which to place the soiled diaper before disposal. If the client's symptoms are lessening and diarrhea is not a major worry, but leaking (associated with passing gas) is a concern, a female sanitary pad placed in the underpants will suffice.

In addition to monitoring the response to medication and resolution of disease, the visiting nurse should evaluate (1) diarrhea; (2) weight loss; (3) hydration and nutritional status; (4) skin surfaces in the perianal region; and (5) development of another opportunistic disease. Enteric precautions should be established at home, and the client and significant others should be taught how to avoid environmental contamination when using public toilet facilities.

Candidiasis. The majority of *Candida albicans* infections are endogenous and are related to the severe immunodeficiency seen in HIV disease and AIDS. Although the only candidal infection considered indicative of AIDS is *Candida* esophagitis, chronic *Candida* infection in other parts of the body is common in HIV disease. These *Candida* infections are exacerbated when clients are taking antibiotics for opportunistic infections. A client with severe *Candida* infection may need assistance with chores. Clients with *Candida* esophagitis and severe thrush need special dietary considerations (see Chapter 4). All clients with AIDS receiving home care services should have frequent evaluations by the visting nurse for (1) the presence and severity of thrush, (2) dysphagia and odynophagia, (3) *Candida* vaginitis, (4) intertrigo, and (5) development of another opportunistic disease. Established regimens of mouth and skin care should be instituted for all HIV-ill clients to prevent or control *Candida* infection. Instructions to "swish and swallow" oral antifungal agents should be clearly explained to the client, since many expectorate the medication because of the unpleasant taste.

Cryptococcosis. Clients with cryptococcosis usually have fatigue and weakness related to constitutional symptoms, and some have residual cognitive impairment related to brain infection. In addition to requiring assistance with chores and personal care, clients need careful evaluation of ability to self-administer medication. The visiting nurse should monitor clinical response to medication, resolution of residual neurologic problems, and possible development of another opportunistic disease. Arrangements for someone to accompany the client to physician visits and to provide physical and emotional support may be necessary, especially if repeated lumbar punctures are being performed to evaluate the client's response to therapy.

Histoplasmosis. The constitutional symptoms related to histoplasmosis leave the client profoundly fatigued and in need of assistance with chores, personal care, and trips to and from appointments. Clients with chorioretinitis and vision impairment need additional assistance and usually longer hours of in-home service, as well as a care plan designed to assist in adjusting to vision loss. Occupational therapy in the home should be requested as part of the plan of care. In addition to monitoring the client's response to therapy, the visiting nurse should assess the client for the development of another opportunistic disease.

Coccidioidomycosis. The constitutional symptoms of the client with coccidioidomycosis result in fatigue, and home care needs include assistance with both chores and personal care. In addition to monitoring the client's responses to therapy, the visiting nurse should assess for the development of another opportunistic disease.

Pneumocystosis. The significant advances in treatment and prevention of *Pneumocystis carinii* pneumonia (PCP) have led visiting nurses to focus on prophylaxis against pneumonia. However, the nurse should keep in mind that pentamidine aerosol therapy may result in the development of extrapulmonary sites of *P. carinii* infection (see Chapter 3). For clients receiving home care after an episode of PCP, the service needs are related to the severity of illness. If the client had some form of PCP prophylaxis and zidovudine before the development of PCP, the episode of acute illness is usually less severe and easily treated with a good clinical response. Such a client may need only assessment and teaching from the visiting nurse.

For clients who received no HIV-related therapy before the diagnosis of PCP, the residual deficits of shortness of breath, dyspnea, and fatigue may necessitate chore services, personal care services, and assistance to and from appointments. In addition to monitoring the client's pulmonary status, the visiting nurse should assess (1) activity tolerance, (2) ability to pace activities, (3) initiation or continuation of PCP prophylaxis, and (4) development of another opportunistic disease.

Cryptosporidiosis. A client returning home with cryptosporidiosis requires extensive home care services, especially if response to the limited available therapy has been poor. Many clients can walk only short distances in the home because of the profound weight and fluid loss combined with malabsorption. Since energy conservation is a primary goal, the client will need to have someone else perform all routine chores. Another person will have to perform personal care rather than just assisting the client. Unless the client can be close to the bathroom and toilet at all times, a commode is recommended. A client who is bedbound or incontinent requires significant amounts of disposable care items such as incontinence pads and diapers. This should be addressed in the initial plan of care, since keeping up with ordering supplies can be a problem. Enteric precautions should be carried out at home.

In most cases the visiting nurse can expect to see a decline rather than progress in a client with cryptosporidiosis. This disease requires intensive nursing care, careful assessment, and planning not only for physical comfort measures but also for the devastating psychologic responses to loss of control and alterations in body image. In addition, the visiting nurse should assess for the development of another opportunistic disease.

Toxoplasmosis. Planning for home care of the client with toxoplasmosis will have to take into account residual focal neurologic deficits and, in some clients, residual psychobehavioral problems as a result of brain infection. For example, a client with hemiparesis that affects the dominant side of the body requires much more assistance at home than a client who has hemiparesis on the nondominant side. Both clients will benefit from physical and occupational therapies. In addition to monitoring the client's response to therapy and ability to perform activities of daily living, the visiting nurse should assess for the development of another opportunistic disease. The nurse should maintain contact with the designated significant others, especially if the client has cognitive impairment or psychobehavioral problems.

Isosporiasis. Clients with AIDS usually respond well to therapy for isosporiasis. Although the initial home care services may include the provision of chore services and minimal assistance with personal care, the quantity of service provided should, barring any complications, decrease over time. Even when diarrhea abates, the client may still be apprehensive about soiling clothing based on experience with the disease. Options such as adult diapers or wearing female sanitary pads in the underpants should be offered. Suppressive therapy is usually ordered, since many clients experience recurrence of isosporiasis. In addition to assessing clinical progress, the visiting nurse should montior (1) nutrition and hydration status, (2) skin problems in the perianal region, and (3) the development of another opportunistic disease.

Herpes Simplex Virus. Problems with recurrent herpes simplex virus (HSV) infection usually occur as the client becomes severely immunodeficient and usually appear before the diagnosis of AIDS. HSV is a common, often chronic infection seen in persons with HIV infection. The visiting nurse should assess the client regularly for the development of HSV lesions. Examination for perianal lesions is especially important, since the client cannot see that eruptions are occurring. Typically the only clue is a sensation of itching and tingling, which invites scratching and can lead to extension of lesions or autoinoculation of other parts of the body. Poor oral hygiene or skin care can lead to secondary infection at the site of lesions, especially with *C. albicans* (see Chapter 3).

Drainage and secretion precautions should be instituted at home. A client with chronic HSV infection limited to small areas usually does not require home care services. However, HSV often accompanies other opportunistic diseases, so it becomes an additional clinical consideration. Clients with HSV encephalitis or disseminated infection may need extensive home care services depending on their functional status and response to therapy. In addition to monitoring the clinical response to therapy, the visiting nurse should assess for the development of other opportunistic diseases.

Cytomegalovirus. Home care service needs for the client with symptomatic cytomegalovirus (CMV) infection are usually related to the primary site of infection. Clients with CMV colitis and retinitis, for example, usually require chore services and assistance with personal care. Clients with vision loss must be reeducated in self-care activities, and occupational therapy should be included in the plan of care. The visiting nurse must be aware that treatment for CMV retinitis may not prevent total vision loss (see Chapter 3). Although the CDC (1983) does not recommend a disease-specific isolation category for CMV infection, wearing gloves and handwashing should be emphasized for all caregivers handling the client's secretions and excretions. In addition to monitoring the client's clinical response to therapy, the visiting nurse should assess for the development of other opportunistic diseases.

Progressive Multifocal Leukoencephalopathy. Although prolonged survival (more than 30 months) associated with partial recovery has been reported in persons with AIDS and progressive multifocal leukoencephalopathy (PML), this is rare (see Chapter 3). Most PWAs with PML exhibit a progressive decline in cognitive and motor function that requires a concomitant increase not only in home care services but also in assistive devices. Since no effective standard therapy is available, the nurse must focus on palliative and supportive care rather than rehabilitative or restorative goal setting. Loss and grieving on the part of the significant others should be anticipated and included in the plan of care. In addition to monitoring the increasing physical and protective needs of the client, the visiting nurse should assess for the development of another opportunistic disease.

Kaposi's Sarcoma. Planning for home care for the client with Kaposi's sarcoma (KS) is less predictable than with the other AIDS-indicator diseases. The spectrum of KS varies from a few lesions that are essentially a cosmetic problem to extensive organ involvement such as pulmonary KS, which may cause profound dyspnea and shortness of breath necessitating extensive in-home services. Service determination is therefore related to progression and extension of disease. As with other AIDS clients, the visiting nurse must assess for the development of other opportunistic diseases.

Non-Hodgkin's Lymphoma. The common sites of non-Hodgkin's lymphoma (NHL) are the central nervous system and gastrointestinal tract. The prognosis for response to therapy and survival is poor. Decline in mental and physical status combined with effects of cytotoxic agents usually necessitates rapid increases in home care services. Most clients eventually require chore services and complete provision of personal care. Monitoring for the development of other opportunistic diseases is required.

COMMUNITY-BASED ISSUES

As survival increases in persons with HIV infection, clients commonly ask questions about all aspects of their care. For example, many persons with HIV disease seek alternative therapies. Entering a research protocol and evaluating the risk versus benefit requires careful consideration by the client. Planning for the final stages of illness, although often clear cut in the client's mind, may be beset by legal and ethical issues. The nurse should have some familiarity with these issues to understand the client's concerns.

Alternative Therapies

Alternative therapies, also known as complementary (Strawn, 1989), dubious and rip-off (Monaco, 1989), or unproven (Kane, 1987), include a variety of interventions. The label chosen to identify these numerous strategies may reflect the person's underlying philosophy about them. Psychoneuroimmunology theory proposes the complex interactions of psychologic factors such as emotions and behavior, the central nervous system, and the immune system (Solomon & Temoshok, 1987). It is believed that changes in one area can influence other systems. Alternative therapies may cause people to feel more powerful, autonomous, and in control of their lives and their illness. These positive feelings may, in turn, strengthen the immune system. Proponents of alternative therapies stress that healing occurs within the individual but admit that healing may not be the same as cure (Strawn, 1989). Critics of alternative therapy argue that placing responsibility for healing with the client rather than with a specific treatment or physician may result in guilt and depression for the client (Monaco, 1989).

Alternative therapies focus on a holistic perspective rather than on the disease process. The client is an active participant in the treatment. Some holistic healing programs combine several alternative therapies (Glazier & Glazier, 1990). For example, traditional Chinese medicine uses acupuncture, massage therapy, breathing techniques, and herbal formulas (Zhang & Ziolkowski, 1990). Alternative therapies include homeopathy, acupuncture, chiropractic body work (e.g., massage, yoga, and therapuetic touch), nutrition (e.g., megavitamin therapy and macrobiotic diet), and mind work (e.g., meditation, visualization, and guided imagery). Table 7–4 presents a description of each of these approaches. Nurses use many

TABLE 7–4. Major Categories of Alternative Therapies

METHOD	DESCRIPTION
Homeopathy	Minute doses of substances such as herbs and minerals are used to stimulate a physiologic response.
Acupuncture	Needles are inserted into any one of more than 365 acupuncture points along 12 meridians to free energy blockages. Shiatsu or acupressure is the application of pressure rather than insertion of needles along these points.
Chiropractic therapy	Concerned with the alignment of the 24 vertebrae because stress results from misalignments.
Body work	Involves a variety of interventions, all of which include some physical and energy interactions. Therapeutic touch, for example, is the intentional transfer of energy through the provider to the client.
Alternative nutrition	Emphasizes raw consumption of seasonal fruits, grains, and vegetables. Between 50 and 200 g/24 hr megadoses of vitamin C may be suggested, but these doses often exceed a normal person's bowel tolerance. Macrobiotic diet promotes longevity through balancing foods in terms of yin and yang. Yin foods are acid forming, whereas yang foods are alkaline forming. Steamed grains and vegetables form the bulk of the macrobiotic diet.
Mind work	Fosters self-love, which leads to positive thinking and the forgiveness of self and others.

Data from Glazier, D., Glazier, R. (1990). *AIDS Medical Report*, 3(7), 77-86; Newshan, G. (1989). *Holistic Nursing Practice*, 3(4), 45-51.

alternative therapies for persons with HIV infection, including therapeutic touch and acupuncture (Newshan, 1989; Sanders, 1989).

Research has yet to support the impact of emotions on the immune system of persons with HIV infection as psychoneuroimmunology theory proposes. Nokes and Kendrew (1990a) found no relationship between degree of loneliness and development of infections in PWAs over a 6-month period. However, anecodotal evidence supports the claim that clients who use alternative therapies feel more in control over their lives and powerful. An alternative therapy such as keeping a diary can help clients begin to recognize their emotions and work through anger (Lindemer, 1990).

Four factors that are important in judging alternative therapies are cost, safety, effectiveness, and exclusiveness. Exclusiveness refers to the situation in which the provider insists that the client stop all other interventions and use only the methodology advocated by the alternative therapist. The nurse needs to help the client weigh each of the four factors to decide about the appropriateness of a specific therapy. When cost is reasonable, adverse effects are minimal, effectiveness is uncertain, and combinations with other standard approaches are encouraged, the nurse may support the client in choosing the therapy. As with any other intervention, the risk involved in the treatment needs to be weighed carefully against the benefit that may be achieved.

Clients with HIV infection often use alternative therapies (Irish, 1989). In a recent study, 76 HIV-positive military veterans completed the Alternative Therapies Check List developed by Nokes and Kendrew (1990b). Subjects identified how frequently they used 55 different therapies. Table 7–5 lists the kinds of alternative therapy used by greater than 10% of the sample, a brief description of the method chosen, total number of veterans who used that therapy, and the percentage of subjects who answered that question. Forty-six percent of these subjects identified their transmission behavior for HIV as male-to-male sex, while 34% admitted to a history of IV drug use. These subjects represented different ethnic groups and age groups.

Irrespective of personal opinion about the use of alternative therapies, the nurse needs to create an environment in which the client can share information about strategies being used to cope with HIV infection. The nurse need not condone any intervention, but a comprehensive assessment can be achieved only in a caring environment. Once information about different interventions is learned, health teaching about how the alternative therapy may interact with the standard approach can be tailored to the client's needs. Nurses should also communicate with other health care providers about the different strategies the client is using. Documentation on the clinical record should be as comprehensive as

TABLE 7–5. Alternative Therapies Used by Greater Than 10% of 76 HIV-Positive Veterans

TYPE OF THERAPY	DESCRIPTION	PERCENT*
Alternative nutrition	Multivitamins	76
	Orthomolecular (vitamins)	39
	Vitamin C	34
	Nutritional therapy	38
	Minerals	29
	Chinese herbs	12
	Detoxification	12
	Wheatgrass	11
Mind work	Relaxation	70
	Laughter and humor	63
	Meditation	54
	Visualization	22
	Affirmations	14
	Spirituality†	14
Body work	Massage	30
	Yoga	15
	Therapeutic touch	14

Data from Nokes, K., Kendrew, J. (1990). *Archives of Psychiatric Nursing*, 4(4), 271-277.
*Not all subjects answered every question.
†Not initially on alternative therapies checklist; written in by subjects.

possible in describing the alternative therapy(ies) in use and should indicate the client's preferences for alternative and standard interventions.

Consumer groups often help clients with HIV infection gain access to alternative therapies. These groups may hold meetings, publish newsletters, and offer hotlines. All the major AIDS epicenters in the United States have such groups where PWAs can learn about different alternative therapies and share information about reactions and strategies. Information is available to anyone, and nurses working in the field should try to learn about this treatment network from the client's perspective.

Participating in Research

HIV-positive clients may debate about whether to participate in a clinical drug or treatment trial at any point during the course of illness. The nurse can assist the client to reach a realistic decision about whether to participate. Clinical research trials may be established to study the efficacy of a drug or HIV-related treatments that are psychologic, social, or epidemiologic in nature. The nurse's role in these types of research could be as principal investigator, collaborator, or data collector. The nurse clinician should be prepared to offer clients information about clinical trials and help them enroll if they so decide. Although all research has similarities, the risk/benefit ratio is greater in drug trials and therefore the need for safeguards is greater.

A clinical trial is a study that tests new drugs and other treatments to determine safety and effectiveness (Department of Health and Human Services [DHHS], 1989). The drug approval process occurs through the cooperation of the Food and Drug Administration (FDA), the National Institutes of Health (NIH), and the pharmaceutical manufacturer. The FDA reviews the data supplied by NIH and the pharmaceutical manufacturer and requests additional information until it is certain that the drug is safe and effective. NIH consists of 13 institutes, one of which is the National Institute of Allergy and Infectious Diseases (NIAID). Table 7–6 lists the departments within NIAID involved with HIV infection and AIDS and a brief description of their purposes.

TABLE 7–6. National Institute of Allergy and Infectious Diseases: Departments of AIDS Research

DEPARTMENT	PURPOSE
Extramural Division	Conducts basic research and development and treatment research programs
AIDS Clinical Trials Group	Conducts clinical trials in major medical centers
Community Programs for Clinical Research	Conducts clinical trials in community settings
National Cooperative Drug Discovery Groups	Framework for collaborations between scientists from academe, industry, and government
National Cooperative Vaccine Development Groups	Conceptualizes and develops candidate vaccines for prevention of AIDS
NIAID Vaccine Evaluation Units	Tests vaccines under controlled conditions
Centers for AIDS Research	Promotes development of new scientific knowledge about AIDS within university settings
International Efforts in AIDS Research	Supports international studies about the natural history, epidemiology, clinical immunology, and etiology of AIDS
AIDS Epidemiology Studies	Supports cohort studies such as the Multicenter AIDS Cohort Study, San Francisco Men's Health Study, and Woman and Infants Transmission Study
Genetic Sequence Database and Analysis Unit	Collects and disseminates knowledge of genetic information about HIV
NIH AIDS Reagent Repository	Supplies biologic materials such as clones of HIV-1, which scientists can use to conduct cellular research
NIAID Intramural AIDS Research	Conducts basic biomedical and clinical research on HIV and AIDS
AIDS Outreach and Technology Transfer Program	Provides health care workers with the latest information on AIDS

In 1987 NIAID established the AIDS Clinical Trial Group (ACTG) to conduct collaborative clinical trials for AIDS therapies. By 1990 there were 47 ACTG centers, usually located in major medical centers in geographic areas where the incidence of HIV infection is high. In 1989 NIAID created 18 Community Programs for Clinical Research on AIDS (CPCRAs) to test AIDS-related drugs and vaccines. The expressed purpose of the CPCRAs is to "reach out to population groups that have been underrepresented in AIDS research" (NIAID, 1990, p. 11).

In some communities there is also a growing movement to test drugs in other community settings such as the Community Research Initiative (CRI) (AIDS Treatment Resources, 1990). CRI offers HIV-positive clients the opportunity to take drugs that have uncertain effectiveness and probably have not yet been tested within the formal FDA approval mechanism. Drugs with some demonstrated effectiveness can also be made available to a private physician for clients who cannot participate in a clinical trial or who have failed approved therapies; this process may be considered a parallel track.

Despite the extensive network of clinical trials, activist community groups such as the AIDS Coalition to Unleash Power (ACT-UP) charge that many clients with HIV infection are routinely excluded from drug trials because of life-style, gender, or pregnancy status. These charges seem founded when the demographics of the subjects participating in clinical trials are examined. The overwhelming majority of the subjects are white, gay men living in urban settings (Perryman, 1990); the numbers of persons with HIV infection in those geographic areas do not proportionately reflect this same distribution.

Before a drug reaches the marketplace for general distribution, it must pass through numerous steps. The overall goal of this process is to ensure that the drug is safe and effective. Hundreds and sometimes thousands of chemicals must be made and tested to find one that can achieve the desirable results without too serious side effects (Cohn, 1988). Table 7−7 depicts new drug development from initial synthesis to postmarketing surveillance (Young, 1988). The clinical stage of new drug development

TABLE 7−7. New Drug Development

PRECLINICAL	CLINICAL	POSTMARKETING
Research and development	Research and development	Surveillance
Initial synthesis	Phase 1	Adverse reaction reporting
Animal testing	⟶	Surveys and sampling testing
	Phase 2	Inspections
	⟶	
	Phase 3	
	⟶	

has three phases. Table 7–8 illustrates how experimental drugs are tested in humans by comparing the number of patients, length of testing, and purpose and percentage of drugs successfully completing each phase.

Phase I trials are concerned with learning more about the safety of the drug. These trials are usually conducted with healthy volunteers who are paid for their services. The subjects submit to a variety of tests to determine what the drug does in the human body: how it is absorbed, metabolized, and excreted; its effect on different body parts; and what side effects occur as the dose is increased. A main reason that drugs fail to proceed to phase II is evidence of toxicity at doses too small to produce any beneficial effects (Flieger, 1988).

The purpose of phase II trials is to determine whether the drug is effective in treating the disease or condition for which it is intended. These studies recruit a few hundred patients and attempt to determine short-term side effects and risks in people whose health is impaired. Most of the phase II trials are randomized, controlled trials that are often double blinded. When this methodology is used, subjects are randomly divided into two groups with one group (experimental group) receiving the experimental drug and the other group (control group) receiving a placebo. When the research is double blinded, neither the patients nor the health care providers know which patient is receiving the placebo and which is receiving the experimental drug. By the end of phase II trials, the researchers know whether the drug has a therapeutic effectiveness and its short-term side and adverse effects (Flieger, 1988). The FDA can quickly terminate phase II trials when there is evidence that the experimental

TABLE 7–8. How Experimental Drugs Are Tested in Humans

PHASE	NUMBER OF PATIENTS	LENGTH	PURPOSE	PERCENTAGE OF DRUGS SUCCESSFULLY COMPLETING*
I	20-100	Several months	Mainly safety	70
II	Up to several hundred	Several months to 2 years	Some short-term safety, but mainly effectiveness	33
III	Several hundred to several thousand	1-4 years	Safety, effectiveness, dosage	25-30

From Flieger, K. (1988). Testing in "real people": from test tube to patient. In *New drug development in the United States*. DHHS Publication No. (FDA) 88-3168; Rockville, MD: Department of Health and Human Services.

*For example, of 100 drugs for which investigational new drug applications are submitted to FDA, about 70 will successfully complete phase I trials and go on to phase II; about 33 will complete phase II and go to phase III; 25 to 30 will clear phase III (and, on average, about 20 of the original 100 will ultimately be approved for marketing).

group is receiving major benefit over the control group. This is the situation that occurred when zidovudine was tested.

Phase III studies are designed to provide information about optimum dose rates and schedules. Since thousands of patients are enrolled, more information about the drug's safety and effectiveness is also learned. Although phase III studies are controlled, they more closely approximate the conditions of ordinary medical practice. Not all drugs go through all of the phases (ATR, 1990). The evidence of safety and effectiveness of zidovudine (formerly known as AZT) was so great that phase III studies were not required before the FDA approved the drug for general use. During the 4- to 6-month period of phase II testing, only one patient with AIDS died while being treated with zidovudine, whereas 19 died while being given a placebo. Consequently, zidovudine was prematurely approved (without completion of phase III trials) for compassionate reasons and made widely available.

Several categories of drugs are being investigated for HIV-infected individuals. These include (1) antivirals such as dideoxyinosine (ddI) and dideoxycytidine (ddC) specifically indicated for HIV; (2) antivirals such as ganciclovir to treat CMV infection; (3) cytokines such as alpha interferon for KS and recombinant human erythropoietin for anemia; (4) immunomodulators such as human serum globulin and thymopentin; (5) antiinfectives to treat or prevent opportunistic infections such as aerosol pentamidine; (6) vaccines such as Salk HIV for early HIV infection; and (7) other pharmaceuticals such as megestrol acetate for HIV wasting (Pharmaceutical Manufacturers Association, 1990).

The nurse as health teacher must be knowledgeable about the categories of drugs and phases of clinical trials to answer clients' questions. Since 1974 the rights of human subjects involved in research are protected by institutional review boards (Schaefer, 1988). No clinical trials can begin until the institutional review board within the organization has approved the project and the client freely gives informed consent. The nurse as advocate must ensure that questions are answered and that institutional policies are followed. The nurse as caregiver must refer potential clients to clinical trials that may benefit them.

Patients and health care providers have identified five major benefits of clinical trials. These are (1) having a chance to help others; (2) obtaining access to top-quality health care; (3) gaining power for oneself by taking positive action; (4) being helped by a new drug; and (5) receiving financial assistance (most drugs are provided without charge by the pharmaceutical company, and associated laboratory and other diagnostic tests are usually covered by the agency funding the research study). Three major risks are associated with participating in clinical trials: (1) the treatment may not have benefits; (2) it may actually be harmful; and (3) the drug may have harmful side effects (DHHS, 1989). In addition, in many studies participants are not allowed to take other drugs while they are subjects. A comprehensive checklist of questions the client needs to have answered before making a decision about participating in research is included in Appendix IV.

After drugs are approved for general use, postmarketing surveillance continues. The FDA and the pharmaceutical firm must monitor adverse reactions to drugs. To help track the performance of their products, many drug firms rely on their sales personnel (Ackerman, 1988). The nurse should communicate with these salespersons by sharing ideas and seeking information about the drugs. The FDA has an "adverse drug reaction" form that should be completed whenever a health care provider notices an unusual or adverse reaction to a drug or treatment. However, physicians and other health care providers are not legally required to report these adverse drug reactions to the FDA. It is estimated that less than 10% of adverse drug reactions are reported by physicians and an even smaller percentage by other health care providers. To increase the number of adverse reaction reports, the FDA is educating physicians, pharmacists, and nurses about how reactions should be reported. Reporting has been made easier by the creation of hotlines and more rewarding by the provision of significant information about the drug by the manufacturer (Ackerman, 1988).

Many pharmaceutical firms encourage open communication by providing scientific information about their product. Anecdotal reports may result in the discovery of new uses for established drugs. For example, naltrexone, a drug approved for treating heroin addicts, may be effective for KS and has been used by physicians for KS without the knowledge of the FDA or formal testing. This is legal, since once the FDA has released a drug into the marketplace, no law requires that physicians dispense it only for approved uses (Ackerman, 1988). However, information about results in KS would be useful to other physicians who are not aware of this application for naltrexone.

Legal Decisions and Health Care

Community health nurses need to assist clients in making decisions about their health care and planning for the stage of illness right before death. Because the course of HIV infection is characterized by episodes of acute illness, sometimes accompanied by increasing mental confusion, ideally these decisions should be made while the client feels relatively well and unpressured. Many HIV-positive persons are eager to discuss their treatment preferences ahead of time (Zuger, 1990). By discussing issues such as resuscitation and living wills with clients in an ambulatory setting, the community health nurse and physician can promote a thoughtful analysis of all of the risks and benefits of both action and inaction (Havlir, Brown, & Rousseau, 1989). The health care provider should be careful not to allow personal beliefs to enter unduly into discussions about treatment decisions. Decisions made in an unpressured environment may better reflect the client's wishes.

Although every person has the legal right to give informed consent before any treatment is rendered, the specific details of the law can vary widely. State law has an impact on treatment decisions, especially during the terminal stages of illness. Advance directives are particularly important in situations in which clients may become unable to express their own wishes. Traditionally family members are expected to know what the client would desire if the client were competent to decide. Family members include legal spouses and parents. Clients with HIV infection may be estranged from these family members for a variety of reasons, and a friend or significant other may better understand the client's wishes. However, in the absence of advance directives, the decisions of legally recognized family will prevail.

To give clients with HIV infection appropriate anticipatory guidance, the nurse should be familiar with four advance directives. These legal options inform health care providers and significant others about the client's wishes. The four areas are (1) durable power of attorney, (2) health care proxy, (3) living wills, and (4) do-not-resuscitate orders.

Durable power of attorney is legal in all 50 states and the District of Columbia (McCarrick, 1990). A durable power of attorney is given to a person who can make proxy decisions to carry out the client's wishes when the client is incompetent. This person has the full authority to act as if he or she were the patient making the decisions. The client should consult a lawyer to designate a durable power of attorney.

A health care proxy is a person who has durable power of attorney specifically for making health care decisions. The client can name anyone to make health care decisions in the event that the client is incompetent or chooses not to make those decisions. Health care proxy legislation has been passed in at least 18 states, and nurses need to know the specifics of the law in the state in which they are practicing. However, in some states health care professionals (e.g., physicians and nurses) who are not related to the patient are expressly forbidden or excluded from serving as proxies for either health care or other decisions. In most cases forms for naming a health care proxy are available and consulting a lawyer is not necessary. Witnesses are usually required.

Legislation supporting living wills exists in 42 states (Table 7–9). Although the specifics vary from state to state, living wills are usually alike in that they must be executed by competent adults and witnessed

TABLE 7–9. States and Districts with Living Will Legislation

Alabama	Hawaii	Minnesota	Tennessee
Alaska	Idaho	Missouri	Texas
Arizona	Illinois	Montana	Utah
Arkansas	Indiana	Nevada	Vermont
California	Iowa	New Hampshire	Virginia
Colorado	Kansas	New Mexico	Washington
Connecticut	Kentucky	North Carolina	West Virginia
Delaware	Louisiana	North Dakota	Wisconsin
District of Columbia	Maine	Oklahoma	Wyoming
Florida	Maryland	Oregon	
Georgia	Mississippi	South Carolina	

(Killian, 1990). Living wills direct treatment decisions related to heroic and life-sustaining interventions for terminally ill persons. Although the definition of terminally ill varies, it usually refers to a person who has a life expectancy of less than 1 year. Both the Society for the Right to Die and Concern for Dying provide sample living wills.

Do-not-resuscitate (DNR) orders are medical directives indicating that the client should not receive cardiopulmonary resuscitation. All other treatment is given irrespective of a DNR order. Again, state law varies greatly and the physician should frequently evaluate and renew a DNR order. In some states the law is silent on DNR orders when the client is not in a hospital or nursing home, and this can result in a conflict for the client, significant others, and the community health nurse.

The U.S. Supreme Court decided the Nancy Cruzan case during the summer of 1990. In this decision the highest court of the United States said that a person whose wishes are clearly known has a constitutional right to discontinue life-sustaining treatment. However, in the absence of clear advance directives, the treatment must continue (Greenhouse, 1990). This decision is applicable in every state and reinforces the need for competent adults to plan for periods of incompetency. Clients with HIV infection need assistance in making their wishes clear and naming the person of their choice to make health care decisions for them. When a client does not have a significant other to identify, the community health nurse can serve as an advocate for that person through clear documentation of the client's expressed wishes.

During the last days of illness the community health nurse should explain to the family or significant others that a call to emergency personnel indicates a desire for resuscitation efforts. The nurse should clarify that bringing a client to the emergency room often results in unwanted heroic treatment efforts. By assisting significant others to plan for the hours before death and the days immediately following, the nurse can help to give this period the dignity it deserves.

INSTITUTIONAL LONG-TERM CARE

Progress achieved in clinical research, drug development, and accumulated experience by health care professionals has increased the survival of persons with HIV disease. Most clinicians today view HIV disease as a chronic illness rather than thinking of it as a terminal disease, a viewpoint that dominated the clinical approach to care in the early 1980s. Therefore, as with any chronic illness, planning for long-term care is an absolute necessity.

Throughout the HIV epidemic, home care has played by far the most significant role, not only because care at home is often preferred by consumers, but also because the service has so much potential for flexibility (Wyatt, 1990). However, as with any chronic disease, variables associated with the life of the affected individual may necessitate care in a setting other than the home. These variables range from the lack of a suitable home in which to provide care to the lack of a significant other who can provide the needed care. Options to home care include skilled nursing facilities (SNFs, often referred to as nursing homes), day care, and residential care with supportive services. While the demand for these alternatives has been self-evident and is increasing, the supply has remained pitifully low and in some areas nonexistent.

Care in a Skilled Nursing Facility

According to Benjamin and Swan (1989), when case managers explore the option of nursing home care for persons with HIV disease, they find not a solution but a service gap, since many skilled nursing facilities are reluctant to provide care to this client population. Reasons frequently cited for refusal of nursing homes to accept persons with HIV disease include (1) increased costs for infection control measures and staffing, (2) poor Medicaid reimbursement levels, (3) an unprepared work force, (4) a philosophic orientation to geriatric care, (5) homophobia among administrators or staff members, (6) already high occupancy rates, and (7) possible loss of referrals of non-HIV-infected residents (Taravella, 1990).

To illustrate the short supply further, by March 1990 in New York City, with 9602 persons living with AIDS, approximately 130 dedicated AIDS skilled nursing beds were available at three facilities (New York City Department of Health, 1990; Taravella, 1990). The plans for the future are not promising. Through 1993 there will be an anticipated 1513 skilled nursing beds for persons with HIV illness in the entire United States (Taravella, 1990).

One of the first skilled nursing facilities in the United States to admit a PWA was the Human Resources Health Center in Dade County, Florida.

According to Diana Liebisch, the director of nursing at that time, admission of PWAs to the facility was considered part of its mission and the staff struggled through fear and confusion, changing care regimens as new information became available and adjusting policies to meet the challenge (Harvard AIDS Institute, 1989). By 1989 the facility had served 169 PWAs, and there are plans to expand its capabilities.

Kane and Smith (1989) were the first to study the integration of persons with AIDS into nursing homes. The study was conducted in 16 nursing homes in Minnesota, equally divided between 8 SNFs willing to take or already having admitted PWAs and 8 SNFs that did not have plans to admit PWAs. Kane and Smith interviewed 100 nursing home residents, 100 family members of residents, and 100 nursing home staff members. They also interviewed the administrator, director of nurses, and director of social work at each of the 16 facilities, as well as 4 PWAs who were residents in the SNFs studied.

In facilities receptive to admitting PWAs, the staff was more knowledgeable and held more positive attitudes about integration of PWAs into nursing homes than the staff in comparison homes. The SNFs that had admitted PWAs did not experience negative reactions of residents or family members, and staff members did not resign as anticipated. An interesting finding was the fear among the residents and their families and the staff about the reactions of the others. The residents and their families were fearful that the staff would quit and the staff was fearful that families would move the residents to other SNFs; neither fear materialized. The universal concerns over contagion and infection control practices were also noted but were certainly not limited to the nursing home setting given the nature of HIV infection.

In interviews with PWAs in nursing homes, Kane and Smith (1989) reported that the most significant concerns were (1) lack of training or familiarity of some staff with high-tech equipment, (2) quality of meals, (3) quality of activities, (4) lack of telephones, (5) routines that prohibited sleeping late, and (6) concern about the reactions of non-AIDS residents. The concerns of the PWAs regarding a lack of skill with particular equipment are understandable, but the same problem can occur in other health care settings as well. Complaints about meals, schedules, and activities are common among elderly nursing home residents as well as PWAs (Kane & Caplan, 1990).

The clinical needs of clients with HIV infection remain the same regardless of the setting. For example, clients with toxoplasmosis require suppressive therapy to prevent recurrence, assistance with personal care, and physical and occupational therapy whether they are in a hospital, in a nursing home, or at home. Dementia is the primary clinical condition that requires the supportive and protective environment of a skilled nursing facility (Benjamin & Swan, 1989; Kator & Cunningham McBride, 1990).

The dementia seen in many of the clients with AIDS can result in bizarre behavior, violent acting-out, decline in self-care skills, and delusional thinking (Dunn, 1990). Both staff and residents should be informed about these behaviors as a consequence of disease and taught how to respond appropriately.

As in other health care settings, nursing home staff need preparation to meet the clinical needs of HIV-infected persons with specific opportunistic diseases. They must be trained in such techniques as infusion therapy to suppress opportunistic infections and prophylaxis to prevent infections. Flexibility must be introduced into a system of care traditionally dominated by exclusionary rules.

Based on 8 years' experience admitting PWAs to the Palm Beach County Home and General Care Facility, in Palm Beach County, Florida, Dunn (1990) recommends that planning for skilled nursing facility care includes (1) developing procedures specific to the needs of PWAs, (2) increasing social services, (3) providing support group therapy, (4) offering addiction recovery therapy or meetings at the facility, (5) developing policies and plans for handling substance abuse in the facility, and (6) providing necessary education and support groups for staff.

The concerns and needs of the nursing staff in nursing homes are the same as those expressed by their colleagues in other settings. As history has demonstrated, with education and experience these fears can be decreased.

Day Care

An underdeveloped option for long-term care of persons with HIV infection is a day care and treatment program. In August 1988 the Village Nursing Home in New York City opened the first day care program designed specifically for PWAs. The goals of the program are rehabilitation, socialization, and recreation (McNally & Mason-Beck, 1989). The program also provides meals and respite for the family and significant others.

Day care for clients with AIDS dementia complex can be an important part of the plan of care because of the socialization experience. Including cognitive stimulation and exercise therapy can also improve mental and motor dysfunction associated with the neurotropic effects of HIV. Supervision of medications in this type of program can help ensure compliance. Infusion therapy can be provided at a reduced cost, since the nurse can care for several clients at one time.

For clients who have no significant others, live in substandard housing, and have difficulty providing for themselves, the day care program can function as a coordinator of care and case manager for a variety of services (Wyatt, 1990). Combining day care with home care in the evenings and on weekends for clients with high-level care needs is another option for a plan of care.

In addressing the need for flexibility in the continuum of long-term care, the Village Nursing Home, in addition to its day care program, has plans to implement a home care program and open a skilled nursing facility dedicated to caring for persons with AIDS. This will provide a true "system" of long-term care, allowing clients to move from one service level to another as needed.

Residential Care

In July 1983, the gay community and health care professionals in San Francisco opened the world's first AIDS residence (Harvard AIDS Institute, 1989). Today this program, known as the Shanti Project, operates 14 residences in San Francisco. The program's chief goal is to provide high-quality, long-term, low-cost housing for displaced persons with AIDS or severe HIV disease who are able to live independently and cooperatively with needed support services in a group setting. The staff works closely with other AIDS agencies to provide the medical and social services needed by the residents. Residents requiring home care receive services from the Hospice of San Francisco and Visiting Nurse Association.

In New York City in 1983 members of the gay community recognized the need for housing that was supportive of the needs of PWAs. They formed the AIDS Resource Center, which initially offered donations to individuals for rent, food, and so forth. Today the AIDS Resource Center operates two types of supportive housing programs for persons with AIDS, a congregate living facility and scatter-site apartments.

The congregate living facility, known as Bailey House, has 44 private rooms for clients. Case management, support groups, and on-site health supervision by a professional nurse and visiting physician are provided. The scatter-site housing program is a series of apartments throughout the boroughs of New York City. Services are similar to those at Bailey House except that no on-site health supervision is offered. Clients in both settings who require home care receive services from the Visiting Nurse Service of New York.

The AIDS Housing of Washington is a unique facility being planned in the Seattle area. The 35-bed facility will provide housing, assistance with personal care, 24-hour skilled nursing care, hospice care, respite care, and day care (McInturiff, 1990). Construction is expected to be completed by the fall of 1991. The Sisters of Providence will operate the facility.

One of the most prevalent case management problems in residential programs is substance use, including alcohol, crack and cocaine, marijuana, heroin, and LSD. The problem becomes obvious when the resulting behaviors are property destruction, physical and verbal abuse of residents and staff, and unsafe sex. The problem of substance use is not limited to self-identified drug users. In fact, many of the problems of substance use may not be addressed until after the client takes residence in the facility. Case management should include nondiscriminatory rules regarding behaviors that are not allowed and clear communication of the consequences of breaking the rules. Above all, the staff must be willing to enforce the prearranged limits and must do so consistently. To vacillate and make exceptions gives mixed messages to the client population and encourages them to test the rules.

A recurrent issue encountered by clients in congregate living facilities is constant reminders that they have HIV infection. Clients must deal with grieving, both actual and anticipatory, which in most situations is handled through support groups. Volunteers and a program of recreation as well as the availability of religious and spiritual counseling is an important adjunct to quality living for the residents. Other case management issues to be considered include (1) residents bringing guests back to their rooms to have sex, (2) homophobia and fear of IV drug users among residents, (3) managing and supervising clients with progressive dementia, and (4) both staff and residents receiving and giving preferential treatment.

Hospice Care

Since the opening of St. Christopher's Hospice in England in 1967, hospice care has received considerable attention worldwide. By 1980 the Health Care Finance Administration (HCFA) had approved 26 hospice demonstration programs to study the efficacy and economics of hospice care in the United States. Since then, hospice care has become integrated into the schema of health care in the United States.

Hospice care in the United States has emerged as a model of home care for terminally ill individuals. A prevalent misconception is that a hospice is a place to institutionalize a dying person. Although all certified hospice programs are required to have inpatient beds available, their use is limited to short periods for respite care and symptom control. This basic lack of understanding led to demands, early in the AIDS epidemic in the United States, to place PWAs in hospices.

The major appeal of hospice care is the concept of interdisciplinary and holistic case management as the ideal health care model. Hospice care emphasizes the quality of life for terminally ill individuals through symptom control (palliative care) and expert psychologic and spiritual care. Most clinicians would agree that this ideal approach to care should be applied to all health care settings. Taking this one step further, all health care professionals should emphasize quality of life issues through symptom control and expert psychologic and spiritual care. Although most health care professionals have formally studied death and dying, few have formally studied, with hospice experts, the basics of symptom control, especially pain control. Therefore they are limited in applying symptom control to client care, irrespective of the clinical setting.

Until 1983 the etiology of AIDS remained unknown, and until March 1987 no treatment for HIV infection was available. Consequently, in the early years of the epidemic, AIDS was viewed as a rapidly progressing terminal illness. Through clinical research, the development of antiviral agents, and improved methods of treating and preventing opportunistic infections, the clinical picture has changed dramatically. Today the needs of the HIV-ill person can be more appropriately described as a continuum of care for chronic illness. This is not meant to imply that hospice care is not needed; it should be available to those individuals who wish it. However, barriers to hospice care for PWAs remain. First, federally established reimbursement rates do not reflect the actual costs associated with case management and clinical needs of HIV-infected individuals. Second, national, state and local hospice organizations have had to redefine palliative care as it relates to AIDS. Among the issues are (1) allowing the continuation of IV therapy for palliative reasons, for example, ganciclovir to prevent blindness with CMV retinitis; (2) periodic transfusions to correct anemia; and (3) continuation of expensive suppressive medicines specific for HIV-related illnesses. Third, hospice staff members usually do not have the technical preparation to provide the high-tech services that this client population may need.

Hospice care, regardless of the stage of HIV illness, is unacceptable to many PWAs because they are young and because they believe that a cure is imminent (Ungvarski, 1988). They often choose to pursue aggressive medical treatment and to participate in research protocols (Ungvarski, 1989). Commenting on knowledge, self-determination, and decision making, Derek Hodel (1990), executive director of the People with AIDS Group, summarizes, "The truth is, a lot of people with AIDS don't want to be 'self empowered.' They want to stay alive" (p. 30). Consequently, although the care providers and significant others may clearly see the benefits and need for hospice care, they should not be surprised if the PWA rejects this model of care.

Hospice care focuses on the quality rather than the quantity of life. Therefore the foundation of hospice care is symptom control, that is, taking control of a particular symptom and preventing its recurrence rather than allowing the symptom to control and detract from the individual's life (MacFadden, 1988). Pomerantz and Harrison (1990) identified symptoms common in end-stage HIV illness as (1) pain; (2) diarrhea; (3) nausea and vomiting; (4) dehydration; (5) urinary incontinence; (6) fever; (7) respiratory problems including chest pain, cough, and hypoxemia; (8) decubitus ulcers; (9) delirium and dementia; (10) weight loss; and (11) depression, anxiety, and fear. Chapter 4 includes nursing management information that incorporates symptom control, and Chapter 6 covers the psychosocial aspects of care, including grief and bereavement. The following discussion is limited to medical interventions that may be employed to control symptoms of end-stage HIV illness.

Schofferman (1988) identified pain resulting from peripheral neuropathy as the most commonly encountered pain requiring palliative treatment. Price and Brew (1990) described the pain, thought to be related to HIV infection of nerve or dorsal root ganglion, as painful paresthesias and burning, especially in the feet. It may prevent walking in some individuals and is not generally relieved with zidovudine. Treatment is with tricyclic antidepressants, such as desipramine or imipramine, and analgesics. Newer antiretroviral nucleoside drugs, such as dideoxyinosine (ddI) and dideoxycytidine (ddC), also cause axonal neuropathies, and individuals with underlying neuropathy may be particularly vulnerable to this adverse affect of ddI and ddC (Price & Brew, 1990).

Pain assessment is extremely important to determine the specific plan of care for PWAs. For example, if pain is related to tumor such as KS compressing bone, nerve or hollow viscus, management may include chemotherapy to reduce tumor size. Likewise, if pain is due to extensive lesions, such as esophageal lesions associated with HSV infection, the plan of care should include antiviral therapy for HSV in addition to analgesia. According to Schofferman (1988) treatment of pain in PWAs follows the same general guidelines as in patients with cancer. Constipation, a common side effect of narcotic analgesics, is seen less often in AIDS because of the high incidence of diarrhea (Pomerantz & Harrison, 1990; Schofferman, 1988).

Nausea and vomiting may be the consequence of opportunistic diseases or their treatment. Initial control of these symptoms may be achieved by parenteral administration of medication or use of suppositories. Metodopramide, prochlorperazine, or trimethobenzamide may be used to control nausea and vomiting (Pomerantz & Harrison, 1990). A more recently approved antiemetic is dronabinol. It is classified as a cannabinoid, or synthetic form of active substances found in marijuana.

The assessment of diarrhea should include such causes as side effects of drugs, malabsorption, lactose intolerance, and development of a gastrointestinal opportunistic infection. If none of the preceding is identified as the cause of diarrhea, such agents as loperamide and diphenoxylate with atropine may be administered. Dehydration accompanying diarrhea requires oral fluid replacement to the extent tolerated.

In addition to fluid intake, Pomerantz and Harrison (1990) recommend controlling fever with two tablets of aspirin alternated with two tablets of acetaminophen every 2 hours. In the presence of low platelet counts or idiopathic thrombocytopenic purpura, commonly seen in HIV infection, aspirin administration is contraindicated. In the presence of severe anemia and neutropenia in persons taking zidovudine, acetaminophen may be contraindicated.

Respiratory problems may be alleviated by oxygen administration for air hunger, analgesia for chest pain, and antitussive agents for cough. Although placement of a Foley catheter may result in urosepsis, its benefit for a patient with urinary incontinence may outweigh the risk. Although prevention of decubitus ulcers is every nurse's priority, they may occur. The primary focus is prevention of ulcer extension and secondary infection, since in most cases little healing will take place.

Delirium and dementia may be the result of advanced HIV infection, sepsis, and fever, or in some cases the result of adverse drug effects. Pomerantz and Harrison (1990) suggested that effective treatment can be achieved with the combination of haloperidol and diazepam.

Symptom control is an art as well as a science, and health care professionals who lack the education and experience are strongly encouraged to seek consultation for their clients from hospice staff. This is especially true with pain control. According to Rogers (1989), many studies have demonstrated that patients suffer needlessly because of undermedication, which occurs because health care professionals have insufficient knowledge of the pharmacology of analgesics and because they fear they may be fostering narcotic abuse. Bohnet (1986) pointed out that until the symptoms are controlled or managed, no other concern of the client can be realistically addressed by nursing assessment or intervention.

SUMMARY

Planning for the long-term care needs of the client with HIV disease ranges from primary care with scheduled follow-up in the early phase of diagnosis to provision of home care, long-term residential care, or hospice care in the later stages. Health care professionals responsible for case management can improve access to these services if they are familiar with the capabilities and limitations of the various service providers.

In August 1990 the National Commission on AIDS submitted its first annual report to the President and Congress. Among their findings were that (1) the belief that Medicaid will pay for health care needs of persons with HIV infection is a "Medicaid fantasy"; (2) for people who are medically disenfranchised and unable to pay, no system of care exists; and (3) health care in the United States has been unresponsive to the needs of HIV-infected people. The report emphasizes that at the end of the first decade of the HIV-AIDS epidemic in the United States, there is still no national policy or plan and no national voice.

Unquestionably the health care professionals intimately involved in HIV-AIDS education, care, and research have made great strides in addressing the clinical needs of this client population and have clearly articulated what needs to be done to address the problems of care. The federal government must take a more active role. "The development of a comprehensive system with linkages to research protocols, existing community-based services, hospitals, drug treatment programs, local health departments, and long term care facilities, based on a foundation of adequate support, is long overdue and should be a top priority for the federal government" (National Commission on AIDS, 1990, p. 167).

References

Ackerman, S. (1988). Watching for problems that testing may have missed. In *New drug development in the United States* (pp. 51–53). DHHS Publication No. (FDA) 88–3168. Rockville, MD: Department of Health and Human Services.

AIDS Treatment Resources (1990). *Deciding to enter an AIDS/HIV drug trial* (6th Ed.). New York: AIDS Treatment Resources, Inc.

American Nurses' Association (1980). *Nursing: a social policy statement.* Kansas City, MO: The Association.

American Nurses' Association (1988). *Nursing case management.* Kansas City, MO: The Association.

Benjamin, A.E., Swan, J.H. (1989). Nursing home care for persons with HIV illness. *Generations, 13*(4), 63–64.

Bohnet, N.L. (1986). Symptom control. In M. O'Rawe Amenta & N.L. Bohnet (Eds.), *Nursing care of the terminally ill* (pp. 67–80). Boston: Little, Brown.

Centers for Disease Control (1983). CDC guidelines for isolation precautions in hospitals. In J.S. Garner & B.P. Simmons (Eds.), *Guidelines for prevention and control of nosocomial infections* (pp. 47–78). Atlanta: CDC (U.S. Government Printing Office No. 747-459).

Centers for Disease Control (1990). Screening for tuberculosis and tuberculosis infection in high-risk populations and the use of preventative therapy for tuberculosis infection in the United States. *Morbidity and Mortality Weekly Report, 39*(RR-8), 1–12.

Cohn, J. (1988). The beginnings: Laboratory and animal studies. In *New drug development in the United States* (pp. 8–11). DHHS Publication No. (FDA) 88–3168. Rockville, MD: Department of Health and Human Services.

Dunn, S. (1990). Providing care in a county nursing home AIDS unit. In V.E. Fransen (Ed.), *Proceedings: AIDS prevention and services workshop* (pp. 116–119). Princeton, NJ: Robert Wood Johnson Foundation.

Flieger, K. (1988). Testing in "real people." In *New drug development in the United States* (pp. 13–14, 17). DHHS Publication No. (FDA) 88–3168. Rockville, MD: Department of Health and Human Services.

Gebbie, K.M. (1989). The President's Commission on AIDS: What did it do? *American Journal of Public Health, 79*(7), 868–870.

Glazier, D., Glazier, R. (1990). Understanding alternative therapies often used to fight HIV infection. *AIDS Medical Report, 3*(7), 77–86.

Grau, L. (1984). Case management and the nurse. *Geriatric Nursing, 5*(8), 372–375.

Greenhouse, L. (June 26, 1990). Justices find a right to die, but the majority sees need for clear proof of intent. *New York Times*, pp. 1, 13.

Harvard AIDS Institute (1989). *Alternatives to hospital care for people with HIV infection.* (Invitational Conference, Nov. 8–10, 1989). Cambridge, MA: Harvard School of Public Health.

Havlir, D., Brown, L., Rousseau, K. (1989). Do not resuscitate discussions in a hospital based home care program. *Journal of the American Geriatrics Society, 37*(1), 52–54.

Hodel, D. (1990). All fired up or just all fired. *Outweek, 70,* 30–31.

Irish, A. (1989). Maintaining health in persons with HIV infection. *Seminars in Oncology Nursing,* 5(4), 302–307.

Kane, N. (1987). Unproven methods of cancer treatment. In C. Ziegfeld (Ed.), *Core curriculum for oncology nursing* (pp. 257–259). Philadelphia: W.B. Saunders.

Kane, R.A., Caplan, A.L. (1990). *Everyday ethics: Resolving dilemmas in nursing home life.* New York: Springer.

Kane, R.A., Smith, D. (1989). *Multiple perspectives on AIDS and the nursing home: A pilot study and recommendations for research.* Report No. PB 90-101320. Rockville, MD: Agency for Health Care Policy and Research.

Kator, M.J., Cunningham McBride, L. (1990). Developing a long term care facility program for AIDS patients. *Pride Institute Journal of Long Term Home Health Care,* 9(1), 15–19.

Killian, W. (1990). Knowledge of living will laws essential. *American Nurse, 22*(7), 33.

Lindemer, S. (1990). Writing as therapy. *Coping, Living with Cancer,* 4(1), 31.

Lundberg, G.D. (1991). National health care reform: An aura of inevitability is upon us. *Journal of the American Medical Association, 265*(19), 2566–2567.

MacFadden, D.K. (1988). Symptom control in AIDS. *Journal of Palliative Care,* 4(4), 42–45.

McCarrick, P. (1990). Living wills and durable powers of attorney: Advance directive legislation and issues. In *Scope Note 2.* Washington, DC: National Reference Center for Bioethics Literature, Kennedy Institute of Ethics, Georgetown University.

McCormick, W.C. (1990). Clinical characteristics of persons with AIDS who are appropriate for community care settings. In Agency for Health Care Policy and Resources Conference Proceedings. *Community-based care of persons with AIDS: Developing a research agenda* (pp. 65–73). DHHS Publication No. PHS 90–3456. Washington, DC: U.S. Government Printing Office.

McInturff, P.I. (1990). A comprehensive approach to AIDS housing in a secondwave city: the Seattle–King County Model. In V.E. Fransen (Ed.), *Proceedings: AIDS prevention and services workshop* (pp. 120–127). Princeton, NJ: Robert Wood Johnson Foundation.

McNally, L., Mason-Beck, L. (1989). Day treatment for persons with AIDS. *Generations,* 13(4), 69–70.

Monaco, G. (1989). Counseling patients about dubious and rip-off remedies for AIDS and ARC. *PAACNOTES,* 1(3), 80–84.

Morrison, C. (1990a). Case management and the determination of appropriate care settings. In Agency for Health Care Policy and Resources Conference Proceedings. *Community based care of persons with AIDS: Developing a research agenda* (pp. 75–82). DHHS Publication No. PHS 90–3456Y. Washington, DC: U.S. Government Printing Office.

National Commission on AIDS (1990). *Annual report to the President and the Congress.* Washington, DC: U.S. Government Printing Office.

National Institute of Allergy & Infectious Diseases (1990). *NIAID AIDS Research.* Bethesda, MD: The Institute.

National Institutes of Health. (1989). *AIDS clinical trials: Talking it over.* Bethesda, MD: Department of Health and Human Services.

Newshan, G. (1989). Therapeutic touch for symptom control in persons with AIDS. *Holistic Nursing Practice,* 3(4), 45–51.

New York City Department of Health (1989). *HSA/New York City AIDS Task Force report.* New York: The Department.

New York City Department of Health (1990, February). *AIDS Surveillance Update.* New York: The Department.

Nokes, K., Kendrew, J. (1990a). Loneliness in veterans with AIDS and its relationship to the development of infections. *Archives of Psychiatric Nursing,* 4(4), 271–277.

Nokes, K., Kendrew, J. (1990b). *Health beliefs and use of alternative therapies in HIV positive veterans.* Unpublished manuscript.

Perryman, S. (1990). AIDS: Perspective of a black woman as an epidemic among the myriads. *Body Positive,* 3(7), 37–38.

Pharmaceutical Manufacturers Association (1990, Summer). *In development, AIDS medicines, drugs and vaccines.* Washington, DC: The Association.

Pomerantz, S., Harrison, E. (1990). End-stage symptom management. *AIDS Patient Care,* 4(1), 18–20.

Presidential Commission (1988). *Report of the Presidential Commission on the Human Immunodeficiency Virus Epidemic.* Washington, DC: U.S. Government Printing Office.

Price, R.W., Brew, B. (1990). Management of the neurologic complications of HIV-1 infection and AIDS. In M.A. Sande & P.A. Volberding (Eds.), *The medical management of AIDS* (2nd Ed.) (pp. 161–181). Philadelphia: W.B. Saunders.

Rogers, A.G. (1989). Analgesics: The physician's partner in effective pain management. *Virginia Medical, 116*(4), 164–170.

Sanders, P. (1989). Acupuncture and herbal treatment of HIV infection. *Holistic Nursing Practice, 3*(4), 38–44.

Schaefer, K. (1988). Research review board opportunities. *Dimensions of Critical Care Nursing, 7*(3), 178–182.

Schofferman, J. (1988). Pain: Diagnosis and management in the palliative care of AIDS. *Journal of Palliative Care, 4*(4), 45–46.

Solomon, G., Temoshok, L. (1987). A psychoneuroimmunologic perspective on AIDS research: Questions, preliminary findings and suggestions. *Journal of Applied Social Psychology, 17*(3), 286–308.

Strawn, J. (1989). Complimentary therapies: Maximizing the mind-body connection. In J. Meisenholder & C. La Charite (Eds.), *Comfort in caring, nursing the person with HIV infection* (pp. 181–198). Glenview, IL: Scott, Foresman.

Taravella, S. (1990). Who will provide long-term care for AIDS patients? *Modern Health Care, 20*(12), 38–39.

Ungvarski, P.J. (1987). AIDS and long-term care. *Caring, 6*(10), 44–47.

Ungvarski, P.J. (1988). Testimony on home care. In *The Presidential Commission on the Human Immunodeficiency Virus Epidemic: Hearing on care of HIV infected persons, January 13–15, 1988.* Washington, DC: U.S. Government Printing Office.

Ungvarski, P.J. (1989). Developing long-term plan of care for the HIV epidemic. *Caring, 8*(11), 4–8.

Wyatt, A. (1990). AIDS and the long-term care continuum. *Pride Institute Journal of Long Term Home Health Care, 9*(1), 6–14.

Young, F. (1988). The reality behind the headlines. In *New drug development in the United States* (pp. 4–5). DHHS Publication No. (FDA) 88–3168. Rockville, MD: Department of Health and Human Services.

Zhang, Q., Ziolkowski, H. (1990). Treating HIV disease with Chinese medicine. *Focus, A Guide to AIDS Research and Counseling, 5*(10), 1–2.

Zuger, A. (1990). Ethical decision making in AIDS. *AIDS Clinical Care, 2*(6), 51–52.

8

Cofactors of HIV and Public Health Education

Jacquelyn Haak Flaskerud

The causal agent in AIDS is commonly recognized to be a retrovirus known as human immunodeficiency virus type 1 (HIV-1). Groups of persons whose behaviors and circumstances put them at risk for contracting HIV infection and potentially acquiring AIDS have also been identified: homosexual and bisexual men, intravenous (IV) drug users, hemophiliacs and blood product recipients, persons who have sexual contact with these groups, and infants born to mothers with HIV infection. Ever since AIDS was first recognized, however, it has been apparent that the rate at which members of these groups become immunodeficient or contract complicating diseases when exposed to HIV varies considerably. Within groups of infected individuals (i.e., persons who have antibody to HIV), it is still uncertain in whom and when AIDS will develop. This variable expression of pathogenic properties is true of all but a few microorganisms infecting humans (Osborn, 1986; Siegel, 1986).

Based on observed data, the proportion of people with HIV antibody who will develop AIDS cannot be determined. Available data suggest that in the absence of therapy or treatment, signs or symptoms of illness will develop eventually in most HIV-infected persons (Gerstoft et al., 1987; Goedert et al., 1987; Hessol et al., 1989; Kaplan et al., 1988; Lifson et al., 1988; Moss et al., 1988; Pedersen et al., 1989). These findings have been reported for cohorts of homosexual men studied in the United States and Europe. Several mathematical models predict that in 100% of infected persons AIDS will develop after several years of infection (Lemp et al., 1988; Lui et al., 1988; Rees, 1987). However, among homosexual and bisexual men with long-term HIV seropositivity in the San Francisco City Clinic Cohort Study, some individuals have remained immunologically and clinically normal after 8 or more years of infection (Hessol et al.,

314

1988). Prospective studies and estimates have shown that the incubation period is longer (median of 9.8 years) than originally thought. How much longer is not yet known (Osmond, 1990). Therefore the important questions become: Why do some people not become immunodeficient or contract disease? and What is there about the risk behavior groups that makes them susceptible to infection and disease progression? Something in addition to HIV exposure seems to be required both to acquire the virus and to become ill from it. One or more cofactors must exist.

Several factors might influence the progression to disease (Hessol et al., 1989; Lifson et al., 1988). First, if behavioral cofactors such as sexual or drug use practices exist, behavioral change might reduce the likelihood of disease progression. Second, host factors such as infection with or reactivation of microbial agents or genetic characteristics might influence disease progression. It is also possible that the pathogenicity of HIV varies. Third, antiviral agents such as zidovudine (azidothymidine [AZT]) have been shown to increase the survival time of persons with AIDS (PWAs) and may slow or halt the progression to disease in HIV-infected asymptomatic persons (Lemp et al., 1990; Rothenberg et al., 1987). Finally, the use of prophylactic antibiotics might alter the virulence of the opportunistic infections (such as *Pneumocystis carinii* pneumonia) most commonly associated with mortality in PWAs.

Prospective studies are rapidly identifying specific environmental or behavioral components of life-style that might predict positive or negative outcomes of established HIV infection. Other cofactors being studied are those that would suppress immunity because of either a loss of protective natural defenses or undeveloped protective natural defenses. Cofactors associated with a loss of protective natural defenses include coinfection with pathogens associated with immune suppression, malnutrition, the use of certain drugs and alcohol, HIV strain type, exposure characteristics, a deficient natural resistance system, and genetic parameters such as human leukocyte antigen (HLA) type and familial tendency (Hessol et al., 1989; Hoff & Peterson, 1989; Jason et al., 1989; Lifson et al., 1988; van der Graaf & Diepersloot, 1989). These factors may be operating in some of the current transmission groups: homosexual and bisexual men, drug users, adult recipients of whole blood and blood products, and the sexual partners of the preceding groups. One cofactor associated with undeveloped or underdeveloped natural defenses is age: infants and adults over 50 years of age might be at increased risk.

COFACTORS AND HIV

Several cofactors appear to be involved in determining the pathogenesis of HIV disease. These cofactors might be viewed as occurring in two categories: exposure factors and trigger factors (Table 8–1). Exposure factors are cofactors that might affect acquisition of HIV infection. Trigger factors are cofactors that either increase a person's likelihood of being infected during exposure to HIV or contribute to HIV disease progression in those who have been infected. Cofactors might also be involved in the development of certain manifestations of AIDS such as Kaposi's sarcoma (Hessol et al., 1989; Lifson et al., 1988; Schechter et al., 1985).

Exposure Cofactors. Numerous studies in the United States and Europe have documented the relationship between specific sexual and lifestyle practices and exposure to HIV infection (Goedert et al., 1987; Hessol et al., 1989; Kingsley et al., 1987; Moss et al., 1987; Rietmeijer et al., 1989; Schechter et al., 1985; van der Graaf & Diepersloot, 1989; van Griensven et al., 1987; Winkelstein et al., 1987). Receptive anal intercourse, multiple anonymous sexual partners, douching or rectal enemas before receptive anal intercourse, the presence of genital ulcers, and not being circumcised are all cofactors associated with the acquisition of HIV infection. These cofactors expose a person to HIV by increasing the probability of sexual contact with an infectious partner, providing a route for transmission, causing trauma to the rectal mucosa, and producing membrane disruption that permits access of the viral agent to the bloodstream. However, recent evidence suggests that the virus probably can pass an intact mucous membrane (Rietmeijer et al., 1989; van der Graaf & Diepersloot, 1989). As a cofactor, not being circumcised may be explained by the larger surface of mucosal epithelium of the penis of uncircumcised men.

Other cofactors for acquisition of HIV infection have been associated with various aspects of drug and alcohol use (Hessol et al., 1989; Lifson et al., 1988; Schilling et al., 1989). The disinhibiting effects on behavior caused by alcohol and other drugs are well known and possibly allow more frequent and anonymous sexual exposure to the virus. Some drugs also blunt the sensation of pain, permitting or extending sexual practices that might not ordinarily be tolerated. The most obvious association of drugs and HIV infection is the direct transmission of the virus through the sharing of hypodermic needles, syringes, and other paraphernalia among parenteral drug users. The risk of seropositivity increases with increasing numbers of persons with whom needles are regularly shared and with more frequent injections. In addition, a consistent relationship has been shown between the use of "shooting galleries" and seropositivity (Des Jarlais et al., 1988; Schilling et al., 1989; Schoenbaum et al., 1989). These cofactors produce exposure by increasing the probability of contact with the virus.

Other exposure factors exist for hemophiliacs and blood recipients. The risk of seropositivity for hemophiliacs increases as the number of exposures to factor VIII concentrate increases. Among all blood recipients, exposure to plasma-rich blood components and the number of blood trans-

TABLE 8–1. Cofactors for HIV Infection

Exposure Cofactors

Anal receptive sex
Rectal douching
Multiple sexual partners
Presence of genital ulcers
Needle and syringe sharing
Use of "shooting galleries"
Frequency of injection
Use of recreational drugs
Receipt of factor VIII concentrate
Blood transfusions
Needlestick
Parent with HIV infection

Trigger Cofactors
Noninfectious

Malnutrition
Use of intravenous and recreational drugs
Prescribed drugs
Allergic conditions
Genetics
Emotional stress
Age
Pregnancy
Gender

Infectious

Antigenic overload from multiple infectious diseases (e.g., sexually transmitted diseases, soft tissue infections, bacterial endocarditis, tubercular infections)
Coincident viral infection and immune suppression (e.g., cytomegalovirus, hepatitis B virus, Epstein-Barr virus, herpesviruses)

fusions received are significant risk factors for HIV seropositivity (Blumberg & Heal, 1989; Perkins et al., 1987).

Trigger Cofactors. Trigger cofactors exert an effect on the expression of disease that is independent of any role in producing exposure to HIV. These cofactors augment or accelerate immunodeficiency. They increase the likelihood of being infected during exposure or contribute to the expression of active disease in those who are HIV positive. Trigger cofactors may have additive, deterministic, synergistic, or facilitative roles in the cytopathic effects of HIV on the immune system (Schechter et al., 1985).

The most prominent immunologic feature of AIDS is a drastic reduction in the number of circulating T-helper cells (T4 cells). At the same time the number of circulating T-suppressor cells (T8 cells) often remains at normal levels and in some cases increases, leading to a reversal of the usual T4/T8 (H/S) ratio of around 2:1 (Pederson et al., 1989). Cofactors are postulated to contribute to T cell immunodeficiency and immunologic abnormality through a variety of mechanisms.

Both noninfectious and infectious cofactors are involved in the etiology of and susceptibility to HIV infection and AIDS. Noninfectious cofactors include dietary factors; use of IV, recreational, or prescription drugs; genetics; allergic disorders; stress; age; gender; and pregnancy. The most common cause of T cell immunodeficiency worldwide is protein-calorie malnutrition. Malnutrition reduces the total number of T lymphocytes and helper and suppressor cells, impairs cell-mediated immunity and secretory immunity, reduces complement secretion, alters phagocytic function, and decreases killer cell activity. In addition, malnourishment leads to significant mineral, trace element, and vitamin deficiencies that affect overall immune function (Hickey & Weaver, 1988). Both poor nutrition secondary to drug use and the use of drugs to control appetite can lead to a chronic state of malnutrition that ultimately compromises the body's immune system (Mondanaro, 1987).

Alcohol, nitrites (poppers), amphetamines, marijuana, tobacco (cigarettes), and IV drugs (heroin, cocaine, and morphine) have all been suggested as possible factors in immunosuppression (Des Jarlais et al., 1988). Lymphocyte function is suppressed by the presence of clinically detectable alcohol (Siegel, 1986). In vitro, nitrites have been shown to depress various leukocyte functional parameters associated with host defense (Newell et al., 1985a). Nitrite use has been associated with a transient immunosuppression that may weaken the normal defenses against infection (Goedert et al., 1987; Moss et al., 1988; Newell et al., 1985b). However, cohort studies of PWAs have failed to support this association (Lifson et al., 1990; Rietmeijer et al., 1989). Use of cigarettes and marijuana has been associated with lower T-helper cell counts (Newell et al., 1985b; Schechter et al., 1985). In addition, cigarette smoking, marijuana use, and nitrite inhalation could predispose the lungs to opportunistic infections. IV drug users inject substances that have intrinsic immunosuppressive properties and are associated with chromosomal damage. Both IV and non-IV drugs have been associated with a reduction in numbers of T-helper cells and an increase in T-suppressor cells (Des Jarlais et al., 1988; Siegel, 1986).

Frequent use of antibiotics has also been associated with immunosuppression (McKenna et al., 1986). Chemical immunosuppression, whether from physician-prescribed or self-prescribed antibiotics, has been shown to occur in populations at high risk for sexually transmitted diseases (STDs) and soft tissue infections.

Exposure to allogeneic semen and sperm has been suggested as a possible cofactor in HIV disease (Hoff & Peterson, 1989; Schechter et al., 1985). Immunosuppression could result from exposure to allogeneic cells in passive partners during anogenital sex if sperm and semen can reach the lymphatics and vascular system. This could occur by way of rectal and lower bowel lesions resulting from trauma caused by sexual practices or from viral infections.

Emotional stress has been persistently associated with reactivation of herpes simplex infection and with the abrupt onset of malignancy (Kiecolt-Glaser & Glaser, 1988; Osborn, 1986). An immunologic component of emotional stress has been hypothesized to contribute to the progression of symptomatic disease. However, one study of HIV-infected men demonstrated that a stress reduction program significantly lowered the number of sexual partners but did not affect lymphocyte numbers or function (Coates et al., 1989).

Age is related to immunologic status. Infants are an immunologically incompetent group, and the more premature they are, the more immunologically abnormal they are. Infants have undeveloped natural resistance systems, which makes them susceptible to multiple infections, including HIV (Osborn, 1986). Older adults have an age-related loss of natural resistance, which could make them more susceptible to HIV and other infections (Sandor et al., 1986). Age has been related to HIV infection in homosexual men, hemophiliacs and other blood transfusion recipients, and heterosexual IV drug users. In homosexual men the incidence of HIV infection correlates with younger age at which regular intercourse with a male partner is initiated (Rietmeijer et al., 1989). However, among heterosexual men seropositivity is associated with older age (Chiasson et al., 1990). Among hemophiliacs and other blood transfusion recipients, older age is strongly related to disease progression (Darby et al., 1989; Eyster et al., 1987). In two large cohorts (New York City, n = 5833; San Francisco, n = 4323) that included both homosexual and heterosexual PWAs, survival was significantly related to age: increasing age reduced survival (Lemp et al., 1990; Rothenberg et al., 1987).

Pregnancy is another cofactor that contributes to immunosuppression. Gestational immunosuppression occurs naturally in the second and third trimesters and can be measured by depressed lymphocyte numbers and functions, which return to normal 1 month post partum (Hoff & Peterson, 1989; Nanda & Minkoff, 1989). A relationship between pregnancy and disease progression in seropositive women has been hypothesized. However, the current evidence suggests that pregnancy exerts no influence or only a minor one on the course of HIV disease (Ellerbrock & Rogers, 1990; Nanda & Minkoff, 1989).

Gender differences in response to HIV infection have been noted among IV drug users in New York City (Des Jarlais & Friedman, 1988; Des Jarlais et al., 1988). Although seroprevalence studies found a higher seroprevalance rate among female than male IV drug users, females lost T4 cells at a lower rate than males and had a slower progression to disease (AIDS). This gender cofactor appears to extend to pediatric cases of AIDS as well. Male children with AIDS in New York City have a higher cumulative mortality than do female children (Des Jarlais & Friedman, 1988).

Genetics may also play a role in HIV disease progression and the likelihood that specific disease manifestations will develop. In studies of persons with hemophilia and homosexual men, HLA type has been associated with clinical disease progression (Lifson et al., 1988; Meropol et al., 1989).

Finally, of the possible noninfectious cofactors to HIV, allogeneic blood and blood products may be immunosuppressive, especially plasma-rich blood components such as fresh frozen plasma (FFP), whole blood, and platelets. The transfer of allogeneic blood and blood products could compromise the immune system of recipients. In persons with hemophilia, immunosuppression may result from infusion of factor VIII as replacement therapy (Blumberg & Heal, 1989). The transfusion of stored anticoagulated plasma has been suggested as one factor that may affect host immune defenses and facilitate expression of clinical HIV disease.

Infectious cofactors are also involved in the etiology of and susceptibility to AIDS. In an immunosuppressed person, infection that leads to antigenic overload and stimulation can contribute to the progression to AIDS (Osborn, 1986). If the immune system is continually overstimulated by a high antigenic load in association with various chronic infections, this overstimulation may interfere with the host's capacity to eliminate infectious agents. A history of multiple infectious diseases, among them syphilis, giardiasis, gonorrhea, chancroid, and parasitic diseases, has been suggested as a cofactor in the acquisition of HIV infection (Jason et al., 1989; Lifson et al., 1988; Moss et al., 1987; Osborn, 1986; Rietmeijer et al., 1989; van der Graaf & Diepersloot, 1989). Soft tissue infections, as well as such infections as viral hepatitis and bacterial endocarditis, may result from the IV use of drugs dissolved in nonsterile water, mixed with contaminated diluents and impure narcotics, and self-administered through needles and syringes contaminated by blood and dirt (Chiasson et al., 1990; Osborn, 1986). These infections are thought to produce sufficient insult to the immune system to enhance the pathologic effects of HIV on the host.

Another infectious cofactor that might be operative in the progression from asymptomatic infection to overt disease is coincident immunosuppression caused by viruses other than HIV. Chief among those suggested as playing an additive or synergistic role in potentiating the cytopathic effects of HIV are chronic infections with cytomegalovirus (CMV), Epstein-Barr virus (EBV), hepatitis B virus (HBV), and herpesviruses (herpes simplex virus [HSV] and herpes zoster or varicella zoster virus [VZV]) (Bentwich et al., 1988; Collier et al., 1987; Latchman, 1987; Lifson et al., 1988; Melbye et al., 1987; Osborn, 1986; Quinn et al., 1987). These viruses significantly impair the immune system and may facilitate the progression of HIV infection. The effect of infection with other viruses might be simply immunosuppressive, providing opportunities for reactivation of HIV, or the viruses may activate cells that carry HIV, resulting in the full expression of cytopathologic effects (Quinn et al., 1987).

Finally, both stage of HIV infectivity and HIV strain type may be cofactors in acquisition of HIV infection and progression to clinical disease. The stage of infectivity determines the amounts of circulating virus and antibody. Transmission of the virus to others may vary depending on the amount of circulating virus or stage of infection in an HIV-infected individual (van der Graaf & Diepersloot, 1989). Furthermore, several investigators working with HIV-infected cohorts of hemophiliac and homosexual men have hypothesized that HIV strain type may differ between persons and between populations (Jason et al., 1989; van der Graaf & Diepersloot, 1989). If strains of HIV vary in their virulence, strain type may be related to HIV disease course and clinical outcome.

The various cofactors discussed here play a role in exposure to the virus, transmission of the virus, immunosuppression of the host, and activation or facilitation of the virus. Depending on their combination, they can increase or decrease the risk of HIV infection and the risk of expression of disease.

COFACTORS AND TRANSMISSION GROUPS

Cofactors tend to cluster in the different transmission groups for HIV infection, producing groups more or less at risk for infection by the virus. It is important to note that behaviors and circumstances put people at risk, not the groups with whom they are associated. However, these behaviors and circumstances occur more or less frequently in some groups than others, and therefore the term "risk groups" has emerged. Identification of risk groups has the possible negative result of stigmatization of these groups. A possible positive effect is the opportunity to design health education programs specific to the life-style, practices, and circumstances of a group at risk. Each of the groups defined by the Centers for Disease Control (CDC) as transmission groups for HIV infection and AIDS has specific cofactors associated with group members' risk of acquiring the virus and the progression to clinical disease.

Homosexual and Bisexual Men. The majority of studies identifying cofactors have been conducted with samples of homosexual and bisexual men. Many studies have been carried out in all U.S. cities where AIDS is prevalent and in comparable European cities. These studies are remarkably alike in their identification of cofactors for exposure to HIV in the homosexual and bisexual male transmission groups.

Researchers overwhelmingly agree that the greatest risk of exposure to HIV in the homosexual and bisexual male transmission group comes from anal receptive sexual intercourse and sexual practices (fisting, rectal douching) with multiple sexual partners. These risk factors are found to be associated with HIV seropositivity, generalized lymphadenopathy, AIDS-related complex (ARC), and AIDS (Des Jarlais et al., 1988; Goedert et al., 1987; Kingsley et al., 1987; Moss et al., 1987; Newell et al., 1985b; Rietmeijer et al., 1989; Schechter et al., 1985; van der Graaf & Diepersloot, 1989; Winkelstein et al., 1987). Such sexual practices are implicated not only in exposure to the virus, but also in transmission of the virus via rectal cells or trauma to the rectal mucosa, and in the presence of numerous noninfectious and infectious cofactors of HIV in the homosexual and bisexual transmission group.

Among the noninfectious cofactors, the use of alcohol, marijuana, and volatile nitrites (poppers) in conjunction with sex has been reported among homosexual men with AIDS (Des Jarlais et al., 1988; Goedert et al., 1987; Newell et al., 1985a, 1985b; Siegel, 1986; van Griensven et al., 1987). These drugs are used to heighten sexual arousal, to relax the anal sphincter during anal receptive intercourse, and to prolong duration of intercourse. The use of these drugs may also prolong the duration of exposure to the virus.

In addition, both volatile nitrites and alcohol may act as cofactors to HIV infection because of their immunosuppressive effects. Possibly the suppression of normal lymphocyte function in persons using volatile nitrites and alcohol acts as a facilitator of HIV infection or, in the presence of the virus, contributes to rapid disease progression (Hessol et al., 1989).

Anal receptive sexual practices resulting in trauma to the rectum and bowel provide the route for exposure to allogeneic semen and sperm. Sperm has been suggested as a possible cofactor in AIDS because of its immunosuppressive characteristics (Hoff & Peterson, 1989; Schechter et al., 1985).

Among the infectious cofactors of HIV for the homosexual and bisexual transmission group are several infectious diseases that are transmitted sexually and are facilitated by anal receptive sexual activity. These include gonorrhea, syphilis, and chancroid. These diseases are thought to cause antigenic overstimulation or overload in the host and to act as cofactors that augment or accelerate the pathogenesis of immunodeficiency (Moss et al., 1987; Osborn, 1986; Quinn et al., 1987; Rietmeijer et al., 1989; van der Graaf & Diepersloot, 1989). The physician-prescribed or self-prescribed use of antibiotics by homosexual and bisexual men with multiple infectious diseases has also been associated with immunosuppression (McKenna et al., 1986).

Other infectious cofactors of HIV for homosexual and bisexual men are concomitant chronic infections with other viruses: hepatitis A and B, herpesviruses, EBV, CMV, and human T cell lymphotropic virus types I and II (HTLV-I and HTLV-II). These infections cause coincident immunosuppression with HIV and could be operative in the progression from asymptomatic infection to overt disease (Bentwich et al., 1988; Collier et al., 1987; Friedman-Kien et al., 1986; Getchell et al., 1987; Goedert et al., 1987; Latchman, 1987; Melbye et al., 1987; Osborn, 1986; Quinn et al., 1987; Rietmeijer et al., 1989; Sandor et al., 1986; Schechter et al., 1985).

Some of the similarities and differences in homosexual and heterosexual sexual transmission of the virus should be noted. Heterosexuals who practice anal receptive sex and have multiple sexual partners are considered to be at increased risk for HIV infection (Johnson et al., 1989). However, the virus can be transmitted through vaginal receptive sex, and both male-to-female and female-to-male transmission has been documented (van der Graaf & Diepersloot, 1989). Questions have been raised concerning whether female-to-male transmission is as efficient as male-to-female and whether vaginal transmission is as efficient as anal transmission.

Heterosexual acts that are vaginal receptive and vaginal insertive may be less facilitative of transmission of the virus because of differences in the epithelial lining of the rectum and the vagina (Johnson et al., 1989; Karan, 1989). The susceptibility of the rectum and bowel to trauma and lesions could facilitate the transmission not only of HIV but also of other sexually transmitted infectious diseases, as well as of allogeneic sperm and semen. Both sperm and semen are considered cofactors in the pathogenesis of AIDS. However, anal receptive sex is not a requirement for exposure; bidirectional heterosexual transmission of HIV infection and disease has been documented in studies of female sexual contacts of males with AIDS, in studies of spouses of patients with ARC and AIDS, and in reports from Africa (Quinn et al., 1987; van der Graaf & Diepersloot, 1989).

The similarities and differences between homosexual and heterosexual groups mentioned earlier, as well as other similarities and differences in socioeconomic characteristics and risk factors, are presented in Table 8–2 (Rietmeijer et al., 1989; Rothenberg et al., 1987; Schoenbaum et al., 1989).

Intravenous Drug Users. The most obvious exposure factor in the IV drug user transmission group is the sharing of hypodermic needles, syringes, and equipment. The risk of seropositivity rises with increases in the number of persons with whom needles are shared regularly, the number of injections, the use of parenteral cocaine, and the use of shooting galleries (Des Jarlais et al., 1988; Friedman et al., 1987; Novick et al., 1989; Schoenbaum et al., 1989). Chief among the cofactors of HIV in IV drug users are the intrinsic immunosuppressive properties of the drugs used.

TABLE 8–2. Comparison of Sociodemographic Characteristics and Cofactors in Heterosexuals and Homosexuals Who Are HIV Infected

SOCIODEMOGRAPHIC CHARACTERISTICS AND COFACTORS	SEXUAL GROUP AND DIRECTION OF ASSOCIATION WITH HIV INFECTION	
	HOMOSEXUAL	HETEROSEXUAL
White	↑	↓
Education	↑	↓
Age	↓	↑
Income	↑	↓
Married	↓	↑
Survival	↑	↓
Intravenous drugs	↓	↑
Inhaled cocaine	↑	↓
Inhaled nitrites	↑	↓
Number of sexual partners	↑	↓
Rectal trauma	↑	↓
Exposure to feces or semen	↑	↓
Gonorrhea	↑	↓
Syphilis	↑	↓
Soft tissue infections	↓	↑
Cytomegalovirus	↑	↓
Hepatitis B	↑	↓
Kaposi's sarcoma	↑	↓
Pneumocystis pneumonia	↓	↑

↑, Direct relationship; ↓, inverse relationship.

IV drug users have many immunologic abnormalities (Des Jarlais et al., 1988; Karan, 1989; Novick et al., 1989; Siegel, 1986). The combined effect of drug use and HIV infection on the immune system may facilitate disease expression.

Other cofactors of HIV among IV drug users are the possibility of antigenic overload and the consequent immunosuppression resulting from multiple infections (e.g., cellulitis, abscesses). Such infections are related to the use of nonsterile water, contaminated diluents, impure narcotics, and blood- and dirt-contaminated needles (Des Jarlais et al., 1988; Karan, 1989). Other infections common to IV drug users are the viral hepatitides and bacterial endocarditis, as well as the traditional sexually transmitted diseases of gonorrhea, syphilis, trichomoniasis, and chlamydia (Mondanaro, 1987; Osborn, 1986; Selwyn et al., 1989). Chemical immunosuppression could also be operating among IV drug users because of their physician-prescribed and self-prescribed use of antibiotics for their numerous infections (Mckenna et al., 1986).

Malnutrition may also be a cofactor of HIV in substance users (Karan, 1989; Mondanaro, 1987). Drugs suppress the appetite and alcohol can lead to impaired absorption of food. Malnutrition is exacerbated by inadequate assimilation of vitamins and amino acids owing to damaged liver cells. Ultimately, chronic malnutrition compromises the body's immune system. As noted earlier, malnutrition is the most common cause of T cell immunodeficiency in the world.

Finally, coincident viral infections such as HBV can act as cofactors of HIV in IV drug users (Conte et al., 1987; Des Jarlais et al., 1988). Increased HTLV-I and HTLV-II infections, respectively causing an aggressive lymphoma and hairy cell leukemia, coincident with HIV infection have been observed in IV drug users in an AIDS-endemic area in New York (Robert-Guroff et al., 1986). A high antibody prevalence for HIV was seen in this group (41%). In addition, 9% had antibody to HTLV-I and 18% to HTLV-II. The antibody prevalence for HTLV-I and HTLV-II in the general population is about 1%. HTLV has been shown to impair functioning of the immune system. Chapter 9 addresses HIV infection and IV drug use in depth, including the nursing care of IV drug users.

Transfusion Recipients. The exposure factor for HIV for persons with hemophilia in the United States was the blood supply before 1983. The virus was introduced into the blood supply by infected donors and was transferred to hemophiliacs during transfusion. Persons with hemophilia receive blood that is concentrated from the pooled plasma of literally thousands of donors. The virus was evidently able to survive the fractionation procedures then in use, and about 80% to 90% of an estimated 15,000 to 20,000 hemophiliacs became seropositive. Persons with severe hemophilia receive an average of 122,000 units of clotting factor concentrate annually (Haverkos, 1987; Osborn, 1986).

Hemophiliacs who are dependent on clotting factor VIII concentrate (hemophilia A) and clotting factor IX concentrate (hemophilia B) might have been measurably immunosuppressed before infection (Eyster et al., 1987; Osborn, 1986). Immunosuppression resulting from clotting factor concentrate might be a cofactor in susceptibility to infection in persons with hemophilia. Likewise, in recipients of multiple blood transfusions, the transfer of allogeneic blood (especially plasma-rich blood components) and possibly blood products causes at least temporary immunosuppression, making them susceptible to HIV infection when the virus is present in the blood supply. In persons with hemophilia the risk for seropositivity reflects severity of their disease as measured by dosage of concentrate used and exposure to pooled plasma components. In blood transfusion recipients the number of blood transfusions received, number of donors to whom a recipient is exposed, and exposure to plasma-rich blood components such as FFP, whole blood, and platelets are significant cofactors for HIV seropositivity (Blumberg & Heal, 1989; Perkins et al., 1987).

Hemophilia is the clearest example of the presence of cofactors that might augment or accelerate the pathogenesis of immune deficiency (Osborn, 1986). Other than the alloantigens represented in clotting factor concentrate, the infectious and noninfectious risk factors of persons with hemophilia are not extraordinary. One cofactor reported consistently for progression to disease among hemophiliacs is older age (Darby et al., 1989; Eyster et al., 1987; Perkins et al., 1987). Age has also been identified as a cofactor to disease expression among recipients of blood components. Both younger age and older age have been significantly related to the development of AIDS in seropositive transfusion recipients (Perkins et al., 1987). Thrombocytopenia, a marker for chronic liver disease in persons with hemophilia, is another cofactor associated with disease progression (Eyster et al., 1987). Chronic liver disease may be the result of prolonged use of factor VIII concentrate, which is also associated with older age. Finally, hemophiliacs may have a familial tendency to serious complications of HIV infection related to HLA type (Meropol et al., 1989).

Despite the presence of these cofactors and the fact that persons with hemophilia have the highest rate of transmission of HIV infection of any risk group, they have the lowest rate of progression to AIDS. Several investigators have reported a lower rate of progression to AIDS among hemophiliacs than among other transfusion recipients, homosexuals, and IV drug users. The cumulative incidence reported in the United Kingdom, Sweden, and the United States ranges from 2% to 11% over a 5- to 6-year period (Darby et al., 1989; Eyster et al., 1987; Medley et al., 1987; Vetrosky et al., 1987). This rate of progression differs significantly from the other transmission groups. However, one study reports opposite findings (Jason et al., 1989). These investigators found no difference in the rate of progression to AIDS comparing a cohort of homosexual and hemophiliac men who were HIV seropositive. They cautioned against generalizing their findings, but it should be noted that their findings conflict with the epidemiologic data thus far.

Women. Exposure factors to HIV infection for women include IV drug use (52%) and sexual contact with infected men (29%), principally IV drug users and bisexuals (Connor et al., 1989; Mondanaro, 1987; Willoughby, 1989). Women are discussed separately here because they have some different cofactors for HIV infection. Women who engage in anal receptive sex may be at greater risk for infection than other women (Henrion, 1988; Johnson et al., 1989; Landesman, 1989). Anal receptive sex has been identified as an exposure and transmission factor of HIV infection in numerous studies. In addition, because of trauma to the rectal mucosa, anal receptive sex facilitates multiple bacterial infections that may act as cofactors to HIV infection.

All the cofactors of HIV implicated in IV drug users in general apply to women IV drug users as well. These cofactors include poor nutrition, use of drugs known to suppress the immune system, repeated bouts of infection, and high stress. In addition to the concerns raised about nutrition earlier in the discussion of IV drug users, women are known to compound their nutritional problems by purposely using drugs to lose weight. In some women drug dependence coexists with eating disorders. They use a combination of drugs and starvation to control weight (Karan, 1989; Mondanaro, 1987).

Another cofactor of HIV infection is multiple chronic infections in some transmission groups. Women drug users experience more medical problems than their male counterparts (Karan, 1989; Mondanaro, 1987). Drug-dependent women are vulnerable to sexually transmitted diseases and their sequelae, urinary tract infections, soft tissue infections, endocarditis, hepatitis, anemia, and diabetes. Furthermore, drug-dependent women experience much higher levels of stress than do either male drug users or non-drug-using women (Karan, 1989; Mondanaro, 1987). The reasons for increased stress include low income, education, and financial resources; living alone and being responsible for children; partners who use drugs; more dysfunction and pathology in the family of origin; higher levels of anxiety and depression; greater number of recent life change events; and lower self-esteem.

Pregnancy has not been demonstrated conclusively to be a cofactor of HIV infection in women (Henrion, 1988; Landesman, 1989). Immunosuppression occurs naturally in the second and third trimesters of pregnancy. The synergistic effects of immunosuppression and pregnancy on HIV infection may exacerbate the pace and rate of clinical disease in seropositive women, possibly resulting in death. The information on the adverse effect of pregnancy on HIV infection is limited and equivocal. Some studies have demonstrated that not only do a high percentage of the children of these pregnancies become HIV infected, but more than 50% of the women become sick with AIDS, and of those more than half die of AIDS within a few months of delivery (Minkoff et al., 1987; Scott et al., 1985). This represents a higher rate of disease progression than has been seen in other transmission groups. More recent evidence from controlled studies suggests that pregnancy may have only a minor effect or no effect on the progression of HIV disease. Further prospective, long-term studies are needed before the impact of pregnancy is clearly delineated (Ellerbrock & Rogers, 1990; Karan, 1989; Nanda & Minkoff, 1989). Chapter 10 focuses specifically on HIV disease in women. It includes information on the differences in the course of HIV infection in women, their nursing care needs, and the optimal approach to prevention and treatment of opportunistic infections and neoplasms in women.

Infants. HIV infection is transmitted to infants through transplacental spread from mother to fetus in utero, at delivery, or after delivery through breast feeding and through blood or platelet transfusions (Connor et al., 1989; Henrion, 1988; Landesman, 1989). The majority of infants with HIV were infected by their mothers during pregnancy rather than during birth or afterward. Approximately 20% to 50% of infected women give birth to an infected child (Landesman, 1989).

Chief among the cofactors of HIV infection for infants is their undeveloped natural resistance systems, which make them susceptible to many infections, including HIV. Because the immune system does not develop fully until after birth, infants can be considered immunosuppressed. Premature infants have even greater immunologic abnormality (Osborn, 1986). Whereas the average incubation period of AIDS is 2 years or more, in infants it is less than a year (Connor et al., 1989; Henrion, 1988; Landesman, 1989).

Other possible cofactors of HIV infection in infants are the multiple other infectious agents their mothers could pass on to them in utero. These include the viruses with which women in high risk groups are infected (e.g., HBV, EBV, CMV, HSV), bacteria (e.g., syphilis and tuberculosis), and protozoa. Fetal infection by these agents could result in prematurity, low birth weight, developmental anomalies, congenital disease, and persistent postnatal infection (Connor et al., 1989; Lifson et al., 1988). All of these conditions could compromise the infant's ability to survive. In addition, these and other organisms (e.g., *Streptococcus* A and B, *Escherichia coli, Neisseria gonorrhoeae, Chlamydia*) can be transmitted at delivery and are associated with neonatal disease. Chapter 5 addresses the course of HIV infection in infants and children and their unique nursing care needs.

Another age-related kind of immunologic abnormality worthy of concern is the loss of natural resistance or immunity that occurs with aging and may make older adults more susceptible to HIV infection and disease progression (Catania et al., 1989; Osborn, 1986). In women, postmenopausal vaginal changes could act as a factor in HIV transmission. Tears in the vaginal wall might provide additional sites for viral entry (Catania et al., 1989). As noted earlier, older age has been correlated with disease progression in hemophiliacs and blood transfusion recipients and with reduced survival rates in both homosexual and heterosexual PWAs (Darby et al., 1989; Lemp et al., 1990). Age has been shown to be operative in herpes zoster infection, which has an increased incidence in the geriatric population (Sandor et al., 1986). Although the geriatric age group is not currently considered at high risk of exposure to HIV, age-related loss of immunity could operate as a cofactor in HIV-infected asymptomatic persons as they become older. Impaired immunity could also make older adults more susceptible to other noninfectious cofactors.

Ethnic and Racial Subgroups. Latinos and African-Americans are overrepresented among persons with AIDS (43%) compared with their numbers in the general population (20%), and their proportion of total AIDS cases is rising. Other nonwhite groups (Asians and American Indians) account for less than 1% of total cases, although some members of these ethnic groups believe that Asian and Indian cases of AIDS are underreported (Staff, *Optimist*, 1989). Of homosexual and bisexual PWAs, 16.5% are black and 10.5% are Hispanic. Among IV drug users with AIDS 50% are African-American and 30% are Hispanic. Among women with AIDS, 52% are black and 20% are Latina, and among children with AIDS, 52% are black and 25% are Hispanic (Bakeman et al., 1987; CDC, 1991; Faltz & Madover, 1986; Flaskerud, 1988). Blacks and Hispanics are represented in all the transmission groups discussed previously. For reasons that have not been determined, their cofactors for acquisition of HIV and for progression to disease appear to differ from those of whites.

Of the nonwhites who are HIV infected, a greater percentage than whites were exposed to the virus through IV drug use. It would seem that the cofactors for HIV infection in IV drug users should have the same explanatory value in the occurrence of seropositivity in African-Americans and Latinos as they do in whites, but this does not appear to be true. In a study of heterosexual male and female drug users in San Francisco, HIV seropositivity was significantly more prevalent in blacks and Hispanics (14%) than in whites (6%) (Chaisson et al., 1989). This difference could not be explained by behavioral characteristics (number of persons with whom needles were shared, duration of drug use, number of persons rinsing and cleaning needles) or sociodemographic characteristics (age, sex, history of prostitution, type of drug program). However, HIV infection was significantly associated with cocaine use; cocaine injection commonly occurred in shooting galleries and involved needle sharing by a greater number of people. The same racial and ethnic difference has been reported in New York and New Jersey with much higher rates of seropositivity (39% for nonwhites and 11% for whites, and 48% for nonwhites and 17% for whites, respectively) (Novick et al., 1989; Schoenbaum et al., 1989). Whites and nonwhites did not differ significantly with respect to age, sex, frequency of drug taking, or place of origin of drugs. HIV seropositivity was significantly related to cocaine use and to African-American and Latino race or ethnicity in one study (Novick and colleagues), and to cocaine injection, frequency of injection, use of shooting galleries, and African-American or Latino race or ethnicity in the other (Schoenbaum and colleagues). Injecting drugs in shooting galleries, injecting cocaine, and sharing needles with both strangers and acquaintances are more common among African-Americans and Latinos than among whites (Friedman et al., 1987; Schoenbaum et al., 1989). A study of female IV drug users in San Francisco found that black women had higher seroprevalence rates (21%) than white women (7%) (Lewis & Watters, 1989). Although this study failed to identify significant risk factors associated with HIV infection, trends in the data suggested that black women were less likely to use condoms than were white women and that black women may have an unrecognized exposure to bisexual men. Both of these factors would increase the likelihood of exposure to HIV through sexual contact.

It would seem to be true also that in the homosexual and bisexual transmission group, established risk behaviors should have similar power in explaining the occurrence of seropositivity and disease for whites and blacks. Again this does not appear to be the case. In a large prospective study of homosexual and bisexual men in San Francisco, the seropositivity of blacks (65.5%) was significantly greater than that of whites (48.7%) and the seroconversion over 2 years was significantly greater for blacks (20%) than for whites (6.4%). These differences could not be explained by three established risk factors; receptive anal intercourse, multiple sexual partners, and needle sharing did not differ significantly between the groups (Samuel & Winkelstein, 1987).

In addition to higher rates of HIV seropositivity, blacks and Hispanics have a faster rate of disease progression and a shorter survival time. Black female IV drug users have the worst prognosis and the shortest survival time (Friedman et al., 1987; Lewis & Watters, 1989; Rothenberg et al., 1987). Rapid disease progression and shorter survival are not related to initial diagnosis, date of diagnosis, transmission group, or sex (Rothenberg et al., 1987). Cofactors hypothesized for the faster rate of disease progression among nonwhites are delay in seeking medical care; lower quantity and quality of medical facilities; higher probability that sexual or needle-sharing partners are infected; worse health conditions before HIV exposure; greater drug injection frequency and use of shooting galleries; and less knowledge of AIDS and risk-reducing behaviors (Friedman et al., 1987; Novick et al., 1989; Schoenbaum et al., 1989).

To explain the differences in ethnic and racial groups, future studies will need to examine more carefully the other cofactors of HIV infection discussed in this chapter: malnutrition, use of recreational drugs, antigenic overload, and coincident immunosuppression by other viruses. One study of coincident viral infection with HTLV-I, HTLV-II, and HIV (HTLV-III) in IV drug users in New York demonstrated that blacks (46%) were more likely than whites (11%) to be seropositive for HTLV-I or HTLV-II (Robert-Guroff et al., 1986). In this study 73% of blacks were antibody positive for HTLV-I, II, or III (HIV), compared with 26% of whites. While possibly an artifact of sampling, 100% of persons studied with soft tissue infections (mostly caused by *Staphylococcus* and *Streptococcus*) were black. Since both multiple infections resulting in antigenic overstimulation and coincident immunosuppression by other viruses have been identified as possible cofactors in HIV infection, these merit more intensive study in determining differences among racial and ethnic groups.

COFACTORS AND RISK REDUCTION

The identification of cofactors can reduce the risk of exposure to HIV infection in the general population and in the transmission groups and may reduce the rate of progression from asymptomatic infection to AIDS in those infected. Furthermore, defining the cofactors of susceptibility might permit the identification of additional groups at risk and allow the initiation of early preventive steps. Finally, if cofactors can be demonstrated to contribute to susceptibility to AIDS, perhaps concern among the public and health care workers can be reduced.

Identification of the most common exposure and transmission factors in HIV infection has become the focus of public health education programs to prevent HIV infection in all segments of the population, but particularly among transmission groups. Assessment and identification of cofactors for progression of disease is equally urgent: an estimated 1 million asymptomatic HIV-infected individuals in the United States alone now live under the threat of a lethal disease. The likelihood that the disease will occur or progress may be influenced by cofactors specific to a particular group. These cofactors may prove easy to control through public health education campaigns. It may be possible through health education to define life-styles that facilitate continued well-being for many years.

A multifactorial approach to cause, prevention, and cure is needed to control the spread of HIV infection. A multifactorial approach considers changes in the host, the agent, and the environment in order to combat disease. Public health education programs can be designed with these factors in mind. Host factors are behaviors that individuals can engage in or change to prevent exposure to HIV or progression to disease expression. Agent factors include identifying the virus, finding antiviral treatments, and developing a vaccine against the virus. Environmental factors involve HIV infection control in hospitals and the community and decreasing the risk of opportunistic infections. All of these factors should be included in public health education campaigns. Health education should inform the public about the prevention of infection and disease, the treatments and services available to those infected and diseased, and environmental control of and reduction of infection.

The remainder of this chapter focuses on changes in host behavior to prevent the spread of infection and disease. Identification and control of the agent are considered more fully in Chapters 2 and 3, respectively.

Control of environmental factors is discussed in Chapters 3, 4, 7, and 11. Nursing care as it relates to host, agent, and environmental factors is discussed in depth in Chapters 3, 4, 5, 9, and 10.

PRIMARY PREVENTION: EXPOSURE TO HIV

Persons who are HIV antibody negative can protect their negative status by avoiding certain behaviors and practices most closely associated with infection. These include behaviors associated with sexual transmission, IV transmission, and perinatal transmission.

No risk of sexual transmission exists for those who practice sexual abstinence. Likewise, there is no risk of infection if neither partner is infected. This would be true of couples who have been mutually monogamous since the introduction of HIV in the United States (mid-1970s) and of mutually monogamous couples who have been shown to be HIV antibody negative in serologic testing (Becker & Joseph, 1988; Francis & Chin, 1987).

For persons outside of these situations, the risk can be decreased by limiting the number of sexual partners and by selecting partners from groups at low or no risk of infection. The prevalence of infection varies by sex, geography, and sexual practices. Risk of infection is lower in women, outside the AIDS endemic areas (large urban areas in New York, California, Florida, Texas, New Jersey, Illinois, Puerto Rico, Pennsylvania, Georgia, Massachusetts, Maryland, and the District of Columbia), in those not practicing anal receptive intercourse, and in those with few sexual partners (Becker & Joseph, 1988; Francis & Chin, 1987).

Finally, the risk of infection is decreased in those who practice protective sex. Protective sex is sexual activity in which no semen, vaginal secretions, or blood is exchanged between partners. Such practices involve kissing, hugging, caressing, genital manipulation (all in the absence of open lesions), and vaginal and anal intercourse provided a condom is worn and a spermicide is used. The risk of sexual transmission of HIV for various practices is given in Table 8–3.

Homosexual men can reduce their risk of infection by avoiding specific practices. These include anal receptive intercourse, rectal douching, and multiple sexual partners. In combination these practices produce the highest risk for HIV infection in the United States (Becker & Joseph, 1988; Francis & Chin, 1987; Kingsley et al., 1987; van der Graaf & Diepersloot, 1989). Avoidance of anal intercourse is the principal focus of efforts to reduce risk in the male homosexual community.

Among heterosexual men and women, reducing the number of sexual partners and practicing protective sex at all times can reduce the risk of infection. Anal receptive intercourse is also a danger among women with

TABLE 8–3. Risk of Sexual Transmission of HIV

Absolutely Safe

Abstinence
Mutually monogamous sex with noninfected partner

Very Safe

Noninsertive sexual practices

Probably Safe

Insertive sexual practices with the use of condoms and spermicide

Risky

Everything else

---

heterosexual and bisexual partners and among prostitutes, both male and female.

IV transmission of HIV can be prevented both in recipients of blood and blood products and in IV drug users and experimenters. Infection through donated blood and blood products can be prevented by donor exclusion, serologic testing for HIV antibodies, and heat inactivation of products such as factor VIII concentrate. Donor exclusion can be facilitated by education of donors, interviews at blood banks, and confidential post-donation self-exclusion (Ascher & Francis, 1987; Menitove, 1990). Serologic testing of donors for HIV antibody uses both the enzyme-linked immunosorbent assay (ELISA) or enzyme immunoassay (EIA) techniques and the confirmatory Western blot assay. Recently the indirect immunofluorescence assay (IFA) has provided an external standard against which ELISA performance can be judged. The recent addition of HBV antibody-core testing of blood donors might further eliminate donors at risk for HIV infection, since a substantial proportion of those at risk for HIV infection are also at risk for HBV (Ascher & Francis, 1987). Finally, preliminary reports of heat inactivation of factor VIII concentrates suggest that this approach can protect hemophiliacs receiving factor VIII from acquiring HIV infection. Another recommendation is the use of cryoprecipitate instead of concentrated products, since a product from only one individual should be safer than pooled blood products (Haverkos, 1987; Vetrosky et al., 1987). These precautions in combination would virtually eliminate the risk of HIV infection from transfusion of blood and blood products. Worst scenario estimates indicate that 1 of 36,000 to 1 of 300,000 (with a best guess of 1 of 68,000) components may be collected from donors who have false-negative test results (Kleinman & Secord, 1988; Menitove, 1990).

The risk of HIV infection from IV drug use differs by geographic region, social setting (e.g., shooting galleries) of injection, and frequency of injection (Hahn et al., 1989). IV drug users can eliminate their chance of exposure to HIV infection by stopping the use of IV drugs. For this to occur, addicted persons need referrals to rehabilitation programs. Health care workers, local and federal governments, and the general public will have to take a greater interest in the welfare of drug users, who currently arouse little sympathy or interest. Health care workers put little effort into promoting health or preventing illness in this group. Public health education efforts directed at the rehabilitation of drug users or at the prevention of AIDS among drug users are not extensive. Little encouragement to enter treatment programs is given to drug users. In addition, the number of rehabilitation programs available is inadequate to the need if the goal is to stop drug use or if all drug users wish to enroll in such a program. A massive infusion of government and public support is necessary for a major rehabilitation effort (Des Jarlais et al., 1988). Since several observers have noted that HIV infection affects more black and Hispanic parenteral drug users than whites, much of this effort and money will have to be concentrated in minority communities (Friedman et al., 1987; Novick et al., 1989).

If IV drug use cannot be stopped, exposure to HIV infection can be prevented by ending the sharing of unsterilized injection paraphernalia. At a minimum, persons who use IV drugs should clean their equipment with bleach. Another possibility is to provide sterile needles and syringes for IV drug users. To decrease their risk of seropositivity through parenteral drug use, IV drug users should stop using shooting galleries for injection and decrease the frequency of injection (Table 8–4).

Outside the addicted population is a substantial number of persons who experiment with drugs. Educational programs for teenagers, for communities in which drug use is high, and for the staff of drug clinics must emphasize the danger of sharing needles and equipment.

IV drug users will likely serve as the major entry of HIV infection into the heterosexual population, especially in poor urban communities (Hahn et al., 1989; Leukefeld et al., 1990; Lewis et al., 1990). An aggressive prevention effort is required to prevent further spread of HIV into social and ethnic minority communities. Finally, drugs are implicated in a broader sense in the spread of HIV infection. The use of drugs in conjunction with sexual practices is prevalent in many groups, including homosexual men, teenagers, and prostitutes, and has a disinhibiting effect on sexual practices. A public health education campaign, similar to the one linking drinking and driving, can link substance abuse to the possibly lethal consequences of sexual activity.

Perinatal transmission of HIV can be avoided if infected women do not become pregnant. Pregnancy is associated with a high risk of infection to infants and acceleration of the development of AIDS in HIV-infected mothers. Women in high-risk behavior groups (IV drug users, prostitutes,

TABLE 8–4. Risk of Transmission Through Intravenous Drug Use

Absolutely Safe
Stop the use of intravenous drugs

Very Safe
Use sterilized injection paraphernalia

Probably Safe
Clean injection paraphernalia with bleach

Risky
All other activities

---

and women with multiple sexual partners, with STDs, or with sexual partners at high risk) should be encouraged to undergo testing for HIV infection. Those who are infected should be encouraged to postpone pregnancy until more is known about the risks to themselves and their infants. Women who are HIV infected and become pregnant should be given abortion counseling in the first trimester (Francis & Chin, 1987; Guinan & Hardy, 1987; Nanda & Minkoff, 1989; Stein, 1990; Wofsy, 1987) (Table 8–5).

SECONDARY PREVENTION: PREVENTION OF DISEASE EXPRESSION

Persons who are HIV antibody positive and asymptomatic can engage in a number of activities that might slow or prevent progression to clinical disease. These activities center on minimizing or eliminating the effects of both infectious and noninfectious cofactors. Disease progression cofactors were identified earlier in this chapter as risk factors that augment or accelerate immunodeficiency; that is, they contribute another factor besides HIV to immunosuppression of the host. Through public health education, HIV-infected persons can become aware of the particular cofactors to HIV that might be operating in their lives. Through life-style changes, persons with HIV infection can also minimize or eliminate immunosuppressant factors and emphasize factors that promote immune functioning.

The noninfectious cofactors identified earlier are malnutrition, use of recreational drugs and alcohol, pregnancy, stress, age, and exposure to allogeneic sperm and semen. Regular medical evaluations and follow-up are advised for HIV-infected persons. Health maintenance efforts, including proper nutrition, abstinence and sobriety, stress management, safer

TABLE 8–5. Risk of Perinatal Transmission

Absolutely Safe	*Probably Safe*
Abstinence	Use of condoms
Sterilization	
	Risky
Very Safe	Pregnancy
Birth control measures and abortion	

sex practices, and not sharing needles, may be influential in slowing the rate of disease progression.

Calorie-protein malnutrition is a major cause of immunosuppression. HIV-infected persons can be taught to eat an adequate diet with essential nutrients including protein, carbohydrates, fat, vitamins, and minerals. Persons who are HIV infected need to ensure that their daily intake of calories and protein is adequate and that their vitamin intake is sufficient. Information on nutrition and meal planning is an important aspect of public health education for several of the transmission groups. Homosexual men and heterosexual women may have eating disorders or may diet excessively in an effort to be exceptionally thin to enhance their physical attractiveness. Information on the dangers of this kind of dieting and on what constitutes adequate nutrition may be needed (Karan, 1989).

Another group that may need nutrition information is the urban poor. Even when diets are adequate in calories in this group, they are often deficient in protein, vitamins, vegetables, and fruit and high in fat. Among the urban poor are the IV drug users and substance abusers, who often are poorly nourished because of the appetite suppressant effects of drugs, toxic effects of alcohol on the gastrointestinal tract, and inadequate assimilation of vitamins and amino acids as a result of damaged liver cells (Karan, 1989; Mondanaro, 1987).

The use of alcohol, recreational drugs, and IV drugs is another cause of immunodeficiency (Siegel, 1986). Persons who are HIV infected should be taught the effects of substance abuse on the immune system and should be encouraged to give up the use of alcohol, nitrites, marijuana, cigarettes, and IV drugs. Possibly removal of such potential precursors or determinants will slow or prevent disease progression in HIV-infected individuals (Hessol et al., 1989; Siegel, 1986).

Women who are HIV infected must be informed of the effects of pregnancy on the progression of disease. Pregnancy itself has an immunosuppressant effect; it is possible that pregnancy accelerates the pace of disease expression. Evidence on this point is conflicting. However, seropositive women should be cautioned against pregnancy; they should use a reliable method of birth control. Other information that women need to know about pregnancy and AIDS is that more than 80% of pediatric AIDS is attributed to maternal transmission, that they do not need to be sick to pass HIV to the fetus, that there is no way to prevent the fetus from becoming infected if the mother is infected, and that the virus may be contracted through breast milk (Karan, 1989; Mondanaro, 1987; Wofsy, 1987). Counseling on birth control, pregnancy, and abortion should be part of any health education program for women.

Emotional stress has been shown to activate latent herpesviruses, presumably by immunosuppression (Kiecolt-Glaser & Glaser, 1988). The effects of stress can be mitigated or reduced through regular exercise, adequate and regular amounts of rest and sleep, relaxation techniques, and effective coping. Persons in some of the transmission groups have inadequate or inaccurate knowledge of the benefits of exercise, thinking that exercise should be avoided if a person has the chance of becoming sick. Acceptable and feasible exercise programs might have to be designed for members of some groups. Walking is an exercise available to all and is not overtaxing. Similarly, the importance of adequate regular rest and sleep might need to be explained to persons who believe that they can catch up on rest and sleep or that sleep deprivation has no effect. Teaching relaxation techniques is probably necessary for all groups at risk, since information about these methods is relatively new.

Finally, coping response may have a role in immunologic function through the moderation of stress (Locke et al., 1984). Coping responses to stress occur in three ways: (1) manipulation of the stress-producing situation, (2) reinterpretation of the situation, and (3) action to control the stress resulting from the situation. Good copers are those who use all three coping responses. A person's typical coping response can be assessed, and alternative or additional responses can be taught to help the person deal with stress. For example, persons who cope effectively with the stress of HIV infection are able to (1) change their behaviors in the face of HIV infection, for example, their nutrition, their use of drugs and alcohol, their sexual activity, and their needle-sharing activity; (2) interpret their HIV status as an opportunity to practice health maintenance rather than as a death sentence; and (3) engage in stress-reducing activities such as exercise, relaxation techniques, and rest and sleep.

All persons who are HIV infected need information on the meaning of infection. They cannot assume that they will or will not develop clinical disease. They should be informed that they are probably infected for life and probably contagious for life. This information means that they should not engage in unsafe sexual practices or needle sharing, nor should they donate blood, plasma, body organs, or other tissue. They can thus help to prevent the spread of HIV to noninfected individuals. However, they should not engage in unsafe sexual practices or share needles with other seropositive persons, since repeated exposures to the virus may increase the likelihood of progression to AIDS. Unsafe (unprotected) anal sexual practices also expose the person to allogeneic sperm and semen. As noted earlier, repeated exposure to sperm and semen through the rectum can have immunosuppressant effects, which HIV-infected persons need to avoid.

The infectious cofactors of HIV infection also contribute to immune suppression and can be avoided by changes in behavior that could result in more competent immune functioning. Unsafe sexual practices, anal receptive sex in particular, and IV drug use and needle sharing result in many infections besides HIV. These infections are believed to lead to antigenic stimulation and overload, causing a burden on the immune system, a chronic coincident immunosuppression, or both (Lifson et al., 1988). In the presence of HIV infection these other infections act as cofactors in the development of disease expression. Many of the infectious cofactors of HIV infection can be prevented by the same changes in sexual practices that could prevent HIV infection: avoiding anal intercourse and multiple sexual partners. Anal receptive intercourse is associated not only with HIV infection but also with other STDs that present a health threat to male homosexuals and male and female prostitutes: HBV, CMV, HSV, amebiasis, syphilis, and gonorrhea (Bentwich et al., 1988; Kingsley et al., 1987). Whether through the ability of immunosuppression to provide opportunity for activation of HIV, or through actual activation of cells carrying HIV, coincident chronic infections have significant effects on the immune system and on the progression of HIV infection. Avoiding anal intercourse should be the principal focus of any public health education program because it reduces the risk of HIV infection, the number of repeated exposures to the virus, the risk of other sexually transmitted diseases, and thereby the effects of infectious cofactors. Short of that, condoms should be used for all insertive sexual practices to reduce the risk of infection.

Evidence suggests that public health education and the fear of AIDS have caused homosexual and bisexual men to reduce the number of sexual partners and change to safer sexual practices. These changes have coincided with significantly reduced rates of gonorrhea and syphilis between 1982 and 1986 in London, Stockholm, Seattle, New York, Denver, and San Francisco (Becker & Joseph, 1988; Carne et al., 1987). However, a recent study of homosexual men in San Francisco found a relapse in safer sex practices, which makes it clear that education and prevention programs must be ongoing and innovative to sustain changes in behavior (Stall et al., 1990). Rates of syphilis and gonorrhea have decreased in the heterosexual population as well, although the decline has not been as dramatic as among homosexuals. It seems apparent fear of AIDS is the major factor motivating a change to preventive measures in homosexual men. The motivation for heterosexuals is less apparent, but no other reason is evident. In London, Baltimore, Chicago, Los Angeles, Pittsburgh, and Washington, D.C., seroconversion rates were significantly lower in men who reduced or stopped receptive anal intercourse than in men who continued the practice with at least two or more partners (Kingsley et al., 1987). Clearly, modification of this high-risk behavior can have a substantial impact on risk, both as an exposure factor and as a cofactor of HIV disease progression.

IV drug users can eliminate or significantly reduce the risks of infectious cofactors by stopping the use of IV drugs, using disinfected needles and syringes, stopping needle and equipment sharing, decreasing the number of injections, and avoiding the use of shooting galleries for injection. All of these practices, uncorrected, result not only in HIV infection but also in other infections among IV drug users. Chief among these infections are frequent and chronic soft tissue infections (cellulitis, abscesses), bacterial endocarditis, and the viral hepatitides. In addition, IV drug users who use prostitution to support their drug habits are frequently infected with all of the STDs described previously. These chronic multiple infections can play a role as cofactors in the progression of disease in HIV-infected individuals. Stopping the use and sharing of dirty and infected needles and syringes could reduce HIV infection, the number of exposures to the virus, the risk of other infections, and thus the effects of infectious cofactors. The focus of public health education for drug users should be on stopping the use of drugs, stopping the sharing of dirty needles and syringes, and encouraging safer sex (use of condoms, cessation of anal receptive intercourse, and reduction in number of sexual partners).

There is evidence that IV drug users in the United States are beginning to change their needle-sharing habits out of fear of AIDS or are cleaning needles and syringes with bleach (Becker & Joseph, 1988; Des Jarlais et al., 1989). In the Netherlands, England, and Italy the threat of AIDS combined with the availability of clean equipment through needle exchange programs has reduced the number of addicts using contaminated and dirty needles and syringes (Becker & Joseph, 1988; Staff, *NIDA Notes*, 1987). Although needle sharing has decreased, more drug rehabilitation and AIDS education programs are needed for IV drug users in the United States. Three groups should be targeted for AIDS prevention, and three different program approaches are needed. First, drug users who want to stop the IV use of drugs should be treated. Second, drug users not likely to stop should be taught safe injection methods or be given sterile needles and syringes in exchange for used ones. Third, persons not yet injecting should be educated about the risks of this behavior.

Distressingly, some other groups show little evidence of behavior change. Little change has been documented among potentially vulnerable adolescent and young adult heterosexuals. The limited data available suggest that urban black and Hispanic populations are also experiencing less behavioral change (Becker & Joseph, 1988). Longitudinal studies of women indicate little change in sexual practices in response to the AIDS epidemic (DeBuono et al., 1990). Some studies suggest that women's sexual behavior over the last 5 years has changed in ways that might promote the spread of AIDS and other venereal diseases (Biggar et al., 1989). These data clearly show that public health education campaigns must be directed toward adolescent and young adult heterosexuals, ethnic and racial minorities, and women. All of these groups evidence a persistent belief that AIDS is a disease of gay white men and fail to recognize their own vulnerability to HIV infection.

TERTIARY PREVENTION: ENHANCING IMMUNOCOMPETENCE

For persons in whom clinical disease has developed, elimination of all risk factors, both exposure factors and cofactors to disease progression discussed previously, is necessary to prevent immunosuppression from sources other than HIV. Therapies other than drugs for enhancing immunocompetence are being tested.

Nutrition. As yet no widely accepted method exists for nutritional management of HIV disease. Nutrition education and management are aimed at improving nutritional status, alleviating symptoms, and enhancing quality of life throughout the course of the disease. More is known about malnutrition. Many aspects of malnutrition have been shown to affect cellular immunodeficiency (Hessol et al., 1989; Hickey & Weaver, 1988; Task Force on Nutrition Support in AIDS, 1989). This has been evident in studies of an association between nutritional status and development of infectious processes, and the outcome of infectious processes and functioning of major organs such as the heart, liver, and gastrointestinal (GI) tract (Chandra, 1983; Chlebowski, 1985; Hickey & Weaver, 1988; Task Force on Nutrition Support in AIDS, 1989). Profound muscle wasting is evident in heart and respiratory muscle atrophy and in impaired digestion secondary to inadequate production of pancreatic enzymes and flattened intestinal villi (Bentler & Stanish, 1987).

In a body composition study of 33 PWAs, whose total body potassium, fat, concentrations of serum proteins and albumin, and water volume were recorded, Kotler and associates (1985) found that patients with AIDS were significantly underweight and depleted of potassium, body fat content, serum protein concentrations, and intracellular water volume. The development of malnutrition was related to impaired intestinal absorption, intestinal damage caused by bacterial parasites or viral infections, intestinal malfunction as a result of malnutrition itself, or decreased pancreatic secretion and intestinal brush border enzyme activities. Other factors contributing to malnutrition include GI manifestations such as oral and esophageal candidiasis and herpes gingivostomatitis, vomiting, and persistent diarrhea and fever (DaPrato & Rothschild, 1986; Hickey & Weaver, 1988).

The latter course of HIV disease is most frequently influenced by malnutrition (Kotler et al., 1985; Task Force on Nutrition Support in AIDS, 1989). In particular, protein-energy malnutrition significantly affects the immune system and the ability to deal with infection (Chandra, 1987). Evidence of impaired immunity has been the absent or reduced delayed cutaneous hypersensitivity response to common microbial antigens, decreased number of thymus-dependent T lymphocytes, reduced capacity of neutrophils to kill ingested bacteria, reduced activity of various complement proteins, decreased concentration of IgA antibody, decreased ability to bind antigen, and decreased total number of T lymphocytes, particularly the T-helper lymphocyte population (Hickey & Weaver, 1988). These changes in the immune defense lead to the development of infectious diseases such as tuberculosis, bacterial diarrhea, herpes, *Pneumocystis carinii* pneumonia (PCP), and candidiasis.

Therapies to reverse or alter the progressive weight loss associated with AIDS may be critical (Chlebowski, 1985). Assessment of nutritional status is a necessary first step in supporting HIV-infected individuals, particularly in a syndrome whose treatment has yet to be established. Assessment and follow-up should include anthropometric measures and evaluation of visceral proteins (serum albumin, total iron-binding capacity, a complete blood cell count, and serum potassium). Blood urea nitrogen, creatinine, and liver function tests should be performed as indicated. Weight should be assessed at least weekly, and frequent assessment of appetite is recommended (Bentler & Stanish, 1987; Hickey & Weaver, 1988).

Special high-calorie, high-protein, low-fat, lactose-free oral diets in combination with a full-strength food supplement are recommended as the first line of nutritional therapy (Hickey & Weaver, 1988). These diets are associated with few complications, require limited nursing management and pretherapy education, and do not restrict daily activities. A detailed nutritional plan is important to provide guidance in meal preparation (Hickey & Weaver, 1988; Klug, 1986).

When diarrhea is a problem, replacement therapy, antidiarrheal agents, diet modification, or bowel rest may be indicated (Hickey & Weaver, 1988; Koter, 1987; Schietinger, 1986). If oral intake is limited, GI tube feeding may provide nutrients if the GI system is functioning (Bentler & Stanish, 1987). If the patient has severely compromised bowel function and if oral or GI tube feedings are inadequate or contraindicated, a short course of either peripheral parenteral nutrition (PPN) or total parenteral nutrition (TPN) should be considered (Hickey & Weaver, 1988). When the patient returns to an oral diet, it should be high in protein and calories to maintain and nourish the existing functioning immune system.

Zinc Supplementation. Zinc deficiency has been associated with depressed cellular immunity, particularly decreased T4 function, decreased killer T cell function, and thymic involution (Chandra, 1987; DaPrato & Rothschild, 1986). However, investigators disagree about the use of zinc supplements by HIV-infected individuals. Some investigators believe that oral zinc supplements improve immune responses by increasing numbers of circulating lymphocytes, intracutaneous delayed hypersensitivity reactions, and specific antibody IgG responses to ingested antigens (Chandra, 1987; DaPrato & Rothschild, 1986; Fabris et al., 1988). In addition, they propose that zinc administration offers significant protection against formed mycotoxins and heals intestinal mucosal lesions. Other investigators believe that advocating the routine use of zinc supplements by HIV-infected persons is premature (Falutz et al., 1988). They note that although zinc does play an important role in maintaining cell-mediated immune function, excessive zinc intake may be detrimental to normal immune function.

Vitamins. Vitamins are essential for optimum immune functioning. Deficiencies in vitamins A, B_6, and E have reportedly led to reduced lymphocyte response to mitogens and antigens, decreased antibody responses, and impaired cellular immunity (Chandra, 1987). In addition, malnourished persons develop significant mineral, trace element, and vitamin deficiencies that adversely affect overall immune function (Hickey & Weaver, 1988; Hutchin, 1987).

Since significant nutritional deficiencies develop during the course of HIV disease, the role of vitamins in enhancing immunocompetence is under investigation. In a clinical study of six patients given ascorbate, patients reportedly had considerable improvement in their condition (remission of biopsy-proven Kaposi's sarcoma) (Cathcart, 1984). The reason proposed for the improvement was that ascorbate suppresses the symptoms of disease and reduces the tendency for secondary infection; it is superior to any other free radical scavenger because it is better able to saturate every cell of the body. Ascorbate in concentrations of 10 to 20 g per day was found to neutralize the suppressor factor in patients with AIDS. Some consider this amount far too toxic to use in humans and note that the role of vitamins and other micronutrients in slowing the progression of disease has not yet been established (Lifson et al., 1988).

To assimilate vitamins and amino acids, the body must have a fully functioning liver. For this reason persons with HIV disease should eliminate the use of alcohol, recreational drugs, and IV drugs, which have a negative effect on nutrition. These substances not only suppress appetite but also irritate the GI tract and lead to impaired absorption of food.

Damaged liver cells resulting from substance abuse can be responsible for inadequate assimilation of vitamins and amino acids and can lead to malnourishment. Damaged liver cells have other negative effects for persons with clinical disease. Many of the therapeutic drugs used to treat the opportunistic infections have toxic side effects. A well-functioning liver is necessary to metabolize these toxins. Finally, alcohol and drugs have immunosuppressant effects and create even greater difficulties for persons whose immune systems are compromised by HIV.

Preventing Polymicrobial Enteric Infection. Other factors recognized as potent immunosuppressants are the polymicrobial enteric infections (Matossian, 1986). Toxins produced by the microbial organisms compromise the individual's immune functioning to the point at which the AIDS virus can express itself in an opportunistic manner (DaPrato & Rothschild, 1986). The pathogenesis of this outcome has been found to include an increase in mucosal cyclic adenosine monophosphate, depression of mucosal immunity leading to diarrhea and consequent nutrient and electrolyte loss, altered macrophage phagocytosis, and T cell immunologic unresponsiveness.

Nurses can play a crucial role in preventing enteric infections. They must teach individuals to reduce microbes in the diet by using canned, bottled, and pasteurized foods, broiling and cooking meat well, scrubbing and washing fruits and vegetables, and avoiding prepared foods such as tuna and egg salads and cold meats (Ungvarski, 1985). The number of microbes in the home can be reduced by using a dilute solution of household bleach to clean surfaces that may come in contact with food. Persons with pets should wear rubber gloves when emptying litter boxes or trays and cleaning bird cages.

Chapters 3, 4, 5, 9, and 10 address in detail the nursing care needs of persons with HIV disease. These chapters include information on nutrition, vitamins, and microbial enteric infections for various patient populations.

Reducing Psychologic Stress. Psychologic stress can be immunosuppressive and is thought to increase the individual's vulnerability to disease (Kiecolt-Glaser & Glaser, 1988; Locke et al., 1984). Research supports this hypothesis, documenting associations between stress and immune system changes. However, clear evidence of the relationship between stress-induced immunosuppression and *illness* has not been reported. One interesting study of stress and immune function suggests that how a person reacts to the stressor (ability to cope) has a greater impact on immunologic impairment than how much stress is experienced (Locke et al., 1984). In a study of the correlation of self-reported life stress and distress symptoms with natural killer cell activity in 114 healthy undergraduate volunteers, Locke and associates (1984) found that "good copers" (subjects who reported major life stressors but few distress symptoms) had significantly higher natural killer cell activity than "poor copers" (those experiencing high levels of distress and life stresses). A study with opposite implications found that stress management training and practices had no effect on the number of T-helper cells, helper-to-suppressor ratio, or immune functioning in men with HIV infection (Coates et al., 1989). However, experimental group subjects did significantly decrease their number of sexual partners in comparison with control subjects in response to a stress reduction program.

Stress can affect health either by causing direct physiologic changes or by causing changes in behavior that affect health or immunity independently (e.g., use of tobacco, alcohol, multiple sexual partners). Although recommending stress reduction programs for persons with HIV infection may seem premature based on current evidence, probably at least two reasons exist for doing so. Such programs may provide more information about stress and immune function in general and especially in HIV-infected populations. Also, if the possibility exists that stress reduction may affect immune status and HIV disease state among infected persons, it would be unthinkable not to offer such programs, especially since they involve no adverse side effects and have a psychologic benefit.

Unquestionably, the diagnosis of HIV infection leads to major psychologic problems. The psychologic and social stress experienced and its impact on immunologic function may play a role in progression of HIV disease. Moreover, personal characteristics of the individual, such as depression, may alter immunologic responses. Furthermore, the presence or absence of social support may influence the effects of stress. In addition to the stress management approaches discussed earlier in this chapter (exercise, health habit changes, sleep and rest, relaxation techniques), psychosocial nursing interventions can benefit the person with HIV disease and are discussed in detail in Chapter 6.

SUMMARY

Cofactors play a major role not only in exposure to HIV infection but also in disease expression and progression. Identifying these cofactors and making them a focus of public health education programs are crucial. Changes in behaviors related to known cofactors have been demonstrated to improve health at all stages of HIV infection. This information must be communicated to the transmission groups and to the public at large. As new cofactors are identified, they must become a part of health education in the prevention of HIV infection. Since health education is a major nursing intervention, nurses must make themselves aware of developments in the area of risk factors, cofactors, and HIV infection.

References

Ascher, M.S., Francis, D.P. (1987). Is the blood supply safe from AIDS? *California Physician,* 4(7), 18–19.

Bakeman, R., Lumb, J.R., McCray, E., et al. (1987). The incidence of AIDS among blacks and Hispanics. *Journal of the National Medical Association, 79*(9), 921–928.

Becker, M.H., Joseph, J.G. (1988). AIDS and behavioral change to reduce risk: A review. *American Journal of Public Health, 78*(4), 394–410.

Bentler, M., Stanish, M. (1987). Nutrition support of the pediatric patient with AIDS. *Perspectives in Practice, 87,* 488–491.

Bentwich, Z., Burstein, R., Berner, Y., et al. (1988). Immune changes in male homosexuals— predisposing factors for HIV seroconversion. *Leukemia, 2*(12), 241S–247S.

Biggar, R.J., Brinton, L.A., Rosenthal, M.D. (1989). Trends in the number of sexual partners among American women. *Journal of Acquired Immune Deficiency Syndrome, 2*(5), 497–502.

Blumberg, N., Heal, J.M. (1989). Transfusion and recipient immune function. *Archives of Pathology and Laboratory Medicine, 113,* 246–253.

Carne, C.A., Johnson, A.M., Pearce, F., et al. (1987). Prevalence of antibodies to human immunodeficiency virus, gonorrhoea rates, and changed sexual behavior in homosexual men in London. *Lancet, 1*(8534), 656–658.

Catania, J.A., Turner, H., Kegeles, S.M., et al. (1989). Older Americans and AIDS: Transmission risks and primary prevention research needs. *Gerontologist, 29*(3), 373–381.

Cathcart, R. (1984). Vitamin C in the treatment of acquired immune deficiency syndrome (AIDS). *Medical Hypothesis, 14,* 423–433.

Centers for Disease Control (1991, April). *AIDS Weekly Surveillance Report.* Atlanta: AIDS Program.

Chaisson, R.E., Bacchetti, P., Osmond, D., et al. (1989). Cocaine use and HIV infection in intravenous drug users in San Francisco. *Journal of the American Medical Association, 261,* 561–565.

Chandra, R.K. (1983). Nutrition immunity and infection: Present knowledge and future directions. *Lancet, 1,* 688–691.

Chandra, R. (1987). Nutrition and immunity: I. Basic considerations. II. Practical applications. *Journal of Dentistry for Children, 54*(3), 193–197.

Chiasson, M.A., Stoneburner, R.L., Lifson, A.R., et al. (1990). Risk factors for human immunodeficiency virus type 1 (HIV-1) infection in patients at a sexually transmitted disease clinic in New York City. *American Journal of Epidemiology, 131*(2), 208–220.

Chlebowski, R. (1985). Significance of altered nutritional status of acquired immune deficiency syndrome. *Nutrition and Cancer, 7,* 85–91.

Coates, T.J., McKusick, L., Kuno, R., et al. (1989). Stress reduction training changed number of sexual partners but not immune function in men with HIV. *American Journal of Public Health, 79*(7), 885–887.

Collier, A.C., Meyers, J.D., Corey, L., et al. (1987). Cytomegalovirus infection in homosexual men. *American Journal of Medicine, 82,* 593–601.

Connor, E., Bardeguez, Apuzzio, J. (1989). The intrapartum management of the HIV-infected mother and her infant. *Clinics in Perinatology, 16*(4), 899–908.

Conte, D., Ferroni, G.P., Lorini, G.P., et al. (1987). HIV and HBV infection in intravenous drug addicts from Northeastern Italy. *AIDS Targeted Information Newsletter, 1*(10), 9.

DaPrato, R., Rothschild, J. (1986). The AIDS virus as an opportunistic organism inducing a state of chronic relative cortisol excess: Therapeutic implications. *Medical Hypotheses, 21*(3), 253–266.

Darby, S.C., Rizza, C.R., Doll, R., et al. (1989). Incidence of AIDS and excess of mortality associated with HIV in haemophiliacs in the United Kingdom: Report on behalf of the directors of haemophilia centres in the United Kingdom. *British Medical Journal, 298,* 1064–1068.

DeBuono, B.A, Zinner, S.H., Daamen, M., et al. (1990). Sexual behavior of college women in 1975, 1986, and 1989. *New England Journal of Medicine, 322*(12), 821–825.

Des Jarlais, D.C., Friedman, S.R. (1988). Gender differences in response to HIV infection. *Psychological, Neuropsychiatric, and Substance Abuse Aspects of AIDS, 44,* 159–163.

Des Jarlais, D.C., Friedman, S.R., Novick, D.M., et al. (1989). HIV-1 infection among intravenous drug users in Manhattan, New York City, from 1977 through 1987. *Journal of the American Medical Association, 261*(7), 1008-1012.

Des Jarlais, D.C., Friedman, S.R., Stoneburner, R.L. (1988). HIV infection and intravenous drug use: Critical issues in transmission dynamics, infection outcomes, and prevention. *Reviews of Infectious Diseases, 10*(1), 151–158.

Ellerbrock, T.V., Rogers, M.F. (1990). Epidemiology of human immunodeficiency virus infection in women in the United States. *Obstetrics and Gynecology Clinics of North America, 17*(3), 523–544.

Eyster, M.E., Gail, M.H., Ballard, J.O., et al. (1987). Natural history of human immunodeficiency virus infections in hemophiliacs: Effects of T-cell subsets, platelet counts, and age. *Annals of Internal Medicine, 107*(1), 1–6.

Fabris, N., Mocchegiani, E., Galli, M., et al. (1988). AIDS, zinc deficiency, and thymic hormone failure. *Journal of the American Medical Association, 259*, 839–840.

Faltz, B.G., Madover, S. (1986). AIDS and substance abuse: Issues for health care providers. *Focus, 1*(9), 1–2.

Falutz, J., Tsoukas, C., Gold, P. (1988). Zinc as a cofactor in human immunodeficiency virus–induced immunosuppression. *Journal of the American Medical Association, 259*(19), 2850–2851.

Flaskerud, J.H. (1988). Prevention of AIDS in Blacks and Hispanics: Nursing implications. *Journal of Community Health Nursing, 5*(1), 49–58.

Francis, D.P., Chin, J. (1987). The prevention of acquired immunodeficiency syndrome in the United States—an objective strategy for medicine, public health, business, and the community. *Journal of the American Medical Association, 257*(10), 1357–1366.

Friedman-Kien, A.E., Lafleur, F.L., Gendler, E., et al. (1986). Herpes zoster: A possible early clinical sign for development of acquired immunodeficiency syndrome in high-risk individuals. *Journal of American Academy of Dermatology, 14*, 1023–1028.

Friedman, S.R., Sotheran, J.L., Abdul-Quader, A., et al. (1987). The AIDS epidemic among Blacks and Hispanics. *Milbank Quarterly, 65*(2), 455–499.

Gerstoft, J., Petersen, C.S., Kroon, S., et al. (1987). The immunological and clinical outcome of HIV infection: 31 months of follow-up in a cohort of homosexual men. *Scandinavian Journal of Infectious Diseases, 19*, 503–509.

Getchell, J.P., Heath, J.L., Hicks, D.R., et al. (1987). Detection of human T cell leukemia virus type I and human immunodeficiency virus in cultured lymphocytes of a Zairian man with AIDS. *Journal of Infectious Diseases, 155*(4), 612–616.

Goedert, J.J., Biggar, R.J., Melbye, M., et al. (1987). Effect of T4 count and cofactors on the incidence of AIDS in homosexual men infected with human immunodeficiency virus. *Journal of the American Medical Association, 257*(3), 331-334.

Guinan, M.E., Hardy, A. (1987). Epidemiology of AIDS in women in the United States—1981 through 1986. *Journal of the American Medical Association, 257*(15), 2039–2042.

Hahn, R.A., Onorato, I.M., Jones, T.S., et al. (1989). Prevalence of HIV infection among intravenous drug users in the United States. *Journal of the American Medical Association, 261*(18), 2677–2684.

Haverkos, H.W. (1987). Epidemiology of AIDS in hemophiliacs and blood transfusion recipients. *Antibiotics and Chemotherapy, 38*, 59–65.

Henrion, R. (1988). Pregnancy and AIDS. *Human Reproduction, 3*(2), 257–262.

Hessol, N.A., Lifson, A.R., Rutherford, G.W. (1989). Natural history of human immunodeficiency virus infection and key predictors of HIV disease progression. In P. Volberding & M.A. Jacobson (Eds.), *AIDS Clinical Review 1989* (pp. 69–93). New York: Marcel Dekker, Inc.

Hessol, N.A., Rutherford, G.W., Lifson, A.R., et al. (1988). The natural history of HIV infection in a cohort of homosexual and bisexual men: A decade of follow-up [abstract 4096]. In: *Programs and abstracts of the Fourth International Conference on AIDS*. Stockholm: Swedish Ministry of Health and Social Affairs.

Hickey, M.S., Weaver, K.E. (1988). Nutritional management of patients with ARC or AIDS. *Gastroenterology Clinics of North America, 17*(3), 545–561.

Hoff, C., Peterson, R.D.A. (1989). Does exposure to HLA alloantigens trigger immunoregulatory mechanisms operative in both pregnancy and AIDS? *Life Sciences, 45*(23), iii-ix.

Hutchin, K.C. (1987). Thiamine deficiency, Wernicke's encephalopathy and AIDS. *Lancet*, *23*, 2100.

Jason, J., Lui, K., Ragni, M.V., et al. (1989). Risk of developing AIDS in HIV-infected cohorts of hemophilic and homosexual men. *Journal of the American Medical Association*, *261*(5), 725–727.

Johnson, A.M., Petherick, A., Davidson, S.J., et al. (1989). Transmission of HIV to heterosexual partners of infected men and women. *AIDS*, *3*, 367–372.

Kaplan, J.E., Spira, T.J., Fishbein, D.B., et al. (1988). A six year follow-up of HIV infected homosexual men with lymphadenopathy. *Journal of the American Medical Association*, *260*, 2694–2697.

Karan, L.D. (1989). AIDS prevention and chemical dependence treatment needs of women and their children. *Journal of Psychoactive Drugs*, *21*(4), 395–399.

Kiecolt-Glaser, J.K., Glaser, R. (1988). Psychological influences on immunity: Implications for AIDS. *American Psychologist*, *43*(11), 892–898.

Kingsley, L.A., Kaslow, R., Rinaldo, C.R., Jr., et al. (1987). Risk factors for seroconversion to human immunodeficiency virus among male homosexuals. *Lancet*, *1*(8529), 345–349.

Kleinman, S., Secord, K. (1988). Risk of human immunodeficiency virus (HIV) transmission by anti-HIV negative blood: Estimates using the lookback methodology. *Transfusion*, *28*(5), 499–501.

Klug, R. (1986). Children with AIDS. *American Journal of Nursing*, *86*, 1126–1132.

Kotler, D.P. (1987). Diarrhea in AIDS—diagnosis and management. *Research, Staff, Physician*, *33*, 30–41.

Kotler, D., Wang, J., Pierson, R. (1985). Body composition studies in patients with the acquired immunodeficiency syndrome. *American Journal of Clinical Nutrition*, *42*, 1255–1265.

Landesman, S.H. (1989). Human immunodeficiency virus infection in women: An overview. *Seminars in Perinatology*, *13*(1), 2–6.

Latchman, D.S. (1987). Herpes infection and AIDS. *Nature*, *325*, 487.

Lemp, G.F., Hessol, N.A., Rutherford, G.W., et al. (1988). Projections of AIDS morbidity and mortality in San Francisco using epidemic models [abstract 4682]. In: *Programs and abstracts of the Fourth International Conference on AIDS*. Stockholm: Swedish Ministry of Health and Social Affairs.

Lemp, G.F., Payne, S.F., Neal, D., et al. (1990). Survival trends for patients with AIDS. *Journal of the American Medical Association*, *263*(3), 402–406.

Leukefeld, C.G., Battjes, R.J., Amsel, Z. (1990). Community prevention efforts to reduce the spread of AIDS associated with intravenous drug abuse. *AIDS Education and Prevention*, *2*(3), 235–243.

Lewis, D.K., Watters, J.K. (1989). Human immunodeficiency virus seroprevalence in female intravenous drug users: The puzzle of black women's risk. *Social Science and Medicine*, *29*(9), 1071–1076.

Lewis, D.K., Watters, J.K., Case, P. (1990). The prevalence of high-risk sexual behavior in male intravenous drug users with steady female partners. *American Journal of Public Health*, *80*(4), 465–466.

Lifson, A.R., Darrow, H.W., Hessol, N.A., et al. (1990). Kaposi's sarcoma in a cohort of homosexual and bisexual men: Epidemiology and analysis for cofactors. *American Journal of Epidemiology*, *131*(2), 221–231.

Lifson, A.R., Rutherford, G.W., Jaffe, H.W. (1988). The natural history of human immunodeficiency virus infection. *The Journal of Infectious Diseases*, *158*(6), 1360–1367.

Locke, S., Kraus, L., Leserman, J., et al. (1984). Life change stress, psychiatric symptoms, and natural killer cell activity. *Psychosomatic Medicine*, *46*(5), 441–453.

Lui, K.J., Darrow, W.W., Rutherford, G.W. (1988). A model-based estimate of the mean incubation period for AIDS in homosexual men. *Science*, *240*, 1333–1335.

Matossian, M. (1986). Did mycotoxins play a role in bubonic plague epidemics? *Perspectives in Biology and Medicine*, *29*, 244–256.

McKenna, J.J., Miles, R., Lemen, D., et al. (1986). Unmasking AIDS: Chemical immunosuppression and seronegative syphilis. *Medical Hypotheses*, *21*, 421–430.

Medley, G.F., Anderson, R.M., Cox, D.R., et al. (1987). Incubation period of AIDS in patients infected via blood transfusion. *Nature*, *328*, 719–721.

Melbye, M., Goedert, J.J., Grossman, R.J., et al. (1987). Risk of AIDS after herpes zoster. *Lancet*, 1(8535), 728–731.

Menitove, J.E. (1990). Current risk of transfusion-associated human immunodeficiency virus infection. *Archives of Pathology and Laboratory Medicine*, 114, 330–334.

Meropol, N.J., Krause, P.R., Ratnoff, O.D., et al. (1989). Tendency to serious sequelae of infection with the human immunodeficiency virus in sibships with hemophilia. *Archives of Internal Medicine*, 149, 885–888.

Minkoff, H., Nanda, D., Menez, R., et al. (1987). Pregnancies resulting in infants with acquired immunodeficiency syndrome or AIDS related complex. *Obstetrics and Gynecology*, 69 (3 Pt 1), 285–287.

Mondanaro, J. (1987). Strategies for AIDS prevention: Motivating health behavior in drug dependent women. *Journal of Psychoactive Drugs*, 19(2), 143–149.

Moss, A.R., Bacchetti, P., Osmond, D., et al. (1988). Seropositivity for HIV and the development of AIDS or AIDS related condition: Three year follow up of the San Francisco General Hospital cohort. *British Medical Journal*, 296, 745–750.

Nanda, D., Minkoff, H.L. (1989). HIV in pregnancy — transmission and immune effects. *Clinical Obstetrics and Gynecology*, 32(3), 456–466.

Newell, G.R., Mansell, P.W.A., Spitz, M.R., et al. (1985a). Volatile nitrites—use and adverse effects related to the current epidemic of the acquired immune deficiency syndrome. *American Journal of Medicine*, 78, 811–816.

Newell, G.R., Mansell, P.W.A., Wilson, M.B., et al. (1985b). Risk factor analysis among men referred for possible acquired immune deficiency syndrome. *Preventive Medicine*, 14, 81–91.

Novick, D.M., Trigg, H.L., Des Jarlais, D.C., et al. (1989). Cocaine injection and ethnicity in parenteral drug users during the early years of the human immunodeficiency virus (HIV) epidemic in New York City. *Journal of Medical Virology*, 29, 181–185.

Osborn, J.E. (1986). Co-factors and HIV: What determines the pathogenesis of AIDS? *Bio Essays*, 5(6), 287–289.

Osmond, D. (1990). Progression to AIDS in persons testing seropositive for antibody to HIV. In P.T. Cohen, M.A. Sande, P.A. Volberding (Eds.), *The AIDS knowledge base* (pp. 1-1.1.6 to 8-1.1.6). Waltham, MA: Medical Publishing Group.

Pedersen, C., Kolby, P., Sindrup, J., et al. (1989). The development of AIDS or AIDS-related conditions in a cohort of HIV antibody-positive homosexual men during a 3-year follow-up period. *Journal of Internal Medicine*, 225, 403–409.

Perkins, H.A., Samson, S., Garner, J., et al. (1987). Risk of AIDS for recipients of blood components from donors who subsequently developed AIDS. *Blood*, 70(5), 1604–1610.

Quinn, T.C., Piot, P., McCormick, J.B., et al. (1987). Serologic and immunologic studies in patients with AIDS in North America and Africa: The potential role of infectious agents as cofactors in human immunodeficiency virus infection. *Journal of the American Medical Association*, 257(19), 2617-2621.

Rees, M. (1987). The sombre view of AIDS. *Nature*, 326, 343–345.

Rietmeijer, C.A.M., Penley, K.A., Cohn, D.L., et al. (1989). Factors influencing the risk of infection with human immunodeficiency virus in homosexual men, Denver 1982–1985. *Sexually Transmitted Diseases*, 16(2), 95–102.

Robert-Guroff, M., Weiss, S.H., Giron, J.A., et al. (1986). Prevalence of antibodies to HTLV-I, -II, and -III in intravenous drug abusers from an AIDS endemic region. *Journal of the American Medical Association*, 255(22), 3133–3137.

Rothenberg, R., Woelfel, M., Stoneburner, R., et al. (1987). Survival with the acquired immunodeficiency syndrome: Experience with 5833 cases in New York City. *New England Journal of Medicine*, 317(21), 1297–1302.

Samuel, M., Winkelstein, W. (1987). Prevalence of human immunodeficiency virus infection in ethnic minority homosexual/bisexual men. *Journal of the American Medical Association*, 257(14), 1901–1902.

Sandor, E.V., Millman, A., Croxson, T.S., et al. (1986). Herpes zoster ophthalmicus in patients at risk for the acquired immune deficiency syndrome (AIDS). *American Journal of Ophthalmology*, 101, 153–155.

Schechter, M.T., Boyko, W.J., Jeffries, E., et al. (1985). The Vancouver lymphadenopathy-

AIDS study. 4. Effects of exposure factors, cofactors and HTLV-III seropositivity on number of helper T cells. *Canadian Medical Association Journal, 133*, 286–292.

Schietinger, H. (1986). A home care plan for AIDS. *American Journal of Nursing, 86*(9), 1021–1028.

Schilling, R.F., Schinke, S.P., Nichols, S.E., et al. (1989). Developing strategies for AIDS prevention research with black and Hispanic drug users. *Public Health Reports, 104*(1), 2–11.

Schoenbaum, E.E., Hartel, D., Selwyn, P.A., et al. (1989). Risk factors for human immunodeficiency virus infection in intravenous drug users. *New England Journal of Medicine, 321*(13), 874–879.

Scott, G.B., Fischl, M.A., Klimas, N., et al. (1985). Mothers of infants with the acquired immunodeficiency syndrome. *Journal of the American Medical Association, 252*, 363–366.

Selwyn, P.A., Hartel, D., Wasserman, W., et al. (1989). Impact of the AIDS epidemic on morbidity and mortality among intravenous drug users in a New York City methadone maintenance program. *American Journal of Public Health, 79*, 1358–1362.

Siegel, L. (1986). AIDS: Relationship to alcohol and other drugs. *Journal of Substance Abuse Treatment, 3*, 271–274.

Staff (1987). International experts discuss needle sharing and AIDS. *National Institute on Drug Abuse Notes, 2*(3), 1–2.

Staff (1989). Native Americans confront AIDS. *Optimist, 1*(2), 1, 7–8.

Stall, R., Ekstrand, M., Pollack, L., et al. (1990). Relapse from safer sex: The next challenge for AIDS prevention efforts. *Journal of Acquired Immune Deficiency Syndromes, 3*, 1181–1187.

Stein, Z.A. (1990). HIV prevention: The need for methods women can use. *American Journal of Public Health, 80*, 460–462.

Task Force on Nutrition Support in AIDS (1989). Guidelines for nutrition support in AIDS. *Nutrition, 5*(1), 39–46.

Ungvarski, P. (1985). Learning to live with AIDS. *Nursing Mirror, 160*, 20–22.

van der Graaf, M., Diepersloot, R. (1989). Sexual transmission of HIV: Routes, efficiency, cofactors and prevention; A survey of the literature. *Infection, 17*(4), 210–215.

van Griensven, G.J.P., Tielman, R.A.P., Goudsmit, J., et al. (1987). Risk factors and prevalence of HIV antibodies in homosexual men in the Netherlands. *American Journal of Epidemiology, 125*(6), 1048–1057.

Vetrosky, D.T., Schmidt, B.A., Sobio, H. (1987). AIDS and the hemophilia patient. *Physician Assistant, 11*, 19–31.

Willoughby, A. (1989). AIDS in women: Epidemiology. *Clinical Obstetrics and Gynecology, 32*(3), 429–436.

Winkelstein, W., Jr., Lyman, D.M., Padian, N., et al. (1987). Sexual practices and risk of infection by the human immunodeficiency virus—the San Francisco men's health study. *Journal of the American Medical Association, 257*(3), 321–325.

Wofsy, C.B. (1987). Human immunodeficiency virus infection in women. *Journal of the American Medical Association, 257* (15), 2074–2076.

9

Chemical Dependency

Jo Anne Staats

As the epidemic of HIV infection enters its second decade, the demographics of the epidemic are changing. Although the infection was originally thought to affect primarily homosexual and bisexual men, it is now clear that intravenous (IV) substance use is a major risk factor accounting for an increasing number of individuals with HIV infection.

In the United States IV drug use is the major means of transmission of HIV infection to the heterosexual and thus the perinatal population. HIV-infected IV drug users (IVDUs) have unprotected sex with women who subsequently become HIV infected. These women, as well as women infected through IV drug use, pass the virus to the fetus during pregnancy or the perinatal period.

EPIDEMIOLOGY

The National Institute on Drug Abuse (NIDA) has estimated that in the United States there are approximately 1.1 to 1.3 million IVDUs (Coutinho, 1990). About half of these individuals may be actively using drugs at any given time (Friedland & Selwyn, 1990). IVDUs account for the second highest number of persons with AIDS (PWAs) in the developed countries (Stimson, 1990). IVDUs in New York City probably first became infected with HIV in the early 1970s, and since then infection has moved rapidly through the IVDU population (Des Jarlais et al., 1989).

As of April 1991, according to the Centers for Disease Control, 22% of total AIDS cases had been reported in individuals whose only risk factor was IV drug use. Of these PWAs 77% were men and 23% were women. There were also 2772 (2% of total AIDS cases) women with AIDS whose only risk factor was having sex with an infected IVDU (Table

350

9–1). The incidence of HIV infection is higher among non-Caucasian IVDUs than among Causcasians.

New York City has the highest number of AIDS cases and the highest seroprevalence rate of HIV infection of any city in the world. Table 9–2 illustrates the geographic differences in HIV infection rates among IVDUs nationwide. The highest incidence is on the Eastern Seaboard, with a lower incidence in the Midwest and far West. However, the incidence of HIV infection is expected to increase in areas that currently have low rates. The history of HIV infection in New York City shows a zero seroprevalence rate in 1978, a 44% rate in 1980, and a 56% rate in 1984, with a stabilization in 1987 to between 55% and 60% (Des Jarlais et al., 1989; Evans et al., 1989).

TRANSMISSION OF HIV INFECTION IN INTRAVENOUS DRUG USERS

HIV infection is transmitted from one IVDU to another by the sharing of syringes and other drug paraphernalia. When IVDUs insert a needle into a vein, but before they inject the drug into the bloodstream (mainlining), they draw blood back into the syringe to ensure they are in a vein (booting) and then inject (Table 9–3). Traces of blood always remain in the syringe and the needle. When uncleaned syringes and needles are shared, the blood is injected into the next user. HIV-infected blood is easily passed from one individual to another in this manner. The equipment (cooker) used to prepare the drugs may also be contaminated with infected blood and when shared with another individual may facilitate transmission. Transmission of HIV through semen from an infected IVDU occurs when condoms are not used.

Among the IV drug–using population, transmission of HIV is associated with a number of factors (Marmor et al., 1987; Schoenbaum et al., 1989). More frequent injections and more injections with used needles per month increase the likelihood of contracting HIV infection. IVDUs who inject cocaine, which has a shorter half-life than heroin and requires more frequent injections, are at higher risk than heroin users. The sharing of needles with either acquaintances or strangers facilitates HIV transmission. For women, having frequent sex with heterosexual IVDUs is an additional risk factor. Schoenbaum and colleagues (1989) also found that the presence of HIV antibody was independently associated with being black or Hispanic, having recently used drugs, frequenting shooting galleries, having a sex partner who uses drugs, and having a low income.

Crack is a purified form of cocaine that is smoked by inhaling the vapors given off when it is heated. It is readily available and inexpensive. Its use has also been associated with transmission of HIV (Schoenbaum

**TABLE 9–1. Adult and Adolescent AIDS Cases in the
United States by Sex, Exposure Category, and Race or
Ethnicity Reported through August 1990**

EXPOSURE CATEGORY	WHITE, NOT HISPANIC		BLACK, NOT HISPANIC	
	NO.	(%)	NO.	(%)
Male				
IV drug use (heterosexual)	4,826	(6)	11,492	(35)
Male homosexual or bisexual contact and IV drug use	5,703	(7)	2,624	(8)
Sex with IV drug user	311	(1)	628	(2)
Other/undetermined*	66,038	(86)	17,896	(4)
SUBTOTAL:	76,878	(100)	32,640	(100)
Female				
IV drug use	1,483	(40)	4,118	(57)
Sex with IV drug user	552	(15)	1,360	(19)
Other*	1,661	(45)	1,743	(24)
SUBTOTAL:	3,696	(100)	7,221	(100)
TOTAL:	80,574		39,861	

From Centers for Disease Control (1990, September) *HIV/AIDS Surveillance*. Atlanta: CDC.
IV, Intravenous.
*Male homosexual or bisexual contact, hemophilia, blood transfusion, undetermined.

et al., 1990). Since 1981, New York City researchers have been studying
behaviors that may be associated with HIV transmission at sexually transmitted disease clinics (Chiasson et al., 1990). One of their findings was
that 4% of infected males and 6% of infected females had no identifiable
risk factor. In this group, however, they did identify independent variables
of crack use and crack-related sexual behavior.

SUBSTANCE ABUSE DEFINED

Substance abuse is a chronic, progressive disease that may be fatal if
untreated. "The central dynamic of addiction is the loss of self-control
evidenced by compulsive repetition of a dysfunctional behavior with negative consequences for the user, family members, friends, or associates"
(American Nurses' Association, 1987, p. 4). Chemical dependency is characterized by an inability to control use of a substance, continued use of
a substance despite the negative consequences, and development of tolerance to the substance and withdrawal (abstinence syndrome) when the
substance is discontinued. Phases of chemical dependency include the
first stage, recreational use when there are no physical abnormalities; the
second stage, purposeful but controlled use when physical abnormalities

HISPANIC		OTHER		TOTAL	
NO.	(%)	NO.	(%)	NO.	(%)
7,611	(39)	43	(4)	24,045	(18)
1,393	(7)	42	(4)	9,766	(7)
176	(1)	4	(1)	1,119	(1)
10,396	(53)	902	(81)	95,474	(74)
19,576	(100)	991	(100)	130,414	(100)
1,428	(52)	28	(72)	7,069	(51)
835	(30)	16	(16)	2,772	(20)
493	(18)	56	(56)	3,966	(29)
2,756	(100)	100	(100)	13,807	(100)
22,332		**1,091**		**144,221**	

become apparent; and the final stage, binge use (Cartter et al., 1989). Rebound occurs when the effects of the drug begin to wear off. The phenomenon of rebound begins at baseline when the drug enters the body. As the drug takes effect, the high is reached, but when the amount of drug in the body diminishes, the user starts to "come down." Baseline is reached, and then the user bottoms out below baseline. The user takes in additional drug to prevent the extreme discomfort associated with rebound.

Patterns of drug use change with time. Before the 1970s heroin use in the United States was largely contained within the ghettoes. The early 1970s found some of those involved in the psychedelic drug culture turning to heroin (Casey, 1989). Then the Vietnam war introduced many middle-class men to the use of heroin and brought it into mainstream America.

Cocaine has seen increasing abuse in the past two decades. This is partially the result of its decreased cost. In the past, it was viewed as a drug of the affluent, jazz musicians, and movie stars. A survey by the NIDA in 1974 revealed that approximately 5 million Americans had used cocaine at least once (Weiss & Mirin, 1987). By 1986, 22 million individuals had used cocaine.

Of increasing concern is the phenomenon of polydrug use: using two or more substances for the purpose of counteracting the negative effects of each substance. When heroin is injected with cocaine (speedball), the

TABLE 9–2. Geographic Differences in HIV Infection Among Intravenous Drug Users

CITY OR AREA	RATE OF INFECTION IN IVDUs (%)
New York City	61
Puerto Rico	59
Jersey City	50
Newark	50
Baltimore	29
Boston	28
Philadelphia	19
Other areas	10 or less

Data from Evans, C.A., Beauchamp, D.E., Deyton, L., et al. (1989). *Illicit Drug Use and HIV Infection.* In: Report of the Special Initiative on AIDS of the American Public Health Association. Washington, D.C.: The Association.
IVDU, Intravenous drug user.

calming effect of the heroin balances the intense euphoria of the cocaine. Alcohol used with methadone potentiates the effects of methadone. The implications for treatment of polydrug use are more complicated than for single drug use.

Social problems—poverty, family dysfunction, lack of educational opportunities—have long been thought to be the cause of chemical dependency. Current research maintains that some substance users have inherited chemical imbalances that make them vulnerable to depression, anxiety, or intense restlessness (Goleman, 1990). They use heroin, cocaine, and alcohol as a type of self-medication to alleviate these symptoms. An estimated one third to one half of chemically dependent individuals have this biologic abnormality. A biologic predisposition to substance use may explain why some individuals can dabble with drugs and never become addicted whereas others become addicted almost immediately.

Researchers have identified a key gene linked to alcoholism in 77% of the subjects studied (Goleman, 1990). The gene is linked to the receptors for dopamine, a neurotransmitter involved in the sensation of pleasure. When alcohol use is stopped, depression secondary to dopamine depletion occurs. It is postulated also that cocaine floods the brain with dopamine and that chronic use of cocaine causes depletion of dopamine, leading to severe depression when cocaine use is stopped (Henneberger, 1990). Dopamine depletion may also be associated with heroin withdrawal.

If chemical dependency has a biologic component, drug therapy offers another treatment option. The NIDA has been working with the drug mazindol, an appetite suppressant that prompts release of small amounts of dopamine and may help block the craving for cocaine. Methylphenidate (Ritalin), an amphetamine derivative, also increases dopamine levels and

TABLE 9–3. Drug-Related Street Terminology

mainlining   injecting drugs directly into the vein

skin-popping   injecting drugs intradermally

snort   short inhalation of heroin through the nose

sniff   short inhalation of cocaine through the nose

booting   process of drawing blood back into the syringe and mixing it with the drug before injecting

spike   needle

works   syringe, needle, and cooker

cooker   spoon or metal soda top that is used to prepare heroin for injection; the heroin is mixed with water, heated over a flame to dissolve it, cooled, then drawn into the syringe through a piece of cotton

shooting gallery   place, frequently an abandoned building, where drugs are sold and bought along with the equipment needed for injecting; sex for drugs and money is also frequently available

tracks   needle marks on the skin

speedball   heroin and cocaine taken together

freebase   kit used to remove impurities from cocaine so the fumes can be inhaled

freeze   cold feeling in throat after sniffing cocaine

line   cocaine powder or flakes placed in a line on a smooth, hard surface so that it may be sniffed

Adapted from Narcotic and Drug Research, Inc. (1989). *AIDS: Medical management of the HIV infected/chemically dependent client*, New York: The Company.

has helped some individuals to withdraw from cocaine. Desipramine, an antidepressant, has been used to treat the depression resulting from the cessation of cocaine.

PHYSIOLOGIC EFFECTS OF HEROIN, COCAINE, AND ALCOHOL

Heroin, an opiate, is a central nervous system depressant. It can be snorted, smoked, or injected intradermally or intravenously. The effects of heroin are most intense after IV administration. Heroin is one of the most physically addicting of all drugs (Table 9–4). Users inject themselves three to five times during a 24-hour period. IV injection of heroin produces a euphoric feeling, a "rush," followed by relaxation that lasts several hours. During this period users are described as having a "nod."

Opioids, including heroin, produce suppression of the cough reflex and respiratory depression (Arif & Westermeyer, 1988). Other physical effects include miosis, constipation, and peripheral vasodilatation. Rapid IV administration causes histamine release, resulting in itching, flushing, and sweating. Tolerance and physical dependence develop with chronic heroin use.

TABLE 9–4. Substance Abuse Terminology

addict   person who is physically dependent on one or more psychoactive substances, whose long-term use has produced tolerance, who has lost control over his or her intake, and who would manifest withdrawal phenomena if discontinuation were to occur

drug abuse   any use of drugs that causes physical, psychologic, economic, legal, or social harm to the individual user or to others affected by the user's behavior

physical dependence   physiologic state of adaptation to a drug or alcohol, usually characterized by the development of tolerance to drug effects and the emergence of a withdrawal syndrome during prolonged abstinence

polydrug abuse   concomitant use of two or more psychoactive substances in quantities and with frequencies that cause the individual significant physiologic, psychologic, or sociologic distress or impairment

psychologic dependence   emotional state of craving a drug either for its positive effect or to avoid negative effects associated with its absence

relapse   recurrence of alcohol- or drug-dependent behavior in an individual who has previously achieved and maintained abstinence for a significant time beyond the period of detoxification

tolerance   physiologic adaptation to the effect of drugs, so as to diminish effects with constant dosages or to maintain the intensity and duration of effects through increased dosage

withdrawal syndrome   onset of a predictable constellation of signs and symptoms involving altered activity of the central nervous system after the abrupt discontinuation of, or rapid decrease in dosage of, a drug

Data from Rinaldi, R.C., et al. (1988). Clarification and standardization of substance abuse terminology. *Journal of the American Medical Association, 259*, 556–558.

Cocaine is a central nervous system stimulant that produces heightened energy and self-esteem. It can be used intranasally (sniffed), smoked as freebase or crack, or injected intravenously (Evans et al., 1989). Cocaine is rapidly absorbed from the bloodstream when it is smoked or injected. The effect, a rapid euphoria, lasts 20 to 40 minutes and is followed by a crash. Binges, episodes of frequent use, maintain the euphoria and prevent the depressive crash. Psychologic and possibly physical addiction develops rapidly with the continued use of cocaine.

The stages of cocaine abuse include euphoria, dysphoria, paranoia, and cocaine psychosis (Shaffer & Costikyan, 1988). A person with cocaine psychosis may have depression, delusional thinking, visual and auditory hallucinations, and paranoia. Typically the symptoms resolve 1 to 2 days after discontinuation of cocaine.

Alcohol is a central nervous system depressant and is important in the discussion of IV drug use because it is frequently used in combination with heroin and cocaine. Alcohol affects social behavior, cognition, motor performance, sexuality, and respiration (Arif & Westermeyer, 1988). Use of alcohol leads to disinhibition of behavior. Continued drinking can lead to depression, somnolence, coma, and death. Tolerance and physiologic dependence develop with long-term alcohol use.

WITHDRAWAL

Few individuals can stop using heroin, cocaine, or alcohol without some type of treatment or support. The abrupt discontinuation of any of these substances results in withdrawal. The treatment approach may vary depending on the substance being used.

Discontinuation of heroin leads to symptoms of withdrawal 4 to 24 hours after the last dose. The symptoms worsen and peak in about 24 to 72 hours. The acute symptoms lessen after 4 or 5 days. Symptoms of heroin withdrawal include anxiety, restlessness, irritability, lacrimation, generalized body aches, insomnia, perspiration, dilated pupils, gooseflesh, hot flushes, nausea and vomiting, diarrhea, fever, increased heart rate, and elevated blood pressure. Dehydration and weight loss may occur during this period. These symptoms are prevented by giving the drug of dependency or, in the case of heroin, administering another opiate in diminishing doses until withdrawal is accomplished.

Although discontinuation of cocaine causes less physical discomfort than occurs with heroin or alcohol, prolonged sleep, lethargy, and an abrupt depressive reaction sometimes occur. This depressive reaction is a powerful motivator for continued use of cocaine. This state of depression has been postulated to be proof of a cocaine withdrawal syndrome (Casey, 1989). As discussed earlier in this chapter, drug therapy research for cocaine withdrawal is being investigated.

Withdrawal from alcohol can be far more dangerous than heroin or cocaine withdrawal. The severity of the symptoms depends on the length of alcohol use and the degree of intoxication. Typically, symptoms begin within 24 hours of alcohol cessation, peak within 2 to 3 days, and resolve within 1 to 2 weeks. Headaches, anxiety, involuntary twitching of muscles, tremor of hands, weakness, insomnia, and nausea are common early symptoms of withdrawal. Hypotension, fever, delirium (as evidenced by disorientation, delusions, and vivid visual hallucinations), and convulsions characterize more advanced withdrawal. IV diazepam or a similar tranquilizer is used during the early stages of alcohol withdrawal, followed by tapering doses of oral medications.

TREATMENT OF SUBSTANCE ABUSE

Various options exist for the treatment of chemical dependency. Some of the more common ones are detoxification programs, therapeutic communities, methadone maintenance programs, and self-help groups. Acupuncture, an alternative to current biomedical therapy, is gaining acceptance as a viable treatment option for chemical dependency.

Detoxification Programs. Detoxification programs may be affiliated with a hospital or may be independent. The length of stay varies from 3 days to more than 30 days depending on the substance involved and the program. In New York City, for example, many inpatient cocaine detoxification programs last 3 days, whereas alcohol detoxification programs typically last 28 days. Programs requiring longer treatment offer counseling in addition to medical management of withdrawal.

Therapeutic Communities. Therapeutic communities (TCs) provide structured environments that are run by and for substance users. Synanon, the first TC, was founded in California in 1958 by Charles E. Dederich, a former alcoholic and active member of Alcoholics Anonymous (Sugarman, 1974). He developed the style of TCs: the confrontational groups, the verbal reprimand, and the principle of joint residence. Before entry into the community, individuals had to agree to conform to all rules and demonstrate their commitment to the community by doing something diffcult but meaningful (such as yelling for help in front of other residents). In 1963 Daytop Village, modeled after Synanon, was started on the East Coast. Many TCs, based on these two early communities, have since been developed.

TCs require a lengthy time commitment (possibly up to 2 years). The theory of TCs maintains that the problem is not just one of addiction but rather a personality problem that leads to addiction. On admission to a TC, the individual is viewed as an infant who needs to learn adult ways, in place of addictive ways, to cope. Through a process of confrontational groups, sharing of chores, and increasing responsibilities and freedom, a personality restructuring is believed to occur.

With the advent of the AIDS epidemic, TCs have had to confront the problem of caring for members who are HIV infected or have AIDS. Many communities allow asymptomatic HIV-infected members but believe they are not equipped to manage persons with HIV-related symptoms. Substance users who are HIV infected, with or without symptoms, find it difficult to gain entrance to a TC if this is the type of treatment they choose. In response to this problem, Project Samaritan, Inc., opened a 66-bed health-related modified TC in New York City for HIV-positive substance users.

Methadone Maintenance. Methadone maintenance is used to treat heroin addiction. Methadone's effectiveness for this purpose was discovered in the early 1960s by Drs. Marie Nyswander and Vincent Dole. Critics of methadone maintenance therapy contend that one addictive drug, methadone, is being substituted for another addictive drug, heroin. However, as one of the few treatments available for heroin addiction, methadone is widely used. The major advantage of methadone maintenance therapy is that it allows individuals to function normally in society.

Methadone is a synthetic drug that has properties similar to those of morphine. It can provide analgesia (when used for this purpose it is prescribed as dolophine), suppress withdrawal symptoms from heroin, and remain effective with repeated administration (Gilman et al., 1985). Since methadone is efficiently absorbed from the gastrointestinal tract, it can be administered by mouth. The effects of a maintenance dose of methadone last up to 30 hours, necessitating only once a day dosage.

Unlike other medications used to treat disease, the dispensation of methadone is controlled by the Food and Drug Administration and state regulations. Guidelines exist for daily dosage, frequency of clinic visits, dispensation of take-home methadone, and provision of counseling. Physicians cannot legally prescribe methadone for the treatment of chemical dependency (Newman, 1987; Novick et al., 1988). Publicly funded methadone maintenance treatment programs (MMTPs) were started in the 1970s (Wesson, 1988).

The goal of methadone maintenance is to prevent withdrawal symptoms and to block the effects of other opiates. If an individual on methadone maintenace should take any opiate in any form, he or she would not experience a high. On entering a methadone program, a person is assessed for the level of heroin use and then started on 10 to 40 mg of methadone per day. The dose is gradually increased, usually by increments of 10 mg, until a maintenance dose is reached, usually after 4 to 6 weeks. A maintenance dose of 60 to 80 mg per day is often sufficient (Dole, 1988). Rarely is more than 100 mg per day required. During this period the goal is to keep the person free of withdrawal symptoms. Symptoms of mild overdosage, which usually are eliminated with dose reduction, include sedation, sweating, and decreased libido (Arif & Westermeyer, 1988). Constipation is a frequent side effect that may not abate with dose change or length of therapy. The blood level of methadone for maintenance should be in the range of 150 to 600 ng/ml, although monitoring of methadone dosage is usually based more on subjective reports than blood levels (Dole, 1988). Miosis may be evident shortly after the methadone is taken and lasts several hours. Persons taking methadone feel a high about 20 to 30 minutes after administration but should not subsequently go into a nod as occurs with heroin.

The use of cocaine by individuals on methadone maintenance has increased recently. The use of other substances (e.g., amphetamines, tranquilizers, and alcohol) is not uncommon. Urine testing as part of the program detects the presence of these substances.

Certain medications can interfere with the metabolism of methadone and necessitate a methadone dose increase when treatment with one of these drugs is initiated. Rifampin, used in the treatment of tuberculosis, and phenytoin (Dilantin), an anticonvulsant, are frequently used in PWAs. Either of these drugs may cause patients to complain that their methadone is "being eaten up." If an individual's methadone dose is not increased when one of these medications is initiated, symptoms of withdrawal will begin several days later. The methadone dose should be increased by 10 mg on the first day of rifampin or phenytoin therapy and then by 10 mg every 1 to 2 days thereafter until oversedation is achieved. Patients may require a methadone dose up to 50% higher than their previous dose (Friedland & Selwyn, 1990). Other opiates, central nervous system depressants, tricyclic antidepressants, and anxiolytics also interfere with methadone metabolism to a lesser degree and require a dose adjustment.

Methadone maintenance does not control pain. Individuals receiving methadone, regardless of the dose, as treatment for heroin addiction are still able to experience pain. They require pain medication in higher and more frequent doses than a narcotic-naive individual would. In addition, adequate pain control is difficult to achieve when the methadone dose is more than 50 mg per day (Gayle Newshan, personal communication). In this circumstance, if long-term pain management is needed, the person should be weaned to 50 mg of methadone per day. When a person on methadone maintenance is admitted to the hospital, the hospital must confirm the patient's methadone dose with the methadone program, since the patient will require methadone while in the hospital. Hospital workers must not assume that the patient is too sick for methadone; without the daily dose the patient will experience withdrawal symptoms regardless of his or her medical condition.

Withdrawal from methadone maintenance is possible. This may be considered when an individual has been stabilized on methadone for a period of time and wants to be drug free. Depending on the maintenance dose of methadone, withdrawal should occur over a period of weeks to months and requires a gradual tapering of the dose (Arif & Westermeyer, 1988). Individuals who withdraw in this manner should be able to function normally and should experience no untoward effects.

Self-Help Groups. Self-help groups involve individuals who have a common problem, chemical dependency, and whose goal is to live drug and alcohol free. The best-known of these groups is Alcoholics Anonymous (AA), from which Narcotics Anonymous (NA) and Cocaine Anonymous (CA) have evolved. Bill Wilson started AA in 1935 to help alcoholics achieve and maintain sobriety. Members of AA must admit they are alcoholics and recognize that they will always be alcoholics. They believe that recovery is a lifelong process. "'Living in Recovery' is a commitment to adopting a drug and alcohol free life-style that consists of a daily adherence to the values and concepts as set forth in the 12 step programs" (Narcotic & Drug Research, Inc., 1989, p. 104) (Table 9–5).

Chapters of AA, NA, and CA have been organized worldwide. In meetings attendees share their experiences with drugs or alcohol and through this process and with the help of a sponsor obtain mutual support to remain drug or alcohol free. When an individual is in the early stages

TABLE 9–5. Twelve-Step Program of Alcoholics Anonymous

1. We admitted we were powerless over alcohol—that our lives had become unmanageable.
2. Came to believe that a Power greater than ourselves could restore us to sanity.
3. Made a decision to turn our will and our lives over to the care of God *as we understood Him.*
4. Made a searching and fearless moral inventory of ourselves.
5. Admitted to God, to ourselves and to another human being the exact nature of our wrongs.
6. Were entirely ready to have God remove all these defects of character.
7. Humbly asked Him to remove our shortcomings.
8. Made a list of all persons we had harmed, and became willing to make amends to them all.
9. Made direct amends to such people wherever possible, except when to do so would injure them or others.
10. Continued to take personal inventory and when we were wrong promptly admitted it.
11. Sought through prayer and meditation to improve our conscious contact with God, *as we understood Him,* praying only for knowledge of His will for us and the power to carry that out.
12. Having had a spiritual awakening as the result of these steps, we tried to carry this message to alcoholics, and to practice these principles in all our affairs.

of recovery, daily meetings are strongly recommended. Because AA, NA, and CA are based on the premise of being drug and alcohol free, individuals on methadone maintenance or PWAs receiving long-term pain medication may be excluded from these meetings. In some cities there are now meetings where such individuals are welcome. In addition, meetings are held for those who speak a language other than English and for gay and lesbian people in recovery. Al-Anon and Al-Ateen are groups for families of people who are actively using drugs or alcohol or are in recovery.

Acupuncture. Acupuncture is a form of Chinese medicine that was developed more than 2500 years ago to relieve pain and stress. It involves insertion of slender needles into specific body points that control organ and body functioning. In the early 1970s Dr. Michael Smith discovered that acupuncture could be used to treat heroin withdrawal and help individuals remain drug free. As a result, he started an acupuncture detoxification clinic at Lincoln Hospital in the South Bronx area of New York City. The program has been so successful that it has been replicated in many other countries.

Western scientists are not certain how acupuncture works. Possibly the needle insertion stimulates the body to produce endorphins, which are natural pain killers. Regardless of its mode of action, acupuncture is now being used to treat alcohol and cocaine addiction with the same reported success rates as with heroin. In the Lincoln Hospital program, patients are encouraged to receive daily acupuncture treatment for the initial 2 weeks of therapy and then maintenance treatments approximately three times a week indefinitely. Treatments involve inserting four or five needles in designated points on each ear and leaving them in place for 30 to 45 minutes. Many patients report a feeling of relaxation and diminished desire to use after treatments. Counseling, along with NA, AA, or CA, is encouraged. Urine screening is done randomly.

The treatment of cocaine addiction by acupuncture is viewed as generally successful, and since few other treatment options exist, New York City has plans to establish acupuncture treatment clinics for cocaine addiction in a number of its municipal hospitals.

CHEMICAL DEPENDENCY AND HIV INFECTION

Even without the addition of HIV infection, chemical dependency has multiple negative effects on the body. Malnutrition, infectious diseases, trauma, and psychiatric disorders are common in substance users and may make disease processes secondary to substance use difficult to differentiate from those secondary to HIV infection. Table 9–6 lists more specific medical conditions that result from substance use.

A dual diagnosis of psychiatric disorders and chemical dependency is not uncommon among the IVDU population. Three patterns of dual diagnosis exist (Batki, 1990). In the first pattern the drug use causes the psychiatric problem. For example, cocaine psychosis is a result of cocaine use. In the second pattern a psychiatric condition predates substance use. Possibly substance use is a form of self-treatment for the psychiatric condition. In the third pattern it is unclear which came first, the substance use or the psychiatric condition. The addition of HIV infection creates, in effect, a triple diagnosis. A dual or triple diagnosis involves a myriad of social, psychologic, and medical problems that complicate the provision of services. Differentiating the cause of the psychiatric symptoms will guide the treatment. HIV-related neuropsychiatric problems are discussed in Chapter 4.

HIV infection is associated with different opportunistic infections and malignancies in IVDUs. The incidence of Kaposi's sarcoma, cytomegalovirus infection, and herpes simplex virus infection is lower among IVDUs; *Pneumocystis carinii* pneumonia, cryptococcal disease, histoplasmosis, and extrapulmonary tuberculosis are more common (Friedland & Selwyn, 1990). Bacterial pneumonia, sepsis, and tuberculosis lead to

TABLE 9–6. Medical Conditions Resulting from Substance Abuse

MEDICAL PROBLEM	COMMENTS
Heart and Lungs	
Cardiomegaly, cardiomyopathy	Direct toxicity of alcohol from thiamine
Congestive heart failure	deficiency
Endocarditis	Results from IV drug use
Increased respiratory infections	Results from immunosuppression
Blood	
Anemia, leukemia, thrombocytopenia	Result from bone marrow suppression, vitamin deficiencies
Immune System	
Increased incidence of infection, AIDS	Results from IV drug use; direct toxicity to bone marrow and white blood cells, increased life-style stress and risk
Nervous System	
Withdrawal symptoms: seizures, tremors, hallucinations, DTs, irritability, depression, paranoid ideation	Direct toxicity and rapid decrease in drug blood levels
Cerebral atrophy and diminished functioning	Direct toxicity and vitamin deficiency are contributing factors
Psychiatric disorders	
Cerebellar degeneration	
Neuropathies, palsies, gait disturbances	
Visual problems	
Digestive System	
Liver diseases (alcoholism leading to hepatitis B, fatty liver, cirrhosis)	Direct toxicity of alcohol; parenteral injection of hepatitis B virus
Pancreatitis	
Ulcers and inflammations of the gut, Mallory-Weiss syndrome, peptic ulcers, diarrhea, constipation	Alcohol directly irritates intestinal mucosa
Nutritional Deficiencies	
Pellagra	Niacin deficiency
Wernicke's encephalopathy	Thiamine deficiency
Dermatitis, cheilosis, stomatitis	Riboflavin deficiency
Anemia	Pyridoxine and folic acid deficiencies
Scurvy	Vitamin C deficiency
Endocrine System	
Hypoglycemia	Secondary to pancreatitis and inhibition of gluconeogenesis
Hypercalcemia	From magnesium deficiency

From Narcotic and Drug Research, Inc. (1989). *AIDS: Medical management of the HIV infected/chemically dependent client.* New York: The Company.

increased non-AIDS mortality among HIV-infected IVDUs. The incidence of sexually transmitted diseases, human papillomavirus, and cervical abnormalities on Papanicolaou smears also is higher among HIV-infected IVDU women (Friedland & Selwyn, 1990). Studies show that HIV infection is a predictor of death from these non-HIV infections (Des Jarlais & Friedman, 1988).

IVDUs are at high risk for tuberculosis (TB). Frequently extrapulmonary TB is the first AIDS-indicator disease in IVDUs. In New York City the incidence of pulmonary TB among IVDUs is increasing. It was found that 57% of patients with both HIV infection and TB in New York City were IVDUs (Friedland & Selwyn, 1990). A study of 169 homeless men in a congregate shelter in New York City found a high correlation between HIV seropositivity, intravenous drug use, and active TB (Torres, 1990). Among these men 22% had active pulmonary TB and 54% reported current active drug use.

TB screening is essential for any individual who is an IVDU and therefore at risk for HIV infection. Drug treatment programs are required by federal regulations to perform tuberculin skin testing before admission. Further evaluation for clinical TB is recommended for an IVDU with HIV infection who has a skin reaction of greater than or equal to 5 mm or for an IVDU who is HIV negative but has a skin reaction of greater than or equal to 10 mm (CDC, 1990a). If these individuals are found to have no evidence of clinical disease, preventive therapy for TB should be instituted. The CDC recommends isoniazid at a maximum adult dose of 300 mg daily. The duration of therapy should be from 6 to 12 months; those with HIV infection should receive 12 months of therapy.

When compliance might be an issue, health care personnel should if possible watch the patient taking the medication. This has been successfully done in methadone maintenance treatment programs and congregate shelters (Selwyn et al., 1989; Torres et al., 1990). If daily observation is not possible, isoniazid may be administered twice weekly in a dose of 15 mg/kg (up to 900 mg) (CDC, 1990c). For individuals who do not regularly attend a program, compliance is of greater concern and may necessitate referral to a community health agency for the purpose of monitoring medication.

RISK REDUCTION

Transmission of HIV infection may be prevented by the cessation of substance use and by abstinence from high-risk sexual activities. Failing these goals, IVDUs need to know how to reduce the risk of transmitting HIV infection. Needle exchange programs, cleansing syringes and needles with bleach, and using condoms are highly effective ways to prevent HIV transmission.

Studies have shown that IVDUs are generally aware of the risk of needle sharing. In one methadone maintenance program and large detention facility in New York City, 97% of subjects interviewed recognized needle sharing as an AIDS risk factor (Selwyn et al., 1987).

Significant controversy surrounds needle exchange programs and instructing users how to clean their works with bleach. Many maintain that these programs encourage substance use, whereas others believe that these measures encourage risk reduction until the individual can enter a treatment program. In the United States, where 80% of active IVDUs are not in treatment, too few treatment slots are available for the number of persons needing and wanting treatment, resulting in a wait for those who ask for it (CDC, 1990b).

The United States has few legal needle exchange programs but several illegal, although tolerated, programs. Studies from Europe, where legal programs exist, and the United States demonstrate that needle exchange programs do not encourage the use of drugs and in fact decrease the number of times IVDUs use drugs with shared needles (Dolan et al., 1990; Keffelew et al., 1990). An integral part of these programs is counseling regarding general risk reduction, including safer sex practices and the distribution of condoms. The same studies show that although needle-sharing behavior can be changed, changing sexual practices is much more difficult. Many participants in these programs share needles fewer times but continue to engage in unsafe sex despite counseling and easy availability of condoms.

Where needle exchange programs are illegal or unavailable, programs that instruct in the use of bleach for cleaning one's works and distribute individual bleach kits have been established. In many of these community-based organizations, recovered IVDUs go into the community to teach and counsel active IVDUs. This nontraditional type of outreach is believed effective in changing behavior with this group of individuals, who have little contact with a more traditional social service and medical care system (Stimson, 1990; CDC, 1990b).

If a patient has no access to any of these programs, a health care worker may give instructions on the cleaning of syringes and needles. The user should be instructed to soak the needle, syringe, and cooker in a mixture of 1 cup household bleach to 10 cups water for 10 minutes and then rinse them under running water. If the IVDU purchases syringes on the street, he or she should be instructed to buy only syringes in unopened packages.

The correct use of condoms (reviewed in Chapter 10) should be discussed with all IVDUs and their partners. It should be stressed that entering drug treatment programs or cleaning their works does little to prevent the transmission of HIV infection unless safer sex is practiced also.

PAIN MANAGEMENT

Substance users have as great a need for adequate pain control as other patients. A study to define the pain syndromes and their management in PWAs found little difference in the complaints of pain between IVDUs and homosexual patients (Newshan et al., 1990). Abdominal and neuropathic pain occurred in approximately 50% of the patients, with equal frequency in IVDU and homosexual patients. Pain from esophagitis, headaches, Kaposi's sarcoma, postherpetic neuralgia, and backache was also reported.

It is important to remember that IVDUs usually require higher and more frequent doses of opiates to manage pain. Every patient with chronic pain should be given medication on a regular basis rather than on an as-needed (PRN) basis. This is particularly important with IVDUs. An adequate amount and frequency of pain medication helps to relieve the anxiety experienced when patients with pain are made to wait for medication. Anxiety increases the pain experience, but anxiolytics, because of their potential for abuse, should be used with care in this population. The anxiety experienced may be relieved with appropriate pain medication, relaxation exercises, therapeutic touch, acupuncture, or counseling.

Of concern to many practitioners is the issue of abuse of pain medication by IVDUs. Some individuals with a substance use history seek medication for this purpose, and distinguishing between real pain and pain reported by those seeking drugs can be difficult. Usually individuals who are not in pain, when questioned as to the location of their discomfort, refer to a general area rather than a specific area. Physical examination may not elicit a pain response. In addition, many of the signs and symptoms of pain, that is, tachycardia, diaphoresis, tachypnea, nausea, and vomiting, are not evident. When they are unaware of observation, these persons may be observed performing tasks they claim are compromised by the pain. If pain medication is prescribed, they may seek inordinately frequent medication renewals.

At Bailey House/AIDS Resource Center (a 44-room residence in New York City for homeless persons with AIDS, of whom the majority have a substance use history) the majority of substance users requesting pain medication have appeared to have a real need for it. However, if it becomes evident that a pattern of abuse is developing, several measures have been found useful. On some occasions a contract has been made with individuals that their prescription will be renewed at the appropriate interval and the staff will not assist with renewal if they run out of their medication. Their physician must be contacted and agree to this contract as well. In extreme circumstances, emergency rooms can be contacted and instructed not to prescribe narcotics for an individual. Other circumstances have warranted the enrollment of the individual in a methadone maintenance treatment program.

RELAPSE PREVENTION AND MANAGEMENT

Relapses frequently occur with IVDUs and should be anticipated. When relapse occurs, the goal is to get the client back to recovery as soon as possible. Relapse may mean one time only use (slip), repeated uses within a short period of time (binge), or a return to frequent or continual use. The most effective approach is to support the individual's desire to be drug free and to minimize the guilt he or she may feel about using. Those who relapse should be confronted about their use in a nonjudgmental manner as soon as use is suspected.

Part of the initial treatment plan should include how a person will remain "clean" and what the person will do if he or she "slips." Table 9–7 lists events and situations that might lead to a relapse. The client may identify some of these during the initial assessment or during the course of treatment. Part of the plan should include discussion of how to avoid, reduce, or manage the triggering events or situations.

HIV TESTING AND COUNSELING

Chapter 6 discusses issues and mechanisms for testing and counseling individuals at risk for HIV infection. Individuals with a history of IV substance use, crack or alcohol use, or multiple, frequent sexual partners are considered at risk for HIV infection. These individuals may enter the health care system when they begin drug treatment, are hospitalized for an acute illness, or receive services from an outreach program. As with any person at risk, all the issues and implications of testing should be reviewed. Regardless of the person's HIV status, emphasis should be placed on discontinuing the risky behavior. Studies show that substance users enrolled in methadone maintenance treatment programs are interested in and seek HIV screening (Carlson & McClellan, 1987; Curtis et al., 1989). This information, and the knowledge that many IVDUs are aware of risky behaviors, should encourage health care providers to discuss counseling openly.

TABLE 9–7. Events and Situations That Could Lead to Relapse

Parties	Rejecting help
Old friends	Not attending Alcoholics Anonymous
Old relationships	or Narcotics Anonymous
Fighting with family	Rationalizing problems
Isolation	Lying consciously
Pressures becoming unmanageable	Feeling self-pity
Guilt	Losing confidence
Being oversensitive	"I can do it by myself" attitude
Living in past	Projecting
Anger becoming unmanageable	High expectations
Daily routine	Taking on too many projects at once
"Don't care" attitude	Cravings

From Narcotic and Drug Research, Inc. (1989). *AIDS: Medical management of the HIV infected/chemically dependent client.* New York: The Company.

ASSESSMENT

The development of a nursing care plan (refer to Chapter 4 for discussion of nursing care plans for the HIV-infected adult client) for an HIV-infected IVDU depends on an assessment of the individual's substance use. The health care worker must find out what drugs are used and in what amounts, the length of time of usage, the route, and what other risk behaviors are present. Without this information, adequate planning for care of the drug problem or the HIV infection is impossible.

A drug history should be taken in a thorough and nonjudgmental manner. The interviewer should explore his or her feelings about drug use before interacting with a client. The interviewer should not ask questions in a hurried manner that might imply that the interviewer is embarrassed or wants to get the session over with. Genuine interest, concern, and a desire to help should be evident.

Table 9–8 presents a drug history questionnaire that has been used with a high degree of success at Bailey House. Not only does the history elicit which substances have been used, but also it explores the motivation to stop using. Without some idea of this, the health care worker cannot discuss treatment options with the client. In addition, a complete health history as outlined in Chapter 4 will help to identify other risk factors and drug-related health problems.

Asking about the use of nonprescribed antibiotics and AIDS-related medications such as zidovudine, acyclovir, or ketoconazole is important. IVDUs commonly purchase antibiotics on the street and use them for self-medication when not feeling well. Selwyn (1989) reported that after an episode of high-risk behavior, IVDUs may obtain AIDS treatment drugs on the street for "preventive" use.

The physical examination as discussed in Chapter 4 should support information obtained in the history. During the physical examination the nurse should be observant for recent injection marks (tracks). The most obvious locations are the arms and legs. Less obvious places are the neck, breasts, groin, feet, and dorsal vein of the penis. Urine toxicologic examination, which can detect opiates, cocaine, benzodiazepines, barbiturates, amphetamines, marijuana, and tricyclic antidepressants, should be an integral part of the health assessment. This should be done as soon as possible, since only the most long-acting substances are evident after several days.

PLANNING

Individuals with chemical dependency and HIV infection require a plan of care that addresses both problems. Many nurses have less difficulty developing a plan for HIV infection than for chemical dependency. Chapter 4 illustrates the development of a nursing care plan for HIV infection. The goal of a nursing care plan for substance use should be to encourage the individual to enter treatment or, if he or she is in treatment, to prevent relapse. A review of treatment options should be followed by a discussion of what might be the best choice for the client based on the drugs being used.

The nursing care plan should include short-term goals that are reasonably attainable. Most substance users are easily frustrated and require fairly immediate gratification. The first, easily measurable part of the plan should be that the client either calls for an appointment or goes in person to the treatment program. This should not be done for the client, but he or she might be accompanied. Once the substance user decides to seek treatment, this step may be the most difficult. Many view the first visit to a treatment program as an admission of having a problem. If the plan of care is being developed in the clinic where the person receives care for the HIV disease, more frequent clinic visits might be scheduled to monitor success and offer encouragement. It is essential that strategies to cope with and prevent relapse be discussed. Individuals need to be reminded that no matter how sure they are that their problem is controlled, they are always at risk for relapse. Encouragement to "take one day at a time" is helpful.

Individuals with a substance use problem must want to stop using. A number of motivating factors can bring them to this point. Occasionally rejection by family makes substance users seek treatment. A hospitalization in which access to drugs is limited (remember it is easy for many substance users to get drugs while hospitalized) and the person stops using for a period of time might encourage him or her to enter treatment.

TABLE 9–8. Sample Drug History Questionnaire

History of Substance Use

When did you start using drugs? What did you start with? How did you take it (i.e., sniffing, smoking, IV)? What did you start using next? How did you take that?

Over the last 5 years have you used: heroin, cocaine, crack, pills, PCP (angel dust), alcohol, methadone? How much of each, how often, and by what route?

Do you take Valium/Xanax/Ativan/Restoril/Halcion/sleeping pills/"nerve" pills? How many and how often?

Where do you get the pills?

Did you ever share your works? Have you ever used in a shooting gallery? Have you ever shared with anyone you know was HIV infected?

How have you paid for your drugs? Did you ever sell drugs? Steer (direct people) to dealers?

Have you ever been arrested? When? For what?

Treatment History

Have you ever detoxed? How many times? When? Where? (jail, hospital, at home)

Why did you detox? (voluntarily or not; also, motivation)

Have you ever been in a therapeutic community? When? Where? How long was the program? Did you complete the program? If not, why did you leave?

Have you ever been involved in after-care? Counseling?

Have you ever attended NA/AA/CA meetings? When? How often?

Life Without Drugs

What was the longest time you have been clean? When was that?

How do you define clean?

Did you drink during that time? How much? How often?

What was the situation in your life at that time (job, girl/boyfriend/wife/husband, where were you living, with whom)?

Same as the above for the second longest time you have been clean.

Did you get any kind of help from anyone to stay clean during those times?

From Bailey House/AIDS Resource Center, New York. Used with permission.

Many residents of Bailey House claim they stopped or decreased their use when their HIV infection was diagnosed. Some see the time from diagnosis to illness as a chance to "get it together." Having never thought they would live long enough to die of anything other than drugs, they see this time as extra time.

Contracts may be useful in encouraging clients to discontinue drugs and remain drug free. Anyone with an active drug problem who seeks admission to Bailey House must agree to enter some form of drug treatment and to attempt to remain drug free while a resident of Bailey House. Probation agreements are used to deal with relapses. The agreements, which must be signed by the resident, state how the relapse will be managed: detoxification progam, increased attendance at 12-step programs, daily pickup at methadone maintenance program if the resident has been on a less frequent pickup schedule, or enrollment in a methadone main-

TABLE 9–8. Sample Drug History Questionnaire *Continued*

Methadone (if applicable)

Have you ever been on methadone? Are you in a program now?
If started and stopped, why did you stop? When was this? How did you stop? (cold turkey, detoxed through a program, detoxed in a hospital)
Have you been clean while in the program? If not, how often do you have dirty urines?
If not in a program now, would you consider being in a program again? Why or why not?

Support

If you attend NA/AA/CA, how often do you go? Do you have a sponsor?
If you do not attend, what do you know about NA/AA/CA?
Do you attend any kind of support group? What kind? Where? How often?
If not, what do you know about support groups?
Whom do you talk to about your problems (drug or others)?
Do your friends or family use drugs or alcohol?
Do you know anyone who is clean?

Insight

What are some of the things that cause you to use?
Do you consider yourself a drug addict? An alcoholic?
Why or why not?
Were you using when you were diagnosed with AIDS?
Have you used since you were diagnosed?
Do you want to be/stay clean?
What do you think is the best way for you to stay clean?
What would you do if you relapsed?
How have you been feeling while talking with me about your drug history?

tenance program if not in one already. If the drug use continues, discharge of the resident may be necessary. It is imperative that the individual understand all ramifications of a contract from the beginning.

Hospitals with specialized AIDS units might make contracts with substance users who are admitted to these units. The contract might state that the person will be allowed to remain on the unit if no substance use occurs while he or she is a patient there. Alternatively, the patient may have certain privileges, such as visitors and cigarette smoking, curtailed if he or she is using.

Contracts cannot be made unless treatment is being offered. In New York City many hospitals do not offer inpatient treatment for substance use for individuals who are not admitted to a unit for that purpose. Individuals who have been active in a 12-step program will have no meetings to attend unless the hospital sponsors meetings. Visits by the patient's sponsor or other friend from the program can usually be arranged when necessary. Enrollment in a methadone maintenance program cannot occur until patients are discharged. However, heroin users can start to receive methadone while in the hospital and can be referred to a methadone maintenance program when discharged. The first visit to the program must occur the day of or the day after discharge so the individual has no days without methadone. Also, if the individual has been in a program before admission, the program must be contacted before discharge so the patient can pick up methadone the day after discharge. A prescription for methadone will not suffice.

The most difficult plan of care to develop is for individuals who do not want to stop using drugs. It is hard to encourage an active user to stop when the user has no motivation to do so. When the user will be discharged back to the same environment he or she came from, it is hard to give a good reason for discontinuing use. However, users cannot be ignored; they deserve and require medical treatment for their other problems. If they cannot be convinced to enter treatment, risk reduction should be discussed and encouraged. If a community-based group that counsels active users is available, a referral should be considered. Nurses also need to be aware of housing and community support services. Sometimes an appropriate referral provides the motivation to stop using. When chemically dependent individuals are treated in a nonjudgmental way and encouraged to keep clinic appointments, the possibility always exists that at some point they may seek treatment.

EVALUATION

Evaluating the plan of care determines its effectiveness and need for changes. If the first step has been enrollment in a treatment program, confirmation may be made by having the patient return with a letter verifying attendance. All treatment programs require a signed letter requesting release of information before they will even acknowledge attendance by an individual at the program. Communication with the program is generally a good idea because it provides easy verification of attendance and compliance and more coordinated care. Many programs perform routine urine drug screening, which also helps to determine the success of treatment. When relapse is suspected, the individual should be confronted with the suspicion and the nursing care plan should be altered accordingly. When confronting persons, the nurse must be very specific about why he or she thinks they are using: they appear high based on their behavior; physical examination reveals evidence of recent use; someone has reported that they have been using. The plan for coping with the relapse should be delayed until the individual is no longer high.

When risk reduction for a person who does not want treatment has been discussed, follow-up visits should involve questioning about specific measures taken by that individual.

CONCLUSION

Nurses must recognize that chemical dependency is a disease and requires nursing and medical intervention as does any other disease. The stigma of HIV infection only adds to the stigma of chemical dependency. With knowledge and understanding nurses can greatly enhance the care given to HIV-infected substance users. IVDUs should not be treated as pariahs. They deserve the same respect and dignity accorded other individuals.

References

American Nurses' Association (1987). The care of clients with addictions. Kansas City, MO: The Association.

Arif, A., Westermeyer, J. (1988). *Manual of drug and alcohol abuse.* New York: Plenum Medical Book Company.

Batki, S.L. (1990). Drug abuse, psychiatric disorders, and AIDS. *Western Journal of Medicine,* 152(5), 547–552.

Carlson, C.A., McClellan, T.A. (1987). The voluntary acceptance of HIV-antibody screening by intravenous drug users. *Public Health Reports,* 102(4), 391–394.

Cartter, N.L., Petersen, L.R., Savage, R.B., et al. (1989). Providing HIV counseling and testing services in methadone maintenance programs. *AIDS,* 4(5), 463–465.

Casey, E. (1989). History of drug use and drug users in the United States. In: *AIDS: Medical management of the HIV infected/chemically dependent client.* New York: Narcotic and Drug Research, Inc.

Centers for Disease Control (1990a). Screening for tuberculosis and tuberculous infection in high-risk populations. *Morbidity and Mortality Weekly Report,* 39, 1–7.

Centers for Disease Control (1990b). Update: Reducing HIV transmission in intravenous-drug users not in drug treatment — United States. *Morbidity and Mortality Weekly Report,* 39, 529–538.

Centers for Disease Control (1990c). The use of preventive therapy for tuberculous infection in the United States, *Morbidity and Mortality Weekly Report,* 39, 9–12.

Chiasson, M.A., Stoneburner, R.L., Heldebrandt, D.S., et al. (1990). Heterosexual transmission of HIV associated with the use of smokable freebase cocaine (crack) [Abstract ThC 588]. Paper presented at the Sixth International Conference on AIDS, San Francisco, June 1990.

Coutinho, R.A. (1990). Epidemiology and prevention of AIDS among intravenous drug users. *Journal of Acquired Immune Deficiency Syndromes,* 3(4), 413–417.

Curtis, J.L., Crummey, C., Baker, S.N., et al. (1989). HIV screening and counseling for intravenous drug users. *Journal of the American Medical Association,* 261(2), 258–262.

Des Jarlais, D.C., Friedman, S.R. (1988). HIV infection among persons who inject illicit drugs: Problems and prospects. *Journal of Acquired Immune Deficiency Syndromes,* 1(3), 267–273.

Des Jarlais, D.C., Friedman, S.R., Novick, D.M., et al. (1989). HIV–1 infection among intravenous drug users in Manhattan, New York City, from 1977 through 1987. *Journal of the American Medical Association,* 261(7), 1008–1012.

Dolan, K., Stimson, G.V., Donoghoe, M.C. (1990). Differences in HIV rates and risk behavior of drug injectors attending syringe-exchanges in England [Abstract FC 108]. Paper presented at the Sixth International Conference on AIDS, San Francisco, June 1990.

Dole, V.P. (1988). Implications of methadone maintenance for theories of narcotic addiction. *Journal of the American Medical Association, 260*(20), 3025–3029.

Evans, C.A., Beauchamp, D.E., Deyton, L., et al. (1989). *Illicit drug use and HIV infection.* In: Report of the Special Initiative on AIDS of the American Public Health Association. Washington, D.C.: The Association.

Friedland, G., Selwyn, P. (1990). Intravenous drug use and HIV infection. *AIDS Clinical Care, 2*(4), 31–32.

Gilman, A.G., Goodman, L.S., Gilman, A. (1985). *The pharmacological basis of therapeutics.* New York: Macmillan Publishing Co., Inc.

Goleman, D. (1990). Scientists pinpoint brain irregularities in drug addicts. *New York Times* (June 26), B5.

Henneberger, M. (1990). Drug research surges after lull. *Newsday* (August 24), 8.

Keffelew, A., Clark, G., Bacchetti, P., et al. (1990). Use of needle exchange programs by San Francisco drug users in methadone treatment [Abstract FC 107]. Paper presented at the Sixth International Conference on AIDS, San Francisco, June 1990.

Marmor, M., Des Jarlais, D.C., Cohen, H., et al. (1987). Risk factors for infection with human immunodeficiency virus among intravenous drug abusers in New York City. *AIDS, 1*(1), 39–44.

Narcotic and Drug Research, Inc. (1989). AIDS: Medical management of the HIV infected/ chemically dependent client. New York: The Company.

Newman, R.G. (1987). Methadone treatment. *New England Journal of Medicine, 317*(7), 447–450.

Newshan, G.T., Wainapel, S.F., Turino, G.M., et al. (Submitted for publication). Pain syndromes and their management in persons with acquired immunodefiency syndrome: Final report.

Novick, D.M., Pascarelli, E.F., Joseph, H., et al. (1988). Methadone maintenance patients in general medical practice. *Journal of the American Medical Association, 259*(22), 3299–3302.

Schoenbaum, E.E., Hartel, D., Friedland, G.H. (1990). Crack use predicts incident HIV seroconversion [Abstract ThC]. Paper presented at the Sixth International Conference on AIDS, San Francisco, June 1990.

Schoenbaum, E.E., Hartel, D., Selwyn, P.A., et al. (1989). Risk factors for human immunodeficiency virus infection in intravenous drug users. *New England Journal of Medicine, 321*(13), 874–879.

Selwyn, P.A. (1989). Issues in the clinical management of intravenous drug users with HIV infection. *AIDS, 3*(suppl 1), S201-S208.

Selwyn, P.A., Feiner, C., Cox, C.P., et al. (1987). Knowledge about AIDS and high-risk behavior among intravenous drug users in New York City. *AIDS, 1*(4), 247–254.

Selwyn, P.A., Feingold, A.R., Iezza, A., et al. (1989). Primary care for patients with human immunodeficiency virus. *Annals of Internal Medicine, 111*(9), 761–763.

Shaffer, H.J., Costikyan, N.S. (1988). Cocaine psychosis and AIDS: A contemporary diagnostic dilemma. *Journal of Substance Abuse, 5*(1), 9–12.

Stimson, G.V. (1990). The prevention of HIV infection in injecting drug users: Recent advances and remaining obstacles. Paper presented at the Sixth International Conference on AIDS, San Francisco, June 1990.

Sugarman, B. (1974). *Daytop Village: A therapeutic community.* New York: Holt, Rinehart & Winston, Inc.

Torres, R.A., Mani, S., Altholz, J., et al. (1990). HIV infection among homeless men in a New York City shelter. *Archives of Internal Medicine, 150,* 2030–2036.

Weiss, R.D., Mirin, S.M. (1987). *Cocaine.* New York: Ballantine Books.

Wesson, D.R. (1988). Revival of medical maintenance in the treatment of heroin dependence. *Journal of the American Medical Association, 259*(22), 3314–3315.

10

HIV Infection in Women

Kathleen M. Nokes

Since HIV infection was first identified in gay men, much of the focus has been on how the infectious process is manifested in men. In the United States, HIV-AIDS is now among the 10 leading causes of death in women of reproductive age and the death rate for HIV-AIDS continues to rise (Chu et al., 1990). AIDS is the leading cause of death among women aged 25 to 34 years in New York City (Allen, 1990). Women are often perceived as vectors of HIV infection—transmitters of the virus to their sexual partners and their unborn children (Mitchell, 1988). This perspective negates the role of women as competent adults and contributes to their feelings of helplessness.

EPIDEMIOLOGY

According to the Centers for Disease Control (CDC) surveillance data reported in November 1990, AIDS has been diagnosed in 14,816 women (CDC, 1990a). The major exposure categories for women are intravenous drug use (51%) and heterosexual contact (32%). The average woman with AIDS is in her late twenties, a period of development that is characterized by stabilizing relationships, growing employment and educational strengths, and childbearing. Seven percent of women with AIDS report having had an other or undetermined risk of infection, whereas only 3% of the men with AIDS had an other or undetermined risk. Thirty-six percent of HIV-seropositive women do not know how they became infected (Allen, 1990).

In the United States the greatest number of cases of AIDS occur in men who engage in unprotected homosexual or bisexual sexual behaviors and then among intravenous drug users (pattern I as defined by the World Health Organization). In pattern II countries most of the reported cases

375

occur through heterosexual sexual contact and the male-to-female ratio is approximately 1:1. Transmission through intravenous drug use or homosexual activity either does not occur or occurs at a low level (CDC, 1990a). Pattern II countries include areas of central, eastern, and southern Africa and some Caribbean countries. AIDS investigators are uncertain whether the epidemic will continue to have different patterns of transmission or become more homogeneous in terms of male/female ratios of transmission. Female exposure category by heterosexual contact and ethnicity is presented in Table 10–1. The last category in Table 10–1 deserves special note: sex with man with HIV infection whose risk is unspecified. This indicates that HIV is being transmitted heterosexually when the male partner has no established risk behavior such as bisexuality or intravenous (IV) drug use. Since the man has no established risk behavior, the woman would have no reason to suspect that he was HIV seropositive.

States with the highest number of women with AIDS are New York, New Jersey, Florida, and California ranked in order from highest to lowest incidence (Willoughby, 1989). The areas with the highest cumulative incidence per 100,000 are New Jersey, New York, Washington, D.C., and Florida (Shapiro et al., 1989). A woman living in an inner-city area following a conventional life-style of monogamy, raising a family, and not using drugs runs a high risk of becoming infected through her male HIV-seropositive partner (Anastos & Marte, 1989).

The number of women with HIV infection is unknown. One common way of estimating this number is through testing umbilical cord blood. As of 1989, 43 states and territories had completed, were conducting, or were planning to conduct their first annual survey of childbearing women by testing blood samples from their newborns (Pappaioanou et al., 1990). This testing is blinded, which means that the mother does not consent to testing nor does she learn the results of the test. In one study in New York City, 2.7% of the women delivering their babies at a voluntary hospital tested positive for HIV antibodies (Sperling et al., 1989). All 224 of these women had received prenatal care, and none was identified through a voluntary screening program based on the woman's perception of risk for being infected with HIV. Although some persons raise ethical questions about the rights of the individual woman to consent to testing, this position is countered by the argument that society needs to sense the scope of the epidemic. Since virtually all babies of HIV-infected mothers are born with antibodies to HIV, HIV infection in women can be indirectly inferrred from the blood of the baby.

In a study of blood drawn from the umbilical cord immediately after birth of women in New York City, the highest seroprevalence rates were among Latina women (2.65%) and black women (1.36%), no samples positive for HIV were found in white women in this study (Shapiro et al., 1989). Compared with white women, black women have a 13.2 times

TABLE 10–1. AIDS Female Heterosexual Exposure Category and Ethnicity Reported Through October 1990, United States (n = 4810)

HETEROSEXUAL CONTACT	WHITE NO. (%)	BLACK NO. (%)	HIS-PANIC NO. (%)	ASIAN/ PACIFIC ISLANDER NO. (%)	AMER-ICAN INDIAN/ ALASKAN NO. (%)	TOTAL
Sex with IVDU	595(19)	1480(49)	924(30)	11(—)	5(—)	3026
Sex with bisexual male	260(54)	150(31)	53(11)	9(1)	1(—)	474
Sex with man with hemo-philia	62(87)	6(8)	2(2)	1(1)	—	71
Born in pattern II country	3(—)	532(98)	3(—)	1(—)	—	541
Sex with man born in pattern II country	6(12)	42(84)	1	—	—	50
Sex with transfu-sion recipient with HIV infec-tion	66(69)	11(11)	16(16)	1(—)	—	95
Sex with HIV-in-fected man: risk not speci-fied	167(30)	259(46)	120(21)	5(—)	2(—)	553

Data from Centers for Disease Control (1990, November). *HIV/AIDS weekly surveillance report.* Atlanta: CDC. *IVDU,* Intravenous drug user.

greater incidence of AIDS and Latina women have an 8.1 times greater incidence. The major exposure categories for black women are IV drug use and heterosexual contact (57% and 32%, respectively), whereas in Latinas the rates are 51% for exposure through IV drug use and 37% through heterosexual contact.

KNOWLEDGE, ATTITUDES, AND PRACTICES

Because HIV infection is such a problem among black and Latina women, research on the knowledge, attitudes, and practices within these groups is beginning. Flaskerud and Nyamathi (1989) interviewed poor black (n = 51) and Latina (n = 56) women about their knowledge, attitudes, and sexual and drug use practices related to AIDS. They found significant differences in knowledge and attitudes between the two groups; blacks had more knowledge and positive attitudes than Latinas, and La-tinas were more uncomfortable talking about AIDS than blacks. No statistically significant differences were found between groups on sexual and drug use practice. These investigators also noted that the majority from both groups denied IV drug use or having multiple sexual partners and that only 23% used condoms.

Increased fear about AIDS and negative attitudes regarding sexuality and drug use were associated with safer sexual and drug use practices among Latina women (Flaskerud & Nyamathi, 1989). This raises a question about a possible undesirable side effect of changing attitudes about AIDS in the Latina population: more favorable attitudes may increase the risk of adopting behaviors associated with becoming infected with HIV. Latina women may hold traditional beliefs about culturally specific gender roles. Traditionally in Latin cultures the male holds a dominant and protective role in family relationships. Communication regarding sex may be minimal or nonexistent. Women may define themselves primarily through their role as childbearer or mother (Karan, 1989). Attractiveness is associated with sexual purity (Worth & Rodriguez, 1987).

Twenty-two poor black women were interviewed about their beliefs regarding the cause of AIDS (Flaskerud & Rush, 1989). A majority of respondents believed that AIDS was a result of breaking religious and moral laws, a punishment for sin. Since 1% to 1.4% of the black population may be infected with HIV compared with 0.3% to 0.5% of the white population, black women having sexual relationships with black men are more likely to become infected with HIV through unprotected sex with an infected man (Lewis & Watters, 1989). The nurse should assess whether the specific client holds traditional beliefs about the causes of illness and whether interventions can be adapted so they are consistent with cultural practices yet decrease the risk of acquiring HIV infection.

INTRAVENOUS DRUG USE

At present most AIDS cases among women of childbearing age are related to IV drug use, either directly or indirectly through sexual contact with an IV drug user (Gayle et al., 1990). Chemically dependent women generally have low self-esteem, are not independent and autonomous, and are often in traditional roles in their relationships with men (Mitchell, 1990). They have more obstacles to overcome in protecting themselves from HIV infection. Alcohol and other drugs may relax inhibitions and result in unsafe needle-sharing and sexual practices (Karan, 1989). Cocaine use is associated with the acquisition of both HIV and syphilis, since women may trade sex for drugs. Women using cocaine may fail to use prenatal services (Minkoff et al., 1990b). Drug users are more susceptible to rape and physical abuse. Unlike sexual partners of male drug users, the women drug user's sexual partner probably also uses drugs. Female drug users often have irregular menses, which they may incorrectly interpret to mean that they are not fertile. These women often come from dysfunctional, abusive families. Their children often experience the effects of their drug use in utero and after birth may be hyperirritable and sickly. This heightens the difficulty in achieving adequate parenting skills and bonding between mother and baby.

Women in the black and Latina communities who use IV drugs are different from women in these cultural groups who do not use drugs. Worth and Rodriguez (1987), in a study of poor Puerto Rican women in New York City who used IV drugs, found that many were introduced to drug use between 12 and 14 years of age by men, by their parents, or in school. Most of these women had begun with the use of marijuana and pills and progressed to IV drug use by 15 or 16 years of age. When comparing black and white heterosexual IV drug users, Lewis and Watters (1989) found that white women were more likely to (1) share needles with a larger number of partners, (2) have four or more sexual partners, and (3) engage in anal intercourse. Black women were significantly less likely than white women to use any form of contraception. The nurse working with HIV-positive women who may currently use or previously have used drugs needs to intervene with respect to both the drug use and HIV problems. Consultation and referrals are the hallmarks of these services. Chapter 9 addresses the problems and treatments for IV drug users in detail.

SEXUAL PRACTICES

To paraphrase the former surgeon general, C. Everett Koop, barring abstinence, a condom is the only effective way to prevent the transmission of HIV infection. Since condoms are used to cover the penis and require the consent of the male sexual partner, women are often left with only one choice: abstinence. Even this choice is often unrealistic because of a variety of sexual, economic, cultural, and religious issues that may have an impact on a woman's decisions about her sexual behavior. Resistance to condom use is related to negative associations with promiscuity (Worth, 1989). In some cultures only prostitutes use condoms. For women who are socialized to believe that sex is natural, condom use may imply a decision to have unnatural or undesirable sex.

During sexual activity, HIV is transported by infected lymphocytes or macrophages in the seminal fluid into the mucous membrane of the vagina. Spermatozoa proceed to the cervical opening of the uterus in the attempt to fertilize the ovum. Barriers at the cervix, such as the diaphragm or spermicidal sponge, do not prevent contact of the infected semen with the vaginal walls. Withdrawal before ejaculation is ineffective, since HIV is in the clear fluid that often precedes male ejaculation (New York City

Department of Health, 1989). Douching after intercourse may facilitate movement of the infected semen into the uterus, so women should be counseled to avoid douching.

In one study of heterosexuals in San Francisco, men reported not using a condom during their last intercourse if (1) they had used alcohol or other drugs, (2) they were "in love" with their partners, (3) they experienced difficulty in communicating with their partners about condoms, and (4) their partners did not want to use condoms (Lindan et al., 1990). In the same study a lower incidence of condom use was associated with (1) being black, (2) the perception that condom use decreased sexual pleasure, (3) being "in love" with a partner, and (4) partners being unwilling to use condoms.

College-age women attending a large private university in the Northeast were asked about their sexual practices in 1975, 1986, and 1989 (DeBuono et al., 1990). Despite public health announcements suggesting that women limit their sexual partners and avoid anal intercourse, these behaviors did not change over the 14-year period. Condom use did increase from 21% in 1986 to 41% among sexually active college women in 1989. Thus safer sex messages have influenced the choice of contraceptive method in women of college age.

Women in preexisting relationships are particularly resistant to introducing condom use. Condoms for many individuals are symbols of sexual activity outside the relationship (Worth, 1989). A woman who does not use drugs and has one steady partner may not believe that she is at risk. This belief may be erroneous. Although the woman may be monogamous, her male sexual partner may live according to a different standard. In one study of male IV drug users with steady female partners, 83% reported multiple partners, 15% reported male-to-male sexual contact, 38% reported heterosexual anal intercourse, and 73% never used condoms (Lewis et al., 1990).

Even when the couple knows that one partner is HIV seropositive, condom use may be infrequent. In one United Kingdom study of heterosexual risk transmission when one partner was HIV positive, most vaginal intercourse occurred without the use of a condom (Johnson et al., 1989). In this study the HIV-positive person was male in 78 couples and female in 18 others. In two of the seropositive women, seroconversion was documented after one act of unprotected sexual intercourse.

To use or insist on the use of a barrier such as a condom, a woman needs to perceive that she is at risk of HIV infection. In New York City during 1988 and 1989, 1850 women between the ages of 15 and 44 years were interviewed and 89% of this sample of women assessed their personal risk of AIDS as very small or none at all (Stoneburner et al., 1989). A different study examined women living in a shelter for homeless single women in Brooklyn, New York. The overriding issues for these women were powerlessness, addiction (alcohol, drugs, and gambling), and violence and not personal risk for HIV infection. They reacted to the topic of AIDS by focusing on a search for the source of the infection: "there was a lot of accusation, blaming, and anger" (Kenny et al., 1990).

PREVENTION

To change behaviors in the community, educational and prevention programs must be culturally relevant to the community they serve (Flaskerud & Rush, 1989). Women with HIV infection are a diverse group. Many are poor, but others are not; many are black or Latina, but others are from different cultural groups; most are heterosexual, but some are lesbians; urban living is common, but HIV infection is growing in rural areas. The nurse should avoid generalizations in dealing with a woman who has HIV infection and should evaluate whether intervention is appropriate for that particular client.

Pretest and posttest measures indicated that one educational intervention was successful in changing knowledge about AIDS over time in a group of poor black and Latina women (Flaskerud & Nyamathi, 1990). In this program, either a black or a Latina nurse educator presented a 12-minute English or Spanish slide-tape educational program on AIDS. Participants also received a brochure on AIDS and a community resource guide that described AIDS service organizations. This educational program was initially successful at changing attitudes and practices related to AIDS, but these changes regressed somewhat over a 3-month period. This educational program was short and didactic; an experiential format may be more successful in retaining change over time.

Forty percent of a large sample of women in New York City reported changes in behavior in response to the AIDS epidemic (Stoneburner et al., 1989). These changes included (1) being more selective in their choice of sex partner, (2) reducing their number of sex partners, (3) starting or increasing the use of condoms, (4) establishing a mutually monogamous relationship, and (5) refraining from any sexual activity. Factors associated with changing behaviors to reduce HIV risk were higher socioeconomic status, having been tested for HIV antibody, knowing someone infected with AIDS, and perceiving themselves at risk for HIV. Fourteen percent of the women attributed occasional use or nonuse of condoms to a partner's refusal.

A woman trying to introduce condom use may be physically abused or abandoned. Even though the man's behavior may place the dyad at risk for HIV infection, he may blame her for infecting him if she is the first person in whom HIV is diagnosed. Contact notification of partners is an important way of slowing HIV transmission. Table 10–2 outlines some of

TABLE 10–2. Resistance to Condom Use in Heterosexual Relationships

Cultural

Belief that condoms are a symbol of promiscuity
Passive role of women in sexual decision making
Embarrassment associated with obtaining condoms

Economic

Fear of loss of financial support from sexual partner for self and children
Expense involved in buying condoms and contraceptives

Mechanical

Feelings of vaginal and urinary irritation both from condom and from nonoxynol 9
Creates artificial barrier during intimate behaviors
Condom failure secondary to (1) improper application, (2) breakage, and (3) slipping off
as penis is removed

Psychologic

Denial of risk since not aware of behaviors of sexual partner
Reluctance to introduce with steady partners because of implication of mistrust
Feelings of powerlessness when partner refuses to use
Uncertainty about whether condom will truly protect against HIV transmission

the problems and resistance women may experience related to the use of condoms.

Little attention has been given to barriers in HIV transmission that depend on the woman for their use (Stein, 1990). Some possibilities of barrier protection methods applied by the woman are the female condom, dental or latex dams, and topical agents inserted into the vagina. The female condom (Fig. 10–1) consists of a soft polyurethane sheath with two flexible rings. The ring at the closed end is inserted into the vagina and anchored under the pubic bone, similar to the diaphragm. The ring at the other end is much bigger and covers the labia and base of the penis (Rispin, 1989). Dental or latex dams are flat squares of latex, often 6 inches by 6 inches, that come in different colors and may have fruit or candy flavors. These squares are held in place over the external genitalia during oral sex by either partner. Both the female condom and dental dams are difficult to buy. They are not usually sold at the local drugstore. Some consumer groups have advocated the use of plastic wrap such as Saran Wrap during oral sex (New York City Department of Health, 1989), but the pores within the plastic wrap may allow passage of HIV. Both the female condom and the latex dam require consent from the sexual partner, since the external genitalia are covered.

Spermicides or topical creams and foams that are inserted into the vagina are usually available at the drugstore and do not necessarily require consent of the woman's sexual partner. Barriers that depend exclusively on the woman may not be as efficacious as condoms but may be better

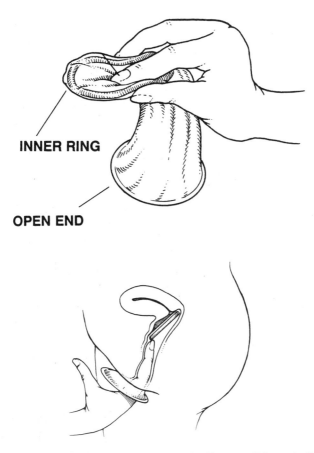

FIGURE 10–1. Insertion of the Reality vaginal pouch. (Courtesy Wisconsin Pharmacal Company, Chicago, Ill.)

than no barrier at all. Some contraceptive creams and foams contain non-oxynol 9, which is known to be effective in killing HIV. The barrier or the spermicide can irritate the penis or vagina, especially if one partner is allergic to the substance being used (Schaaf et al., 1990). No in vivo research exists at present as to the effectiveness of using a contraceptive vaginal cream or foam with nonoxynol 9 versus no protection. In vitro research had demonstrated that nonoxynol 9 kills the virus and therefore may be considered effective on its own. Research is needed to address the question of the effectiveness of a vaginally inserted spermicide containing nonoxynol 9 used with a condom versus without any other barrier.

Since theoretically the spermatozoa could proceed to the cervical os without being surrounded by infected seminal fluid, a virucide that would be inserted in the vagina has been proposed (Stein, 1990). This virucide would kill HIV without killing the sperm, thus allowing the possibility of pregnancy while preventing transmission of HIV. No vaginal virucides currently exist, and whether development of one is planned is not known.

Artificial insemination is another source of infection for women. Transmission of HIV through artificial insemination has been documented (CDC, 1990b). In one case a woman was inseminated three times with semen from her HIV-seropositive hemophiliac husband. His semen had been treated to remove HIV. No other risk behavior existed in this case, since the couple reported protected sex and did not engage in oral or anal intercourse. However, the woman became HIV seropositive. Since there is no procedure that reliably eliminates HIV from semen, the CDC (1990b) advises against artificial insemination when the donor is HIV positive.

HIV is also transmitted by blood. Infected women should be counseled about safely disposing of their menstrual products and using bleach solutions to remove blood from their underpants. Like men, they should be advised to keep their toothbrushes and razors separate from those of other family members and reassured that HIV is not spread through casual contact.

Prevention of HIV transmission for lesbians has a different focus. Lesbians are particularly at risk for HIV infection during oral sex if one partner is menstruating. Barrier protection is recommended for all oral sex and unprotected hand or finger to vagina or anus contact if cuts are present on the hand. Lesbians should be instructed to use barriers to the exchange of vaginal secretions, urine, feces, menstrual blood, or breast milk (Women's AIDS Network, 1988).

The issues surrounding prevention of HIV in women are not simple ones. Nurses need to be clear about their personal beliefs and open to hearing about the situation from the woman's perspective. This can be challenging when the woman is acting in ways the nurse believes are irresponsible. Judging the behaviors of others and giving advice are easy, but it is much more difficult to respect the client by helping her make realistic changes within her existing constraints. The nurse does not have to agree with the woman's choice but rather to create an environment in which the woman can feel safe to explore alternatives.

CLINICAL MANIFESTATIONS IN WOMEN

Literature and research on the presentation of HIV infection in women are sparse (New Jersey Women & AIDS Network, 1990). This lack of reliable information poses formidable burdens for the health care provider. Anecdotes and misinformation provide an insufficient data base on which to build appropriate interventions. As an illustration of the confusion about HIV infection and its manifestations in women, contrast "women with AIDS most frequently present with Pneumocystis carinii pneumonia" (Poole, 1988, p. 33) with "PCP is significantly less likely in women than in men with AIDS" (Carpenter et al., 1989, p. 775). Providers need to check research findings against clinical data and question any inconsistencies.

Women with other sexually transmitted diseases, such as syphilis, should be considered at risk for HIV infection and presented with the issues surrounding the decision about taking the HIV antibody test. Evidence suggests that genital ulcer diseases such as genital herpes, chancroid, genital warts, syphilis, and possibly *Chlamydia* infection and gonorrhea increase the risk of HIV transmission during sexual activity (New Jersey Women & AIDS Network, 1990).

HIV infection should be considered as a differential diagnosis in women with persistent or unusually severe pelvic inflammatory disease (PID), herpes simplex virus (HSV), *Candida* vaginitis, or human papillomavirus and neoplasia. When any of these conditions is characterized by unusual severity, resistance to treatment, or frequent recurrences, a concurrent HIV infection is a possibility.

PID includes endometritis, salpingitis, tuboovarian abscess, and pelvic peritonitis. Symptoms of PID include bilateral sharp, cramping pain in the lower quadrants; fever; chills; purulent vaginal discharge; irregular menstrual bleeding; malaise; and nausea and vomiting. In some cases the women may have normal laboratory findings and no symptoms (Schober, 1986). Many cases of PID are associated with *Neisseria gonorrhoeae* infections, but *Chlamydia* should also be considered. PID is confirmed by laparoscopy, but since this diagnostic procedure is often unavailable, women are frequently treated empirically with antibiotics. Depending on the severity of the case, women should be advised that hospitalization with parenteral antibiotics is the strategy of choice, especially if the woman is interested in future pregnancies. However, some providers are reluctant to treat PID aggressively in HIV-seropositive women. Sterility is a common sequel to untreated PID, and the health care provider may perceive this as a desirable outcome in HIV-positive women.

Recurrent or persistent HSV infection is associated with an increased risk of HIV infection. Higher doses of acyclovir may be needed to control the infection and achieve remission. Symptoms often recur when the medication is discontinued, and the drug may not be effective when it is resumed. Suppressive therapy may be necessary for chronic HSV.

HIV infection should be considered a possibility in all women with recurrent or persistent vaginal candidiasis. *Candida* is part of the normal flora of the mouth, intestines, and vagina in healthy women. Infection occurs when there is overgrowth (Schober, 1986). Fungal overgrowth causing infection seems widespread in HIV-positive women. Antifungal treatment provides only temporary relief even when medications are continued for long periods. Some women with recently diagnosed HIV infection report months of unsuccessful treatment for *Candida* vaginitis. These women also report that the health care provider never discussed the possibility of HIV infection with them and never suggested HIV antibody testing. Although severe vaginal candidiasis may be associated with advanced HIV infection, the CDC does not consider this presentation to be an AIDS-indicator disease (Anastos & Marte, 1989). Consequently, AIDS may be grossly underdiagnosed in women. Vaginal candidiasis may precede oral thrush. Table 10–3 presents assessment and intervention strategies for women with *Candida* vaginitis.

A strong association exists between HIV infection and abnormal Papanicolaou (Pap) smears (CDC, 1990c). HIV-infected woman have a high prevalence of cervical and vaginal cytologic abnormalities (Schrager, 1990). HIV enters cervical and vaginal secretions by sloughing of HIV-infected cells from the cervix. HIV-infected women often have mild, chronic cervicitis (Allen, 1990). They may be at significant risk of cervical cancer because they have a high prevalence of cervical intraepithelial neoplasia and human papillomavirus (McCann, 1990). More study is needed before this relationship can be established definitively (Schrager et al., 1989). The nurse should instruct women with abnormal Pap smears about the importance of repeating this test every 4 to 6 months (Allen, 1990) to rule out cervical cancer. When the Pap smear shows abnormalities, the possibility of HIV infection should be considered.

A retrospective chart review of 24 women with AIDS in Rhode Island during June 1982 and June 1988 yielded interesting data about AIDS in women. In this small sample the most common (38%) AIDS-defining event was *Candida* esophagitis; 25% had constitutional disease or wasting and 13% had *P. carinii* pneumonia (Carpenter et al., 1989). *Candida albicans* infections were the most frequent fungal infections and were documented in 23 of the 24 patients. Viral infections occurred in 20 of the 24 patients; the most frequent were genital and perianal herpes infections. Kaposi's sarcoma did not develop in any of the women in this study. The authors compared survival rates in men and women with AIDS and concluded that "the clinical course of AIDS in women is no worse, and may be better, than that in men" (p. 774). This conclusion is different from that offered by another author: "Clearly, women with AIDS, especially pregnant women with AIDS, have a more fulminant course than men" (Allen, 1990, p. 558).

Kaposi's sarcoma in women is probably related to infection through sexual activity with bisexual partners. Kaposi's sarcoma is four times more common in women with bisexual partners than in women with partners in other HIV risk groups (Beral et al., 1990). This evidence lends support to the proposal that Kaposi's sarcoma may be caused by a sexually transmitted infectious agent.

Since the presentation of HIV is different in women, treatment strat-

TABLE 10–3. *Candida* Vaginitis

Medical diagnosis: *Candida* vaginitis
Nursing diagnosis: Alteration in comfort related to recurrent vaginal *Candida* infections

Assessment

1. Assess for the presence of symptoms.
   a. Thick, white, curdy, cottage cheese–like discharge
   b. Vaginal pruritus
   c. Vaginal wall inflammation
   d. Discharge with pH of 4.5 or lower
   e. No vaginal odor (Schaaf et al., 1990)
2. Determine prior response to treatment.
3. If HIV positive, determine CD4/CD8 counts and ratio.
4. Assess whether other risk factors are present such as the use of birth control pills or antibiotics, pregnancy, or diabetes.
5. Determine whether symptoms are related to menstrual cycle, especially menstrual period.
6. Determine whether partner also has symptoms because treatment of both will then be indicated.

Planning and Intervention

1. Provide safe environment in which woman can describe her symptoms.
2. Obtain vaginal discharge for culture.
3. Discuss self-help strategies.
   a. Wearing cotton underpants
   b. Avoiding tight-fitting clothing
   c. Avoiding spreading anal secretions to vaginal area both during sex and after bowel movement
   d. Avoiding douching and use of feminine hygiene products
   e. Minimizing sugar, sweets, and refined foods in diet
   f. Killing yeast on underpants by boiling, bleaching, ironing, or if damp, microwaving for 5 minutes (Hackney, 1990)
4. Determine whether woman wants to use alternative therapies such as vinegar rinse; garlic vaginal suppositories; acidophilus vaginal suppositories, or 2 acidophilus tablets daily for 1 week starting after the course of antibiotics is completed; yogurt tablets into vagina or plain, unsweetened yogurt with applicator into vagina; golden seal and myrrh douche (Gardner, 1989).
5. Discuss prescriptive therapies with physician, such as miconazole intravaginal cream 2% or suppository (100 mg) every day for 7 days; nystatin intravaginal cream or tablet (100,000 units) twice a day for 7 days; clotrimazole intravaginal cream (1%) or tablet (100 mg) every day for 7 days; ketoconazole 200 mg po twice a day for 5 to 7 days (Bartlett, 1990); and fluconazole.
6. Teach woman how to insert suppository or applicator and make sure that she understands technique.

Evaluation

1. Woman shares feedback about the effectiveness of different strategies.
2. Sexual partner does not reinfect the woman.
3. Barriers are used during sexual activity to prevent transmission of HIV and other organisms.

egies may need to be adapted accordingly. Medication doses may need to be decreased in women, who often have smaller body surface areas than men. The CDC should examine its diagnostic criteria for AIDS and determine whether female-specific conditions should be included. An AIDS diagnosis, although often devastating, can result in access to a variety of social services and entitlements that may be denied to an HIV-infected person who does not meet the established criteria.

HIV INFECTION AND PREGNANCY

According to the CDC (1990a), 81% of women with AIDS are between the ages of 20 and 44 years. Decisions about pregnancy assume great importance during those years. A woman infected with HIV should avoid using oral contraceptives because they may hasten disease progression. Intrauterine devices should be discouraged because they may increase transmission of the virus to the woman's sexual partner (Allen, 1990). HIV-AIDS has further complicated an already complex issue.

Pregnancy may be associated with a decrease in cell-mediated immunity (Nanda & Minkoff, 1989). Research has demonstrated a significant decrease in relative and absolute number of T-helper lymphocytes (CD4 cells) during pregnancy, with a return to normal levels by the fifth postpartum month (Nanda & Minkoff, 1989). HIV also decreases the number of T-helper cells, and therefore it was initially believed that pregnancy would adversely affect the health of an HIV-positive woman (Minkoff, 1987). However, more recent studies do not support the claim that HIV infection progresses more rapidly during pregnancy (Coyne & Landers, 1990).

Many women seek confirmation and treatment from the health care system when they suspect that they are pregnant. The CDC recommends HIV testing of women who are at risk of infection through IV drug use or unprotected sexual contact with an HIV-infected partner. Nonspecific symptoms such as fatigue, anorexia, and weight loss are common in both pregnancy and HIV infection. A woman may not know that her sexual partner engaged in behaviors that placed her at risk. The impact of learning of HIV infection during pregnancy is unique and overwhelming (Minkoff, 1987). The health care provider needs to be sensitive to the issues that are important to the client.

Health care providers should be aware of their own values about continuing or terminating pregnancy in HIV-seropositive women and of how these values may influence their relationship with the client. When a pregnant woman learns that she is positive for HIV early in the pregnancy, she may choose to terminate the pregnancy. Since many women with HIV are poor and only 12 states in the United States provide Medicaid funds to poor women seeking abortions (Mitchell, 1988), this option may be severely limited.

Other factors also influence the decision to continue the pregnancy. Sixty-four infected and HIV-positive women with a history of IV drug use were asked about their decision to continue or terminate pregnancy (Selwyn et al., 1989). Half of the women infected with HIV chose to have an abortion. Neither perceived personal risk of becoming sicker nor concern about AIDS was associated with terminating pregnancy. The most compelling reasons were financial problems, conflicts with work or school, and family concerns. The most important reasons for continuing the pregnancy were the desire for a child and religious beliefs. These researchers found that IV drug users may perceive pregnancy as a symbol of self-esteem, an affirmation of life, and an opportunity to leave behind a legacy.

Timing is crucial in the decision to terminate a pregnancy. In one study 27 of 82 pregnant HIV-positive women learned their test results early enough in pregnancy to consider abortion (Holman et al., 1989). All were counseled about the issues surrounding HIV and pregnancy. Four of these women chose to abort, citing concern about their health, reluctance to risk having an infected child, or both these reasons. One of the four women was unable to secure an abortion. She wanted the abortion performed on an outpatient basis, but available facilities had policies against doing outpatient abortions on women who were taking methadone.

Health care for a pregnant HIV-infected woman depends on her stage of HIV infection. For the most part management of pregnancy in an asymptomatic or mildly symptomatic woman does not differ from standard prenatal care (Connor et al., 1989). Case finding for other infectious and bloodborne diseases such as gonorrhea, syphilis, or infection with hepatitis B virus, *Chlamydia*, HSV, cytomegalovirus, or papillomavirus should be done because of similar routes of transmission. Infection with *Mycobacterium tuberculosis* should always be considered in an HIV-positive person. Since pregnancy may depress immune function, reactivation of latent infections such as HSV, cytomegalovirus, and *Toxoplasma* can be a problem. Baseline antibody titers of the last two should be obtained to assist in diagnosis if symptoms appear (Minkoff, 1987).

Medications are limited during pregnancy because of potential adverse effects on the fetus. Acyclovir during pregnancy may not be safe (Minkoff, 1987). Zidovudine (Retrovir) rapidly crosses the placenta (Lopez-Anaya et al., 1990). Zidovudine probably has toxic effects on the fetus similar to those reported in young infants (Nicholas et al., 1989). However, whether zidovudine causes fetal harm is not known. Zidovudine should be given to a pregnant woman only if clearly needed (Burroughs Wellcome, 1990).

Prophylaxis against *P. carinii* pneumonia during pregnancy may decrease the risk of hypoxic damage to the fetus (Landesman, 1989), but the use of teratogenic drugs such as trimethoprim and most antiviral agents should be avoided unless the mother has a life-threatening illness (Rutherford et al., 1987). Pentamidine isethionate (NebuPent) should not be given to a pregnant woman unless the potential benefits are judged to outweigh the unknown risk. Whether pentamidine isethionate can cause fetal harm is not known (Lyphomed, 1989).

Monitoring the woman's medication blood levels during pregnancy is essential because the physiologic changes of pregnancy alter the excretion and sometimes the metabolism of drugs (Mitchell, 1990). Most pregnant women are routinely excluded from research clinical trials of new drugs because of the potential adverse effect on the fetus. These facts should be presented to the woman so that she can understand why medications are not being offered.

Both European and American studies have shown that complications of pregnancy in HIV-positive women are similar to those in noninfected women (Henrion, 1988). Studies with matched samples of HIV-infected and noninfected pregnant women have found that factors other than HIV infection, such as drug use and poverty, have adverse effects on pregnancy. Numbers of CD4 cells decrease in both infected and HIV-negative women during pregnancy and then increase at delivery. However, the numbers of CD4 cells are about 10% to 20% lower in the HIV-positive women (Landesman, 1989).

Current thinking is that pregnancy may be complicated in women with advanced cases of HIV disease. Women with T4 lymphocyte counts of fewer than $300/mm^3$ have a much greater risk of serious infections during pregnancy (Minkoff et al., 1990a). In a longitudinal study of 16 women, five had serious problems during pregnancy, including opportunistic infections, pneumonia, and a postpartum abscess requiring two operations (Landesman, 1989). A retrospective review of data from state health departments, state maternal mortality study committees, and the national surveillance programs for AIDS at the CDC, as well as national mortality data from the National Center for Health Statistics, identified 20 unpublished cases of women who died of AIDS during pregnancy or within 1 year after termination of pregnancy (Koonin et al., 1989). All of the pregnancies had obstetric complications, two resulted in stillbirths, and all live-born infants were delivered prematurely. Four women died undelivered during pregnancy. Sixteen (80%) died of P. carinii pneumonia. These findings highlight the importance of both identifying HIV-positive women and staging their infection to manage their health care during pregnancy with careful attention to preventing problems.

Gloeb and colleagues (1988) conducted a retrospective chart review of 50 pregnant women with HIV infection. Two women became pregnant twice, accounting for 52 births studied. Fifteen mothers had uncomplicated antenatal courses, three died of complications from AIDS either during pregnancy or 4 months after delivery, and three experienced fetal death. Preterm labor occurred in 35% of the women. There were 36 vaginal deliveries among 34 patients; the remaining women had cesarean deliveries of which 12 were primary sections for complications and 4 were repeat sections. Fourteen women experienced postpartum complications.

As HIV infection advances, the woman may experience more complications during delivery because of concurrent infections and body system damage. Pulmonary, cardiac, renal, and liver dysfunction caused by progressive HIV infection complicates the use of medications during delivery, fluid management, and the physical capabilities of the woman to tolerate the stress of labor (Connor et al., 1989). If the woman has HIV-associated dementia, her decision making will be impaired. Anemia is common in HIV-positive persons, and thrombocytopenia may increase the impact of blood lost during delivery. Monitoring of the fetus during labor is more difficult, since use of internal scalp electrodes and measurement of scalp pH is avoided to maintain the integrity of the fetus' scalp as a barrier to infected vaginal secretions. External fetal monitoring devices should be used when feasible (Minkoff, 1987). Table 10–4 presents a summary of some of the issues surrounding HIV infection and pregnancy.

A major focus during the delivery period should be avoidance of occupational exposure. Suction devices used to clear the neonate's airway, such as the DeLee, which uses mouth suction, should be replaced by mechanisms that use wall or bulb suction. Care should be delivered in a manner that protects both the client and the provider.

During 1989, 5600 HIV-infected women gave birth in the United States (Pediatric, Adolescent & Maternal AIDS Branch, 1990). The percentage of infected babies of HIV-infected mothers seems to be remaining stable at between 30% and 50%. The process of vertical transmission, or transmission of HIV from the mother to the unborn fetus, remains unclear. Three mechanisms have been proposed: transplacental, exposure to maternal blood and vaginal secretions at time of delivery, and breast milk. Intrauterine exposure appears to present the greatest risk by far (Valente & Main, 1990). There is no difference in rates of HIV infection between babies delivered vaginally and those delivered by cesarean section.

That only 30% to 50% of the offspring of HIV-infected women are infected with HIV suggests that some women have a circulating protective factor, such as neutralizing antibodies, that prevents or limits placental involvement (Valente & Main, 1990). Possibly the stage of HIV infection in the woman has an impact on whether the fetus will be infected (Nicholas et al., 1989). Women who are clinically ill are more likely to transmit HIV to their babies. Risk of HIV transmission varies inversely with maternal CD4 T cell count. Other factors such as maternal CD4 + to CD8 + ratio, beta$_2$-microglobulin level, interleukin-2 (IL-2), and serum IL-

TABLE 10-4. Pregnancy in HIV-Positive Woman

ASSESSMENT	FACTORS TO CONSIDER
1. Whether pregnancy is wanted	1. Sociocultural values. 2. Social support, especially from father of child or current sexual partner 3. Presence of other well children
2. Knowledge of HIV and pregnancy	1. Stage of HIV infection 2. Feelings about baby being possibly infected 3. Access to prenatal care 4. Willingness to adopt positive health behaviors 5. Concerns over personal health
3. Decision about continuation or termination of pregnancy	1. Stage of pregnancy 2. Religious beliefs 3. Economic resources 4. Access to abortion services 5. History of previous abortions 6. Feelings about transmitting HIV infection to unborn baby

2R along with the maternal stage of HIV infection and the virulence of a given HIV strain all seem to influence vertical transmission (Coyne & Landers, 1990).

Women who delivered term infants were less likely to transmit HIV to offspring if they had high reactivity of antibody to gp120 (Coyne & Landers, 1990). Ongoing research indicates that premature infants born to infected women are at higher risk for vertical transmission of HIV infection than full-term infants born to these women. Also, pregnant women with high levels of anti-gp120 antibodies were at less risk of transmitting infection to their infants than women with low or absent levels of this antibody against HIV (Pediatric, Adolescent & Maternal AIDS Branch, 1990). If a specific biologic marker can be associated with preventing vertical transmission of HIV, pregnant women could be injected with this substance.

Breast milk has been implicated as a mode of transmission for HIV. In the United States where other sources of infant food are readily available, women should be counseled to avoid breast feeding. In pattern II countries, such as those in Africa, other sources of food are not available, and therefore breast feeding is still encouraged, since otherwise the baby will starve to death long before HIV disease develops.

Many unanswered questions about HIV infection in pregnant women remain. These questions include whether HIV infection has an impact on the overall health of the mother, whether pregnancy influences disease progression, and whether HIV-positive women whose offspring develop AIDS and die experience a faster disease progression than HIV-positive women with healthy offspring and others. The National Institutes of Child

Health and Human Development created the Pediatric, Adolescent, & Maternal AIDS Branch in July 1988 to address some of these issues. This branch is coordinating a multifaceted research program that should provide answers to some of the questions. This is also a fertile ground for nursing research.

CONCLUSIONS

Often HIV infection is not diagnosed in women because many health care providers are reluctant to consider that a specific woman may be infected (Dennenberg, 1990). This reluctance to assess HIV infection in women has had serious consequences for the infected women and has led to "failure to diagnose" malpractice suits against the health care providers involved. Effective treatment depends on accurate diagnosis, and an HIV antibody test is a relatively inexpensive way to arrive at a diagnosis. AIDS in women is often misdiagnosed, and women may die without AIDS being diagnosed.

Failure to diagnose AIDS in women may be related to countertransference, which occurs when the provider identifies with the client (Macks, 1988). Most nurses are women and find it easy to identify with HIV-infected women. They may be in a similar age group or from a similar cultural background. The infected women may engage in behaviors familiar to the provider, such as a monogamous relationship with a man who has not used drugs for many years. Some providers react to the anxieties produced by countertransference by distancing themselves from clients, whereas others overidentify with them. Some female providers feel frustrated or angry with female clients who find it difficult to make changes in their sex lives (Macks, 1988).

Working with women with HIV infection evokes deep feelings and makes health care providers question their values and perspective on life. In order to continue to care for others, providers need to take care of themselves by scheduling time for fun, setting limits, and recognizing that no one has control over another's life or decisions. The issues of women and HIV infection will multiply as more women are infected. Nurses need to pace themselves for the long run.

References

Allen, M. (1990). Primary care of women infected with the HIV. *Obstetrics and Gynecology Clinics of North America, 17*(3), 557–569.

Anastos, K., Marte, C. (1989). Women—the missing persons in the AIDS epidemic. *Health/ PAC Bulletin 19*(4), 6–13.

Bartlett, J. (1990). *Pocketbook of infectious disease therapy.* Baltimore: Williams & Wilkins.

Beral, V., Peterman, T., Berkelman, R., et al. (1990). Kaposi's sarcoma among persons with AIDS: A sexually transmitted infection? *Lancet 335*(8682), 123–128.

Burroughs Wellcome Co. (1990). Product information monograph: Retrovir (zidovudine). Research Triangle Park, NC: The Company.

Carpenter, C., Mayer, K., Fisher, A., et al. (1989). Natural history of AIDS in women in Rhode Island. *American Journal of Medicine 86*(6 Pt. 2), 771–775.

Centers for Disease Control (1990a, August). *HIV/AIDS weekly surveillance report*. Atlanta: CDC.

Centers for Disease Control (1990b). HIV-1 infection and artificial insemination with processed semen. *Morbidity and Mortality Weekly Report, 249,* 255–256.

Centers for Disease Control (1990c). Risk for cervical disease in HIV infected women—New York City. *Morbidity and Mortality Weekly Report, 39*(47), 846–849.

Chu, S., Buehler, J., Berkelman, R. (1990). Impact of the HIV epidemic on mortality in women of reproductive age, United States. *Journal of the American Medical Association, 264*(2), 225–229.

Connor, E., Bardeguez, Apuzzio, J. (1989). The intrapartum management of the HIV infected mother and her infant. *Clinics in Perinatology, 16*(4), 899–908.

Coyne, B., Landers, D. (1990). The immunology of HIV disease and pregnancy and possible interactions. *Obstetrics and Gynecology Clinics of North America, 17*(3), 595–606.

DeBuono, B., Zinner, S., Daamen, M., et al. (1990). Sexual behavior of college women in 1975, 1986, and 1989. *New England Journal of Medicine, 322*(12), 821–825.

Dennenberg, R. (1990). Women and HIV related conditions. *Community Research Initiative, Treatment and Research Forum, 1*(2), 3–5.

Flaskerud, J., Nyamathi, A. (1989). Black & Latina women's AIDS related knowledge, attitudes, and practices. *Research in Nursing and Health, 12*(6), 339–346.

Flaskerud, J., Nyamathi, A. (1990). Effects of an AIDS education program on the knowledge, attitudes and practices of low income Black and Latina women. *Journal of Community Health, 15*(6), 343–355.

Flaskerud, J., Rush, C. (1989). AIDS and traditional health beliefs and practices of Black women. *Nursing Research, 38*(4), 210–215.

Gardner, J. (1989). *The new healing yourself.* Freedom, CA: The Crossing Press.

Gayle, J., Selik, R., Chu, S. (1990). Surveillance for AIDS and HIV infection among black and hispanic children and women of childbearing age, 1981-1989. *Morbidity and Mortality Weekly Report, 39*(SS-3), 23–30.

Gloeb, D., O'Sullivan, M., Efantis, J. (1988). HIV in women, the effects of HIV on pregnancy, *American Journal of Obstetrics and Gynecology, 159*(3), 756–761.

Hackney, A. (1990). Women's health section, *American Journal of Nursing, 90*(9), 17.

Henrion, R. (1988). Pregnancy and AIDS. *Human Reproduction, 3*(2), 257–262.

Holman, S., Berthaud, M, Sunderland, A., et al. (1989). *Seminars in Perinatology, 13*(1), 7–15.

Johnson, A., Petherick, A., Davidson, S., et al. (1989). Transmission of HIV to heterosexual partners of infected men and women. *AIDS, 3*(6), 367–372.

Karan, L. (1989). AIDS prevention and chemical dependence treatment needs of women and their children. *Journal of Psychoactive Drugs, 21*(4), 395–399.

Kenny, M., Leonard, T., Pack, C., et al. (1990). Qualitative methods in AIDS prevention for women in New York City. Paper presented at a meeting of the Society for Applied Anthropology, York, England, Apr. 1990.

Koonin, L., Ellerbrock, T., Atrash, H., et al. (1989). Pregnancy-associated deaths due to AIDS in the United States. *Journal of the American Medical Association, 261*(9), 1306–1309.

Landesman, S. (1989). HIV in women: An overview. *Seminars in Perinatology, 13*(1), 2–6.

Lewis, D., Watters, J. (1989). HIV seroprevalence in female IV drug users: The puzzle of black women's risk. *Social Science Medicine, 29*(9), 1071–1076.

Lewis, D.K., Watters, J.K., Case, P. (1990). The prevalence of high-risk sexual behavior in male intravenous drug users with steady female partners. *American Journal of Public Health, 80*(4), 465–466.

Lindan, C., Kegeles, S., Hearst, N., et al. (1990). Heterosexual behaviors and factors that influence condom use among patients attending a sexually transmitted disease clinic— San Francisco. *Morbidity and Mortality Weekly Report, 39*(39), 685–689.

Lopez-Anaya, A., Unadkat, J., Schumann, L., et al. (1990). Pharmacokinetics of zidovudine (azidothymidine). I. Transplacental transfer. *Journal of Acquired Immune Deficiency Syndromes, 3*(10), 959–964.

Lyphomed Co. (1989). Product information, NebuPent. Rosemont, IL: The Company.

Macks, J. (1988). Women and AIDS: Countertransference issues. *Social Casework, The Journal of Contemporary Social Work, 69*(6), 340–347.

McCann, J. (1990). Anal, cervical cancers increasing in HIV infected. *Oncology & Biotechnology News, 4*(8), 16.

Minkoff, H. (1987). Care of pregnant women infected with HIV. *Journal of the American Medical Association, 258*(19), 2714–2717.

Minkoff, H., Willoughby, A., Mendez, H., et al. (1990a). Serious infections during pregnancy among women with advanced HIV infection. *American Journal of Obstetrics and Gynecology, 162*(1), 30–4.

Minkoff, H., McCalla, S., Delke, I., et al. (1990b). The relationship of cocaine use to syphilis and HIV infections among inner city parturient women. *American Journal of Obstetrics and Gynecology, 163*(2), 521–526.

Mitchell, J. (1988). Women, AIDS, and public policy. *AIDS and Public Policy Journal, 3*(2), 50–51.

Mitchell, J. (1990). Treating HIV-infected women in chemical dependency programs. *AIDS Patient Care, 4*(4), 36–37.

Nanda, D., Minkoff, H. (1989). HIV in pregnancy—transmission and immune effects. *Clinical Obstetrics and Gynecology, 32*(3), 456–466.

New Jersey Women & AIDS Network (1990). *Me first! Medical manifestations of HIV in women.* New Brunswick, NJ: The Network.

New York City Department of Health (1989). *A woman's guide to AIDS.* New York: The Department.

Nicholas, S., Sondheimer, D., Willoughby, A., et al. (1989). HIV infection in childhood, adolescence, and pregnancy: A status report and national research agenda. *Pediatrics, 83*(2), 293–308.

Pappaioanou, M., George, J., Hannon, W., et al. (1990). HIV seroprevalence surveys of childbearing women—objectives, methods, and uses of the data. *Public Health Reports, 105*(2), 147–52.

Pediatric, Adolescent, & Maternal AIDS Branch, Center for Research for Mothers and Children, National Institute of Child Health and Human Development (1990, June). *Report to the National Advisory Child Health and Human Development Counsel.*

Poole, L. (1988). Women and HIV infection. In G. Gee & T. Moran (Eds.), *AIDS: Concepts in nursing practice* (pp. 25–40). Baltimore: Williams & Wilkins.

Rispin, P. (June 8, 1989). Female condom rates high in trials. *Dimensions, V International Conference on AIDS*, p. 3.

Rutherford, G., Oliva, G., Grossman, M., et al. (1987). Guidelines for the control of perinatally transmitted HIV infection and care of infected mothers, infants, and children. *Western Journal of Medicine, 147*(1), 104–108.

Schaaf, V., Perez-Stable, E., Borchardt, K. (1990). The limited value of symptoms and signs in the diagnosis of vaginal infections. *Archives of Internal Medicine, 150*(9), 1929–1933.

Schober, M. (1986). Gynecologic and urinary problems. In J. Griffith-Kenney (Ed.), *Contemporary women's health* (pp. 588–602). Menlo, CA: Addison-Wesley.

Schrager, L. Friedland, G., Maude, D., et al. (1989). Cervical and vaginal squamous cell abnormalities in women infected with HIV. *Journal of Acquired Immune Deficiency Syndrome, 2*(6), 570–5.

Selwyn, P., Carter, R., Schoenbaum, E., et al. (1989). Knowledge of HIV antibody status and decisions to continue or terminate pregnancy among IVDU. *Journal of the American Medical Association, 262*(24), 3567–3571.

Shapiro, C., Schulz, S., Lee, N., et al. (1989). Review of HIV infection in women in the United States. *Obstetrics and Gynecology, 74*(5), 800–808.

Sperling, R., Sacks, H., Mayer, L., et al. (1989). Umbilical cord blood serosurvey for HIV in parturient women in a voluntary hospital in NYC. *Obstetrics and Gynecology, 73*(2), 179–81.

Stein, Z. (1990). HIV prevention: The need for methods women can use. *American Journal of Public Health, 80*(4), 460–462.

Stoneburner, R., Fordyce, J., Balanon, A., et al. (1989). Women and AIDS: A survey of knowledge, attitudes and behaviors; Final report. New York: Kasanjian Consultants.

Valente, P., Main, E. (1990). Role of the placenta in perinatal transmission of HIV. *Obstetrics and Gynecology Clinics of North America, 17*(3), 607–616.

Willoughby, A. (1989). AIDS in women: Epidemiology. *Clinical Obstetrics and Gynecology, 32*(3), 429–436.

Women's AIDS Network (1988). *Lesbians and AIDS: What's the connection?* San Francisco: San Francisco AIDS Foundation.

Worth, D. (1989). Sexual decision-making and AIDS: Why condom promotion among vulnerable women is likely to fail. *Studies in Family Planning, 20*(6), 297–307.

Worth, D., Rodriguez, R. (1987). Latina women and AIDS. *SIECUS Report, 15*(1), 5–7.

11

Infection Control

Nancy B. Parris

HIV infection is transmitted through sexual contact with infected persons and direct inoculation of contaminated blood products. It can also be transmitted perinatally from mother to neonate. AIDS is not casually or easily spread. Although only blood, semen, vaginal secretions, and possibly breast milk have been implicated in the transmission of AIDS by epidemiologic evidence, HIV has been isolated from many other body fluids, such as saliva, tears, cerebrospinal fluid (CSF), and urine. Therefore all body fluids are presumed to be potentially infective in the discussion of precautions that should be taken when caring for HIV-infected persons. This discussion of precautions taken in the workplace, however, refers only to blood and body fluid contact, since sexual contact is not relevant in this setting.

When providing patient care all nurses and other health care workers must consider any patient to be potentially infected with HIV or other bloodborne pathogens. Therefore appropriate and sensible infection control precautions should be taken at all times. This chapter reviews precautions that should be followed with all patients infected with HIV regardless of whether they have clinical AIDS or not. The same precautions should be taken when in contact with *all* body fluids from *all* patients to avoid percutaneous and mucous membrane exposure. Accidental needlestick exposure poses the greatest hazard to health care workers; donning appropriate garb is not adequate protection. Too often a needlestick injury has occurred when the nurse was in full isolation garb, feeling protected and comfortable, but gloves and a gown do not protect against a needlestick. Health care workers should use common sense in following the recommended guidelines but should never become lackadaisical in their approach to infection control, as can occur when they perform procedures by rote.

When caring for any person requiring isolation precautions or when taking precautions with any patient's body fluids, the health care worker must always consider the patient. Observing good infection control prac-

TABLE 11-1. Barrier Precautions

Gloves prevent contact with and exposure to:
  Body fluids
  Articles contaminated with body fluids
  Mucous membranes
  Nonintact skin
Gowns or aprons protect:
  Clothes from soiling with body fluids
Masks and protective eyewear protect:
  Mucous membranes
  Nonintact skin from splashing or spraying
Handwashing prevents or reduces:
  Transient colonization with nonresident microbial flora
  Resident flora

---

tices and thereby minimizing the risk of exposure to infectious diseases is consistent with the objective of providing high-quality patient care.

PRECAUTIONS FOR NURSES

Precautions have been established to protect nurses and other health care workers from exposure to blood and other body fluids from patients with AIDS and HIV infection, thereby preventing the opportunity for transmission of HIV. Exposure refers specifically to percutaneous or mucous membrane contact with infected blood or other body fluids. Distinguishing exposure from routine contact is important, since ample data indicate that there is no risk of transmission of HIV from contact without exposure (Gerberding et al., 1987; Henderson et al., 1986; Hirsch et al., 1985; Kuhls et al., 1987; Weiss et al., 1985). These studies have demonstrated that health care workers having prolonged contact with patients with AIDS did not show evidence of HIV infection.

Blood and body fluid precautions should be followed for all patients with diagnosed disease as well as those with suspected AIDS, AIDS-related complex (ARC), and HIV infection (CDC, 1987a). The Centers for Disease Control (CDC) has suggested further that these protective barriers, referred to as "universal blood and body fluid precautions" or "universal precautions," be used consistently for all patients. "Body substance isolation" is an alternate system of precautions that accomplishes the same objectives as universal precautions. These precautions are described in more detail later in this chapter. Use of precautions is especially important when the infection status of a patient is unknown.

The guidelines that follow in this chapter are similar to the CDC's blood and body fluid precautions, also called "disease-specific isolation precautions for patients with AIDS," and outline the measures to be followed. The recommended precautions are aimed at preventing the transmission of HIV (Besner et al., 1986; CDC, 1985, 1987a, 1987b; Eickhoff et al., 1984; Garner & Hughes, 1987; Gerberding et al., 1986; Harris, 1986; Jackson et al., 1986; Jackson & Lynch, 1989; Martin et al., 1985; Spire et al., 1984).

Since patients with AIDS are often infected with other organisms, appropriate precautions against transmission of those infections must also be taken. For many of the other infections no additional precautions are required because they are transmitted in the same way as HIV (e.g., hepatitis B) or because they are not transmitted from person to person (e.g., toxoplasmosis). If the patient has pulmonary tuberculosis and has not yet received appropriate treatment, additional precautions will be needed to prevent the transmission of tuberculosis. Precautions to be taken with other infections are not discussed here; the appropriate precautions recommended by the CDC should be followed.

GUIDELINES FOR PRECAUTIONS

Gloves. When contact with a patient's body fluids is anticipated, appropriate protective barriers (i.e., gloves, cover gown, mask, and protective eyewear) should be used routinely to prevent percutaneous and mucous membrane exposure (Table 11–1). Disposable examination gloves should be worn when any blood or other body fluids are handled, but they are not necessary for direct care of patients when there is no contact with body fluids. They are also needed when touching mucous membranes and nonintact skin and for handling items or surfaces contaminated with body fluids. For example, examination gloves should be worn when handling feces of an incontinent patient and when cleaning the patient following use of the toilet, but they are not necessary when assessing vital signs of that patient or any other patient.

Gloves should be worn when the nurse is starting an intravenous (IV) infusion because of potential contact with blood. When phlebotomy is performed, gloves should be worn under the following circumstances: when performing heel or finger sticks on infants or children, when exposure to blood is anticipated, when the nurse has cuts, scratches, or other breaks in the skin, and when receiving training in phlebotomy. Gloves are not necessary when the IV bag, bottle, or tubing is changed or when fluid is added to a burette; they are not needed for transport of a patient, since any drainage or secretions should be adequately contained before transport. Gloves are not necessary for ambulating or bathing a patient.

Gloves should be changed after each contact with each patient. Thorough handwashing following removal and disposal of the gloves is essential. Surgical or examination gloves should never be washed or disinfected for reuse. This may enhance penetration of fluids through undetected holes and may cause deterioration of the gloves.

Disposable examination gloves adequately protect the health care worker's skin from exposure to body substances and any microorganisms present as long as the gloves are not torn. Purchasing special gloves exclusively for use with HIV-infected patients is not necessary because they provide no additional protection and serve no practical purpose. The gloves should be properly fitted; rings that might tear through the glove should not be worn and nails should not be so long as to poke through the gloves. No differences in barrier effectiveness between intact latex and intact vinyl used to manufacture gloves have been reported (Bienvenido et al., 1989; CDC, 1988b; Zbitnew et al., 1989); however, some nurses find that latex gloves fit better than vinyl gloves and therefore give them greater dexterity. The type of glove should be appropriate for the task being performed. Otherwise, the choice between vinyl and latex is an individual one that has no bearing on the overall protection of the health care worker (Table 11–2).

Handwashing. Intact skin is an effective barrier against infection for health care workers. Hands should be washed immediately after being soiled with any body fluids, since handwashing is the single most important means of preventing infection. This applies to all occasions of caring for patients with HIV infection, as well as patients with any other problem or illness. Good handwashing, including cleaning underneath fingernails, between fingers, and beneath any allowable rings, is essential between patient contacts and immediately following removal of any type of gloves. During care of patients jewelry should be kept to a minimum, since it hinders good handwashing and use of gloves. Jewelry that has ridges or stones or that may interfere with proper handwashing should not be worn.

Proper handwashing includes use of warm running water, plenty of soap, friction over all surfaces of both hands, thorough rinsing, and paper towels to turn off faucets so as to avoid recontamination of hands. Special antimicrobial soaps are not necessary; most important is having a soap that is acceptable to staff and that they will use.

Gowns. Wearing protective gowns or aprons is recommended only for contact that might cause the health care worker's clothing to become soiled with body fluids. Since AIDS is not transmitted by fomites and therefore not via contaminated clothing, wearing a protective garment is actually more an issue of esthetics than of protection from infection. As with the examples in the section on gloves, a cover gown is not routinely needed when the health care worker is taking vital signs or feeding or ambulating a patient. On the other hand, use of a gown or apron might be desirable for emptying a bedpan, cleaning a patient who is incontinent of urine and feces, changing a dressing that involves a great deal of drain-

TABLE 11–2. Guidelines for the Appropriate Use of Latex and Vinyl Gloves

Gloves are worn to provide a barrier that helps to:
  Protect the health care worker from acquiring infections
  Prevent the health care worker from transmitting infections to patients or others

Nonsterile Gloves

Should be worn when performing procedures that involve the direct contact of the hands
  with the body fluids of a patient, during the care of a patient, or when handling soiled
  articles
Should be procedure specific, that is, the gloves should be worn only *during* the procedure and then discarded

Vinyl Gloves

Applies to most routine procedures requiring gloves
Indications for use include cleaning up a blood spill

Latex Gloves

Applies only to procedures requiring a high degree of manual dexterity
Indications for use are rare; they might include starting a difficult-to-insert intravenous
  line

Specialized Gloves for Chemotherapy

Should be worn only when performing procedures specifically requiring these gloves

Sterile Gloves (Latex)

Should be worn only when performing procedures requiring strict sterile technique
Should *not* be worn by persons who are outside of the sterile field
Applies to all procedures performed in operating and delivery rooms and to specific pro-
  cedures in other patient care areas
Indications for use other than during surgery or delivery include changing a wound
  dressing or inserting a Foley catheter

age, and performing any procedures that may generate splashes of body fluids. Cover gowns are not necessary when a patient is transported because any drainage or secretions should be adequately contained before transport. Some institutions now require their health care workers to wear a water-resistant apron for protection of clothing rather than the traditional cloth or disposable paper long-sleeved cover gown. Either is adequate as long as it protects clothes from contamination. Once worn, a gown should be discarded into the proper receptacle and not reused.

Masks and Protective Eyewear, or Face Shields. Masks and protective eyewear or face shields should reduce the incidence of contamination of mucous membranes of the mouth, nose, and eyes. Since HIV is not transmitted by the airborne route, masks are not necessary as a routine precaution. However, in one documented case a health care worker was infected with HIV when blood from a patient with AIDS splashed into the worker's mouth. To prevent this type of exposure the worker may wear a mask in certain instances as a barrier to cover the mouth and nose from any splashing body fluids. At the same time, protective eyewear or face shields should be worn as a barrier for the eyes. Both should be worn to protect the eyes, mouth, and nose during procedures that may generate droplets of blood or body fluids. Such procedures include suctioning of a patient, assisting with bronchoscopy or endoscopy, and assisting with surgery in which high-powered drills may generate spraying of particles. The masks and eyewear should be worn only during the procedure for which they are indicated. The exception is during surgery, in which masks and protective eyewear are worn at all times, the mask serving to protect both the patient from the health care worker and the health care worker from the patient. The choice between protective eyewear and face shield depends on the nurse's preference. Some favor goggles or glasses, since the optics of the face shield may be slightly distorted because of the curve of the plastic. Others prefer the face shield because it is one barrier item rather than two and allows better visualization of the health care worker's face.

Protective eyewear not only should provide a shield in front of the eyes and be large enough to be worn over prescription eyeglasses, but also should have protective sides and a top shield and be configured so that the bottom of the lenses angle toward the face for maximum protection. Some health care workers prefer goggles, which should be vented, although an eyeglass that satisfies the foregoing criteria is often more acceptable and less offensive to both patients and staff. Masks are worn once and discarded; reusable protective eyewear must be cleaned and disinfected following each use if eyewear is shared among staff. This protects subsequent users of the eyewear not only from any organisms that may splash onto the front of the lenses, but also from any infection the previous wearer may have.

Nurses are involved in several hospital procedures and routines that require special precautions with patients to prevent exposure. Other situations cause concern to nurses regarding the potential for exposure (Table 11–3).

Needles and Sharps Disposal. To date, of the few cases of HIV infection in health care workers, most have resulted from accidents with or improper handling of needles and sharps. Gloves reduce the incidence of contamination of hands, but they cannot prevent penetrating injuries caused by needles or other sharp instruments. Therefore extreme caution should be taken to avoid any accidental injuries caused by needles, scalpels, or other sharp instruments or devices. Needles should never be recapped, bent, or broken and should not be handled in such a manner as to cause a puncture injury. Once used, needles and sharps should be discarded immediately into a rigid puncture-proof container; they should never be left unattended on countertops or other surfaces. Disposal containers should be placed at convenient and accessible sites to encourage

TABLE 11–3. Procedure Precautions

Needles and Sharps

Do *not* recap, bend, or break
Avoid accidental puncture injuries

Cardiopulmonary Resuscitation

Use resuscitation bag or
Use mask with one-way valve

Transport

Standard procedures are adequate

Dishes

Nondisposable dishes and utensils are adequate

Laboratory Specimens

Standard procedures for all infective and potentially infective materials are adequate

immediate disposal of needles and sharps following their use. Once filled, the sharps containers should be closed securely and discarded with no further handling of the contents.

Any accidental needlestick, puncture injury, or exposure to broken skin from articles contaminated with blood or other fluids from any patient should be immediately attended. The site should be bled initially, then washed well with an antimicrobial soap. If the incident involves blood or body fluids splashed into the mucous membranes of the eyes, nose, or mouth, the area should be flushed immediately with water. The incident should be reported to the facility's occupational health department with follow-up according to the CDC's recommended protocol (Table 11–4).

Cardiopulmonary Resuscitation. Although the risk of infection with HIV as a result of performing cardiopulmonary resuscitation (CPR) is minimal and no cases of transmission of infection from mouth-to-mouth resuscitation have been documented, alternatives to direct mouth-to-mouth resuscitation should be available not only for use with patients who have HIV infection but for all patients. The available alternatives are a hand-held resuscitator bag or a protective mask with a one-way valve. This equipment should be readily and constantly available on every unit or in every patient room. Plastic mouth and nose covers with filtered openings may provide a degree of protection against transfer of oral fluids and aerosols. The use of these devices is more important in preventing exposure to other communicable diseases in addition to AIDS, since saliva has not been implicated in HIV transmission (Cummins, 1989; Emergency Cardiac Care Committee, 1989).

Transporting the Patient. No special precautions are required in transporting a patient with AIDS or HIV infection. Any open draining wounds

TABLE 11–4. Postexposure Follow-Up

Protocol for the follow-up of accidental needlestick exposures to biologic specimens of HIV-seropositive individuals:
1. Clinical assessment and determination of HIV infection risk factors
2. Routine postexposure care
3. HIV antibody testing of employee and source patient for confirmation (with consent)
4. Counseling concerning the risk of HIV infection and prevention of its transmission
5. Instructions to report all illness in the next 6 months

If the health care worker does not develop illness consistent with HIV infection:
1. HIV antibody testing 6 months following exposure
2. This may be prolonged if the person has taken zidovudine prophylaxis
3. If seronegative, may stop follow-up

If the health care worker develops illness consistent with HIV infection:
1. Clinical assessment
2. HIV antibody testing (repeat monthly × 3)
3. Complete blood cell and differential counts
4. Consider other laboratory tests to rule out other etiologies of illness
5. Close follow-up

Data from Kuhls, T.L., Cherry, J.D. (1987). Readers' forum: The management of health care workers' accidental parenteral exposures to biological specimens of HIV seropositive individuals. *Infection Control* 8, 211–213.

should be adequately covered before transport. If secretions and drainage are contained, the need for transport personnel to wear a gown or gloves will be alleviated. Transport personnel need not wear a mask or protective eyewear, nor must the patient with HIV infection wear a mask.

Dishes. Patients infected with HIV do not require special dishes, glasses, or flatware for meals. Dishes, glasses, and utensils can be washed following routine procedure used with all other dishes. This should include hot water and detergent and fall within requirements set forth by local health departments for routine dishwashing.

Laboratory Specimens. All blood and body fluid laboratory specimens should be treated as infective, including laboratory specimens from patients with HIV infection. Specimen containers should be well constructed with the lid always securely sealed to prevent leakage during transport. Care should be taken when collecting the specimen to avoid contaminating the outside of the container. The container, once sealed, should be placed in a plastic bag for transport. The laboratory requisition should remain outside the bag so it is not contaminated by the specimen. Once the specimen is bagged, the person transporting the specimen does not have to wear gloves since he or she should have no contact with the contents. Specimens from patients infected with HIV should not be identified as "AIDS specimens." Implementation of universal precautions eliminates the need for warning labels on specimens, since specimens containing blood and body fluids from all patients are handled as if infective.

Precautions for Other Infections. Since AIDS involves a deficiency in the immune system, many HIV-infected patients also have other infections. These infections are often opportunistic, in which event no additional precautions are required. However, certain infections require further precautions. Any additional isolation precautions required for the additional infections must be observed. For example, if the patient has pulmonary tuberculosis, "tuberculosis isolation" or "acid-fast bacilli (AFB) isolation" procedures as recommended by the CDC are indicated. A patient with diarrhea requires "enteric precautions," as described by the CDC, in addition to precautions against transmission of HIV.

Pregnant Women. Many female nurses and health care workers have questioned whether pregnant women should provide direct care for patients with AIDS. The pregnant health care worker is at no greater risk of contracting HIV infection than the nonpregnant health care worker. However, if a pregnant woman is infected with HIV, the infant is at risk of infection through perinatal transmission. Meticulous adherence to the recommended precautionary techniques should be observed to prevent inadvertent exposure during routine patient care and subsequent risk of HIV infection. Furthermore, the pregnant health care worker is at no greater risk than a nonpregnant worker for other infections the patient with AIDS may have (e.g., cytomegalovirus).

UNIVERSAL PRECAUTIONS AND BODY SUBSTANCE ISOLATION

The CDC has recommended infection control and isolation precautions for hospitalized patients for many years. Their most recent guideline for isolation precautions in hospitals provided two alternative isolation systems: one that is category specific and includes the category "blood and body fluid precautions" and another that is disease specific, in which specific barrier precautions are indicated for each disease listed (CDC, 1988b). The purpose of disease-specific precautions is to minimize unnecessary precautions that occur with the category-specific system. In both of these systems, infectious diseases are listed and precautions necessary to interrupt the transmission of each are indicated, either by category or by listing all needed barriers. The concept includes posting a sign on the patient's door or by the bed, indicating precautions to be followed but not the patient's diagnosis. One of the infectious diseases listed in this guideline is AIDS, which falls into the blood and body fluid category of precautions. The specific precautions needed to interrupt the transmission of AIDS and HIV infection are outlined in this chapter.

Because a nurse or caregiver may not be aware that a patient is infected with HIV or some other bloodborne infection such as hepatitis B virus, the CDC recommends that blood and body fluid precautions, or those barrier precautions necessary to interrupt the transmission of HIV and other bloodborne infections, be taken with all patients, or universally. These measures are now commonly known as "universal precautions" or "universal blood and body fluid precautions." Precautions are taken with blood, tissue, and body fluids associated with the transmission of bloodborne pathogens, which includes CSF, pleural fluid, peritoneal fluid, pericardial fluid, synovial fluid, and amniotic fluid. Feces, nasal secretions, sputum, sweat, tears, urine, and vomitus are included only if they contain visible blood, since the risk of transmission of HIV or hepatitis B from these materials is extremely low or nonexistent.

The CDC has always encouraged hospitals to modify and tailor infection control recommendations to meet their own needs, and "body substance isolation (BSI)" is such a system (Lynch et al., 1987). The concept of this system includes treating all blood and other body substances of all patients as potentially infective, including feces, urine, and saliva at all times, which is one way this differs from universal precautions. Signs are not placed on the individual rooms of patients with known infectious diseases notifying persons of barrier precautions necessary in the care of that patient. Instead, a sign reminding all persons of barrier precautions to take with all patients is placed on *each* patient room and health care workers do not know which patients have an infectious disease.

The purpose here is not to debate the merits of the two systems but to describe their basic differences. Both systems protect workers caring for patients both known and not known to have AIDS, HIV, or other infection. Both systems are currently in use at various institutions around the country. The basic concept behind both is the same, that of protecting the health care worker, protecting the patient, ensuring patient privacy, and protecting other patients from cross-infection. Which system is in place in any institution is secondary; more important is understanding the need for following specific barrier precautions outlined herein with all patients, since that concept is truly universal.

ENVIRONMENTAL CONSIDERATIONS

Although no environmentally mediated mode of HIV transmission has been documented, routine procedures and precautions should be followed with all patients (CDC, 1987a). Procedures for cleaning and disinfecting the patient's environment are generally those routinely used for all patients (Table 11–5). Although this section focuses on the hospital

TABLE 11-5. Environmental Precautions

Cleaning the Room
Standard cleaning procedures are adequate

Trash
Standard procedures for infective trash are adequate

Linen
Standard procedures for soiled linen are adequate

Sterilization and Disinfection
Standard procedures are adequate

---

environment, the same principles apply to a long-term care facility or the person's environment at home.

Cleaning the Room. Standard cleaning procedures are recommended both while a patient with HIV infection occupies the room and when the patient leaves the room on discharge, transfer, or death. Neither HIV nor other infections are transmitted as a result of soiled walls, ceilings, floors, countertops, and other environmental surfaces; therefore total decontamination or other extraordinary cleaning is not necessary. Any articles or surfaces visibly soiled with body fluids should be cleaned with a germicide solution as soon as possible after exposure. Disinfectant fogging is neither necessary nor recommended.

Waste. No epidemiologic evidence suggests that improper disposal of hospital waste has caused disease in the community. Therefore identification of wastes for which special precautions are indicated is largely a matter of judgment about the relative risk of disease transmission, as well as compliance with local and state regulations. Trash contaminated with blood and body fluids from HIV-infected patients should be handled in accordance with the facility's policy for all infective waste. This policy must define infective waste or identify waste with the potential for causing infection during handling and disposal and for which special precautions appear prudent. Although any item that has had contact with blood, exudates, or secretions is potentially infective, treating all such waste as infective is not usually considered practical or necessary. Blood, suctioned fluids, excretions, and secretions may be carefully poured down a drain connected to a sanitary sewer (i.e., a hopper, toilet, or utility sink). Sanitary sewers may also be used to dispose of other infectious wastes that can be ground and flushed into the sewer.

Handling waste defined as infective may require the use of two bags, specially marked as infectious or hazardous waste, of sufficient strength to prevent leakage of contents. It is not necessary to use a double-bag procedure (i.e., two nurses removing the bag from the patient's room, one wearing protective garb and the other holding a cuffed outer bag into which the linen or trash bag is placed). Special handling of trash once it leaves the facility may be required by county or state regulations. This generally involves incineration or decontamination by autoclave before final disposal in a sanitary landfill. Disposal of trash from a patient with AIDS or HIV infection is no different from routine handling of trash containing any infective material.

Soiled Linen. Soiled linen from a patient with AIDS does not need to be handled differently or separately from other soiled linen as long as it is properly and safely handled by all personnel coming in contact with it. It should be handled as little as possible and with minimal agitation to prevent gross microbial contamination of the air and of persons handling the linen. Soiled linen should be placed directly into the linen hamper at the location of use, not placed on the floor or on furniture in the patient's room. It should not be sorted or rinsed in the patient care areas. Any linen soiled with blood or other fluids should be placed in a leakproof bag.

Laundry room staff should handle all soiled linen in such a manner as to protect themselves from inadvertent exposure to any organisms contained within it, although risk of disease transmission is negligible. All laundry personnel handling soiled linen must wear protective garb, including gloves and water-resistant aprons. Linen washed with detergent in hot water (at least 71° C [160° F]) for 25 minutes, or in cool water (≤70° C [158° F]) with germicide suitable for low-temperature washing at proper use concentration, is decontaminated during the laundering; therefore the laundered linen can be used for any patient. There is no reason to dispose of or incinerate linen soiled with blood from a patient with AIDS or HIV infection.

The greatest risk of infection to laundry room personnel is from contaminated needles or sharp instruments accidentally left with the linen and subsequently injuring someone. Therefore health care workers must ensure that instruments and articles are not inadvertently sent with the soiled linen.

Sterilization and Disinfection. Standard procedures for disinfection and sterilization of equipment, instruments, and other articles are recommended. No additional steps need be taken, since properly followed disinfection or sterilization procedures destroy HIV. Studies have demonstrated that commonly used germicides rapidly inactivate HIV with routine use and at concentrations much lower than those used in practice (CDC, 1987a; Eickhoff et al., 1984; Garner & Simmons, 1983; Gerberding & University of California, San Francisco, 1986; Martin et al., 1985). It is neither necessary nor recommended that separate equipment or instruments be used exclusively for patients with AIDS or HIV infection.

Instruments or devices that enter sterile tissue or the vascular system of any patient or through which blood flows should be sterilized before reuse. Devices or items that come in contact with intact mucous membranes should be sterilized or receive high-level disinfection whereby all vegetative organisms and viruses are killed, although bacterial spores are not (CDC, 1987a). Hospital policy and manufacturer's specifications regarding use of any particular chemical sterilant should be followed. The chemical germicide or other method chosen for sterilizing or disinfecting a particular medical device depends on the manufacturer's specifications for compatibility of that device with the method or agent. At all times instruments or devices should be thoroughly cleaned before being exposed to a chemical germicide or other method of sterilization or disinfection to ensure that all organic material (e.g., blood and mucus) is removed. Otherwise, sterilization or disinfection may not be achieved. Disposable instruments or devices should never be reused unless guidelines set forth by the manufacturer are followed. The importance of this point was underscored by a recent outbreak of AIDS in hospitalized infants in the Soviet Union where disposable syringes were reused between infants even though the needles were changed.

HIV is extremely fragile and is rapidly inactivated after drying. It has been demonstrated that high concentrations of HIV may survive in the environment for several days under laboratory conditions. Routine cleaning of the environment, proper cleaning of soiled surfaces, and proper cleaning and decontamination of instruments and devices prevent this from being of any significance in the transmission of HIV. This does not create the need for any extraordinary cleaning or decontamination procedures but supports the need for adherence to proper procedures as described.

Blood or Body Fluid Spills. Gloves should be worn during cleanup and decontamination of a blood or body fluid spill. In most instances the proper procedure is removal of visible material, most likely with a paper towel. The area should then be decontaminated, preferably with a solution of 5000 parts per million (ppm) of sodium hypochlorite (a 1:10 dilution of household bleach). For large spills of cultured or concentrated infectious agents in the laboratory, the contaminated area should be flooded with a liquid germicide before cleaning, then decontaminated with fresh germicide.

SPECIAL AREAS IN THE HOSPITAL

Patient care may vary significantly in different areas of the hospital depending on the specific patient population (e.g., surgical units versus pediatrics, inpatient versus outpatient), or procedure or purpose (e.g., operating room versus delivery room versus dialysis unit). Nonhospital settings can also be the sites of health care delivery. Precautions may differ depending on the area under consideration (Table 11–6).

Inpatient Areas. All of the precautions described previously apply to inpatients. As inpatients, persons with AIDS, ARC, or HIV infection do not routinely require a private room to prevent the spread of their disease to other patients. Because of their immunocompromised status, however, they may need to be protected from other patients who have infections. If their condition is such that they cannot contain body fluids, persons with AIDS may be placed in an individual room. For example, the need for a private room may be due to a fulminating diarrhea that causes the patient to be incontinent of stool, or it may be due to central nervous system involvement that interferes with the patient's ability to handle personal secretions and excretions properly and hygienically. There are no special requirements as to positive or negative air balance for the room, since HIV is not airborne. Furthermore, there is no reason to restrict the patient to the room, unless the patient has pulmonary tuberculosis or some other infection requiring such restriction, or cannot contain or control his or her excretions and secretions. Unless restricted to the room for the aforementioned reasons, the patient may walk through the halls and use common lounges, treatment rooms, cafeterias, and lobby areas.

Separate toilet facilities are not required routinely for patients with AIDS, although they may be needed in certain instances, such as when the patient has diarrhea. No special procedure is needed for cleaning the toilet seat following its use by a patient with AIDS. Any toilet soiled with feces or urine should be cleaned using routine cleaning procedures before being used by another person, whether or not the person has AIDS.

Outpatient Departments. Essentially the same precautions apply in the outpatient departments as in the inpatient setting. Patients with AIDS or HIV infection may share a waiting area with other patients and may share bathroom facilities. Nurses should use appropriate barrier precautions; no additional precautions need be taken.

Operating Rooms. No additional preoperative precautions are necessary for patients with AIDS or HIV infection. The patient can be safely admitted to a multipatient preoperative room without risk of HIV infection to other patients. No special room is needed, nor is any special equipment required.

Since surgery involves exposure to large amounts of blood, the use of sharp instruments, and percutaneous and mucous membrane exposures, it is an area of particular concern. During surgery double gloving by the surgeon or other persons scrubbed for surgery is recommended (Gerberding et al., 1989). Puncture-resistant gloves are available, although their bulkiness may result in a loss of dexterity and for that reason they are not widely used. All other protective barriers and precautions de-

TABLE 11–6. Precautions for Special Areas in the Hospital

Special Areas

Inpatient units
Outpatient clinics
Emergency rooms
Operating rooms
Labor and delivery rooms
Dialysis units

Precautions

Universal blood and body fluid precautions
Standard infection control procedures
Availability of manual resuscitation equipment
Special caution in handling sharps
Routine cleaning procedures
Plastic sleeve for dialysis

---

scribed previously also apply to the operating room. For example, a circulating nurse who is counting and handling bloody sponges should wear nonsterile gloves; protective eyewear should be worn by all persons scrubbed for surgery who are at risk of having blood or body fluids splashed into their eyes. Protective eyewear or face shields that protect the eyes from all sides are especially important in the operating room.

Extreme caution with all sharp instruments is important to prevent an accidental puncture injury that may result in exposure to the virus. To prevent accidental puncture injuries to the surgeon and scrub nurse during the operative procedure, surgeons can pick up and set down the instruments from a Mayo stand set up for this purpose rather than having them passed. Since a good portion of needlestick injuries among surgeons involve the index finger of the nondominant hand, protecting this digit may greatly reduce the risk of injury and subsequent infection (Lowenfels et al., 1989). Needlestick is most often due to attempting to grasp a needle or guide its tip, and therefore this practice should be avoided. A torn glove should be removed and replaced as soon as possible.

Postoperatively the patient may be admitted to the postanesthesia room for recovery. Surgical instruments are washed and disinfected per hospital policy for a "contaminated" or infected case; trash and linen are handled according to routine policy for infective trash and linen. Routine procedures for cleaning the room are carried out before the next patient.

Labor and Delivery Rooms. Recommendations similar to those for operating room nurses should be followed in labor and delivery rooms. A patient with AIDS or HIV infection may share a labor room with another patient. During and following delivery, health care workers should wear gloves and a gown when handling the placenta or infant until the blood and amniotic fluid have been removed from the infant's skin. Gloves and gown should also be worn during postdelivery care of the umbilical cord. Meconium should not be aspirated by mouth suction.

Emergency Rooms and Emergency Transport. Emergency room and transport nurses encounter blood and body fluids under uncontrolled and emergent circumstances, causing many opportunities for exposure. Universal precautions must be observed with *all* emergency room patients. Standard emergency room procedures and routines should be carried out with adequate and appropriate barrier precautions taken for patients with infections of any kind, including HIV infection (CDC, 1989; Holloway, 1986). A patient with AIDS or HIV infection in an emergency room or in an emergent situation is treated no differently from one in an inpatient setting. The same precautions are indicated in the same instances. As mentioned previously, manual resuscitation equipment (masks and bags) should be available to staff at all times so that mouth-to-mouth resuscitation of a patient with respiratory arrest is not needed.

Dialysis Units. Patients with HIV infection who have end-stage renal disease and are undergoing maintenance hemodialysis or peritoneal dialysis can be safely dialyzed when infection control precautions are used. When dialyzing all patients, health care workers should routinely follow universal blood and body fluid precautions. A patient with HIV infection need not be isolated from other patients. During dialysis and especially when the patient is being attached to and removed from the dialyzer, there is considerable exposure to blood and accidents that cause blood splashing are not uncommon. Therefore additional protective measures should be taken for dialysis. A clear plastic bag with a hole at each end can be used to cover the arm and dialysis site (Corea, 1987). Then, if blood splashes, it is contained and should not contaminate anyone else. The dialyzer should be similarly covered with a plastic bag, since it may rupture and cause blood to splash. Routine procedures for care and cleaning of the dialysis equipment should be followed, with no additional precautions for persons with HIV infection. The dialysis fluid pathways of the hemodialysis machine are generally disinfected with 500 to 750 ppm of sodium hypochlorite for 30 to 40 minutes, or a 1.5% to 2% solution of formaldehyde overnight. The dialyzer may be discarded after a single use. If the dialysis center has a dialyzer-reuse program in which a dialyzer is issued to a single patient and removed, cleaned, disinfected, and reused several times for that patient, HIV-infected patients can be included in the program. A dialyzer should never be used on more than one patient.

NONHOSPITAL (ACUTE CARE) SETTINGS

Psychiatric Facilities. Many patients with HIV infection are treated in psychiatric facilities for either psychiatric disorders or problems resulting from central nervous system involvement with HIV. In this setting no special restrictions need be placed on patients with HIV infection (Table 11–7). They may share common rooms and dining facilities with other patients and staff. If the facility involves patients in their own food preparation, patients with HIV infection may participate and share responsibilities and duties with other patients. Their laundry can be washed in machines provided for all patients. Patients with HIV infection should not be restricted from group events and activities or from using the facility's swimming pool. As in other health care settings, the patient may need evaluation for the presence of unacceptable behaviors or any changes that result in inappropriate actions such as biting or lack of control of secretions or excretions. A patient demonstrating these behaviors may have to be isolated or segregated from other patients until the behavior subsides or can be controlled. The patient may need further evaluation to determine whether additional precautions are indicated. This should be done on an individual basis with no restrictions placed on any patient unless absolutely necessary.

Long-Term Care Facilities and Nursing Homes. Patients with AIDS or HIV infection can be safely cared for in long-term care facilities. No precautions in addition to those already mentioned are needed. Special attention should be paid to preventing decubiti or infection in patients with AIDS.

Home Care. Home care nurses may not know the HIV status of their clients. They should follow barrier precautions with all patients, as well as precautions similar to those mentioned previously (Bryant, 1986; Lusby et al., 1986; Visiting Nurse Service, 1990). If running water is not available for handwashing, a waterless gel or commercially available solution should be used. The nurse should carry this product at all times. Some situations that may require the use of gloves include working with incontinent patients; changing disposable pads, diapers, dressings, or perineal pads; providing mouth care or urinary catheter care; and irrigating indwelling urinary catheters or cystostomy tubes. Examination gloves should never be reused. Rubber household gloves or general purpose utility gloves used for housecleaning may be reused provided they are washed with soap and water before removal and decontaminated with a 1:10 dilution of household bleach if soiled with blood or body fluids. They should be discarded once they begin to deteriorate. Gowns, masks, and protective eyewear are seldom needed in home care. Some situations in which they may be useful are in removing or replacing dressings on large wounds with copious amounts of fluids; irrigating wounds, indwelling urinary catheters, or cystostomy tubes; suctioning the airway of a patient with copious secretions; or having direct sustained contact with a client who is coughing excessively and is unable to cover his or her mouth.

As mentioned previously, avoiding needlestick injury is of paramount

TABLE 11–7. Precautions for Nonhospital Settings

Settings

Psychiatric facilities
Long-term care facilities
Home care
Schools
Occupational settings

Precautions

Universal blood and body fluid precautions
Standard disinfection and cleaning procedures
Care with sharps
Attention to biting and injuries

---

importance. Needles or sharp instruments contaminated with blood should be disposed of safely. Laws concerning needle and sharp disposal vary among states and should be consulted, but in all instances needles and sharps must be placed in a rigid, puncture-proof, unbreakable container. A coffee can with a lid or a detergent or bleach bottle works well as an improvised container. The lid should be kept on the container, which should be labeled and placed out of the reach of children. When the container is full, a 1:10 solution of household bleach should be poured into it until all contents are covered to decontaminate the contents. The lid should be secured with tape. The container should be placed in a paper bag and discarded on the day of trash collection by being placed directly into the garbage can, in a manner consistent with local public health regulations (Table 11–8).

A plastic leakproof bag can be used for disposal of dressings and other disposable items, excluding needles and sharps. Feces, urine, vomitus, sputum, and other body wastes can be flushed down the toilet. A 1:10 dilution of household bleach is the most practical agent for cleaning environmental surfaces in the home. Additional information on the care of persons with AIDS in community settings can be found in Chapter 7. Chapter 4 presents a detailed account of the nursing management of AIDS in an adult client that is applicable to all settings.

School Settings. As few people as possible should be aware that a child has HIV infection; transmission is not casual and should not occur at the school. Therefore it is not necessary to inform teachers, administrators, parents, classmates, and other students of the child's diagnosis, since they are not at risk of transmission. When the child returns to school, a conference including the child's physician, the local public health officer, school nurse and the child's parents may be helpful. The only purpose of such a conference should be to deal with any special needs the child may have so that the nurse may more readily attend to the child if

TABLE 11-8. Disposal of Wastes for Home Care

Needle Disposal

Place needles, syringes and sharps in a rigid, puncture-proof, nonbreakable container, such as a coffee can or detergent or bleach bottle

Never recap needles or throw them directly into the trash

Keep the lid on the container

Label the container so as not to confuse with original contents

Keep out of reach of children

When full:

Fill container to cover contents with a 1:10 dilution of household bleach

Secure lid and seal with tape

Place in a paper bag

Place directly in garbage can on day of pickup

Disposal of Other Waste Materials

Place dressings, bandages, contaminated tissues, and other disposable items *excluding needles and sharps* in a plastic leakproof bag

For disposal, tie up bag and place in garbage can

Dispose of feces, urine, sputum, and vomitus directly into the toilet and flush

Do not dispose of feces, urine, sputum, and vomitus into a sink or directly into the garbage

---

a problem occurs. The child may participate in regular school activities unless the physician deems restrictions necessary for medical reasons.

Children with poor hygiene who are unable to control their excretions and secretions may need to be restricted from certain classroom activities, but only children with severe illness or those exhibiting certain unacceptable behaviors, such as biting others, should be prohibited from attending school. HIV-infected children must be assessed periodically for changes in mental status that may have an impact on their behavior and hygiene.

If a child with HIV infection sustains an injury, the nurse should take the same precautions as do nurses in other outpatient settings when in contact with the child's blood and body fluids. This includes wearing gloves when handling blood. Any objects contaminated with blood should be cleaned and disinfected immediately with a germicide.

In preschool areas, children should be prevented from sharing toys they might place in their mouths. This is especially important for children infected with HIV, although the role of saliva in the transmission of AIDS is not clear. If toys that the children place in their mouths are used, they should be washed, disinfected, and rinsed well with water before being given to other children. If the toy is made of hard plastic or a similar substance, it can be washed with soapy water, soaked for 10 minutes in bleach or another disinfectant, and then rinsed *well* to remove all traces of the disinfectant. If made of soft cloth, the toy should be washed in hot soapy water with bleach added, preferably in an automatic washing machine. Common sense should prevail when dealing with other similar objects.

Occupational Settings. The barrier precautions previously mentioned should be followed by occupational health nurses handling a company's industrial emergencies and work-related problems for persons with AIDS or HIV infection. Such employees may continue to work without restriction unless their physicians indicate otherwise. Co-workers should not be informed of the person's diagnosis.

RISK OF HIV INFECTION

Because of the high mortality rate associated with AIDS, health care workers working with patients with AIDS and people living with persons with AIDS have concerns and fears about acquiring HIV infection. Many employees (especially health care workers) who might be infected with HIV have fears about the possibility of transmitting the virus to patients or co-workers (Table 11–9). Research on the risk of infection to health care workers and household contacts is ongoing.

Health Care Workers. Several studies, including some in progress, demonstrate that the risk of acquiring HIV infection from occupational exposure is extremely low (Anonymous, 1984; CDC, 1988a; Flynn et al., 1987; Gerberding, 1989; Gerberding et al., 1986; Hadley, 1989; Henderson et al., 1986; Hirsch et al., 1985; Kuhls et al., 1987; McCray & Cooperative Needlestick Surveillance Group, 1986; Marcus & Cooperative Needlestick Surveillance Group, 1988; Neisson-Vernant et al., 1986; Oksenhendler et al., 1986; Stricoff & Morse, 1986; Weiss et al., 1985). By definition, "exposure" means actual percutaneous or mucous membrane exposure to the blood or body fluids of a patient with HIV infection, whereas "contact" refers to virtually any other activity between the health care worker and the patient with HIV. This may involve touching the patient, transporting the patient, performing a bed bath, giving postural drainage or physical therapy, and any other type of activity involved in providing routine care to a patient. No risk of acquiring HIV infection during routine contact with a patient with AIDS has been demonstrated, and a very low risk of infection (<0.4%) is associated with percutaneous or mucous membrane exposure to the blood or body fluids of a patient with HIV infection. To date, more than 1000 health care workers with percutaneous exposures to blood or mucous membranes of open wounds contaminated by blood or body fluids have been prospectively followed. Only a handful have become infected with HIV as a result of this exposure. Each of these individuals denied having risk factors other than the described work exposure. Those who did not have needlestick exposures had not observed barrier precautions at the time of the exposure resulting in infection;

TABLE 11-9. Risk of HIV Infection

Risk of HIV infection to health care workers or household contacts or from employees
  with AIDS or HIV infection requires:
  1. Actual percutaneous or mucous membrane exposure to blood or body fluids or
  2. Sexual contact

barrier precautions offer little protection to a health care worker following
a needlestick exposure. Despite these unfortunate cases, routine patient
contact that does not involve actual exposure cannot result in infection
with a virus transmitted blood to blood.

The risk of HIV infection to health care workers following an exposure
remains low. As stated previously, barrier precautions should prevent
exposure, and infection cannot occur without exposure.

Prophylaxis. No effective vaccine against HIV has been developed,
nor is there a proved prophylactic agent for postexposure treatment. Zidovudine, also known as azidothymidine, AZT, ADV, and Retrovir, is a
thymidine analogue that in vitro has been shown to inhibit replication of
some retroviruses, including HIV, by interfering with the action of viral
ribonucleic acid (RNA)-dependent deoxyribonucleic acid (DNA) polymerase (reverse transcriptase) and possibly also by other mechanisms
(CDC, 1990; Yarchoan et al., 1988). Zidovudine has been used for treatment
of adults with symptomatic HIV infection, including AIDS, and has been
shown to increase the length and quality of life of patients with advanced
HIV infection and AIDS. It may delay disease progression in patients with
less advanced HIV infection. Some institutions and physicians are now
offering this drug for postexposure prophylaxis following occupational
exposure to HIV.

A study to examine the efficacy of zidovudine prophylaxis for humans
after exposure to HIV included 84 health care workers with occupational
percutaneous, mucous membrane, or nonintact skin exposure to HIV-
infected blood (CDC, 1990; Henderson & Gerberding, 1989). None was
seropositive for HIV after at least 6 months of follow-up; 49 had been
given zidovudine, the others a placebo. The absence of seroconversions
in this small group is not unexpected, regardless of whether they took
zidovudine, since the risk of infection is approximately 0.4%. There are
anecdotal reports of a few individuals who took zidovudine following
occupational exposure and subsequently became infected with HIV, although the circumstances surrounding the exposures and period of time
before prophylaxis was given vary so much that no conclusion can be
drawn from these cases (Lange et al., 1990; Looke & Grove, 1990). Data
involving studies of laboratory animals are limited and are thought to be
inadequate to support or reject the hypothesis that zidovudine may be
effective prophylaxis for humans occupationally exposed to HIV. Studies

are examining the toxicity of the agent when used for occupational post-exposure prophylaxis.

Various regimens are followed for zidovudine prophylaxis following occupational exposure. No data are available yet to determine the efficacy or compare the toxicity of dosages. The regimens may vary from a 100 mg to 200 mg dose given every 4 hours either five or six times daily (some protocols elect to skip the 4 AM dose) for 4 to 6 weeks. Some clinicians have used an initial dose of 400 mg; others have prescribed treatment from 4 days to 4 months. The sooner the drug is started, the more chance it has to be effective; some institutions encourage health care workers to initiate treatment within 1 hour after exposure.

Zidovudine has some toxic and adverse effects, including granulocytopenia and anemia as the most frequently reported. Other symptoms include headache, nausea, insomnia, myalgia, diaphoresis, fever, malaise, anorexia, diarrhea, dyspepsia, vomiting, dyspnea, rash, and taste abnormalities. Less commonly reported side effects are polymyositis, peripheral neuropathy, and seizures.

Data from animal and laboratory studies are inadequate to establish the efficacy or safety of zidovudine for prophylaxis after occupational exposure to HIV. Reasons for using zidovudine as postexposure prophylaxis include the severity of the illness that may result from HIV infection, the documented antiviral effect in the treatment of persons with established HIV infection, the apparent reversibility of acute toxic effects when the drug is taken for short periods, and the suggestion from some animal studies that the drug may modify the course of some retroviral infections. Reasons not to use zidovudine for postexposure prophylaxis include a lack of data demonstrating efficacy for this purpose, limited data on toxic effects in uninfected persons, and carcinogenic effects in rats and mice.

Nurses and other health care workers need to be aware of the facts regarding use of zidovudine for postexposure prophylaxis so they can make a timely decision if confronted with this situation. They must take into account the risks and potential benefits. They should consider factors surrounding the exposure incident, including the type and route of exposure (percutaneous versus mucous membrane), the volume of fluid involved, and the concentration of virus in the source fluid (clinical versus research laboratory setting). Furthermore, the individual should be counseled regarding the risks of exposure and rationale for prophylaxis. If the health care worker decides to use zidovudine as postexposure prophylaxis, it should be initiated promptly following the exposure. Follow-up should include evaluating the person for drug toxic effects and HIV seroconversion. Monitoring for servoconversion may have to be extended for a longer period than that of a person with HIV exposure but not taking zidovudine.

Persons taking zidovudine should abstain from sexual intercourse or use an effective contraceptive because of the unknown but possible risk of teratogenesis associated with its use. Throughout the follow-up period, latex condoms should be used or abstinence from sexual intercourse should be practiced to prevent transmission of HIV to sexual partners.

HIV Screening of Patients. Much concern has been expressed about the need to identify patients with AIDS or HIV infection for the benefit of protecting health care workers. Although generally knowing everything possible about a patient's overall medical condition is desirable, nurses do not need to know a person's HIV antibody status to protect themselves, especially since some patients who are infected with HIV have a negative antibody test. In many states HIV antibody testing is illegal without the explicit consent of the patient, and in *all* instances posting a diagnosis on a patient's door breaches confidentiality and a patient's right to privacy. Observing good hygiene, infection control practices, and barrier precautions protects health care workers whether or not they are aware of the patient's diagnosis.

Patients with HIV infection need the same good-quality nursing care provided for all patients. Fear of AIDS does not protect a nurse. Knowledge and understanding of the transmission of HIV help the nurse deal rationally with precautions and offer protection from exposure and subsequent potential infection. The procedure, benefits, and risks of HIV antibody testing for patients are discussed in detail in Chapter 6.

Household Members. Studies have demonstrated that, without sexual contact, household contacts of infected patients have little increased risk of HIV infection, and none at all when a few guidelines are followed (Bryant, 1986; Lusby et al., 1986; Visiting Nurse Service, 1990). Good hygiene should be practiced to prevent transmission of all organisms within the home, especially to prevent infecting a person with AIDS with an opportunistic organism. Razors, toothbrushes, and other personal articles that may come into contact with blood or body fluids should never be shared.

A person with HIV infection need not eat from special dishes or with special utensils; routine washing in a dishwasher or soaking in hot soapy water removes and destroys the virus. As a matter of routine, household members should never eat from the same utensils or drink out of the same glass or cup.

The laundry of a patient with AIDS does not have to be segregated, since HIV is destroyed by hot water and soap in a washing machine. If clothing is soiled with blood or body fluids, bleach should be added to the water. There have been no documented cases of transmission of HIV via fomites (inanimate articles) other than contaminated needles. Even if clothing is soiled with infective blood, transmission of the disease would not occur with such contact.

Employees with AIDS. Much concern has been expressed about workers, especially health care workers, with AIDS or HIV infection. The only instance in which a health care worker could transmit AIDS to a patient would be when the patient has a high degree of trauma that would provide a portal of entry for the virus (e.g., during surgery) and when blood or serous fluid from the infected health care worker has access to the open tissue of the patient. Such a circumstance is rare, as is the chance that a health care worker will infect a patient or another employee. Therefore each situation involving HIV infection in an employee should be handled individually. Precautions to prevent transmission of HIV infection from health care workers to patients are simple. *All* health care workers should wear gloves for direct contact with mucous membranes or nonintact skin of *all* patients. Health care workers who have exudative lesions or weeping dermatitis should refrain from direct patient care and from handling patient care equipment until the condition resolves itself. Termination of the worker's employment is not necessary, and work restrictions are rarely indicated. Protecting the employee's privacy and information about his or her diagnosis is important. Numerous companies and corporations have established policies permitting persons with AIDS to continue working as long as they are physically able; the only limitations are in situations that would increase risk of opportunistic infection to the HIV-infected employee. Recent court cases have resulted in rulings protecting a person with an infectious condition from employee discrimination under certain circumstances. This applies to persons with HIV infection, since it is not casually transmitted or airborne. New CDC recommendations were released July 1991.

The CDC does not recommend work restrictions for personal service workers (e.g., hairdressers, manicurists, or others providing services that involve casual contact with their clients) or food workers solely on account of HIV infection, since no cases of HIV transmission have been documented in these settings. Employees should not be restricted from using equipment and facilities in the workplace, including telephones, toilets, drinking fountains, eating facilities, and office equipment.

Few work situations warrant HIV antibody screening of employees, and such screening is generally inadvisable, since it raises serious questions concerning employees' privacy rights. The primary indications for screening include follow-up of an exposure incident and obtaining and storing blood of persons in laboratories who work with concentrated virus.

Fear of AIDS may cause employees, including health care workers, to refuse to work beside or perform services for persons infected with HIV. Such situations include health care workers who refuse to care for patients with AIDS, office employees who will not work with other employees who are infected, and employees refusing to serve clients who have AIDS. In many of these situations legal action has been taken against the employee. The courts have maintained that the employer has an obligation to inform and educate the employee regarding the transmission of HIV if that employee is to work with clients or patients with AIDS. If an employee does not work directly with persons with AIDS but because of unfounded fear refuses to perform a part of his or her job, education about HIV infection and its transmission should precede any corrective action on the part of the supervisor. An employee who refuses to work is protected from dismissal or other disciplinary action only if the refusal is both reasonable and based on a good faith belief in the existence of an imminent threat of serious injury or death (Bayer, 1986; Matthews & Neslund, 1986; Mills et al., 1986). The most effective way to prevent this from occurring is by education of all employees about the transmission of HIV and methods of prevention in situations where it is possible (e.g., working with infected patients).

SUMMARY

The importance of education when dealing with AIDS and HIV infection cannot be stressed enough. The nurse in practice must know and understand how HIV is transmitted and the simple and practical methods to prevent transmission. Observing universal precautions with all patients is important, but even more important is understanding why the precautions have been established and how they halt transmission. Comprehension of these basic facts alleviates unfounded fears and enables people to deal more effectively and compassionately in any capacity with patients who have HIV infection.

References

Anonymous (1984). Needlestick transmission of HTLV-III from a patient infected in Africa. *Lancet, 1*, 1376–1377.
Bayer, R. (1986). Notifying workers at risk: The politics of the right-to-know. *American Journal of Public Health, 76*, 1352–1356.
Besner, J., Thiessen, M., Sutherland, R., Wiens, R. (1986). Acquired immunodeficiency syndrome (AIDS). *Alberta Association of Registered Nurses, 42*, 25–27.
Bienvenido, G., Yangco, M.D., Yangco, N.F. (1989). What is leaky can be risky: A study of the integrity of hospital gloves. *Infection Control and Hospital Epidemiology, 10*, 553–556.
Bryant, J.K. (1986). Home care of the client with AIDS. *Journal of Community Health Nursing, 3*, 69–74.
Centers for Disease Control (1985). Recommendations for preventing transmission of infection with human T-lymphotropic virus type III/lymphadenopathy-associated virus in the workplace. *Morbidity and Mortality Weekly Report, 34*, 681–695.
Centers for Disease Control (1987a). Recommendations for preventing HIV transmission in health-care settings. *Morbidity and Mortality Weekly Report, 36* (suppl.), 1S–18S.
Centers for Disease Control (1987b). Human immunodeficiency virus infection in transfusion recipients and their family members. *Morbidity and Mortality Weekly Report, 36*, 137–140.
Centers for Disease Control (1988a). Update: Acquired immunodeficiency syndrome and

human immunodeficiency virus infection among health care workers. *Morbidity and Mortality Weekly Report, 376*, 229–239.

Centers for Disease Control (1988b). Update: universal precautions for prevention of transmission of human immunodeficiency virus, hepatitis B virus, and other bloodborne pathogens in health-care settings. *Morbidity and Mortality Weekly Report, 37*, 377–388.

Centers for Disease Control (1989). A curriculum guide for public-safety and emergency-response workers: Prevention of transmission of human immunodeficiency virus and hepatitis B virus. Atlanta: CDC.

Centers for Disease Control (1990). Public Health Service statement on management of occupational exposure to human immunodeficiency virus, including considerations regarding zidovudine postexposure use. *Morbidity and Mortality Weekly Report, 39*, 1–14.

Corea, A. (1987). Discussion of departmental policies. UCLA Dialysis Unit. Unpublished.

Cummins, R.O. (1989). Infection control guidelines for CPR providers [editorial]. *Journal of the American Medical Association, 262*, 2732–2733.

Eickhoff, T.C., Axnick, K.J., Brimhall, D., et al. (1984). A hospitalwide approach to AIDS: Recommendations of the advisory committee on infections within hospitals. *Infection Control, 5*, 242–248.

Emergency Cardiac Care Committee of the American Heart Association (1989). Risk of infection during CPR training and rescue: Supplemental guidelines. *Journal of the American Medical Association, 262*, 2714–2715.

Flynn, N.M., Pollet, S.M., Van Horne, J.R., et al. (1987). Absence of HIV antibody among dental professionals exposed to infected patients. *Western Journal of Medicine, 146*, 439–442.

Garner, J.S., Hughes, J.M. (1987). Options for isolation precautions. *Annals of Internal Medicine, 107*, 248–250.

Gerberding, J.L. (1989). Risks to health care workers from occupational exposure to hepatitis B virus, human immunodeficiency virus, and cytomegalovirus. *Infectious Disease Clinics of North America, 3*, 735–745.

Gerberding, J.L., Bryant, C.E., Moss, A., et al. (1986). Risk of acquired immunodeficiency syndrome (AIDS) virus transmission to health care workers (HCW): Results of a prospective cohort study. Program of the Second International Conference on AIDS, Paris, France, p. 124. Geneva: WHO.

Gerberding, J.L., Bryant-LeBlanc, C.E., Nelson, K., et al. (1987). Risk of transmitting the human immunodeficiency virus, cytomegalovirus, and hepatitis B virus to health care workers exposed to patients with AIDS and AIDS-related conditions. *Journal of Infectious Diseases, 156*, 1–8.

Gerberding, J.L., University of California, San Francisco Task Force on AIDS (1986). Special report: Recommended infection-control policies for patients with human immunodeficiency virus infection—an update. *New England Journal of Medicine, 315*, 1562–1564.

Gerberding, J.L., Littel C., Brown, A., et al. (1989). Predictors of intraoperative blood exposures. Fifth International Conference on AIDS, Montreal, Quebec. Geneva: WHO.

Hadley, W.K. (1989). Infection of the health-care worker by HIV and other blood-borne viruses: Risks, protection, and education. *American Journal of Hospital Pharmacy, 46*, S4–S7.

Harris, L.J. (1986). A safe working environment for hospital nurses. *Quality Assurance, 36*, 237–238.

Henderson, D.K., Gerberding, J.L. (1989). Post-exposure zidovudine chemoprophylaxis for health-care workers experiencing occupational exposures to the human immunodeficiency virus: An interim analysis. *Journal of Infectious Diseases, 160*, 321–327.

Henderson, D.K., Saah, A.J., Zak, B.J., et al. (1986). Risk of nosocomial infection with human T-cell lymphotropic virus type III/lymphadenopathy-associated virus in a large cohort of intensively exposed health care workers. *Annals of Internal Medicine, 104*, 644–647.

Hirsch, M.S., Wormser, G.P., Schooley, R.T., et al. (1985). Risk of nosocomial infection with human T-cell lymphotropic virus III (HTLV-III). *New England Journal of Medicine, 312*, 1–4.

Holloway, N.M., (1986). AIDS awareness in the emergency department. *Critical Care Nurse, 6*, 90–93.

Jackson, M.M., (1986). *Rituals without reason: Updating the curriculum in infection control* pp. 171–187. New York: National League for Nursing.

Jackson, M.M., Healy, S.A., Straube, R.C., et al. (1986). The AIDS epidemic: Dilemmas facing nurse managers. *Nursing Economics, 4,* 109–116.

Jackson, M.M., Lynch, P. (1989). Infection prevention and control in the era of the AIDS/HIV epidemic. *Seminars in Oncology Nursing, 5,* 236–243.

Kuhls, T.L., Viker, S., Parris, N.B., et al. (1987). Occupational risk of HIV, HBV and HSV-2 infections in health care personnel caring for AIDS patients. *American Journal of Public Health, 77,* 1306–1309.

Lange, J.M.A., Boucher, C.A.B., Hollak, C.E.M., et al. (1990). Failure of zidovudine prophylaxis after accidental exposure to HIV-1. *New England Journal of Medicine, 322,* 1375–1377.

Looke, D.F.M., Grove, D.I. (1990). Failed prophylactic zidovudine after needlestick injury. *Lancet, 335,* 1280.

Lowenfels, A.B., Wormser, G.P., Jain, R. (1989). Frequency of puncture injuries in surgeons and estimated risk of HIV infection. *Archives of Surgery, 124,* 1284–1286.

Lusby, G., Martin, J.P., Schietinger, H. (1986). Infection control at home: A guideline for caregivers to follow. *American Journal of Hospice Care, 3,* 24–27.

Lynch, P., Jackson, M.M., Cummings, J., Stamm, W.E. (1987). Rethinking the role of isolation practices in the prevention of nosocomial infections. *Annals of Internal Medicine, 107,* 243–246.

Marcus, R., Cooperative Needlestick Surveillance Group (1988). Surveillance of health care workers exposed to blood from patients infected with the human immunodeficiency virus. *New England Journal of Medicine, 319,* 1118–1123.

Martin, L.S., McDougal, S., Loskoski, S.L. (1985). Disinfection and inactivation of the human T lymphotropic virus type III/lymphadenopathy-associated virus. *Journal of Infectious Diseases, 152,* 400–403.

Matthews, G.W., Neslund, V.S. (1986). The initial impact of AIDS on public health law in the United States—1986. *Journal of the American Medical Association, 257,* 344–352.

McCray, E., Cooperative Needlestick Surveillance Group (1986). Occupational risk of the acquired immunodeficiency syndrome among health care workers. *New England Journal of Medicine, 314,* 1127–1132.

Mills, M., Wofsy, C.B., Mills, J. (1986). Special report: The acquired immunodeficiency syndrome; infection control and public health law. *New England Journal of Medicine, 314:* 931–936.

Neisson-Vernant, C., Afri, S., Mathez, D., et al. (1986). Needlestick HIV seroconversion in a nurse. *Lancet, 2,* 814.

Oksenhendler, E., Harzic, M., LeRoux, J.M., et al. (1986). HIV infection with seroconversion after a superficial needlestick injury to the finger. *New England Journal of Medicine, 315,* 582.

Spire, B., Barre-Sinoussi, F., Montagnier, L., Chermann, J.C. (1984). Inactivation of lymphadenopathy associated virus by chemical disinfectants. *Lancet, 2,* 899–901.

Stricof, R.L., Morse, D.L. (1986). HTLV-III/LAV seroconversion following a deep intramuscular needlestick injury. *New England Journal of Medicine, 314,* 1115.

Visiting Nurse Service Home Care and Administration (1990). Policy on universal precautions—infection control practice for all patient care. New York City. (Unpublished manuscript.)

Weiss, S.H., Saxinger, W.C., Rechtman, D., et al. (1985). HTLV-III infection among health care workers—association with needle-stick injuries. *Journal of the American Medical Association, 254,* 2089–2093.

Yarchoan, R., Thomas, R.V., Grafman, J., et al. (1988). Long-term administration of 3'-azido-2', 3'-dideoxythymidine to patients with AIDS-related neurological disease. *Annals of Neurology, 23* (suppl), S82–S87.

Zbitnew, A., Greer, K., Heise-Qualtiere, J., Conly, J. (1989). Vinyl versus latex gloves as barriers to transmission of viruses in the health care setting. *Journal of Acquired Immune Deficiency Syndromes, 2,* 201–204.

12

Ethical Aspects

Christine Grady

Now, approximately 10 years into an epidemic that came as a surprise, an unprecedented amount of knowledge has been accumulated about HIV: what it is and what it does to human cells, the human immune system, and the person as a whole. However, much remains to be learned and many challenges lie ahead. Perhaps the most difficult challenges of the HIV epidemic are ethical and social ones.

The majority of ethical issues that arise in the context of HIV disease are not new, although there are some unique features. For the most part these are issues that people have struggled with before and not adequately resolved, nor have they agreed on approaches. Some of the HIV-related ethical issues are complex because of the populations in which HIV is predominantly found, that is, in individuals who are generally young, socially ostracized, and misunderstood. In addition, the issues are complicated by the fact that HIV causes an infectious disease with a fatal outcome.

It is imperative to consider some of the difficult ethical issues that nurses confront when working with HIV-infected clients. Normative ethics is a discipline that helps us to determine what "ought" to be done (as distinct from what we can do or know how to do), the "right" way to act in a given situation based on reason and reflection rather than on personal preference or desire (Beauchamp & Childress, 1989; Veatch & Fry, 1987). In biomedical ethics (the ethics of judgments made within the biomedical sciences), several guiding principles are often employed in making ethical decisions about "right" actions. In a moral framework, principles serve as the general foundation for, or justification of, rules that guide our conduct and help us decide what ought to be done in a particular situation (Beauchamp & Childress, 1989).

The bioethical principles used in this discussion include nonmaleficence, beneficence, autonomy, justice, and fidelity. In the following pages these principles are used to provide a rationale for the provision of ethical nursing care to HIV-infected persons. The principle of nonmaleficence obligates us to avoid harming or injuring others. Beneficence is the positive

424

counterpart to nonmaleficence and entails promoting the good of others or contributing to another's welfare. Autonomy is a principle that encompasses the right to self-determination, noninterference, and liberty. There is a corresponding obligation to respect the autonomy, liberty, and rights of others. Justice is a principle of fairness, a principle by which each person gets his or her fair share. It obliges the nurse to provide an equitable distribution of benefits and burdens where patient services are concerned. Fidelity is a principle that entails a moral obligation to follow through on commitments made to others, such as keeping promises and fulfilling contracts (Beauchamp & Childress, 1989; Veatch & Fry, 1987).

ETHICAL CONSIDERATIONS IN DECISIONS ABOUT ACCESS TO CARE

The distribution of health care resources and equitable access to care services are issues that invoke an appeal to the principle of justice. A question we must ask ourselves as a society is, "Are we as a society committed to a just health care system?" Are we willing and able to provide the range and depth of services needed by HIV-infected individuals (as well as people with other illnesses and health care needs)? As Dr. Leroy Walters (1988) writes, "The central ethical question confronting the U.S. health care system was evident long before HIV was discovered or named. . . . Does our society have a moral obligation to provide some level of health care to every one of its members?" (p. 601). Some of the weaknesses and deficiencies in our health care delivery system have shown up as obvious gaps in our ability to provide comprehensive services to HIV-infected people. An integrated, coordinated consortium of services that are cost effective is needed (Kelly, 1987; Report of the Presidential Commission on HIV epidemic, 1988). For HIV-infected persons these services include (1) early diagnosis and counseling; (2) outpatient follow-up, teaching, primary care, and counseling; (3) acute care hospitalization; (4) home care, chronic care, and terminal care; and (5) counseling and supportive services.

People with HIV disease do not currently have equitable access to health care services (Green & Arno, 1990). Some patients with AIDS have been refused care by individual health care practitioners or health care institutions (Cooke, 1990; Eisenberg, 1986; Gillon, 1987; Levine, 1986). Discharge planning and placement of people with AIDS in long-term care facilities are also difficult (see Chapter 7). In addition, an increasing number of HIV-infected persons are ethnic minorities and are poor, inner-city dwellers who traditionally have had limited access to health care. The increasing numbers of homeless people with HIV infection pose a special problem in providing care (Report of the Presidential Commission, 1988).

Getting Medicaid or other forms of public assistance is difficult without an address, and this further compromises the delivery of needed services. A particularly tragic problem is the increasing number of HIV-infected children whose parents are unable to care for them. Placement of these children in foster homes or transitional homes is extremely difficult (Report of the Presidential Commission, 1988).

The cost of caring for a person with AIDS and the consumption of resources are also high (Green & Arno, 1990; Iglehart, 1987). Care of HIV-infected persons is already straining health care resources, especially in high-prevalence areas such as New York City and San Francisco. Unfortunately, many people with AIDS are either uninsured or underinsured, which has a strong negative influence on access to care (Green & Arno, 1990). The uninsured make up a larger proportion of persons with AIDS than the general population (20% versus 16%), and rely much more on Medicaid than the general population (40% versus 9%) (Green & Arno, 1990; Makadon et al., 1988). In New York State almost 70% of people with AIDS are covered by Medicaid. This situation is bound to get worse as the number of intravenous drug users with AIDS rises and as private health insurance companies continue to deny coverage for infected individuals (Green & Arno, 1990).

A striking one third to one half of all poor Americans are excluded from Medicaid because of eligibility criteria (Colburn, 1987). Medicaid eligibility, coverage, and reimbursement vary dramatically from state to state (Green & Arno, 1990). An estimated 23% of persons below the poverty line are covered in South Dakota, while almost 97% of those below the poverty line are covered in California. In 34 states less than 50% of persons below the poverty level are eligible for Medicaid (Makadon et al., 1988). In some states Medicaid coverage for home care or other out-of-hospital care is nonexistent.

Medicaid reimbursement to providers of care also varies from state to state and has generally been believed inadequate for the treatment of persons with AIDS (Green & Arno, 1990; Thompson, 1988). Nationwide, the average inpatient cost of caring for a person with AIDS in 1985 was an estimated $630 a day. While the reimbursement rates in some regions of the country approximated $500 per day, the rate in the South was only $282 per patient day (Iglehart, 1987; Report of the Presidential Commission, 1988; Thompson, 1988). In New York City an intermediate care office visit for a new patient is compensated by private insurance at $84 and by Medicaid at $11; a bronchoscopy is reimbursed by private insurance at $775 and by Medicaid at $60 (Green & Arno, 1990). Only about 2% of people with AIDS have received Medicare benefits. This is because Medicare requires an individual to be classified as disabled for 24 months before being eligible for benefits. This time period exceeds the life span of many people with AIDS (Makadon et al., 1988; Thompson, 1988). Regulatory changes in 1983 provided that individuals with a diagnosis of AIDS would automatically be determined disabled for purposes of eligibility for Social Security Disability Insurance. This provision, however, excludes anyone who is HIV infected but does not have a diagnosis of AIDS. People with HIV infection who are employed and covered by group health insurance are in the best position to cope with the costs of needed health care (Walters, 1988). However, many HIV-infected people lose their jobs and with them insurance coverage. Federal legislation (Consolidated Omnibus Budget Reconciliation Act [COBRA]) extends the availability of group coverage for up to 29 months after termination of employment. Unfortunately, many cannot afford the premiums if unemployed (Green & Arno, 1990; Walters, 1988).

Many people with HIV disease receive care in already overburdened public hospitals. It is estimated that by 1991, 12.4% of all acute care beds in San Francisco and 8.1% in New York City will be occupied by patients with AIDS (Lo, 1990a). The shortage of acute care beds in many cities is exacerbated by the shortage of nurses and by long lengths of stay for patients without homes or families to care for them.

The emphasis is shifting to ambulatory care and home care for people with HIV disease. The primary goals are to reduce costs yet maintain high-quality care. Nurses and volunteers deliver a large percentage of out-of-hospital care. As the number of HIV-infected persons who are actively using drugs or who are homeless or without caregivers increases, the feasibility of these methods of health care delivery is challenged.

A related dilemma that appeals to the principle of justice is access to treatment. Zidovudine is an antiretroviral drug approved for all HIV-infected individuals with fewer than 500 T4 cells/mm^3. Although the price has been reduced, zidovudine for one person still costs approximately $5000 per year plus the cost of tests for monitoring its use (Lo, 1990a). Aerosolized pentamidine, recommended as prophylaxis against Pneumocystis carinii pneumonia for HIV-infected individuals with fewer than 200 T4 cells/mm^3, costs between $100 and $500 per month plus the cost of monitoring laboratory tests (Lo, 1990a). These are major costs that many insurance plans do not cover adequately and that represent impossible expenses for those without insurance.

HEALTH CARE PROVIDERS' OBLIGATION TO PROVIDE CARE

Besides access to care and treatment, there remain questions about access to individual health care practitioners. Are practitioners obligated to care for any or all patients who seek care? If yes, what are the limits to this obligation? A difficult issue facing many nurses in the context of the HIV epidemic is the extent of a nurse's obligation to care for patients. Many nurses had never thought they would be in a position of not wanting to care for certain patients. Anecdotal reports of nurses and other health care providers refusing to care for persons known or suspected to be HIV infected have appeared in the literature (Cooke, 1990; Eisenberg, 1986; Gillon, 1987; Koenig, 1988; Lo, 1990a, 1990b; Walters, 1988). Several surveys describing the attitudes of nurses toward HIV-infected patients conclude that even among those who do not refuse to care for patients, many dislike or disapprove of their patients (Blumenfield et al., 1987; Jacobs et al., 1987; Kelly et al., 1988). How does this attitude affect a nurse's ability to provide impartial care? Recognizing that some nurses have refused to care for HIV-infected patients does not discount the thousands of nurses and other health care providers who may have struggled with fear or dislike but are providing sensitive, high-quality care to people with HIV disease.

How can the extent of a nurse's or other health care provider's obligation to give care be determined? Several of the principles of biomedical ethics can provide guidance with this question. According to the principle of nonmaleficence, the nurse must do no harm to a patient. If refusing to provide care or providing prejudicial care may harm a patient, these actions would be a violation of the principle of nonmaleficence. A good example of this is when refusal to offer nursing care to a patient in an emergency situation results in harm or death to the patient. Beneficence is a principle that promotes the good of others. By virtue of their license and their education, nurses have an *obligation* to benefit patients (American Nurses' Association [ANA], 1985). Nurses are committed to promoting the good of their patients. Fulfillment of this obligation reflects conduct consistent not only with the principle of beneficence, but also with the principle of fidelity. Some ethicists have appealed to the principle of justice in deciding a nurse's obligation and have argued that this principle does not allow discrimination in the allocation of nursing resources (Koenig, 1988).

In addition to the principles of biomedical ethics, nurses can turn to an intermediate source of rules for guidance with respect to obligation to provide care. Intermediate rules of conduct are usually based on ethical principles or theories, and reference to these rules can help a person easily determine how to act in a particular situation. The professional codes of ethics are rules that help guide nurses' behavior. The first tenet of the ANA's Code for Nurses states: "Nurses provide services with respect for human dignity and the uniqueness of the client, unrestricted by considerations of social or economic status, personal attributes, or the nature of the health problem" (ANA, 1985). Reflecting a similar philosophy, the International Council of Nurses' (ICN) Code for Nurses states: "The need for nursing is universal. Inherent in nursing is respect for life, dignity and the rights of man. It is unrestricted by considerations of nationality, race, creed, color, age, sex, politics, or social status" (ICN, 1983). Based on these two professional codes that guide ethical nursing practice, a nurse may not refuse to care for a patient because he or she dislikes the patient's personal attributes, politics, economic status, or illness. In "Guidelines for Nursing Management of HIV infection," published by the ICN and the World Health Organization (WHO) in 1988, it is stated that "nurses are in a position to provide care that respects the dignity of the individual and to model appropriate nonjudgemental attitudes for other health care workers and community members" (ICN, 1988).

Nurses also have rights, and the profession recognizes and respects these rights (Ungvarski, 1988). In 1986 the ANA's Committee on Ethics issued a "Statement Regarding Risk vs. Responsibility in Providing Nursing Care" (ANA, 1986). This document clarifies the circumstances in which a nurse is morally justified to refuse to participate in the care of a patient. These include (1) when the nurse refuses for reasons of patient advocacy (providing care would violate the rights or wishes of the patient) and (2) when the nurse has a moral objection to a specific intervention. This ANA statement further states, "Accepting personal risk which exceeds the limits of duty is not morally obligatory, it is a moral option. . . . The profession does not and cannot demand the sacrifice of the nurse's well-being, physical, emotional, or otherwise, or the nurse's life for the benefit of the patient" (ANA, 1986). Although nursing is a profession with built-in risks, risk to the welfare of the nurse is not mandatory, but a moral option. The ANA statement gives four fundamental criteria for differentiating between benefiting another as a moral duty and benefiting another as a moral option. They are: (1) the patient is at significant risk of harm, loss or damage if the nurse does not assist; (2) the nurse's intervention or care is directly relevant to preventing harm; (3) the nurse's care will probably prevent harm, loss, or damage to the patient; and (4) the benefit the patient will gain outweighs any harm the nurse might incur and does not present more than minimal risk to the nurse (ANA, 1986).

Presumably, any patient would be harmed by not receiving nursing care and helped by nursing interventions that are appropriate and safe. The questions that must be answered then are, "Does the risk of occupationally acquired HIV infection exceed the limits of the nurse's duty?" and "Are there circumstances in which it is ethically acceptable to refuse to care for an HIV infected person because of the risk?" Cumulative data from several prospective surveillance studies of health care providers exposed to HIV via percutaneous injury or mucocutaneous splash indicate that the risk of acquiring HIV infection from a single needlestick exposure is approximately 0.3% (based on six seroconversions from 2042 percutaneous exposures) (Henderson et al., 1990). The risk from a nonpercutaneous exposure is even less (Henderson et al., 1990). The adoption of universal precautions, recommended by the Centers for Disease Control (CDC) in 1987 and subsequently implemented by most health care institutions across the country, minimizes the risk of contracting HIV infection. Nurses have an obligation to comply with recommended precautions, and health care institutions have an obligation to provide the necessary equipment and work conditions to make compliance possible (Creighton, 1986).

Because the risk of occupationally acquired HIV is extremely low, most professional organizations have concluded that it does not justify refusal to provide care. Despite this, considerable fear is still associated with HIV disease. As Freedman (1988) pointed out, "perception, rather than reality, controls the generation and resolution of ethical issues, and the perception is that now, because of the new HIV factor, health care is a potentially risky occupation." Clearly, perception of risk does not always lead to avoidance of risk. Many people do not wear seat belts and continue to smoke cigarettes although these are known to be risky behaviors. Some health care providers who express great fear of acquiring HIV have not received the available vaccine for hepatitis B (HBV), although the risk of occupationally acquiring HBV is 20 to 30 times higher than that of HIV (Goldsmith, 1990). In addition, health care providers express fear of HIV but do not comply with universal precautions. A study at San Francisco General Hospital (Goldsmith, 1990) found that about 50% of all needles were recapped, although recapping needles is explicitly prohibited by universal precautions. In a survey of nurse midwives, Willy and colleagues (1990) reported that only about 55% were using universal precautions, even though exposure to blood during delivery is likely.

In addition to the risk of HIV itself, other risks are associated with caring for persons with HIV disease. Home care workers must often enter homes or neighborhoods where drug use is prevalent and crime is high (Hanley, 1990). Health care providers who administer aerosolized pentamidine may experience some respiratory side effects (Jacobson, 1990). There have been anecdotal reports of discrimination against health care workers because of their work with HIV-infected patients. Professional nursing organizations have concluded that because of the low risk, no justification exists for refusing to care for HIV-infected persons. The nursing profession has yet to define, however, what level or amount of risk is acceptable for nursing practice in general.

ETHICAL CONSIDERATIONS IN DECISIONS ABOUT TESTING AND DIAGNOSIS

Complex ethical issues underlie decisions about testing for antibody to HIV. Although many clinicians have argued that the HIV antibody test should be handled like any other test ordered at the physician's discretion, the reactions of the patient, the health care community, and the society at large to a positive HIV test argue against this. There is general consensus that testing should be voluntary, done with the individual's informed consent, and accompanied by counseling (Cooke, 1990; Lo, 1990a). Obtaining informed consent and providing counseling show respect for the individual's autonomy and promotes his or her welfare. In addition, counseling promotes the welfare of others if it encourages notification of partners and protection of others from transmission (see Chapter 6).

A decision about whether to test a given individual should be the result of a careful risk-benefit analysis. An HIV antibody test is indicated for any individual with a history of behaviors that increase the risk of acquiring HIV or with symptoms or clinical findings that might suggest HIV disease. The benefits of testing include (1) obtaining useful diagnostic information, (2) knowing whether to begin treatment with zidovudine or with prophylactic drugs for opportunistic infections, (3) promoting a change in behaviors that would reduce the possibility of transmission to others, and (4) obtaining information that allows the person to make informed decisions about marriage, childbearing, employment, insurance, and perhaps better self-care. The risks include the possibility of discrimination and stigma, as well as depression, anxiety, or even suicide.

Decisions about testing of groups take on different dimensions. The debate is essentially between respecting the autonomy of the individual and safeguarding the public health. Voluntary HIV testing can have enormous public health benefits (Lo, 1990a). Studies have shown that seropositive individuals, tested voluntarily and with counseling, support, and protection of confidentiality, do reduce their high-risk behaviors and do notify their contacts (Lo, 1990a, 1990b). In protecting the public health, behavior change is the goal. Ironically, data show that some well-intentioned public health measures such as premarital testing, mandatory reporting of HIV results, and contact tracing without consent were counterproductive in that the numbers of people willingly being tested decreased and so did the numbers identified as seropositive (Lo, 1990a, 1990b). In addition, the HIV antibody test has been shown to be less reliable when used in low-prevalence populations (i.e., high number of false positives compared with true positives) (Cooke, 1990). These observations suggest that public health measures designed to change behavior and safeguard the public must be evaluated as to their effectiveness, modified appropriately, and used carefully.

Closely tied to decisions about testing are decisions about who should know the results. From an ethical perspective the individual being tested should always be informed of the results based on respect for autonomy. Yet a recent survey of the HIV testing policies and practices of hospitals in the United States found that one in four hospitals does not require notification of the patient if the test is positive (Lewis & Montgomery,

1990). Does anyone besides the infected individual have an ethical claim to this information if the person tested does not want disclosure? In other words, is there ever justification for overriding the confidentiality of the tested individual?

Confidentiality is a contract, a promise, and an obligation that one makes with another in certain situations when information is provided in confidence (Beauchamp & Childress, 1989; Walters, 1978, 1988). The recipient is expected to protect the entrusted information and to use it appropriately. Confidentiality is based on the concept of respect for persons, which encompasses the principles of autonomy and fidelity (Beauchamp & Childress, 1989; Walters, 1978). Generally thought to be subsumed under the right to autonomy is a right to privacy, or the right to control information about ourselves. Each person has some control over what personal information to share with others and with whom to share it. When personal information is confided to another individual, he or she is expected to maintain the confidentiality of that information in conformity with respect for privacy and respect for persons. According to the principle of fidelity, there is a moral obligation to keep commitments and promises made to others. Requesting personal information from a person in the health care setting entails an explicit or implicit commitment to use that information appropriately or to maintain confidentiality.

Confidentiality is a classic requirement of professional health care ethics. Patients share a great deal of private and sensitive information with their health care providers and trust that it will be used appropriately. Virtually all professional codes of ethics include some form of confidentiality requirement (Beauchamp & Childress, 1989). The ANA's Code for Nurses states, "The nurse safeguards the client's right to privacy by judiciously protecting information of a confidential nature" (ANA, 1985).

When, if ever, can confidentiality be overridden in the setting of HIV infection? The interpretive statements that accompany the ANA Code for Nurses expand on the tenet cited previously: "Clients trust the nurse to hold all information in confidence. This trust could be destroyed and the client's welfare jeopardized by injudicious disclosure of information provided in confidence. The duty of confidentiality is, however, not absolute when innocent third parties are in direct jeopardy" (ANA, 1985). In the case of HIV infection, the consequences of injudicious disclosure or in some cases any disclosure are dramatic. Discrimination and isolation are real phenomena suffered by people known to be HIV positive or to have AIDS (Brown, 1987; Cooke, 1990; Eisenberg, 1986; Koenig, 1988; Levine, 1986; Milliken & Greenblatt, 1988; Ostrow & Gayle, 1986; Walters, 1988). People have unjustly lost their jobs, housing, and insurance. Some infected children have been unable to go to school, and uninfected children of an infected parent or sibling have also been kept out of school. In a well-publicized incident in Florida in 1987, a house was fire-bombed because three hemophilic boys living there were known to be HIV positive. How does the jeopardy to the client's welfare caused by disclosure balance with risk to innocent third parties? Are third parties at risk whose right to know might justify overriding the confidentiality of an individual?

The legal right to information about an individual's serostatus varies from state to state. In some states, such as Colorado and Minnesota, reporting of HIV-positive antibody tests to the public health department is required. These states and many others also have programs to notify the sexual partners that the tested individual has named (Report of the Presidential Commission, 1988). Several states have passed laws that allow physicians at their discretion to inform sexual or needle-sharing partners without the consent of the seropositive individual, but do not require such notification. In the military, HIV antibody testing is required of everyone and the results are reported to the individual's superiors.

Ethicists have argued that overriding confidentiality is justifiable in the interests of a third party at risk, or in "direct jeopardy" (Walters, 1978). Those at risk of acquiring HIV infection from an infected person are the sexual partners of that individual, as well as anyone exposed to the person's blood, for example, caregivers or persons who share needles with the individual (Grodin et al., 1986; Henderson et al., 1990; Milliken & Greenblatt, 1988; Reisman, 1988; Report of the Presidential Commission, 1988). Many people agree that sexual partners should be informed. However, the more controversial question is who should inform them. Ideally, infected individuals should themselves inform their sexual partners. Infected individuals have an ethical duty to notify partners they place at risk (Lo, 1990a). This way the autonomy of partners is respected and they have the power to make informed decisions about testing, medical care, sexual behaviors, and childbearing. With encouragement, guidance, counseling, and sometimes an offer of assistance, most HIV-infected individuals do inform their own partners.

The President's Commission on the HIV Epidemic (1988) recommended that all state and local health agencies develop confidential (i.e., without identification of the infected individual) HIV partner notification programs that include counseling, testing, and supportive follow-up for the notified individual. Where such programs are in place, nurses and other members of the health care team are responsible for identifying infected individuals who are unwilling or unable to notify their partners. These individuals can then be reported to the public health authorities responsible for notifying partners. In all cases it is the responsibility of the nurse, in conjunction with the health care team, to remind infected persons of their obligations to inform their sexual partners and to offer them assistance in doing so.

There is less agreement on whether health care providers have a right to know someone's serostatus. Many believe that with the correct use of universal precautions the risk of exposure to infected blood or body fluids is minimal and therefore that confidential information should not be disclosed to the health care provider without the infected individual's consent (Gostin, 1988). Universal precautions do not depend on determination of antibody status. "A stratified infection control procedure could produce either unacceptably casual attitudes toward the possible transmission of serious infection from antibody-negative patients or the use of inappropriate and ineffective measures to prevent transmissions from antibody-positive patients, or both. Thus screening of hospitalized patients to protect staff does not produce the increase in safety that would justify the intrusion of testing" (Cooke, 1990, p. 1214.3). Interestingly, a survey of 561 U.S. hospitals showed that of 83% with testing policies, the greatest influence to institute testing was staff fears of contagion (Lewis & Montgomery, 1990). An argument could be made for a nurse's need to know so he or she can be an effective patient advocate and a provider of care to the whole person, rather than a nurse's right to know based merely on risk. HIV seropositivity is diagnostic information that enables the nurse to more appropriately plan care, teach, and support the patient and the patient's significant others as a patient advocate. This argument is not based on the concept of direct risk but rather on an understanding of the nurse's role and the information needed to function in that role. Of course, nurses must be expected to use the information appropriately and to protect the confidentiality of the patient from any unnecessary disclosure.

ETHICAL CONSIDERATIONS IN DECISIONS ABOUT TREATMENT

The nurse, as a patient advocate, demonstrates respect for what the patient wants and needs and takes action to help the patient achieve it; in other words, the nurse respects the autonomy of the patient and helps to maximize patient choices. It is generally agreed that the patient has the right to make decisions about treatment and care based on adequate and realistic information from the care provider. The role of advocacy includes ensuring that the patient has adequate information and adequate opportunities to make informed decisions and to make his or her wishes known. The nurse can maximize patient autonomy by ensuring that a patient gives informed consent and by advocating for the patient in decisions about treatment, including those involving life-sustaining therapy or participation in research. In these areas HIV infection presents special challenges.

All competent patients should have the information they need to make their own decisions about treatment, diagnostic tests, care, and research. This is the basis of informed consent. Informed consent has three primary components: (1) adequate information to make rational decisions, (2) mental competence on the part of the decision maker, and (3) uncoerced, freely given consent by a nonvulnerable, autonomous individual (Grodin et al, 1986).

Several potential difficulties are associated with the process of informed consent for HIV-infected persons. First, information about AIDS still has many unknowns, especially in regard to treatment that is still experimental. Since the available information is incomplete, the HIV-infected person must be willing to accept some degree of uncertainty. The nurse can ensure that the patient regularly receives updated information and is given the opportunity to make new decisions based on that information.

Second, a high incidence of neuropsychiatric disease is associated with HIV infection. Between 60% and 70% of people with AIDS have some degree of associated dementia (Price et al., 1988). This dementia, coupled with a high incidence of depression and anxiety, may raise a question about patients' competence to make autonomous decisions (Ostrow & Gayle, 1986). Mental abilities may also be compromised by central nervous system infections, which are common in HIV-infected individuals. In adults competence should always be assumed unless careful evaluation, adjudication, or agreement by all parties, including the patient, deem otherwise (Cooke, 1986, 1990; Veatch & Fry, 1987).

Third, because treatment and care options are limited for people with HIV infection, some may feel unable to make a free choice. They may, in fact, feel desperate or coerced. For example, is there a "free" choice when a person may be able to obtain experimental therapy at no cost by joining a clinical trial if the only other option is no treatment or unaffordable treatment.

Informed consent takes on special dimensions when the individual is considering participation in a clinical trial. This decision may be complicated because of public attention and criticism about the speed and manner in which AIDS clinical trials have been conducted. Clinical trials are necessary to determine whether drugs and other agents are safe and effective. Without this assurance, people may be exposed to harm from unknown or unanticipated side effects without any benefit. In addition, there are potential economic harms, that is, spending of private or public money on ineffective or less effective therapies at the expense of others. Individuals considering participation in a clinical trial must be provided with information about the purpose of the research and the requirements and restrictions involved in participation. Many HIV-infected individuals have chosen alternative therapies or unproven experimental therapies outside of a controlled clinical trial (see Chapter 7).

Because AIDS is ultimately a fatal disease, decisions about life-sustaining therapy commonly arise. Established legal and ethical precedent and guidelines allow informed, competent individuals with any disease to refuse life-sustaining therapies, even if others disagree with their decisions or if life would otherwise be sustained. Again, some facts about the HIV epidemic make decisions about life-sustaining therapy more complicated. First, information is rapidly changing. In 1985, 86% or more of HIV-infected patients with *Pneumocystis carinii* pneumonia (PCP) died, even with mechanical ventilation. In 1990 more than 50% survive to discharge, and with PCP prophylaxis, recurrences are less frequent (Cooke, 1990). Second, because of the common neuropsychiatric disorders associated with HIV infection, many patients become incompetent to make decisions, especially as they approach death. Treatment decisions, including life-sustaining treatment, for an incompetent person are least complicated if the person has previously made his or her wishes known through some form of advanced directive. Examples of advance directives defined by statutes in most states are the durable power of attorney (DPA) and the living will (Cooke, 1986; Koenig, 1988; Levine, 1986; Roy & Tsoukas, 1986; Walters, 1988). A DPA is especially useful because it allows legal designation of a proxy to make decisions of many kinds in the event of the designating individual's incompetence. When stipulated, these decisions can involve treatment, research, and medical care. This type of transfer of authority for decision making is very important when a patient has a lover, friend, or family member who without a legally executed DPA would have no legal standing and thus might be excluded from decision making (Grodin et al., 1986; Steinbrook, 1985). "Nurses show respect for a patient's autonomy by making sure that the appropriate legal documents are available" (Koenig, 1988, p. 291). Providing early opportunities for thinking about, talking about, and planning for difficult decisions such as resuscitation and life-sustaining therapy is helpful and must be done sensitively.

A person can best discuss and decide what he or she wants when not in a crisis situation and when given time for reflection (Cooke, 1990; Roy & Tsoukas, 1986; Veatch & Fry, 1987). Postponing this type of discussion only makes the decisions more difficult and all too frequently leads to a situation in which the patient's wishes are not clearly known and can no longer be ascertained. When knowledge of the patient's wishes is no longer obtainable and no surrogate decision maker is available, health professionals must make decisions in conjunction with family, friends, and others based on the presumed "best interests" of the patient (Cooke, 1990; Koenig, 1988). Decisions about life-sustaining therapy should always be individualized. Blanket policies such as no intensive care for people with AIDS not only are unfair, but also deprive people of their rights to make decisions about treatment and care (Cooke, 1986, 1990; Veatch & Fry, 1987).

Despite the best efforts of health professionals, some patients refuse to participate in discussions about life-sustaining therapy. Such refusal must also be respected. In addition, in the context of HIV disease, discomfort and lack of familiarity with the life-styles of drug users or homosexuals may influence health care professionals in the way they approach discussions about life-sustaining therapy or even cause them to devalue patients' choices (Steinbrook et al., 1986). Discomfort arising from identification with the patient may also be a problem; many patients with AIDS are young men whose age, education, and socioeconomic status are similar to those of many physicians (Steinbrook et al., 1985). Furthermore, some physicians may approach discussions about life-sustaining therapy differently with patients who have AIDS. A study by Wachter and colleagues (1989) reviewed do not resuscitate (DNR) orders for patients with diseases that have similar prognoses: AIDS, lung cancer, cirrhosis with esophageal varices, and severe congestive heart failure with atherosclerotic disease. They found that while 52% of patients with AIDS and 46% of patients with lung cancer had DNR orders, only 16% and 5% of patients with cirrhosis and congestive heart failure, respectively, had a DNR order (Wachter et al., 1989). They concluded that the differences were not explainable by patient preferences, but rather indicated that physicians discussed resuscitation more frequently with patients who have lung cancer or AIDS (Lo, 1990a; Wachter et al., 1989).

An increasingly common phenomenon in the HIV epidemic is the patient who shares with his or her health care worker plans about "rational suicide" or "self-deliverance." Although not unique to persons with HIV infection, "rational suicide" raises difficult issues for the health care provider. Whether or not the health care provider views suicide as a viable option, does he or she have an obligation to protect individuals and try to stop them from following through on their plans? Is this even possible? Should the health care provider just listen and offer advice, encouragement or discouragement, and referral, or should more restrictive steps be taken to protect the individual? Is it clear that the individual is competent and not depressed? If successful, the suicide of a patient, "rational" or otherwise, usually leaves the health care staff with strong feelings of guilt, sadness, and sometimes anger.

SUMMARY

This chapter has discussed some of the ethical issues facing health care practitioners working with patients who have HIV disease. Issues considered included those related to access to care, health care providers' obligation to provide care, testing and diagnosis, confidentiality, and decisions about treatment or refusal of treatment.

During the past few years a large body of knowledge about HIV infection and all of its ramifications has accumulated. Clearly, however, many unanswered questions remain, especially the issue of how one "ought" to act toward HIV-infected persons. HIV disease poses many complex and difficult ethical questions. All health care professionals have a great need for reflection, reexamination of values, and ethical analysis of their behaviors. When the history of the HIV epidemic is written, it will be the responses of health care workers and society as a whole toward those who are infected that will tell the real story.

References

American Nurses' Association (1985). *Code for nurses with interpretive statements.* Kansas City, MO: The Association.

American Nurses' Association Committee on Ethics (1986). Statement regarding risk vs. responsibility in providing nursing care. Kansas City, MO: The Association.

Beauchamp, T., Childress, J. (1989). *Principles of biomedical ethics* (3rd Ed.). New York: Oxford University Press.

Blumenfield, M., Smith, P., Milazzo, J., et al. (1987). Survey of attitudes of nurses working with AIDS patients. *General Hospital Psychiatry 9*, 58–63.

Brown, M. (1987). AIDS and ethics: Concerns and considerations. *Oncology Nursing Forum, 14*(1), 69–73.

Centers for Disease Control (1987). Recommendations for prevention of HIV transmission in health care settings. *Morbidity and Mortality Weekly Report, 36* (suppl. 2s), 3S–17S.

Colburn, D. (1987). Report faults Medicaid fairness, *Washington Post,* December 29, 1987.

Cooke, M. (1986). Ethical issues in the care of patients with AIDS. *Quality Review Bulletin, 12*(10), 343–346.

Cooke, M. (1990). Ethical issues related to AIDS. In P.T. Cohen, M. Sande, & P.A. Volberding (Eds.), *The AIDS knowledge base* (pp. 1214.1–1214.8). Waltham, MA: Medical Publishing Group.

Creighton, H. (1986). Legal aspects of AIDS—part II. *Nursing Management 17*(12), 14–16.

Eisenberg, L. (1986). The genesis of fear: AIDS and the public's response to science. *Law, Medicine and Health Care, 14*(5–6), 243–249.

Freedman, B. (1988). Health professions, codes and the right to refuse to treat HIV infectious patients. *Hastings Center Report, 18,*(2) suppl. 20–25.

Gillon, R. (1987). Refusal to treat AIDS and HIV positive patients. *British Medical Journal, 294*, 1332–1333.

Goldsmith, M. (1990). Even in perspective, HIV specter haunts health care workers. *Journal of the American Medical Association, 263*(18), 2413–2420.

Gostin, L. (1988). AIDS as an occupational disease: whose right to know. *Delaware Medical Journal, 60*(9), 479–483.

Green, J., Arno, P. (1990). The "Medicaidization" of AIDS. *Journal of the American Medical Association, 264*(10), 1261–1266.

Grodin, M., Kaminow, P., Sassower, R. (1986). Ethical issues in AIDS research. *Quality Review Bulletin, 12*(10), 347–352.

International Council of Nurses and World Health Organization (1988). Guidelines for nursing management of HIV infection. *International Nursing Review, 35*(2), 53–54.

Hanley, E. (1990). The impact of caregiving on formal and professional caregivers: One agency's experience. In AHCPR conference proceedings: *Community based care of persons with AIDS: Developing a research agenda.* Rockville, MD: Department of Health and Human Services, (Publication No. PHS 90–3456).

Henderson, D., Fahey, B., Willy, M. et al. (1990). Risk for occupational transmission of HIV-1 associated with clinical exposures. *Annals of Internal Medicine, 113*(10), 740–746.

Iglehart, J. (1987). Financing the struggle against AIDS. *New England Journal of Medicine, 317*(3), 180–184.

International Council of Nurses code for nurses: Ethical concepts applied to nursing. In T. Beauchamp & J. Childress (1983). *Principles of biomedical ethics* (2nd Ed.) (pp. 332–333). New York: Oxford University Press.

Jacobs, J., Oschtega, Y., Grady, C., et al.(1987). Survey of AIDS related knowledge and experiences among oncology nurses. *Unpublished data.*

Jacobson, E. (1990). New hospital hazards: How to protect yourself. *American Journal of Nursing, 90*(2), 36–41.

Kelly, J., St. Lawrence, J., Hood, H., et al. (1988). Nurses' attitudes toward AIDS. *Journal of Continuing Education in Nursing 19*(1), 78–83.

Kelly, K (1987). AIDS and ethics: An overview. *General Hospital Psychiatry, 9,* 331–340.

Koenig, B. (1988). Ethical and legal issues in the AIDS epidemic. In A. Lewis (Ed.), *Nursing care of the person with AIDS/ARC* (pp. 287–305). Rockville, MD: Aspen Publishers.

Levine, C. (1986). AIDS: An ethical challenge for our time. *Quality Review Bulletin, 12*(8), 273–277.

Lewis, C., Montgomery, K. (1990). The HIV testing policies of U.S. hospitals. *Journal of the American Medical Association, 264*(21), 2764–2767.

Lo, B. (1990a). Clinical ethics and HIV-related illnesses: Issues in therapeutic and health services research. *Medical Care Review, 47*(1), 15–32.

Lo, B. (1990b). Ethical dilemmas in HIV infection. *Journal of Podiatric Medical Association, 80*(1), 26–30.

Makadon, H., Seage, G., Thorpe, K., et al., and Harvard Study Group on AIDS-Financing Subgroup (March, 1988). Testimony before the President's Commission on the HIV epidemic.

Milliken, N., Greenblatt, R. (1988). Ethical issues of the AIDS epidemic. In J. Monagle & D. Thomasma (Eds.), *Medical ethics: A guide for health professionals.* Rockville, MD: Aspen Publishers.

Ostrow, D., Gayle, T. (1986). Psychosocial and ethical issues of AIDS health care programs. *Quality Review Bulletin, 12*(8), 284–294.

Price, R., Brew, B., Sidtis, J., et al. (1988). The brain in AIDS: Central nervous system HIV-1 infection and AIDS dementia complex. *Science, 239*(4840), 586–591.

Reisman, E. (1988). Ethical issues confronting nurses. *Nursing Clinics of North America, 23*(4), 789–802.

Report of the Presidential Commission on the HIV Epidemic (1988). Washington, DC: U.S. Government Printing Office.

Roy, D., Tsoukas, C. (1986). AIDS and clinical ethics: Honoring patient's dignity, *Dimensions Health Services, 63*(7), 32–33.

Steinbrook, R., Lo B., Moulton, J., et al. (1986). Preferences of homosexual men with AIDS for life-sustaining therapy. *New England Journal of Medicine, 314*(7), 457–460.

Steinbrook, R., Lo, B., Tirpack, J., et al. (1985). Ethical dilemmas in caring for patients with acquired immunodeficiency syndrome. *Annals of Internal Medicine, 103*(5), 787–790.

Thompson, J. (January, 1988). Cost as an obstacle to care. Testimony before the Presidential Commission on the HIV Epidemic.

Veatch, R., Fry, S. (1987). *Case studies in nursing ethics.* Philadelphia: J.B. Lippincott Co.

Ungvarski, P. (1988). Nursing and HIV infection: Risks, rights, and responsibilities. *Caring, 7*(11), 30–32.

Wachter, R., Luce, N., Hearst, N., Lo, B. (1989). Decisions about resuscitation: Are patients with different diseases but similar prognoses approached equally? *Annals of Internal Medicine, 11*(6), 525–532.

Walters, L. (1987). Ethical aspects of medical confidentiality. In T. Beauchamp & L. Walters (Eds.), *Contemporary issues in bioethics* (pp. 169–175). Belmont, CA: Wadsworth Publishing Co., Inc.

Walters, L. (1988). Ethical issues in the prevention and treatment of HIV infection and AIDS. *Science, 239*(4840), 597–602.

Willy, M., Dhillon, G., Loewen, N., et al. (1990). Adverse exposures and universal precautions practices among a group of highly-exposed health practitioners. *Infection Control Hospital Epidemiology, 11*(7), 351–356.

13

Living with AIDS

W. Carole Chenitz

In this chapter, I'm going to share my personal experience of living with AIDS. In doing so, I am going to present for the first time to a professional audience my personal life, who I am as a person and as your colleague, and my illness and its impact on me and my family. I will focus on the experience of AIDS for women and look at what nurses have done for me and what they haven't. Finally, I'll take a glimpse into the future, a glimpse that's filled with hope not only for treatment but for change.

Writing this chapter means taking a risk, but I have found that survival with AIDS requires a wellness plan, risk taking, and a willingness and openness to change. I have written a fair amount as a nurse researcher; writing this is different. This is about me, the patient. The patient with a disease that even in 1991 we keep secret. This chapter is not a scholarly work. It is written from the heart to give you a glimpse into the world in which persons with AIDS (PWAs) live.

Even though I am no longer a nurse researcher, old habits die hard. I've therefore included at the end of this chapter a reference list on coping with AIDS and other life-threatening illnesses, as well as a list of books written by PWAs, their family members, and caregivers. These lists are meant for nurses and for nurses to give to clients. I find it a great comfort to read others' experiences, and I have learned and grown from this reading. Another benefit from reading and hearing about others' experience is that it helps decrease the sense of isolation and increase feelings of empowerment. Self-empowerment is not just a concept or a lofty ideal if one is to live with AIDS; it's got to be a reality. In addition, I've included a resource list of newsletters and sources of information with which nurses and PWAs should be familiar to keep up with the rapid changes in the epidemic. This list is basic to all PWAs.

A version of this chapter was presented at the meeting HIV/AIDS: 1990, Hilton Head Island, South Carolina, Nov. 15, 1990. The author thanks Angie Lewis, R.N., M.S., FAAN, for her support and encouragement.

440

My family and friends are all I have today. They are what is of value to me now. All the articles and books published, presentations made, studies conducted, classes taught are part of another person in another time. Maybe slowly I'll be able to integrate my professional self with my new self, but that hasn't happened yet. Today I identify myself as a PWA. Making the transition from what was in my life to what is was difficult. I want to tell you what it's like to make that kind of transition and what it's like to live on the other side of it.

PERSONAL AND PROFESSIONAL BIOGRAPHY

In 1968 I graduated from Kings County Hospital Center School of Nursing in Brooklyn, New York. As a new graduate, I worked in a male trauma unit, recovery room, and open heart surgery recovery room. After a year of practice the handwriting was on the wall; if I wanted to make a difference in nursing, I would need a bachelor of science degree. In 1969 I began college, taking a full course load and working full time. In 1970 I married a physician I had met while in nursing school. We moved to South Carolina and then to Boston where we spent several years and had a beautiful baby girl in 1973. The same year I graduated from college. I always worked in nursing, mostly full time.

After moving back to the New York area, my husband and I divorced and I began graduate school. I received a master's degree in psychiatric/mental health nursing from Columbia University in 1976 and a doctorate in education in 1978 also from Columbia. On the doctoral level I focused on research in clinical settings as my functional role. Upon graduation I wanted more training in research methods and was accepted to do a postdoctoral fellowship at the University of California, San Francisco. With my daughter Rebecca, then 5 years old, I moved from the East Coast to the West.

In 1981, upon finishing my fellowship, I began working first as a nurse researcher/assistant chief of nursing service for psychiatry and then after a year as the associate chief of nursing service for research at the Veterans Administration Medical Center in San Francisco. I stayed at this job until October 1989 when AIDS was diagnosed. I loved my job: my boss was supportive, the nurses were enthusiastic, and I was working in a clinical setting that allowed me to maintain clinical practice and be in touch with patient care.

After my divorce I was involved in a long-term relationship that ended in 1983. After the breakup, I dated a man from May to October 1983. I dated one other fellow before getting remarried in 1987. Life was great. I had a beautiful daughter and was guardian of my precious niece Kim who came to live with us when she was 3 years old.

ON BEING HIV POSITIVE

Two years ago I donated blood during a blood drive. Ninety days later, on a cold, gray northern California day, I received a certified, registered letter. It was my day to work the evening shift, as I did every Monday. This enabled me to conduct a seminar for the nurses and to facilitate a multifamily therapy group on the substance abuse inpatient unit. The letter was from the blood bank, informing me that I was HIV positive. My heart stopped as I read the letter. "How can this happen? There must be some mistake. Oh my God, I'm going to die!" I was scared. I felt that I had just walked through a warp in time and space. I was now on the other side of the pale seeing myself and my life as if it belonged to someone else. I felt each breath would be my last. Waves of pain, fear, and sadness washed over me. "What am I going to do? Who can I talk to? What about the children?"

It was time to go to work. I got through the class; I really can't remember any of it except that while I was functioning on one level, I was aware that I was crying inside. My sorrow was palpable, but I couldn't let it show because I couldn't talk about what was happening to me. I got caught up in the nurses' seminar, and later in family group I was able to throw myself in and the pain subsided for a brief time.

Within the next 24 hours, I was able to talk to my wonderful husband, two dear friends, and my sister. The support was like a cold glass of spring water on a hot, muggy summer day. It was life giving. They loved me. They were there for me. They didn't feel that I was less of a person, nor were they ashamed of me. Their love, concern, and steady presence enabled me to put one foot in front of the other and take up my path again.

Instead of feeling better, as time passed, irrational fear took hold of me. I was afraid to use the same shower as my husband. I was worried about sharing the soap with him. What about food and kissing? What about when the kids take a sip of the beverage I'm drinking? Now, I was very knowledgeable about AIDS and HIV transmission. I had several dear friends who had AIDS. I never worried about being infected by them, since we did not have intimate contact. Now that I was infected, however, I felt unclean, like a leper, an outcast afraid of infecting someone else. It took several weeks before my rational mind could overcome the irrational fear. As usual, talking about it helped because I was able to share these fears with my husband and friends.

The next week was a blur. I have no idea what happened or what I did. We were scheduled to go on vacation and visit my mother. The kids were really excited, and my husband and I decided that we couldn't cancel but that we weren't ready to talk about it yet. My mother was the last person I wanted to tell. She has been my role model as a mom and a nurse, and she has always been so proud of me. I knew this would cause her incredible pain, and I couldn't hurt her.

I look at pictures from that trip now, and I see this rather typical American-looking family. We're all smiles as befits a family on vacation. That's not how it felt to me. That week was one of the worst in my life. Each step I took, I thought I would walk over the side of the earth. I would look at people and wonder if they knew, if they could tell. I wanted to scream out, "I have the HIV virus!" I wanted to scream, to cry, to hide. Somehow, my husband and I made it through the week. We would whisper about "it" behind our closed bedroom door and then emerge all smiles ready for the next adventure and fun-filled day.

I decided that I would continue to live life as if nothing had changed. I would not tell people that I was HIV positive until I absolutely had to. Only with a diagnosis of full-blown AIDS would I tell others of my condition. Until then, I wanted to hold onto my life as long as I could. I didn't want my children to be worrying about me when they had their own lives to focus on. I didn't want to cast my AIDS shadow over their lives until it became unavoidable, and until I felt ready in my own heart.

I went into therapy. I cried. I asked, "why me?" I was angry at AIDS, the virus, myself, and my source contact. I was able to get in touch with my sexual partners from the previous decade. They were frightened when they heard why I was calling. Each one except one person called me back. Each one said he tested negative for HIV. One person didn't get back to me, and through his family I discovered that his dearest friend had just died of AIDS. Since then we've been in touch, and indeed, he is HIV positive. Even though I was aware of the low rates of transmission from HIV-positive women to their male sexual partners, each phone call terrified me as I worried about whether I infected them or whether they infected me. Was my husband infected too? He tested negative.

Over the next few months my feelings became more stable and I was even able to feel periods of serenity. I constantly had to remind myself that I was okay today. Sometimes I had to remind myself that I was okay at this moment. I had to stay focused on the here and now. I've learned that if I get caught up in the past and what I should have done or on the future and what I could do, I start sinking emotionally. In the present moment nothing is ever that bad. So life continued, and I was consciously grateful for every moment.

GETTING A DIAGNOSIS

The American Nurses' Association, Council of Nurse Researchers Conference was in Chicago in September 1989. At the meeting I had a poster presentation. It was, as usual, an exciting, packed meeting with lots of good sessions to attend, old friends to see, new people to meet. During the meeting I was very tired. I had three cups of coffee during the poster session, which was very unusual behavior since one cup a day was my limit. Even with the coffee I was tired. I napped frequently, but other than fatigue I felt fine. We went to the Art Institute of Chicago, one of my very favorite museums. We went to a show. All in all, a productive and enjoyable meeting.

Upon returning home I found the usual pile of mail, phone messages, and things to do that had accumulated while I was gone. The week went by quickly. On Friday, after work, Kim had an appointment with her pediatrician for a routine physical. I took her there, and when we came home I was beat. My family rallied and got dinner. The next morning I couldn't get out of bed to take Kim to her swimming lesson. I felt like I had the flu and spent the weekend in bed. On Monday I was still weak but feeling much better. I stayed home from work and at my husband's insistence went in to see my physician.

The physical was fine, my lungs sounded clear, and I was ready to leave. My doctor stopped me. "Carole, as long as you're here, let's get a chest x-ray." I agreed with that, why not? The x-ray was ready within minutes, and we both looked at it. My physician, a young, bright, funny guy, turned to me with grim eyes. There was no laughter in his voice. "Carole, this is scary. Do you see what I see?" I did. Both lungs and both upper lobes were affected. Tuberculosis (TB) or *Pneumocystis* pneumonia? "You're going into the hospital right now. We need to get a sputum and if we can't get that we need a bronchoscopy."

Bronchoscopy produced a diagnosis, but I could not bounce back from the sedation. I started on intravenous (IV) Septra, but I continued to get worse. The most difficult thing to deal with was being unable to breathe. Even with oxygen it was difficult to get enough air. I was sleepy and had chills and fever. I was acutely ill, scared, trying to hold a front for my children, and feeling a deep sense of despair.

No one is ever prepared for an AIDS diagnosis. There is no way to describe the feelings I had when my doctor said with tears in his eyes, "The bronchoscopy report confirms *Pneumocystis*. Carole, you now have AIDS." Again, I started operating on two levels. I was chatting with my doctor about treatment while inside I was screaming, "No, no, not me. This is a big mistake. This can't be happening to me. God, help me." Fear, sorrow, and anger swept through me. I just wanted to pull the covers up over my head and pretend it wasn't happening. I felt dirty, damaged, devalued, a diminished person. I hated the body that was betraying me. I hated myself. I didn't want to die, but I didn't see how I could live.

MY NURSING CARE

Upon entering the hospital I was placed on TB precautions, and that unfortunately really alienated me from the nursing staff. The nurses would scold my children into wearing masks, keeping off the bed, and the like. It seemed to me that for these nurses the form was critically important. That is, they cared more about whether all of the rules were complied with, whether I had the blanket I needed when I rang the call bell, whether my bed was neat and clean, whether I had the oxygen at the proper setting, and not at all about how I was. I was a case, not a person. Shocked and emotionally distraught about my AIDS diagnosis, this dispassionate care fed my sense of unreality. I was in a living nightmare.

I don't know if the nurses felt intimidated by me. I remember one very young nurse was in the room and my doctor came in with, "Good afternoon, Dr. Chenitz." I responded by using his "doctor" title and we joked and laughed for a few minutes. I glanced at the nurse and smiled. She looked frightened and uncomfortable and left the room immediately. Up until that point I had no idea that I might have a chilling effect on the nurses who cared for me. Since I have always identified as a nurse, I feel at home wherever there are other nurses. We share more than a profession. We share a value system and a way of seeing the world. So, I had never thought that my AIDS diagnosis and who I was (a successful nurse) could frighten other nurses. Whatever the reason, when I needed these nurses, they simply weren't there, but my nursing admission interview was done and I'd wager that my nursing care plan was up to date.

Certainly the nurses were polite, respectful, and nice. But no one ever asked me how I felt. The lonely evenings after my family and friends left were very hard for me. The bed was uncomfortable (with that hard plastic ticking that protects hospital mattresses). My fevers would spike and the night would just seem to come down on me. What was to become of my life? What was to become of my children? What was left? How many more hospitalizations would there be? Would I lose my dignity, self-control, eyesight, ability to think? Would my children be forced to see their mother like this? Should I commit suicide?

Every evening I was tormented, and the nights in hospital became what St. John of the Cross called "dark nights of the soul."

I really couldn't talk to my family and friends about this, since they had enough to deal with. I just couldn't burden them with any more. Sadly, through all this, no one in the hospital stopped to ask me how I felt, how I was. They did their job efficiently and moved on.

Not only did the emotional needs I had go unrecognized, but no one touched me. No one in the hospital staff took my hand, rubbed my back, gave me support, or did any of the comfort and care measures that we nurses pride ourselves on. I will never forget how I felt.

Moreover, the effect this had on me was to be overwhelmed with my body's disgrace. I was unclean, untouchable, undesirable, a patient with a disgusting disease. If you get too close, you may get it, too. Obviously, if I were in good health, in my usual role, and felt like me, the impact of this uncaring care would not have affected me, but I was now a person with AIDS. I had crossed from caregiver to care recipient. My choice was to accept this role and go on or to sink into the morass that I felt all around me. Oh, how much easier it would have been if one of these nurses had reached out with a warm hand.

Two things happened for me about this time. The first was an answer to my struggle with the question, "Why me?" One night the answer became crystal clear: "Why not me?" Illness, tragedy, and misfortune can happen to anyone. I was not immune. I had a good life, and I could still have a good life. So, why not me?

A little miracle also occurred about this time, several days into my hospital stay. A nurse came into my room with flowers. She was the discharge planner and had seen my name on the hospital list with the diagnosis. She had heard me speak at a conference and came to tell me how sorry she was about my illness. She told me I had given a great talk when she heard me and that she was very impressed. She gave me the flowers and left. I never saw her again. I don't know what you would call her, but I called her an angel. All of a sudden, I was a person again, I had a history. I was someone. It felt so good to be recognized as the old me again.

The emotional impact of an AIDS diagnosis is compounded by the acute physical illness of the person receiving it. For me, it was the sickest I had ever been in my adult life. My defenses were down, and I was concentrating on maintaining bodily functions. I wasn't improving with Septra. I was vomiting, my liver enzymes were markedly elevated, and I was becoming increasingly lethargic. My shortness of breath was becoming worse, and I was now so weak, I couldn't make it to the bathroom. I was allergic to Septra and started on IV pentamidine. I improved almost immediately. After 5 days, which seemed like eternity, I went home.

Home. What a lovely word. I sat on my couch, looking out the picture window at the grove of redwoods in our yard. The sky was that brilliant robin's egg blue; white clouds were racing by, chased by the wind. I sat there overwhelmed with gratitude at the beauty around me and that I was here to see it. I gave a silent prayer of thanks for this day, for this image, and for my life. Tears came to my eyes at how beautiful everything is, how beautiful life is.

However, things got bad again and very quickly. I couldn't stop vomiting, and nothing touched the diarrhea. I was getting dehydrated. I couldn't keep an IV in, and it was getting increasingly difficult to find a vein. I have very small, frail veins, and only one on one arm is really usable. The others are too small and collapse easily. Another hospitalization was arranged, this time for a venous access device.

It had now been 1½ weeks since my AIDS diagnosis. I was very sick again and back in the hospital. I was still struggling with what it meant to be a person with AIDS. I still felt unclean and untouchable. I was discouraged, and my lack of control over my bowels was a source of deep humiliation. I was readmitted to the same hospital but to a different unit. This unit was a "healing place" created by the nurses who worked there.

I believe now that these nurses saved my life. I was in bed shortly after admission. It was early evening. I was getting an infusion of blood and waiting for an operating room to open up. I couldn't make it to the bathroom. I just couldn't negotiate the IV pole and my body. I was so weak that any movement was a supreme effort. The bathroom was in Europe and I didn't have a plane. Diarrhea was everywhere. I wanted to die. I loathed myself. Further, my bodily fluids were dangerous to others. How could I put others at risk? I put on the call bell, fighting back the tears.

In came Inge, middle aged, blond, composed, with a warm smile. "What's the matter?" she asked kindly. I could feel the compassion in her voice. It made me want to cry, but that would be too much for me. "I'm sorry but I couldn't make it to the bathroom. My bed is a mess. I am so sorry."

"What's there to be sorry about? I'll have it cleaned up in a few minutes. You should have a bedpan or a commode near you. Do you think you could make it to a commode by the bed?" I wasn't sure, so we decided I would get a bedside commode and a bedpan in my bed to hold onto for security. Then we both laughed. She turned to leave the room. Suddenly she turned around and looked into my eyes. She said gently, "All your life you have cared for people, now let us take care of you. It's your turn. It's okay, that's what we do. Let us take care of you for a while."

Simple words from an ordinary woman, but they were magic. All the nurses on this unit were like that. They loved being nurses, and they defined nursing as caring, compassionate, loving, nonjudgmental care. They cleaned, bathed, touched, started IVs, helped me to the commode, and gave me medicine with great efficiency, but what really mattered is that they did it with compassion. I felt my sense of dignity return, the dignity I felt in their care. The unit was a healing place where I knew I would live and be okay. I got a glimmer that there is life after AIDS.

The trip to the operating room was uneventful. I returned to my room receiving fluid infusions through my new Groshong catheter. After a tearful good-bye to my nurses, I went home to put the pieces of my life together, which I was ready to do after my time in the "healing place." My healing had begun.

PEER SUPPORT

I needed other people with AIDS. I needed to identify with others and find role models and mentors in my new life. I called around and joined a support group at the Center for Attitudinal Healing in Tiburon, California, which fortunately was close to my home. It was a group for women with HIV and AIDS. I made an appointment with the Marin AIDS Support Network (MASN). I started ordering newsletters such as the one from Project Inform, the PWA Coalition Newsletter, and AIDS Treatment News. I knew that to develop a healthy identity with AIDS, I had to surround myself with people with AIDS to be my friends. I wanted to be around people who understood what was happening to me.

The group I joined has about 30 women enrolled, and six to seven come on an average week. Interestingly, we are all upper-middle-class and middle-class white women. The group members represent the various professions and a range of occupations. These women are essential to my well-being, and today I count some of my dearest friends among the members of the group. If something happens to one of us, we all know and we are all affected. When I am discouraged, angry, or scared, the women in my group are there either on the phone or in person. We fill each other in on the treatment of the month. We share treatment recipes the way other women share food recipes. We meet weekly, and I try never to miss it. I speak to several group members during the week. I feel so blessed to have this wonderful group of women through whom I was able to let go of my professional identity and assume my identity as a woman living with AIDS.

I am connected with the Marin AIDS Support Network, our local AIDS agency. I had never been a client in a social service agency. I was always on the provider side. Now, I was the client. I went for my intake interview. It was very difficult for me to reach out and ask for help. When I did, wonderful people were there to help me across the chasm from what was to what is.

Michael, my counselor at MASN, is one of them. Michael is tall, blond, handsome, and full of information about services and things I need to consider. As my intake interview was ending, I was getting ready to leave when Michael quietly asked, "Carole, how are you dealing with your disability?"

I whirled around. "My what?" I felt angry. I didn't look like I had AIDS. No one could see my Groshong catheter. "What disability?" I responded coldly.

He looked at me steadily. "The fact that you can no longer do the things you once could. It is one of the biggest problems that people I see with AIDS have."

I felt my breath leave me. I had not articulated this, but it was an issue I was grappling with. That was it: I couldn't do the things I once could. I was too fatigued. I had no stamina. I became upset and unnerved quickly. Was this disability? I was so relieved that my struggle had a name. I had been striving to return to the way things were. I had wanted my life back, although I knew things would never be the same. I had wanted to be the person I once was and to do the things that person could do. That was impossible now, and I had to discover what I could do. This was a whole new ballgame, and I couldn't play by the old rules.

The support group members and Michael's insightful and sensitive words provided the context for a design for change and a new life. My family and friends provided the opportunity to change with their loving support and acceptance. I began to see myself as a person with AIDS. I began to accept who I was. I started to enjoy my new life, which centers around my wellness program (Table 13–1), my family, my friends, and my community. Love is the basic operating principle in my life. Those who can't give it or who are living in fear have no place in my life today.

I developed a protective denial. That is, when I am feeling good, I live as fully as I can. I do everything my energy will allow. I don't ignore AIDS, but I don't dwell on it either. I focus on the wellness and what I can do, rather than my illness and what I can't do. On bad days I become more identified with my body. I focus on just getting through the day. I allow myself to watch television (I didn't have a television in my house for 10 years), stay in bed, read, or just sleep. This was unthinkable to me a year ago. During the bad times I consciously work at remembering that nothing lasts forever. All pain stops. All things pass, the bad times as well as the good times.

DISCLOSURE

While I was putting my internal life together, other things had to be dealt with. One of the first questions that has to be answered in putting one's life together as a person with AIDS is whom to tell, when to tell, and how to tell. People were naturally concerned about what I had. Friends and colleagues were calling, sending cards and flowers, and bringing food to the house. Neighbors and parents of the children's friends wanted to know what I had and when I would be able to work again.

The central question was, "Do I tell them I have AIDS?" Or do I simply say, "I had pneumonia" and leave it at that? If I tell my friends and colleagues, could one of them inadvertently slip and tell my children? I could just hear the conversation, "Hello, Becky, this is Marie. I just heard the news about your Mom and I'm really sorry that she has AIDS. . . ."

I knew I had to tell my children. Should I just tell Becky, who was now 16, or should I also tell Kim, now 10? Was Kim too young to know?

TABLE 13–1. Personal Wellness Program

1. Have contact with at least one person with HIV or AIDS each day.
2. Read articles, newsletters, books, and pamphlets to keep informed about AIDS information and treatment.
3. Start each day with prayer and take time to pray several times a day.
4. Have quiet time each day just to sit and be still.
5. Remember my priorities. Don't let the little things bother me.
6. Avoid people who are not loving and supportive. Cut them off and out of my life.
7. Have family time each day.
8. Take time for periods of introspection, such as retreats for persons with AIDS (PWAs).
9. Talk about AIDS to schoolchildren, high school students, and community groups for disease prevention and to give a face to the epidemic.
10. Volunteer in the community. Help others whenever I can.
11. See friends. "Do lunch" at least once a week with a friend.
12. Try creative projects.
13. Exercise when possible.
14. Go to a physician at any sign or symptom of illness.
15. Follow information on clinical trials.
16. Participate in clinical trials whenever possible.
17. Go to a chiropractor for adjustment at least twice a month.
18. Attend support groups for PWAs.

What would it do to her emotionally? In any event the hospital did not seem the best place to tell them and I wasn't in any shape to help them through their process. I decided I needed a professional's help with the decisions of if, when, and how I should tell my children. In the San Francisco Bay area, resources are available to deal with all aspects of AIDS. I found an agency that specialized in family issues and AIDS.

As a result of consultation with staff in this agency and my therapist, my husband and I made a plan to tell the children. We would take them away for a weekend; we would not tell them at home where they could be distracted. We would answer each and every question, including how I was infected, as honestly and as completely as possible. The weekend was heartbreaking but drew us all closer together. Both of my children have continued to grow and blossom, even with the knowledge of my AIDS. They have made a conscious decision to live one day at a time.

Becky was writing her college applications, and she was able to answer the question, "Describe a significant event in your life and how it has affected you" by describing finding out that her mother had AIDS and what that meant to her. It was a moving, honest essay. She was also able to tell her favorite teacher, her drama teacher. This woman was magnificent and made it safe for Becky to be open with her classmates. Becky found her friends and classmates supportive and loving.

We were very worried about Kimberly and didn't want her to share my diagnosis with her friends. She wasn't ready to either. Children in the fourth grade can be mean. We were afraid that if people found out that I had AIDS, Kimberly would be ostracized by her classmates. So we decided to wait. Kim felt comfortable with this, since many of her classmates had made negative comments about gays and people with AIDS. While we were sure that the overwhelming majority of people in our community would respond with concern and compassion, we were afraid about the one or two who would react from unbridled fear.

Once the children knew my diagnosis, I was much more comfortable. The pressure to keep the secret from them was gone. We were able once again to talk openly, which had always been a family value. The evening dinner is a time for getting together and sharing both major and minor events of the day. Now, these could include open discussions. We now talked about experimental treatments for AIDS, my latest blood report, political issues surrounding AIDS, and anything else related to my illness. We were a family again.

After this hurdle was cleared, I was free to tell others. I knew I didn't want to return to work. I did not feel physically and emotionally able to handle it. So, I had to tell my boss, another heartbreakingly difficult task. She had hired me 8 years before to create a research environment within nursing service. More than that, we had agreed that the research program had to exist within an academic context. Therefore academic values needed to be part of nursing service values. We wanted nurses to feel the satisfaction of publishing their ideas, conducting clinical studies, utilizing research, reading journals, participating as presenters at conferences and workshops, and so forth. For 8 years my boss supported me in this effort. Without her there could be no research nor an environment for research in our setting. Further, I cared deeply about her as a person. Telling her would be like telling a family member.

After I was home for several weeks, we arranged a time to meet. It was difficult to tell her because I knew it would hurt her. I received her love, and like the administrator she is, she told me not to worry about ongoing activities. We discussed these, and she took care of them as efficiently as she ran her service. What a gift to me! What a relief! I could go back and clean out my office, but I didn't have to see a lot of people and talk about what was happening.

It was still a shock to me that my life was evolving this way. Initially I was too sick to think about my life and my goals. Later, when my energy was so low, loss of work wasn't difficult to bear, since I couldn't do it anyway. However, the loss of who I was and what I had done my entire adult life hit after several months: I wasn't a nurse anymore. I still had a license, but I would never practice nursing again. All of the articles published, papers presented, book chapters written, grants developed, and classes taught didn't matter now. It was gone. If I were to survive, I would need to develop new skills. I would have to learn to accept my new life. I needed to learn to relax. Maybe I could salvage something from my old life, but I wasn't sure what.

WOMEN WITH AIDS

All people with AIDS experience, to a greater or lesser degree, physical, social, emotional, and economic changes as a result of the disease. This common shared experience creates a bond between us and is felt in support groups, meetings, parties, or wherever two or more people with AIDS meet. The major group affected by AIDS has been men, particularly gay men. Women, while not newcomers in the epidemic, are sadly taking our place among the groups hard hit by this disease. In my experience and those of the women I know, several issues make this experience different for women than it is for men.

The first and perhaps the most difficult issue for women is related to our children and childbearing. Almost every woman I know, if she has children, asks, "What's going to happen to my children?" Fear for our children and the stigma they may have to bear keeps us silent and invisible. The desire to maintain a normal family life, however that's defined, makes us hesitate to tell them. In addition, the long protracted illness affects them deeply, and we know it but are powerless. The sense of frustration at our inability to fulfill the maternal role can lead to despair.

For many women who have not yet had children, the mourning is for the loss of this dream. The biological clock has wound down, and they are only 24 or 29 or 33 years old. They will never experience the joys of pregnancy, childbearing, and motherhood. Other women decide to have a baby in spite of their HIV-positive status. These women may be judged harshly by others and treated with disdain and scorn by health care providers. "How dare she have a baby when she's HIV positive? Doesn't she know what she's doing? She could infect her own baby." Even among other PWAs there is negative judgment about the decision to have a baby under these conditions. For some women, however, having a child is the fulfillment not only of a life's goal but also of their identity. Who are we to judge?

Another issue that faces women is the curiosity factor. When people find out I have AIDS, the first thing they ask is, "How did you get it?" People presume that they know how a man was infected. However, with women, especially white middle-class women who don't fit some stereotype of PWAs, there's a tremendous sense of curiosity.

I expect curiosity from the community but not from health care providers. I have gotten to the point that I ask for the clinical relevance of this question. "Is my source of infection going to affect my care? If not, then you have no need to know." While this might seem rude, I think satisfying your curiosity is rude. I am a very personal and private person. I have always been reticent about discussing my sexual life with anyone other than very dear friends. Since I have AIDS, there is an assumption that I am willing to discuss my past and present sexual activities with all comers. I find this assumption offensive. I know many PWAs who don't feel this way, who feel quite comfortable discussing their personal sexual lives. I'm not like them. Each PWA is a unique person with his or her own world view and reaction to the disease.

Access to information in the AIDS epidemic is lifesaving. Information about treatments and experimental drugs or clinical trials to prevent opportunistic infections, such as clofazimine to prevent *Mycobacterium avium-intracellulare* infection, is critical. Information gives us the essential facts upon which to make decisions and to act. Without information the individual has very few options for treatment.

The gay community has been very effective at mobilizing in the epidemic. Information about treatments and experimental drugs and clinical trials can be found within this community. Women, however, have two handicaps: we are not part of the community; and many of us do not have the educational background to understand what we need to know or how to access this critical information. The gay community was open, sharing, caring, and positive when I initially made my contacts as a PWA. A woman must be proactive, however. If you are not part of the community in which this information is commonplace, you must approach that community and seek it out. I spend hours every week on AIDS health care news. I wonder with great concern how women without my resources and knowledge manage to get and assimilate this information.

The final issue that women confront is the lack of knowledge about the effects of the virus or the treatments on women. While all PWAs face the ambiguity of the lack of knowledge and lack of treatments, for women the situation is even more abysmal. There is a recent movement to have the Centers for Disease Control definition of AIDS changed to include the vaginal and uterine infections that women manifest. This is only one of the issues.

Clearly discrimination against women exists in the enrollment in research projects and clinical trials. The excuse is that participation in research is too risky because women bear children. A woman's word that she is not going to have a child is not enough. If a women is enrolled and her reaction is different from the others', there is no way to know if the reason is the treatment under study or the virus. Even basic natural history data on women is lacking. The much talked about findings that women with AIDS die sooner may or may not be true in all populations of women, but this remains to be seen. We have so many questions and so few answers.

THE FUTURE

As I look toward the future, I have no doubt that AIDS has changed and will continue to change health care. In the future I believe several things will happen in relation to AIDS and health care.

First, there will be an end to what I call therapeutic nihilism. This attitude of health care professionals is characterized by a lack of assertive or aggressive treatment for PWAs. For some providers it's a form of burnout. They have had so many people die, they no longer have the drive to seek out experimental treatments or to be creative about treatments. For others, it's a way to withdraw and not deal with AIDS. Therapeutic nihilism toward persons with AIDS is demonstrated by providers who ignore minor symptoms: "Don't worry about hair loss (or fungal infections on the feet or face rash or missed menses). At least you're alive and this won't kill you." Another form is, "So what are you worrying about, you're going to die anyway." The more subtle form is not to work to find out about new treatments. If the standard treatment doesn't work, that's it.

I believe therapeutic nihilism also manifests itself in the standard treatment of persons who are HIV infected but without symptoms. The standard is to wait until the numbers of T4-helper cells drop to a certain point and then to initiate treatment. This attitude allows people to be at high risk before treatment is initiated. Once the T-4 helper cell numbers start dropping, I haven't heard of anyone who has been able to restore them to a normal or near normal level for any significant period of time. Why are we waiting for treatment? Immune enhancers should be started immediately. Low-dose antivirals for HIV-infected people with high T4-helper cell counts are being investigated and should be. New methods to prevent Pneumocystis pneumonia and other opportunistic infections need to be tested and used. It is simply not enough to tell people to wait until they are at risk before treatment is begun. That's not treatment, that's a death sentence.

Second, our attitude toward death and dying will change. Like many people with AIDS, I am not afraid of death, I am afraid of dying. The dying process and how that will be handled is of great concern to me. Everyone is going to die. Death is a part of life. However, AIDS brings with it a terribly painful, often humiliating dying process and that terrifies me. Compassion, assurance, and competence is what I need from health care providers. You have not failed me if I die. You have failed me if I die alone, frightened, in pain or distress. It is enlightened help with the dying that I need. I want help to maintain my dignity, keep me pain free, and allow my family and friends to be there. Too often today this type of treatment is not available. Why not? This is nursing care, and for this we are responsible.

Third, the future in health care is a shared partnership in care. Nurses have talked about a partnership with patients for years, but now PWAs and people with other life-threatening illnesses are demanding partnerships. PWAs have organized into highly effective, vocal political lobbies. The generation most affected by AIDS is the baby boomers and those who came after. These are not passive recipients of care. They are demanding partnerships at all levels of the health care delivery system: individual providers, the experts at local, state, and national levels, drug companies, the Food and Drug Administration, and the National Institutes of Health. The long time lag from laboratory testing of new therapeutic agents through the several phases of human testing through data analysis and review to final approval is not acceptable to people whose lives may be extended by these agents. PWAs are demanding representation at all levels of decision making about new treatments and the process for approval of treatments.

It has become clear that the system is not trustworthy. For example, in May 1990 a panel of 16 experts was convened by the National Institute of Allergy and Infectious Diseases to determine whether steroids should be used in the treatment of *Pneumocystis* pneumonia, a major killer of PWAs. They reviewed five unpublished papers whose authors were panel members and reached a conclusion. They then delayed announcing their conclusion until some of the papers had been accepted for publication 5 months later (*San Francisco Chronicle*, 1990). How many people died as the result of this delay? Our lives for their publications. There is something wrong with this system. This type of delay cannot be tolerated when you are dealing with my life and those of others.

In spite of efforts to refute these charges, the foot dragging of federal agencies in approving drugs for use in AIDS care has eroded confidence in the system. To date, 11 years into the epidemic, there is one approved drug to treat AIDS, that is, zidovudine (AZT). Two other promising drugs, didanosine (DDI) and dideoxycitidine (DDC), await review for approval. Six months ago it was evident that I had to discontinue AZT. I was lucky to begin a clinical trial with DDC. How many others are not so lucky? I know many people who can no longer tolerate AZT and have developed neuropathy on DDI or DDC. What antivirals are left to them? Today, there is nothing else in mainstream medicine.

Fourth, AIDS will become a truly chronic disease. AIDS will be the cancer of the next decade. In recent times there has been a great deal of excitement about the prolongation of life in PWAs. Unfortunately, the average life expectancy for PWAs has increased by only 6 months for men. No one is sure about women, since we are so rarely studied.

There is also a danger that we as a society will trivialize the disease. While on one hand we need to eliminate the irrational fear that surrounds AIDS, we need to replace this fear with personal caution and concerned, attentive care. If the disease is trivialized, PWAs will be ignored as they once were by all levels of government and the public, and the virus will spread.

As AIDS becomes more chronic, fear about the virus, the illness, and PWAs will decrease. PWAs will be treated with compassion and concern by all people. The horrible stories of job loss, rejection by family and friends, house burning, and so forth will be a thing of the past.

CONCLUSION

At this writing I have lived with AIDS for 16 months. I have been very fortunate and had not needed to be rehospitalized, nor have I had another opportunistic infection. I have made the transition from my old life as a nurse researcher to my new life as a person with AIDS. Rebecca is now a freshman in college, and our phone bills are enormous as we call each other. I am a volunteer in Kim's school at the lunch bar and a coleader for her Girl Scout troop.

On December 1, 1990, I appeared with the mayor of San Francisco at a press conference to commemorate World AIDS Day. I used my whole name and appeared on local TV and radio news. The word was out in our community, and so far, aside from a few ripples of fear-based concern, the response has been wonderful. The most common thing I hear is, "If there is anything I can do, let me know." This just warms my heart. Kim has had no problems at school; and both the principal and her teacher are watching out for her, but I think our fears were needless.

Periodically, when I least expect it, I feel the pangs of loss and grief: loss of my old life, my goals, my health, even my body, and grief over the loss I continue to experience. My energy never returned to my preillness level, and I have to be cautious about my schedule. I do a fair amount of public speaking at schools and community groups, and I find it exhilarating, scary, and exhausting. I do it because it's my way to contribute to the community. I believe that no one should be infected with this virus in 1991. That means we must reach the groups that are getting infected: women and IV drug users. In addition, there is still the need to give the epidemic a face and to inform people that we are human, too, that we are part of the community.

I follow treatment news and experimental drug news closely. After 10 months, AZT was no longer effective and my T4-helper cells continue to decline. I have been on an experimental antiviral for 4 months now and it doesn't seem to be working. This week, I had four T4 cells per cubic millimeter. We are going to have to make some decisions about treatment again. Each time there's a treatment decision to make I am afraid, but the fear passes. My physician is my partner, and we will negotiate another mutually agreeable plan, in spite of the lack of options. I am truly taking each day one day at a time.

PWAs, individually and collectively, are symbolic representations of society's guilt about sex and moral outrage at certain behaviors (Levine & Ram Dass, 1986). We are modern-day lepers, the outcasts, the outsiders. When you care for one PWA, you are symbolically caring for all of us. This is not a disease that affects us and them. We are them and they are us. AIDS is a human disease.

When history looks back to write the story of AIDS in this country and around the world, there will be heroes recorded. There will also be thousands of unrecorded heroes. Nurses and other health care providers who on a daily basis deliver life-enhancing and life-giving care to PWAs in all settings are the real heroes in this epidemic. While many of you may never be commemorated by name and fame may never be yours, you will be recorded in our hearts and those of our family and friends.

References

Levine, S. & Ram Dass (1986). *Exploring the heart of healing*. Novato, CA: The Access Group.

San Francisco Chronicle (Nov. 14, 1990). AIDS steroid report was delayed by panel.

Resources for Treatment for Persons with HIV Infection and AIDS

The following is not a comprehensive list of resources available to persons with HIV and AIDS. These are national resources and a good place to get started for information. Local AIDS organizations and public health departments should be contacted for specific services.

AIDS Clinical Trials Information Service (ACTIS) operates a free hotline on HIV and AIDS clinical trials funded by the federal government and drug companies. The hotline is open Monday to Friday from 9 AM to 7 PM Eastern time. Hotline number 1-800-TRIALS-A.

AIDS Treatment News, twice monthly newsletter published by John S. James, P.O. Box 411256, San Francisco, CA 94141, (415)255-0588.

AIDS/HIV Experimental Treatment Directory, published by the American Foundation for AIDS Research (AMFAR), lists clinical trials on a quarterly basis and a full directory twice a year. AMFAR, 1515 Broadway, Suite 3601, New York, NY 10036, (212)719-0033.

The Body Positive, monthly newsletter of The Body Positive, an organization for people who are HIV positive. Body Positive, 2095 Broadway, Suite 306, New York, NY 10023, (212)633-1782.

Treatment Issues, monthly newsletter of the Gay Men's Health Crisis, Department of Medical Information, 129 West 20th Street, New York, NY 10011, (212)807-6655 (hotline), (212)807-6664 (office).

PI Perspectives, quarterly newsletter by Project Inform, which focuses on experimental treatment and drug regulation policy. Project Inform, 347 Dolores Street, Suite 301, San Franciso, CA 94110, 1-800-822-7422 (national), 1-800-334-7422 (California), (415)558-8669 (local).

PWA Coalition Newsline, published every other month by People with AIDS Coalition, Inc., 31 West 26th Street, New York, NY 10010, (212)532-0290.

Bibliography

General Reading on Coping with AIDS and Other Life-Threatening Illness

Badgley, Laurence (1986). *Healing AIDS naturally: Natural therapies for the immune system.* San Bruno, CA: Human Energy Press.

Cousins, Norman (1979). *Anatomy of an illness as perceived by the patient.* New York: W.W. Norton Company.

Humphry, Derek (1984). *Let me die before I wake: Hemlock's book of self deliverance for the dying.* Los Angeles: Hemlock Society (distributed by Grove Press).

Kubler-Ross, Elisabeth, with Warshaw, Mal (1978). *To live until we say good-bye.* Englewood Cliffs, NJ: Prentice-Hall, Inc.

Kubler-Ross, Elisabeth, with Warshaw, Mal (1987). *AIDS: The ultimate challenge.* New York: Macmillan, Inc.

Jampolsky, Gerald G. (1983). *Teach only love.* New York: Bantam Books.

Kushner, Harold S. (1981). *When bad things happen to good people.* New York: Schocken.

Lingle, Virginia A. & Wood, Sandra M. (1988). *How to find information about AIDS.* New York: Harrington Park Press.

Levine, Stephen & Ram Dass (1986). *Exploring the heart of healing.* Videotape, parts 1 & 2. The Access Group, 4 Cielo Lane, Novato, CA (415)883-6111.

Martelli, Leonard J, with Peltz, Fran D. & Messina, William (1987). *When someone you know has AIDS: A practical guide.* New York: Crown Publishers, Inc.

McKusick, Leon (Ed.) (1986). *What to do about AIDS: Physicians and mental health professionals discuss the issues.* Berkeley, CA: University of California Press.

Norwood, Chris (1987). *Advice for life: A woman's guide to AIDS risks and prevention.* New York: Pantheon Books.

Serinus, Jason (Ed.) (1986). *Psychoimmunity and the healing process.* Berkeley, CA: Celestial Arts.

Siegel, Bernie S. (1986). *Love, medicine and miracles.* New York: Harper & Row Publishers.

Personal Experiences with AIDS

Callen, Michael (Ed.) (1987). *Surviving and thriving with AIDS: Hints for the newly diagnosed.* New York: People with AIDS Coalition.

Cox, Elizabeth (1990). *Thanksgiving: An AIDS journal.* New York: Harper & Row.

Dreuilhe, Emmanuel (1988). *Mortal embrace: Living with AIDS.* New York: Hill & Wang.

Holleran, Andrew (1988). *Ground zero: Essays.* New York: Morrow.

Landau, Elaine (1990). *We have AIDS.* New York: Franklin Watts.

McCarroll, Talbert (1988). *Morning glory babies: Children with AIDS and the celebration of life.* New York: St. Martin's Press.

Monette, Paul (1988). *Borrowed time: An AIDS memoir.* New York: Harcourt Brace Jovanovich, Publishers.

O'Connor, Tom, with Gonzalez, Ahmed (1987). *Living with AIDS.* San Francisco: Corwin Publishers.

Oyler, Chris (1988). *Go toward the light.* New York: Harper & Row.

Peabody, Barbara (1986). *The screaming room: A mother's journal of her son's struggle with AIDS: A true story of love, dedication and courage.* San Diego: Oak Tree Publishers.

Peavey, Fran (1989). *A shallow pool of time.* San Francisco: Crabgrass Press.

Nungesser, Lon G. (1986). *Epidemic of courage: Facing AIDS in America.* New York: St. Martin's Press.

Reed, Paul (1987). *Serenity: Challenging the fear of AIDS—from despair to hope.* Berkeley, CA: Celestial Arts.

Rieder, Ines & Ruppelt, Patricia (Eds.) (1988). *AIDS: The women.* San Francisco: Cleis Press.

Shilts, Randy (1987). *And the band played on: Politics, people and the AIDS epidemic.* New York: St. Martin's Press.

Tilleraas, Perry (1990). *Circle of hope: Our stories of AIDS, addiction and recovery.* Center City, MN: Hazelden.

White, Edmund (1988). *The darker proof: Stories from a crisis.* New York: New American Library.

Whitmore, George (1988). *Someone was here: Profiles in the AIDS epidemic.* New York: New American Books.

AIDS-Related Fiction and Poetry

Hoffman, Alice (1988). *At risk.* New York: Bantam Books.

Klein, Michael (1989). *Poets for life: Seventy six poets respond to AIDS.* New York: Crown Publishers, Inc.

Monette, Paul (1990). *Afterlife.* New York: Crown Publishers, Inc.

IN MEMORIAM

W. Carole Chenitz, R.N., Ed.D., Assistant Clinical Professor, Department of Mental Health, Community and Administrative Nursing, School of Nursing, University of California, San Francisco, died February 11, 1992, of AIDS-related complications. She was 45 years of age and resided in Greenbrae, California, with her family. She received her Bachelor of Science degree from Boston College and her Master of Education and Doctor of Education degrees from Columbia University Teachers College, New York. She completed a postdoctoral fellowship in nursing and medical sociology at the Department of Social and Behavioral Sciences, University of California, San Francisco. She also attended the Mental Research Institute, Palo Alto, California, where she completed a clinical externship in family therapy. She was formerly Associate Chief, Nursing Service for Research, Veterans Affairs Medical Center, San Francisco, where her research focused on gerontologic nursing, substance abuse, and sexually transmitted diseases including AIDS. Her work was based primarily on the use of the qualitative method, grounded theory. With Janice M. Swanson, she edited *From Practice to Grounded Theory: Qualitative Research in Nursing*, Addison-Wesley, 1986; and with Joyce Takano-Stone and Sally Salisbury, she edited *Clinical Gerontological Nursing: A Guide to Advanced Practice*, W. B. Saunders, 1991, which was named a Book of the Year by the *American Journal of Nursing*. Carole Chenitz was known for her belief in nursing and her dedication to the profession. She will be remembered for her ability to inspire nurses to do research, especially nurses working in clinical settings.

Appendix I

Drugs Used to Treat HIV Infection and AIDS-related Conditions

See following pages for Appendix I table.

Drugs Used to Treat HIV Infection and AIDS-related Conditions

GENERIC NAME (TRADE NAME)	ROUTE OF ADMINISTRATION	INDICATIONS	SIDE/ADVERSE EFFECTS
*Adenine arabinoside (Vidarabine) (Vira-A)	IV	Herpes simplex virus infection, herpes zoster infection, progressive multifocal leukoencephalopathy, varicella infection	Anorexia, nausea, vomiting, diarrhea, tremors, dizziness, confusion, hallucinations, ataxia, psychosis, leukopenia, thrombocytopenia, elevated SGOT and bilirubin levels, anemia
Amikacin (Amikin)	IV, IM	*Mycobacterium avium* complex infection	Increase/decrease in frequency of urination or amount of urine, increased thirst, loss of appetite, nausea, vomiting, muscle twitching, numbness, tingling, any loss of hearing, ringing or buzzing, clumsiness, dizziness, unsteadiness, difficulty in breathing
Amphotericin B (Fungizone)	IV	Candidiasis, coccidioidomycosis, cryptococcosis, histoplasmosis	Fever, chills, hypokalemia (irregular heartbeat, muscle cramps or pain, extreme fatigue), pain at site of infusion, anemia, blurred or double vision, renal failure (increased or decreased urination), paresthesias, impaired hearing, tinnitus, seizures, shortness of breath, skin rash or itching, agranulocytosis or leukopenia, thrombocytopenia
Ampicillin (Omnipen) (Omnipen-N) (Polycillin) (Polycillin-N) (Principen) (Totacillin) (Totacillin-N)	PO, IM, IV	Salmonellosis	Anaphylaxis, serum sickness, neutropenia, platelet count dysfunction, skin rash, fever, hives, itching, pseudomembranous colitis, seizures, diarrhea, nausea, vomiting, thrush, abdominal pain or cramps
*AS-101	IV	HIV infection	Garlic smell of breath, rash, nausea, vomiting, diarrhea, lightening of hair color, Stevens-Johnson syndrome

Drug	Route	Used for	Side effects
Azidouridine (AzdU)	PO	HIV infection	Nausea, headaches, leukopenia
Bleomycin (Blenoxane)	IV	Kaposi's sarcoma, non-Hodgkin's lymphoma	Cough, shortness of breath, pneumonitis, fever, chills, stomatitis, confusion, syncope, diaphoresis, changes in skin color and texture, rashes, swelling of fingers, nausea, vomiting and anorexia, weight loss, hair loss
*CD4, recombinant soluble (Receptin)	IV, IM	HIV infection	Local reactions at injection site, fever
Chloramphenicol (Anocol) (Chloromycetin)	PO, IM, IV	Salmonellosis	Blood dyscrasias, abdominal distention, blue-gray skin color, low body temperature, difficulty breathing, coma, cardiovascular collapse, skin rash, fever, confusion, delirium, headache, loss of vision, paresthesias, extremity weakness, diarrhea, nausea, vomiting, pale skin, sore throat, bleeding
Ciprofloxacin (Cipro)	PO	Mycobacterium avium complex infection	Restlessness, tremors, seizures, crystalluria (blood in urine, dysuria, low back pain), skin rash, itching, redness, swelling of face or neck, joint pains, stiffness, visual disturbances, photosensitivity, dizziness, headache, abdominal pain, diarrhea, nausea, vomiting, insomnia, unpleasant taste in mouth
Clindamycin (Cleocin)	PO, IM, IV	Toxoplasmosis, pneumocystosis	Pseudomembranous colitis, skin rash, neutropenia, thrombocytopenia, abdominal pain, nausea and vomiting, diarrhea, fungal overgrowth

*Investigational as of March 1991.

Table continued on following page

Drugs Used to Treat HIV Infection and AIDS-related Conditions *Continued*

GENERIC NAME (TRADE NAME)	ROUTE OF ADMINISTRATION	INDICATIONS	SIDE/ADVERSE EFFECTS
Clofazimine (Lamprene)	PO	*Mycobacterium avium* complex infection	Colicky or burning abdominal or stomach pain, nausea, vomiting, pink or red to brownish black discoloration of skin (two suicides have been reported as a result of mental depression secondary to skin discoloration), visual changes, gastrointestinal bleeding, hepatitis or jaundice, dry rough scaly skin, anorexia, dizziness, drowsiness, dryness, burning, itching or irritation of eyes, skin rash, photosensitivity
Clotrimazole (Mycelex Troches)	PO	Candidiasis (oropharyngeal)	Abdominal or stomach cramping or pain, diarrhea, nausea or vomiting
Cyclophosphamide (Cytoxan) (Neosar)	PO, IM, IV	Non-Hodgkin's lymphoma	Missing menstrual cycles, darkening of skin and fingernails, loss of appetite, nausea, vomiting, diarrhea, stomach pain, flushing and redness of face, headache, increased sweating, swollen lips, skin rash, hives, loss of hair
Cycloserine (Seromycin)	PO	*Mycobacterium avium* complex infection, *Mycobacterium tuberculosis*	Anxiety, confusion, dizziness, drowsiness, increased irritability, increased restlessness, mental depression, muscle twitching or trembling, nervousness, nightmares, other mood or mental changes, speech problems, skin rash, numbness, tingling or burning pain or weakness in the hands or feet, headache, seizures

Drug	Route	Use	Side Effects
Cytarabine (Ara-C) (Cytosine arabinoside) (Cytosar-U)	PO, IM, IV	Non-Hodgkin's lymphoma, progressive multifocal leukoencephalopathy	Fever, chills, cough, hoarseness, lower back/side pain, difficult urination, diarrhea, sores in mouth or on lips, unusual bleeding/bruising, numbness or tingling in fingers, toes, or face, unusual tiredness, swelling of feet or lower legs, pain at injection site, skin rash, reddened eyes, chest pain, shortness of breath, itching of skin, headache
Dapsone (Avlosulfon) (DDS)	PO	Pneumocystosis	Hemolytic anemia, Stevens-Johnson syndrome, agranulocytosis (fever and sore throat), hepatic damage, methemoglobinemia (bluish fingernails, lips, or skin, fatigue, dyspnea), mood changes, peripheral neuritis
*Didanosine (formerly known as ddI) (Videx)	PO	HIV infection	Diarrhea, abdominal pain, pancreatitis, peripheral neuropathy, seizures, headaches, abnormal bone marrow function, abnormal liver function, electrolyte abnormalities, cardiac arrhythmias, allergic reactions
*Didehydrodideoxythymidine (d4T)	PO	HIV infection	Peripheral neuropathy, elevated liver function tests, headaches, nausea
*Dideoxycytidine (ddC)	PO	HIV infection	Peripheral neuropathy, oral aphthous ulcers, fever, rash, stomatitis
*Diethyldithiocarbamate (DTC) (Imuthiol)	PO, IV	Immunomodulation	Metallic taste, abdominal pain, fatigue, nausea, inability to concentrate, increased energy levels after IV infusion, Antabuse-like effect when alcohol is ingested

Table continued on following page

Drugs Used to Treat HIV Infection and AIDS-related Conditions *Continued*

GENERIC NAME (TRADE NAME)	ROUTE OF ADMINISTRATION	INDICATIONS	SIDE/ADVERSE EFFECTS
Doxorubicin hydrochloride (Adriamycin)	IV	Kaposi's sarcoma, non-Hodgkin's lymphoma	Leukopenia or infection (fever, chills, sore throat), stomatitis, esophagitis, flank, stomach, or joint pain, pain at infusion site, peripheral edema, fast or irregular heartbeat, shortness of breath, gastrointestinal bleeding, thrombocytopenia (unusual bleeding or bruising), changes in skin color, diarrhea, nausea, vomiting, skin rash or itching, hair loss, reddish color to urine
*Eflornithine hydrochloride (DFMO) (Ornidyl)	PO, IV	Cryptosporidiosis, pneumocystosis	Diarrhea, thrombocytopenia, anemia, hearing loss
Epoetin alfa, recombinant (Epogen) (Eprex) (Procrit)	IV, SC	Anemia associated with HIV infection or zidovudine therapy	Chest pain, edema, tachycardia, headache, hypertension, polycythemia, seizures, shortness of breath, skin rash, arthralgias, asthenia, diarrhea, nausea, fatigue, influenza-like syndrome after each dose NOTE: should be temporarily discontinued if the hematocrit reaches or exceeds 36%
Ethambutol (Myambutol)	PO	Mycobacterium avium complex infection, Mycobacterium tuberculosis	Acute gout, chills, pain and swelling of joints, skin rash, fever, arthralgias, numbness, tingling, burning pain, weakness of hands/feet, blurred vision, eye pain, red-green color blindness, any loss of vision, abdominal pain, anorexia, nausea, vomiting, headache, mental confusion

Drug	Route	Uses	Side Effects
Ethionamide (Trecator-SC)	PO	*Mycobacterium avium* complex infection, *Mycobacterium tuberculosis*	Yellow skin/eyes, tingling, burning or pain in hands or feet, mental depression, clumsiness/unsteadiness, confusion, mood or mental changes, coldness, decreased sexual ability, dry puffy skin, weight gain, hyperglycemia, blurred vision or loss of vision, skin rash
Etoposide (VePesid)	IV	Kaposi's sarcoma, non-Hodgkin's lymphoma	Leukopenia, thrombocytopenia, stomatitis, ataxia, paresthesias, tachycardia, shortness of breath or wheezing, pain at site of injection, nausea, vomiting, loss of appetite, diarrhea, fatigue, loss of hair
Fluconazole (Diflucan)	PO, IV	*Candidiasis*, cryptococcosis	Abnormal liver function, Stevens-Johnson syndrome, nausea, headache, skin rash, vomiting, abdominal pain, diarrhea
Flucytosine (Ancobon) (5-Fluorocytosine) (5FC)	PO	*Candidiasis*, cryptococcosis	Anemia, yellow eyes/skin, skin rash, redness, itching, sore throat, fever, unusual bleeding/bruising, confusion, sensitivity of the skin to sunlight, abdominal pain, diarrhea, loss of appetite, nausea, vomiting, dizziness, lightheadedness, drowsiness, headache
*Foscarnet sodium (Foscavir)	IV	Cytomegalovirus infection, herpes simplex virus infection, HIV infection	Increased thirst, headaches, nausea, anorexia, flank pain, muscle twitching, elevated creatinine, mild proteinuria, renal failure, decrease in hemoglobin, both increase and decrease in calcium hyperphosphatemia, fatigue, irritability, tremors, seizures, genital ulcers

Table continued on following page

Drugs Used to Treat HIV Infection and AIDS-related Conditions *Continued*

GENERIC NAME (TRADE NAME)	ROUTE OF ADMINISTRATION	INDICATIONS	SIDE/ADVERSE EFFECTS
Ganciclovir (Cytovene) (formerly known as DHPG)	PO, IV	Cytomegalovirus infection	Granulocytopenia, thrombocytopenia, anemia, mood changes, tremor, nervousness, fever, skin rash, abnormal liver function, phlebitis, abdominal pain, loss of appetite, nausea, vomiting
*Granulocyte, macrophage–colony stimulating factor-E (GM-CSF) (LEUCOMAX) (rGM-CSF)	IV, SC	Neutropenia associated with HIV infection or zidovudine or ganciclovir therapy	Hypersensitivity reactions (urticaria, angioedema, bronchoconstriction, anaphylaxis), fever, chills, rigors, bone pain, arthralgias, adult respiratory distress syndrome, rash, pericarditis, local erythema at site of injection, hypoxia
Interferon alfa recombinant (Intron-A) (Roferon-A)	PO, IM, SC	HIV infection, Kaposi's sarcoma	Parenteral: flulike syndrome (fever, myalgias and malaise), leukopenia, elevation in liver enzyme levels, weight loss, hair loss, fatigue, proteinuria, reversible congestive cardiomyopathy (weight gain and signs of right- or left-sided congestive heart failure) Oral: no side effects have been reported with low-dose oral alfa interferon
*Interleukin-2 recombinant (IL-2) (Proleukin)	IV	HIV infection	Fluid retention, hypotension, fever, chills, elevated creatinine, elevated BUN, oliguria, anuria, azotemia, fatigue, weight gain, tachycardia, nausea, vomiting, transient changes in liver function studies, headache, lightheadedness, dizziness, mental changes, pulmonary symptoms, anemia, leukocytosis, skin rash, myalgia, arthralgia

Drug	Route	Use	Side Effects
Isoniazid (INH) (Izonid) (Laniazid) (Nydrazid) (Teebaconin)	PO, IM	Mycobacterium avium complex infection, Mycobacterium tuberculosis	Loss of appetite, nausea, vomiting, diarrhea, unusual tiredness or weakness, dark urine, yellow eyes/skin, clumsiness or unsteadiness, numbness, tingling, burning or pain in hands or feet, fever, sore throat, unusual bleeding/bruising, skin rash, pain at injection site, arthralgia, seizures, depression, psychosis, blurred vision with or without eye pain
*Intraconazole (Sporanox)	PO	Maintenance therapy for cryptococcosis or histoplasmosis	Nausea, headaches, fatigue, abdominal cramps, rash, loss of potassium, edema
Ketoconazole (Nizoral)	PO	Candidiasis	Hepatitis, nausea, vomiting, diarrhea, dizziness, drowsiness, gynecomastia, headache, skin rash, itching, impotence, insomnia, photophobia
Leucovorin (Citrovorum) (Folinic Acid) (Wellcovorin)	PO, IM, IV	Prophylaxis and treatment of toxicity related to: methotrexate, pyrimethamine, or trimethoprim	Skin rash, hives, itching, wheezing
*Megestrol acetate (Megace)	PO	HIV wasting	Alteration of menstrual pattern with unpredictable bleeding, pain in chest, visual disturbances, headache, insomnia, pain in abdomen, groin, calf or leg, loss of coordination, slurred speech, weakness or numbness in extremities, yellow eyes/skin, depression, skin rashes, peripheral edema, brown spots in skin, acne, increased body hair, increased breast tenderness, loss of scalp hair

Table continued on following page

Drugs Used to Treat HIV Infection and AIDS-related Conditions *Continued*

GENERIC NAME (TRADE NAME)	ROUTE OF ADMINISTRATION	INDICATIONS	SIDE/ADVERSE EFFECTS
Methotrexate (Folex) (Folex PFS) (Mexate) (Mexate-AQ)	PO, IM, IV	Non-Hodgkin's lymphoma	Gastrointestinal ulceration or bleeding, enteritis, intestinal perforation, leukopenia, bacterial infections, septicemia, thrombocytopenia, stomatitis, renal failure, azotemia, hyperuricemia, nephropathy, cutaneous vasculitis, hepatotoxicity, pulmonary fibrosis, pneumonitis, central nervous system toxicity, anorexia, nausea, vomiting, acne, boils, skin rash
Miconazole (Micatin) (Monistat Derm) (Monistat IV)	PO, IM, IV, topical	Candidiasis, coccidioidomycosis, cryptococcosis	Fever, chills, skin rash, itching, redness, swelling at injection site, unusual tiredness, weakness, unusual bleeding/bruising, anorexia, diarrhea, nausea, vomiting
Nystatin (Mycostatin) (Nilstat) (Nystex)	PO	Candidiasis (oropharyngeal)	Diarrhea, nausea, vomiting, stomach pain
*Octreotide (Sandostatin)	SC	HIV-related diarrhea	Hyperglycemia, hypoglycemia, abdominal pain, diarrhea, nausea, vomiting, pain at injection site, headache, fatigue, dizziness, lightheadedness, edema, flushing of face, hepatic dysfunction
*Paromomycin sulfate (Humatin)	PO	Cryptosporidiosis	Nausea, vomiting, diarrhea, renal damage

Drug	Route	Indication	Side Effects
Pentamidine isethionate (Nebupent, inhalation) (Pentam parenteral)	IM, IV, inhalation	Pneumocystosis	Parenteral: blood dyscrasias, rapid irregular pulse, diabetes mellitus, skin rash, hyperglycemia, hypoglycemia, hypotension, pain or tenderness at site of injection, redness or flushing of the face, metallic taste in mouth. Inhalation: chest pain, congestion, coughing, dyspnea, pharyngitis, wheezing, skin rash, metallic taste in mouth, pneumothorax
*Pentosan polysulfate sodium (Elmiron) (PPS)	PO, IV	HIV infection, Kaposi's sarcoma	Bone marrow suppression, bruising, bleeding, headache, dizziness, nausea, diarrhea, dyspepsia, peripheral edema, skin rash, anemia, thrombocytopenia, abdominal pain, appetite change, tremors, night sweats, impaired concentration, fatigue, confusion, stomatitis, shortness of breath, peripheral neuropathy
*Piritrexim isethionate	PO, IV	Mycobacterium avium complex infection, Pneumocystis carinii infection, toxoplasmosis	Mucositis, myelosuppression, anemia, leukopenia, thrombocytopenia, nausea, vomiting, phlebitis
*Polyribonucleotide (Ampligen)	IV	HIV infection	Mild flulike symptoms including transient headache, fever, myalgia, malaise, flushing of face and chest, shortness of breath, nausea, diarrhea, photophobia, rash, transient visual disturbances
Pyrazinamide (PZA)	PO	Mycobacterium tuberculosis	Joint pain, loss of appetite, unusual tiredness or weakness, yellow eyes/skin, swelling of joints, itching, rash
Pyrimethamine (Daraprim)	PO	Pneumocystosis, toxoplasmosis	Folic acid deficiency (loss of taste, glossitis, diarrhea, sore throat, dysphagia, ulcerative stomatitis), fever, bleeding, bruising, fatigue, skin rash, trembling, unsteadiness or clumsiness, seizures, anorexia, vomiting

Table continued on following page

471

Drugs Used to Treat HIV Infection and AIDS-related Conditions *Continued*

GENERIC NAME (TRADE NAME)	ROUTE OF ADMINISTRATION	INDICATIONS	SIDE/ADVERSE EFFECTS
*Rifabutin (Ansamycin)	PO	*Mycobacterium avium* complex infection	Increase in both liver enzymes and creatinine, rash, fever, leukopenia, gastrointestinal distress, hemolysis, arthralgias
Rifampin (Rifadin) (Rifadin IV) (Rimactane)	PO, IV	*Mycobacterium avium* complex infection, *Mycobacterium tuberculosis*	Chills, difficult breathing, dizziness, fever, headache, muscle and bone pain, shivering, rash, itching, skin redness, sore throat, yellow eyes/skin, unusual bleeding/bruising, loss of appetite, nausea, vomiting, unusual tiredness or weakness, bloody or cloudy urine, stomach cramps, diarrhea, sore mouth or tongue, discoloration of urine, feces, saliva, sputum, sweat or tears
*Spiramycin (Rovamycine)	PO, IV	Cryptosporidiosis	Parenteral: paresthesias, irritation at injection site, dysesthesia, giddiness, pain, stiffness, burning sensation, hot flashes Oral: nausea, vomiting, diarrhea, fatigue, indigestion, sweating, heaviness in chest, cool sensation in mouth or pharynx
Sulfadoxine and pyrimethamine (Fansidar)	PO	Pneumocystosis	Stevens-Johnson syndrome, toxic epidermal necrolysis, fulminant hepatic necrosis, agranulocytosis, aplastic anemia, photosensitivity, bleeding and/or bruising, folic acid deficiency (loss of taste, glossitis, diarrhea, sore throat, dysphagia, ulcerative stomatitis), skin rash, fatigue, aching in joints or muscles, hematuria, dysuria, goiter, tremors, seizures, headache, dizziness, nausea, vomiting

Drug	Route	Indication	Side Effects
Sulfamethoxazole and trimethoprim (Bactrim) (Bethaprim) (Cheragan W/TMP) (Cotrim) (Septra) (Sulfamethoprim) (Sulfaprim) (Sulfatrim) (Sulfoxaprim) (Triazole) (Uroplus)	PO, IV	Isosporiasis, pneumocystosis, salmonellosis, toxoplasmosis	Skin rash, itching, Stevens-Johnson syndrome (myalgia, arthralgia, redness, blistering, peeling, or loosening of the skin, extreme fatigue), dysphagia, fever, leukopenia (sore throat), thrombocytopenia (unusual bleeding or bruising), hepatitis (dark urine, pale stools, yellow skin and/or sclera), cystalluria, hematuria, diarrhea, dizziness, headache, anorexia, nausea, vomiting
Sulfamethoxazole (Gantanol)	PO	Toxoplasmosis	Fever, itching, skin rash, hepatitis, photosensitivity, blood dyscrasias, difficulty swallowing, redness, blistering, peeling of skin, hematuria, crystalluria, thyroid dysfunction, dizziness, headache, anorexia, nausea, vomiting, diarrhea
Sulfisoxazole (Gantrisin)	PO	Toxoplasmosis	Fever, itching, skin rash, hepatitis, photosensitivity, blood dyscrasias, difficulty swallowing, redness, blistering, peeling of skin, hematuria, crystalluria, thyroid dysfunction, dizziness, headache, anorexia, nausea, vomiting, diarrhea
Trimethoprim (Proloprim) (Trimpex)	PO	Salmonellosis	Blood dyscrasias (bleeding), headache, methemoglobinemia, skin rash, itching, alteration in taste, sore mouth or tongue, anorexia, diarrhea, nausea, vomiting, abdominal pain, cramping
*Trimetrexate glucuronate	IV	Pneumocystosis	Decrease in neutrophil and platelet counts, nausea, vomiting, diarrhea, reversible liver function abnormalities, skin rash, fever

Table continued on following page

GENERIC NAME (TRADE NAME)	ROUTE OF ADMINISTRATION	INDICATIONS	SIDE/ADVERSE EFFECTS
Vinblastine (Velban) (Velsar)	IV	Kaposi's sarcoma	Fever, chills, cough, hoarseness, lower back pain, side pain, painful or difficult urination, pain or redness at site of injection, sores in mouth and on lips, rectal bleeding, dizziness, difficulty in walking, double vision, drooping eyelids, headache, jaw pain, mental depression, numbness or tingling in fingers and toes, pain in fingers or toes, pain in testicles, weakness, nausea, vomiting, loss of hair
Vincristine (Oncovin) (Vincasar PES) (Vincrex)	IV	Kaposi's sarcoma, non-Hodgkin's lymphoma	Constipation, stomach cramps, bed wetting, decrease or increase in urination, dizziness, lightheadedness, dysuria, lack of sweating, joint pain, lower back or flank pain, visual changes, ataxia, drooping eyelids, headache, jaw pain, numbness or tingling in fingers or toes, pain in testicles, weakness, hyponatremia, leukopenia, thrombocytopenia, stomatitis Syndrome of inappropriate antidiuretic hormone (SIADH) evidenced by agitation, confusion, dizziness, hallucinations, anorexia, mental depression, seizures, insomnia, loss of consciousness

Drug	Route	Indication	Side Effects
Zidovudine (Retrovir) (formerly known as AZT)	PO, IV	HIV infection	Anemia, leukopenia, neutropenia, platelet count changes (either increased or decreased), anorexia, asthenia, diarrhea, dizziness, fever, headache, nausea, insomnia, malaise, myalgia, pain in abdomen, rash, somnolence, taste alteration
Zovirax (Acylovir)	PO, IV, topical	Herpes simplex virus infection, herpes zoster infection, varicella infection	Parenteral: skin rash, hives, hematuria, lightheadedness, headache, diaphoresis, confusion, tremors, abdominal pain, difficulty breathing, decreased frequency of urination, nausea, vomiting, unusual thirst, extreme fatigue Oral: changes in menstrual period, skin rash, diarrhea, dizziness, headache, joint pain, nausea, vomiting, acne, anorexia, somnolence Topical: mild pain, burning, itching, skin rash

Appendix II

Administration of Aerosolized Pentamidine for Pneumocystis carinii *Pneumonia Prophylaxis*

I. *Background information*

Since 1989 aerosolized pentamidine isethionate has been one of the two methods recommended by the CDC to prevent AIDS-related PCP (CDC, 1989d). Based on clinical trials the current recommendation for aerosol therapy is 300 mg of pentamidine isethionate, administered once every 4 weeks via the Respirgard II jet nebulizer (CDC, 1989d).

According to Lyphomed (1989), cough and bronchospasm were the most frequently reported side effects in the trials. In the 277 individuals initially studied, cough developed in 38% and bronchospasm developed in 15%; these symptoms occur primarily in individuals who smoke cigarettes and continue to smoke or who have an underlying disease such as asthma (Conte et al., 1987; Godfrey-Fausett et al., 1988; Montgomery et al., 1987). Administration of an aerosolized bronchodilator such as albuterol, metaproterenol, or terbutaline usually controls such symptoms, and in certain cases the bronchodilator should be administered before treatment to prevent recurrence (Lyphomed, 1989; U.S. Pharmacopeial Convention, Inc., 1990). A hand-held micronebulizer along with a bronchodilator, ordered by the physician, should always be available for all clients treated. The Respirgard II nebulizer should not be used to administer bronchodilator therapy because of the difference between the particle size it delivers and that required to achieve bronchodilation.

Another serious adverse event that has been reported in persons receiving aerosolized pentamidine is spontaneous pneumothorax (Lyphomed, 1989; Martinez et al., 1988; Scannell, 1990). In most cases the clients had a previous documented episode of PCP. Whether the pneumothorax was the result of pulmonary damage from infection or of an increased risk associated with nebulized pentamidine has not been established. However, the possibility of this occurrence indicates a need for supervised inhalation treatments. Should pneumothorax occur while the client is performing

476

the treatment alone at home, the associated chest pain and diminution of voice sounds may make summoning emergency assistance difficult, if not impossible.

Neither animal nor human reproduction studies have been conducted to determine safety in pregnant women, and whether the drug, taken as an aerosol treatment, is excreted in breast milk is not known. No studies have been conducted to determine the effects of pentamidine isethionate on fertility or in relation to mutagenesis or carcinogenesis. No geriatric-specific information is available.

F.E. Young and colleagues (1989) pointed out that aerosolized pentamidine may pose a risk to health care workers administering the drug if the nebulizer is improperly used and large quantities of pentamidine are released into the air through the mouthpiece. This can cause adverse events in health care workers similar to those that may affect the client inhaling the drug. Cutaneous reactions and conjunctivitis have been reported in clients receiving pentamidine aerosol (Conte et al., 1987; Lindley & Schleupner, 1988). Jacobson (1990) cited incidents in which health care workers complained of scratchy throat, burning eyes, reduced lung function, and a drop in carbon monoxide diffusion capacity when administering the drug in poorly ventilated rooms.

Montgomery and associates (1990) conducted studies to measure the ambient concentration of aerosolized pentamidine in an unventilated treatment room and concluded that the risk to health care workers was low and that systemic toxic effects were unlikely. Until long-term occupational studies are performed, health care workers should limit environmental exposure by using nebulizers with expiratory filters (Respirgard II), performing the treatment in adequately ventilated rooms, teaching the client proper equipment use, and wearing tight-fitting face masks (Montgomery et al., 1990).

Both health care workers and clients may be at risk for exposure to TB in settings where cough-inducing procedures such as aerosolized administration of pentamidine are performed (CDC, 1989a). The CDC recommends that all HIV-positive persons be evaluated for the presence of potentially infectious TB with chest roentgenograms and sputum smears for AFB (CDC, 1989c). Only after negative results should pentamidine treatment be initiated. If TB is diagnosed, the client should be started on anti-TB therapy before receiving pentamidine aerosol treatments.

Pentamidine aerosol treatments performed in congregate settings such as clinics, offices, or hospitals should be carried out in rooms or booths with negative air pressure in relation to adjacent rooms or hallways (CDC, 1989a). Air in these rooms or booths should be exhausted directly to the outside of the building and away from intake vents. The number of air exchanges per hour in the room or booth should be sufficient to remove infectious organisms during the time between patients. Ultraviolet lights are also useful in killing airborne tubercle bacilli. Pentamidine aerosol treatments performed at home should be carried out in well-ventilated areas, with windows open to outside air.

Health protection for the person providing the treatment should include barriers to prevent exposure to both pentamidine and TB. Montgomery and colleagues (1990) noted that the greatest occupational risk is exposure to TB and that wearing a tight-fitting face mask such as one meeting NIOSH/MSHA Dusts/Flames/Mists TC-21-C-202 standards would trap most particles and provide some protection against TB. Standard, loose-fitting paper masks are of no value.

Additional protective barriers that may be used by health care workers include protective eyewear that provides a seal around the eyes (goggles), disposable gowns, and disposable gloves. Health teaching for the client should include covering the mouth when coughing, and turning the gas source *off before* removing the mouthpiece. The Respirgard II uses both electrostatic and impact methods of filtration for expired air, which prevents environmental contamination by pentamidine and filters exhaled gases. Conover and colleagues (1988) recommended that pregnant health care workers not administer aerosolized pentamidine, although no risk has been reported.

II. *Preadministration assessment* (to be performed before the first treatment)

  A. Has the client ever received pentamidine isethionate either systemically or via aerosol, and have any adverse events occurred?

  B. Review of the pulmonary system (Smith, 1990; Ungvarski, 1991)

    1. Past history of respiratory infections

    2. Past history of asthma, bronchitis, or emphysema

    3. Current history of AIDS-related pulmonary malignancy or opportunistic infection

    4. Has the client been evaluated for pulmonary TB?

      a. Chest roentgenogram

      b. Sputum collection for AFB

    5. If pulmonary TB has been diagnosed, has sputum been examined for evaluation of treatment response?

    6. History of smoking, including tobacco, marijuana, and crack cocaine

  C. Review of metabolic system, including diabetes and hypoglycemia. The latter, a frequently encountered side effect of systemic pentamidine therapy, is rare in persons receiving aerosolized pentamidine, but it has been reported (Lindley & Schleupner, 1988; Lyphomed, 1989).

   D. Female clients

     1. Are they currently or do they plan on becoming pregnant?

     2. Are they breast feeding?

III. *Equipment needed*

   A. Pentamidine isethionate, 300 mg

   B. One 10 ml vial of sterile water USP for injection (preservative free; do not use bacteriostatic sterile water)

   C. 10 ml syringe with 18-gauge needle

   D. Respirgard II nebulizer system

   E. Hand-held micronebulizer

   F. Unit dose bronchodilator prescribed by client's physician

   G. Gas source (can use compressed air or oxygen or a freestanding air compressor)

     1. If compressed air or oxygen is used, a flowmeter is required to adjust gas flow rate.

     2. If a freestanding air compressor is used, select one with a 40 to 50 pounds per square inch (psi), a pressure-regulating knob, and a psi gauge. In addition, a nipple adaptor is required, and an in-line bacterial filter is needed to filter air going to the client's lungs.

   H. A cup of liquid (selected by client, either hot or cold) to be sipped during procedure to moisten upper airway

   I. Protective wear for the person administering the treatment

IV. *Pretreatment teaching*

   A. Explain the procedure

   B. Breathing instructions

     1. Breathe only through the mouth so that any exhaled drug or microorganisms will be trapped by the nebulizer's exhalation filter. (Some clients may benefit from nose clips to prevent nasal breathing.)

     2. Breathe at a normal rate, but take a deep breath at least once every minute by exhaling all the air from the lungs and then inhaling deeply to fill them. If possible, hold this breath for a few seconds before exhaling.

   C. If the client needs to take a break during the treatment, the gas supply should be turned *off before* the mouthpiece is removed. This minimizes environmental contamination and facial exposure to the drug. Encourage the client to take deep breaths at the beginning of the break. Breathing periodically from residual volume may provide a more equal distribution of the aerosol to the lungs (Sarti, 1989).

   D. Positioning instructions

1. Optimal positioning for the treatment has not been definitively established. In most cases the client assumes an upright
(high-Fowler's) position. Alternatives are having the client lie
in a supine position or take half of the treatment lying on one
side and then switch (Lyphomed, 1989).

2. Baskin and colleagues (1990) evaluated the effects of varying
body position and breathing pattern on the overall lung distribution of aerosolized pentamidine. They concluded that
aerosol distribution was more uniform when the drug was
administered with the client in the supine position.

E. Remind the client to report any problems during the treatment.

V. *Preparation of the medication*
   A. Thoroughly wash hands.
   B. Reconstitute medication by injecting 6 ml of sterile water USP
      to the medication vial.
   C. Shake well until all particles are dissolved.
   D. Withdraw all of the solution into the syringe.

VI. *Preparation of the nebulizer*
   A. Assemble the nebulizer according to the package instructions.
   B. Once the nebulizer is assembled, inject the pentamidine solution
      into the nebulizer reservoir.
   C. Attach the connecting tubing to the selected gas source.
      1. For in-wall oxygen or air, the flow rate should be set between
         5 to 7 liters per minute.
      2. For compressed oxygen or air (in a tank), use the same flow
         rate.
      3. For a freestanding compressor, attach the nipple adaptor and
         in-line bacterial filter first (before attaching the connecting
         tubing); the pressure setting should be 22 to 25 psi.

VII. *Administration of treatment*
   A. The client should perform mouth care before the treatment.
   B. Position the client.
   C. Measure blood pressure, pulse, and respiratory rate and aus-
      cultate breath sounds before the treatment and record the infor-
      mation on the client's record.
   D. Before starting treatment, emphasize that the client should take
      rest periods and should turn off the gas source before removing
      the mouthpiece.
   E. Have the client insert the mouthpiece and then turn on the gas
      source.
   F. Auscultate breath sounds during the procedure to detect rhonchi
      (wheezes) that may indicate ensuing bronchoconstriction. If
      wheezing is detected, turn off the gas source, administer the
      bronchodilator ordered by the physician, and allow the client

to rest briefly. If respiratory symptoms are not relieved, discontinue the therapy and notify the physician.

    G. If the client demonstrates symptoms of dyspnea, chest pain, or fever, discontinue the therapy and notify the physician.

    H. Continue the therapy until the nebulizer's reservoir is dry (about 30 to 40 minutes).

    I. Assess the client's response to treatment, measure blood pressure, pulse, and respiratory rate, and ascultate breath sounds. Record findings on the client's record.

    J. The Respirgard II should not be reused because of the possibility of occluded jet orifices, sticking one-way valves, and bacterial growth.

VIII. *Other adverse experiences*

    A. Fatigue can be minimized by scheduling therapy in the evening rather than at the beginning of the day.

    B. Cough can be minimized by having the client sip liquids during treatment. Antitussive agents may be of benefit.

    C. Shortness of breath can be minimized by rest periods.

    D. Residual metallic taste from the drug can be minimized by having the client perform mouth care after as well as before the treatment. Hard candies (licorice or butterscotch flavors) or breath mints may be of some help.

    E. Appetite change: See the discussion of weight loss in Chapter 4.

    F. Dizziness or lightheadedness is often associated with deep rapid breathing during the treatment. Encourage the client to breathe normally and take rest periods.

    G. Wheezing may indicate bronchospasm and the need for bronchodilator therapy.

    H. Fever or rash may indicate a drug reaction. Stop treatment and notify the physician.

    I. Sudden chest pain, dyspnea, and diminution of voice sounds indicate a spontaneous pneumothorax. Stop treatment and call for emergency medical assistance.

Appendix III

Case Management: Initial Database for Client Assessment

I. Demographics
   A. Personal data: name, age, date of birth, sex, race/ethnicity, marital status
   B. Address, telephone number(s)
   C. Social Security number
   D. Occupation/profession
   E. Country of origin
   F. Immigration status if not a citizen
   G. Language(s) spoken (note primary/preferred language)
   H. Risk behavior/factor for acquiring HIV infection
II. Support person(s)
   A. Person living with client (note relationship)
   B. Person designated by the client to act on the client's behalf in an emergency (telephone number[s])
   C. Person who is willing to participate in the plan of care and to provide care when necessary
      1. Is the person available 24 hours per day, 7 days per week?
      2. If not, who can be designated as an alternative care partner?
   D. Family members
      1. Who is aware of the client's diagnosis?
      2. Where do they live (nearby or in another city, state, or country)?
      3. Are they in agreement with the client's chosen care partner/significant other?
   E. Community-based AIDS services
      1. Is the client receiving services from AIDS organizations?
      2. Types of services
III. Functional status
   A. Physical impairments
      1. Sensory: speech, sight, hearing, or areas of anesthesia and/or paresthesias
      2. Motor: dominant arm/hand dysfunction, hemi, para, or quadriparesis/plegia

    3. Functional limitations because of neurological, cardiovascular, or respiratory disease

    4. Bladder/bowel control: continent, occasionally incontinent, or always incontinent

  B. Mental impairments

    1. Cognitive impairment: disoriented, short-term memory impairment, impaired judgment, calculation problems

    2. Communication: can the client make needs known, and can the client direct others?

    3. Emotional status: anxious, agitated, angry, abusive, depressed, or danger to others

    4. Does the client wander when left unattended?

    5. Any sleep disorder?

    6. Does the client need safety monitoring (e.g., smoking)?

  C. Activities of daily living

    1. Personal care: bathing, grooming, dressing, toileting, ambulation, feeding (independent or needs assistance)

    2. Chore services: cleaning, laundry, shopping, meal preparation, reheating prepared meals (independent or needs assistance)

IV. Clinical needs of the client

  A. Medical diagnoses: include all, noting whether chronic or resolved

  B. Medications

    1. Allergies: allergy and type of reaction

    2. Current drug therapy: names, dosages, routes, and frequency

    3. Client's ability to self-medicate: needs reminding and help with preparation; needs supervision or requires preparation and administration by another person

    4. Can the client be taught to self-administer medications?

    5. What arrangements are needed for medication administration?

  C. Clinical trials

    1. Type

    2. Location of trial

    3. Frequency of visits

    4. Special information on trial

  D. Nutrition

    1. Method: oral, enteral, or parenteral

    2. Is the client independent or in need of assistance?

  E. Rehabilitation therapy

    1. Does the client require occupational, physical, or speech therapy?

    2. What are the goals (i.e., functional, restoration, or maintenance)?

    3. What is the frequency of therapy sessions?

  F. Treatments

    1. Does the client require special treatments, such as decubitus care; turning, positioning, and exercising if bedbound; incontinent care; ostomy care (type); catheter care (type); tube irrigation; oxygen therapy; inhalation therapy (including pentamidine aerosol); suctioning; infusion therapy?

    2. Frequency of special treatments

    3. Who is available to perform treatments, and has this person been taught how to perform the procedures?

  G. Equipment needed for care

    1. Assist devices: cane, crutches, walker, wheelchair, hospital bed with trapeze bar, siderails, commode, bedpan, urinal, bath bar, bath seat, hand-held shower, Hoyer lift, and so on

    2. Disposable supplies: incontinence pads, diapers, dressing supplies, and so on

    3. Infusion and tube-feeding supplies

    4. Respiratory equipment

  H. Medical follow-up

    1. Frequency of physician visits required

    2. Laboratory abnormalities that should be monitored: actual or potential and frequency

  I. Addiction treatment

    1. Does the client wish:

      a. To seek addictions treatment

      b. Needle exchange program (if available)

      c. To continue to use drugs (specify type and route)

    2. Is the client enrolled in an addiction treatment program if needed?

    3. Specify type of treatment program and frequency of contact visits

V. Family data

  A. Has the client's sexual partner been tested for HIV? What were the results?

  B. Is the above person in need of health care?

  C. Is the client pregnant?

    1. How many months?

    2. Is she receiving prenatal care (where)?

    3. Does she want abortion information?

  D. If the client is a parent:

    1. Living with sexual partner?

    2. Single parent?

      3. Children (first names, ages, and HIV status)
      4. Health care problems of the children

VI. Legal data
   A. Has the client legally:
      1. Provided for durable power of attorney
      2. Appointed a health care proxy
      3. Drawn up a:
         a. Living will
         b. Will for estate
      4. Provided for guardianship of children
   B. Does the client wish to complete any of these tasks?

VII. Social data
   A. Living arrangements
      1. Housing
         a. Owns own home
         b. Rents an apartment in the home of another
         c. Rents a room (shares facilities) in a home of another
         d. Rents home
         e. Rents apartment
         f. Hotel
         g. Shelter for the homeless
         h. Special housing: supportive housing for persons with AIDS
         i. Senior citizen housing
      2. Facilities
         a. Wheelchair accessible, both inside and outside
         b. Utilities: heat, hot water, electricity, air conditioner, sink, tub, shower
         c. Toilet: own or shared
         d. Cooking facilities: stove, hot plate, toaster-oven, microwave, refrigerator
         e. Elevator or walkup: can the client manage?
         f. Laundry: appliance in home, in building, or nearby
   B. Community assessment
      1. Safety: does the client live in a neighborhood where in-home services if needed could be provided?
      2. Available services: grocery shopping, pharmacy, etc.
      3. Transportation
         a. Does client own a car and is client able to drive?
         b. Is public transportation available near client's home and can client negotiate public transportation?
   C. Spiritual needs
      1. What are the client's spiritual (religious) preferences?
      2. Does the client participate in religious services (frequency)?

        3. How important is religion to the client?

VIII. Financial

    A. Employment: is the client able to continue?

        1. How many hours per week?

        2. Benefits?

    B. Monthly income versus monthly expenditures

    C. Savings and financial assets

    D. Health care payments: including insurance and payments for service care or drugs not covered

    E. Eligibility for entitlements:

        1. Medicaid

        2. Medicare

        3. Special programs for financial aid to persons with AIDS

IX. Services currently received by client

    A. List all agencies and individuals providing service to client

    B. Identify contact persons and telephone numbers to facilitate case planning and management

Appendix IV

Deciding to Enter an AIDS/HIV Drug Trial

1. About the trial
   a. What is the name of this trial? What kind of trial is it? Phase I? Phase II? Phase III? Double-blind design? Open label? Placebo?
   b. What type of drug is being tested? Antiretroviral? Immunomodulator? Antineoplastic? Treatment or prophylaxis for a specific opportunistic infection or illness?
   c. How often must the drug be taken? How will the drug be given in this trial? Orally? Intravenously? Other?
   d. If the participant is a child, will this affect how the drug is taken? Will any physical restraints be used (for instance, in the case of intravenous drugs)? How will the drug's effectiveness be monitored in children?
   e. Must the drug be taken in the hospital, at a test site, or can I take the drug at home?
   f. Do I need to be in the hospital to be in this trial? For how long?
   g. How often must I visit the test site? What will happen on these visits? How long will each visit take?
   h. Is the trial being conducted at any other locations? If there a location easier for me to get to? Is there a site that may meet my particular needs (for instance, Spanish-speaking counselors, or child care)?
   i. What if I have to miss a visit or forget to take the drug?
   j. When can I start in the trial? How long will the trial last?
   k. Do I have to do any special activities while I am at home? Do I have to write down these activities?
2. About the drug
   a. What other drugs are being used today for my problem? How does the trial drug compare in safety and success? What is the evidence that this substance can be helpful in treating my problem?
   b. Has this drug been used before? For what conditions? What were the results? Were there any risks with taking the drug?
   c. What are the immediate side effects of this drug? What are the long-

---

From AIDS Treatment Resources (1990). *Deciding to enter an AIDS/HIV drug trial* (6th Ed.). New York: AIDS Treatment Resources, Inc.

term effects of my using this drug? Are any of the above effects permanent?

   d. If I have any side effects, how will I be helped to deal with them? Whom can I call?

   e. How will taking the drug affect my day-to-day activities? Are there things I cannot do during the trial? Will I be able to continue working? Exercise? Sex?

   f. Is this drug available outside of this trial? If so, where and how could I get it?

3. Financial concerns

   a. Do I need to have my own doctor in order to get into the trial? If I can't afford my own doctor, will the trial provide one?

   b. Do I need health insurance to be in the trial?

   c. Do I have to pay for laboratory tests or any other costs?

   d. If I experience side effects requiring emergency room treatment, which hospital can I go to and who pays for the treatment?

   e. Will I be given any money for participating in the trial?

   f. Will I be given carfare for traveling to and from my visits?

   g. If I am caring for a child, is child care available?

4. Laboratory tests

   a. What tests will be given before I start? Will I get results of these tests?

   b. What tests will be given during the trials? How often? Will I get the results of these tests?

   c. How often will the researchers tell me how I am doing while I am in the trial?

5. Medical history

   a. What do the researchers need to know about my medical condition to see how the drug may affect my health?

   b. If I am a person with a medical problem, including hemophilia, how will the drug impact on my specific condition?

6. Foods, special diets, and other considerations

   a. If the drug is a pill or capsule, should I take it on an empty stomach? With food? Which foods?

   b. Are there any special foods that I need to eat while in this trial? If I am already on a special diet, may I continue? Can I take vitamins?

   c. Are there any foods or other substances that I shouldn't have while taking this drug? Can I drink alcoholic beverages? Can I take any over-the-counter (nonprescription) drugs? Aspirin? Nonaspirin pain killers (such as Tylenol or other forms of acetaminophen)? Cold tablets? Cough syrup?

   d. Can I use prescription drugs while I am in this trial? Can I use other experimental drugs? Can I take drugs against HIV? Can I take immunomodulators? Can I take prophylaxis or treatment for opportunistic infections, cancers, or any other illnesses I may get?

 e. What type of contraceptives can I use? Are oral contraceptives permitted? Will my use of contraceptives be monitored? Are pregnant women allowed in the trial?

7. Informed consent

 a. Is this trial confidential? Will anyone outside of the trial know about my health condition without my permission?

 b. How will information about me be coded to protect my privacy?

 c. Do the consent papers that I am signing describe all of the risks and benefits of my participating in the trial?

 d. What written information will be given about the trial and the drug?

 e. How often will the institutional review board (IRB) review the trial for any changes?

 f. How will I be informed of those changes? If this trial changes significantly, or if I'm put into another trial, will I receive an updated informed consent form to sign?

8. Leaving the trial/end of the trial

 a. If my condition gets worse while I am on the drug, will I be taken out of the trial? If I am in a placebo group, can I get the drug if my condition gets worse during the trial?

 b. If I develop health problems as a result of being in the trial, will treatment be available to me even if I leave the trial before it is over?

 c. If the trial was successful, can I take the drug once the trial is over? Will the sponsors of the drug supply it to me free until it is marketed and publicly available? If the drug worked for me, can I continue to take the drug even if the trial was declared a failure? How is success of this trial defined by the protocol?

 d. How will decisions about stopping the trial be made? How is failure defined in the protocol?

 e. Will my health continue to be checked after I stop taking the drug? For how long and under what conditions? Will this be done even if I decide to leave the trial before it is over? Even if the entire trial is stopped early by the researchers?

 f. Will there be long-term follow-up on how I am doing? Will this be done even if I leave the trial before it is over? Even if the entire trial is stopped early by the researchers?

 g. How can I find out the results of the trial?

 h. Will I be able to participate in future trials of this drug? Will I receive the results of future trials using this drug?

Index

Page numbers in *italics* refer to illustrations; page numbers followed by t refer to tables.